Mastering
Medical Coding

Third Edition

Mastering
Medical Coding

Third Edition

Marsha S. Diamond, CPC, CPC-H

Department Chair
Health Information Technology
Central Florida College
Orlando, Florida

National Advisory Board Member
American Academy of Professional Coders
Salt Lake City, Utah

Senior Consultant/Auditor
Medical Audit Resource Services, Inc.
Orlando, Florida

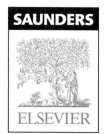

SAUNDERS

ELSEVIER

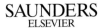

11830 Westline Industrial Drive
St. Louis, Missouri 63146

Notice

Neither the Publisher nor the Authors assume any responsibility for any loss or injury and/or damage to persons or property arising out of or related to any use of the material contained in this book. It is the responsibility of the treating practitioner, relying on independent expertise and knowledge of the patient, to determine the best treatment and method of application for the patient.

The Publisher

Library of Congress Cataloging-in-Publication Data

Diamond, Marsha S.
    Mastering medical coding/Marsha S. Diamond.—3rd ed.
        p.   cm.
    Includes index.
    ISBN 1-4160-2395-X
    1. Nosology—Code numbers.   I. Title.
    RB115.D535 2006
    616.001'2—dc22

Publishing Director: Andrew M. Allen
Executive Editor: Susan Cole
Developmental Editor: Beth LoGiudice
Publishing Services Manager: Patricia Tannian
Designer: Paula Ruckenbrod
Producer: Cindy Ahlheim

Printed in the United States of America

Last digit is the print number: 9 8 7 6 5 4 3 2 1

DEDICATION

If you want to be successful,
KNOW what you are doing,
LOVE what you are doing, and
BELIEVE in what you are doing.
Will Rogers

For those who love what they do, they can only hope to have the opportunity to pass the passion for their profession along to others in the field. By writing about and teaching the field of medical coding, I have achieved that golden opportunity. My special thanks to the many students who have passed through my classroom, who have entered the coding field, and who share that same passion; they are the continuum for the coding profession.

For those outside the classroom who support my endeavors on a never-ending basis:
My constant companions during my endless hours of writing, Charlotte and Cassie, and those companions in the past, Oreo and Charlie, whose wagging tails and sparkle in their eyes have held fast despite the long hours of writing and rewriting.

My grandchildren, Tavious and Jaylen, who, I hope, will one day look at their grandmother as an educator and motivator in the coding profession.

My loving daughter, Jennifer, who understands and shares the work ethic of dedication and perseverance in all her endeavors.

To Stan, who endures it all, assisting in improving the clinical accuracy of the medical information and supplying the endless supply of paper, paper, and more paper.

And, of course,
Mom and Dad, who are my lifelong inspirations of work ethic and perseverance—something I hope I successfully pass along to all who learn from me.

DEVELOPMENT OF THIS EDITION

This book would not have been possible without the following team of educators and professionals, including practicing coders and educational consultants.

Editorial Review Board

Korene Atkins, MS, RHIA, CCS, CPC, CPC-H
Director of Health Information Technology
Assistant Professor
West Virginia Northern Community College
Hopedale, Ohio

Barbara Baran, RN
Instructor
Cambria Rowe Business College
Indiana, Pennsylvania

Dorine Bennett, MBA, RHIA, FAHIMA
Director and Associate Professor
Health Information Management Program
Dakota State University
Madison, South Dakota

Vicki L. Bond, LPN, IV-2, Limited Radiology Certified
Medical Office Technology Program Coordinator &
   Instructor
Pikes Peak Community College
Colorado Springs, Colorado

Vickie Farley, BSN, MA, RN, LPC
Instructor
Virginia College at Birmingham
Birmingham, Alabama

Deborah Forcier, CPC
Health Claims Specialist/Program Instructor
Department Chairperson
Branford Hall Career Institute
Southington, Connecticut

Barbara Goff, MS
Medical Program Coordinator
Education & Life Training Center
Fort Collins, Colorado

Rebecca Hageman, BGS, RHIA, CCS
Instructor
Hutchinson Community College
Wichita, Kansas

Susanna Hancock, RMA, CMA, RPT, COLT, AAS
Medical Assistant Director (Past)
American Institute of Health Technology
Wilder, Idaho

Stacy Horn, CMA, CPC
Advisor for Coding and Transcription
Midstate College
Peoria, Illinois

Karen Levein
Instructor
Monrovia Community Adult School
Monrovia, California

Maryagnes Luczak, BS, AS, CMA, CHUC, CPT
Vice President of Operations
Career Training Academy
New Kensington, Pennsylvania

John Manter, BA, BSN, RN, MS, CCS, CPC, CPHQ
APC Coordinator
DeKalb Medical Center
East Point, Georgia

Anne Martin-Segrini, RHIT, BS
Lead Faculty/Program Director (Retired)
Health Information Management
Santa Fe Community College
Newberry, Florida

Chris Merle, RHIA, BS, MS
Assistant Professor
Health Information Management
Arkansas Tech University
Russellville, Arkansas

Cassandra Perry, RHIT
Instructor
Georgia Perimeter College/Atlanta Area Technical
   College
Atlanta, Georgia

Kimberly Rash, AS
Instructor
Insurance Billing/Coder Certification Program
Gateway Community and Technical College
Edgewood, Kentucky

Assistant Manager
Transcription Department
St. Elizabeth Hospital
Covington, Kentucky

Carol Skelton, CPC
Professional Billing Coordinator
Physicians Practice Group
Hephzibah, Georgia

Donna Thrasher, CPC
Medvance
Cookeville, Tennessee

Lori Warren, MA, RN, CPC, CCP, CLNC
Medical Department Co-Director
Medical Coding/Healthcare Reimbursement Program
  Director
Spencerian College
Louisville, Kentucky

PREFACE

As an experienced instructor of medical coding and billing and having used the medical coding texts that are available in the market, I have come to the conclusion that these texts do not help teach the student HOW to code. Although most of these texts specifically present the many idiosyncrasies of coding for specialty cases, few, if any, explain the actual process of selecting the diagnosis and the corresponding codes.

Mastering Medical Coding provides an accurate picture of the real world of medical coding by illustrating all types of medical records within a medical practice and highlighting the role of the medical coder in the entire reimbursement process. As you will learn, medical chart documentation "drives" the coding process. As a result, this text extensively discusses documentation and provides suggestions for enhancements to maximize coding and reimbursement. Most other texts begin with the introduction of diagnostic and/or procedure coding without offering an explanation of what part of the documentation can be used. *Mastering Medical Coding* provides instruction on the selection of information that is codeable from the documentation, which is perhaps the most important step in the coding process.

Mastering coding is a building-block process. It is building on the knowledge learned from previous steps. The basic rules remain the same, even in the most complex coding scenarios. Coding encompasses a multitude of rules and guidelines; however, they are built from basic ground rules. With basic rules or building blocks, the process of coding becomes much simpler.

Prerequisite Instruction

To learn effectively from this text, you must have a comprehensive knowledge of medical terminology, anatomy and physiology, and disease processes. It is recommended that you complete courses in these areas before undertaking any comprehensive coding education.

Organization of This Textbook

Mastering Medical Coding provides a solid foundation in coding principles with an emphasis on teaching through actual physician documentation that prepares students to tackle any coding scenario, from routine to complex. The 23 chapters are divided into the following seven sections.

Section I, Role of Physician Documentation, emphasizes the unique approach of *Mastering Medical Coding* by discussing the importance of the medical record and medical documentation in the coding and reimbursement process.

Section II, ICD-9-CM Diagnostic Coding, has been expanded from the previous edition to include even more coverage of ICD-9-CM coding. A full chapter on V and E codes is also included, as well as a separate chapter on ICD-10-CM.

Section III, Physician Procedure Coding, covers all aspects of procedural coding, from assigning CPT codes to using modifiers to HCPCS coding. Content is split into short, manageable chapters that can be covered quickly and can be easily reinforced.

Section IV, Hospital Coding, discusses both coding and billing for hospital services, including guidelines for inpatient coding and proper APC and DRG assignment. Thus *Mastering Medical Coding* is a truly comprehensive coding textbook.

Section V, Putting Together Coding Systems, illustrates how proper coding brings together CPT, ICD-9-CM, APCs, and DRGs to provide an accurate picture of a patient's history and visit.

Section VI, The Reimbursement Perspective, focuses on the guidelines and rules of different third-party carriers and promotes a thorough understanding of the effect of coding on all aspects of the reimbursement process.

Section VII, Monitoring/Compliance and Certification Review, reemphasizes the importance of proper medical documentation and discusses the legislation regarding fraud and abuse, as well as a comprehensive monitoring process to ensure compliance.

Also in this section is a certification review that contains review materials, practice examinations, and a 50-question mock certification examination, which is a culmination of the textbook content. These questions provide valuable practice for the actual examination and will give you a chance to test your retention of the information in the textbook.

Distinctive Features

This book was designed to be the start of your coding education, and it has many unique features to assist you.

Learning objectives, numerous examples, chapter reviews, and coding reference tools throughout *Mastering Medical Coding* provide the necessary educational aids to fully master basic and advanced coding concepts. In addition to fully updated content, the new edition has an expanded discussion of the medical record and a simulated medical practice, Godfrey Medical Associates, which is followed throughout the book in different documentation examples. The reinforced focus truly makes it clear that "documentation drives the coding process," and this book contains the tools you need to develop the necessary skills to succeed in the workplace.

Key Features

This book was designed to be the start of your coding career, and it has many key features to assist you through your coursework.

- As stated in Chapter 1, the main emphasis of *Mastering Medical Coding* is on proper review of **actual physician documentation** in the medical record and on application of basic coding rules—the key steps in the coding process.
- **Godfrey Medical Associates,** a simulated medical practice used throughout the text and explained in the Introduction, reinforces the focus of the text by providing a standard list of physicians and records for explanation and understanding.
- **Explanatory illustrations** of different types of medical records and physician documentation provide visual examples and practice opportunities in every chapter.

- Each chapter contains specialized **coding reference tools,** which put together key information from the text discussion into an easy-to-use format for quick reference and everyday use.

RULES FOR SELECTING APPROPRIATE DIAGNOSES
(For Physician Coding)

1. If it is not documented, it did not happen.

2. The condition, problem, or other circumstance chiefly responsible for the health encounter/visit/problem is reported. This will be referred to as **Chief Reason for Encounter.**

3. Unconfirmed diagnoses described as "possible," "probable," "questionable," "rule out," "ruled out," "suspect(ed)," CANNOT be utilized for physician diagnoses or physician coding.

4. Code the condition to the **highest level of specificity.** In some cases, this may be the sign, symptom, abnormal test, or reason for visit/encounter.

5. If the physician does not identify a definite condition or problem at the conclusion of the patient visit/encounter, the coder should select the documented chief complaint or chief reason for the encounter.

6. Never code a diagnosis not listed by the physician. In the event the coder feels the physician has not listed an appropriate diagnosis, the coder must check with the physician.

If the physician believes the information has been omitted in error, the provider may add an addendum to the original medical record, and, at that time, the coder may code accordingly.

- **Key terms, learning objectives,** and **coding reference tools** are listed at the beginning of every chapter to highlight important information to improve comprehension when reading the material.
- In-text *Stop & Practice* exercises appear in every chapter to provide immediate reinforcement of concepts and procedures just discussed in the text.

CONSULTATIONS

Indication for consultation:
Ventricular tachycardia

History:
54-year-old with known history of cardiac disease who was undergoing outpatient arthroscopy of the knee. Patient's cardiac rhythm was noted to have multiple runs of non-sustained ventricular tachycardia. Patient remained asymptomatic stable.
Status post MI 15 years ago.
FAMILY/SOCIAL HISTORY:
Non-contributory

Exam:
PHYSICAL EXAM:
Head: Normocephalic, atraumatic
Neck: Supple, w/o evidence of JVP, mass or bruit
Chest: Clear to auscultation
Cardiac: Normal carotid upstroke with normal contour
Abdomen: Soft, nontender, no evidence of mass
Extremities: Showed no evidence of clubbing, cyanosis, or edema
Neurologic: Grossly intact, nonfocal
EKG: Ectopic atrial rhythm with delayed precordial transmission

Diagnosis/assessment:
IMPRESSION:
Known history of coronary atherosclerotic heart disease and atrial fibrillation, now presents with run of nonsustained V tach per report. It would be prudent to continue patient on his current medications and allow him to follow-up with his primary cardiologist.

We appreciate the opportunity to participate in the overall evaluation and management of this patient.

Patient name: _____
Date of service: _____
GODFREY MEDICAL ASSOCIATES
1532 Third Avenue, Suite 120 • Aldon, FL 77713 • (407) 555-4000

STOP AND PRACTICE

Code the following hypertension exercises.

ICD-9-CM Code(s)

1. Hypertension
2. Postoperative hypertension
3. Elevated blood pressure
4. Postpartum hypertension
5. Pulmonary hypertension

6. Myocarditis due to hypertension _____
7. Hypertension with chronic renal failure _____
8. Hypertension due to brain tumor _____
9. Gestational hypertension _____
10. Hypertension, possibly malignant _____

- **Chapter Review Exercises** at the end of each chapter provide more reinforcement and practice for chapter concepts by several different types of questions, including sample medical charts for practical application of the skills learned.
- Concepts necessary for you to know and understand in preparing for the coding **certification examination** are included at the end of the chapter in a bulleted list.
- The **Student Study Guide** at the end of each chapter lists suggested activities for continued success while the textbook and its ancillaries are used.

CHAPTER IN REVIEW

CERTIFICATION REVIEW

- The Table of Drugs and Chemicals located in ICD-9-CM is intended to simplify the assignment of adverse effects.
- Each drug or chemical is assigned a code based on the diagnostic statement as to whether the injury is the result of poisoning, overdose, wrong substance given or taken, or intoxication.
- Some adverse effects require two ICD-9-CM codes: one for the poisoning and an additional E code for the external cause.
- When the cause of adverse effects is not stated by the physician, the coder must use the Undetermined category. This is particularly important in potential suicide cases in which the physician does not or will not state that the adverse effects were intentionally inflicted.
- Adverse effects from therapeutic use occur only when the correct substance is administered correctly as prescribed.
- Accidental poisoning codes are used only when accidental overdose of a drug, wrong substance, drug taken in error, or accidents in the use of drugs or biologicals are identified.
- Drugs and chemicals listed in the Table of Drugs and Chemicals in the ICD-9-CM codebook are listed alphabetically; generic names are used for prescription drugs.
- A neoplasm is defined as any new and abnormal growth. That growth may be malignant, benign, or undetermined.
- Masses are not coded or classified as neoplasms unless the physician states "neoplasm" or "neoplastic" in the diagnostic statement.
- When secondary or metastatic neoplasms are coded, the primary site should always be coded. If the site is known, use the appropriate code. If the site is not known but is known to exist, use 199.0 or 199.1. If the site no longer exists, use history of malignant neoplasm codes.
- Carcinoma in situ refers to malignant neoplasms that stay confined to the point of origin without invading surrounding areas.

STUDENT STUDY GUIDE

- Study Chapter 5.
- Review the Learning Objectives for Chapter 5.
- Complete the Stop and Practice exercises.
- Complete the Certification Review for Chapter 5.
- Complete the Chapter Review exercises to reinforce concepts learned in this chapter.

CHAPTER REVIEW EXERCISE

Code the following:

	Code Assigned
1. Essential hypertension	
2. Suicide attempt by cocaine	
3. Open wound of abdomen due to shotgun blast to abdomen	
4. Overdose of phenobarbital, prescribed by physician, taken as directed	
5. Hypertensive heart and renal disease	
6. Attempted homicide by rat poison	
7. Hypertension in pregnancy, antepartum	
8. Secondary hypertension due to pulmonary edema	
9. Allergic reaction to spider bite	
10. Asbestos poisoning	
11. Secondary hypertension	
12. Pulmonary hypertension	
13. Transient hypertension of pregnancy	
14. Accidental overdose, doxycycline	

Extensive Supplemental Resources

Student Workbook

The Workbook for *Mastering Medical Coding* provides extra practice with medical record documentation with exercises and medical records. All the content has been fully updated to reflect the latest coding information, and the cases have been tailored to the new edition of the textbook.

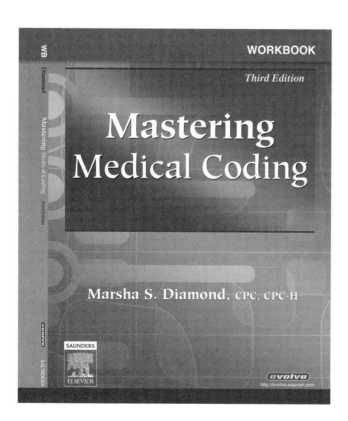

The simulated medical practice, Godfrey Regional, is carried through the workbook to provide consistency with the text and offer the opportunity for fully integrated assignments. For all the coding concepts to be brought together with simulated practice, the workbook contains all the documentation you need to see a full "Day in the Life of Godfrey Medical." By completing these activities, you will see how information flows in the medical office and will be required to code multiple cases for multiple physicians with a variety of responsibilities. Critical thinking and self-assessment questions are also included to stimulate discussion and make the difference between a good coder and an excellent coder.

Instructor's Resource Manual with CD-ROM

This combined printed and electronic Instructor's Resource Manual for *Mastering Medical Coding* includes answers to *Stop and Practice* and Chapter Review text sections, plus a discussion of workbook exercises that provides suggestions for eliminating future errors. The CD-ROM, bound free with this item, includes all printed content, a collection of PowerPoint slides, and a test bank in ExamView. The slides can be easily customized to support lectures or formatted into overhead transparencies or handouts for student note taking. The ExamView test generator will help you quickly and easily prepare quizzes and examinations, and the test bank can be customized to meet any teaching method.

Evolve Resources

The Evolve Resources that accompany *Mastering Medical Coding* offer helpful material that will extend your studies beyond the classroom. Important links and industry news provide information necessary to stay current in the coding field, and content updates for the book will keep your study material current too. Instructors can also download all the material from the Instructor's Resource Manual for easy use in any classroom.

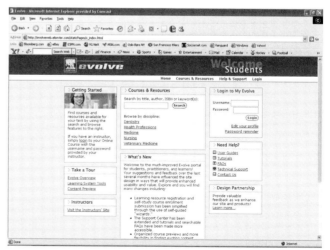

A course management system is also available as an option for instructors who adopt the textbook. This Web-based platform gives instructors yet another resource to facilitate learning and to make medical coding content accessible to students. In addition to the standard Evolve Resources, instructors who choose this option can manage their entire course online, with online assessments, chat functionality, threaded discussions, and an online grade book.

To access this comprehensive online resource, simply go to the Evolve home page at http://evolve.elsevier.com and enter the user name and password provided by your instructor. If your instructor has not set up a course management system, you can still access the free Evolve Resources as http://evolve.elsevier.com/Diamond/.

TEACH Lesson Plan Manual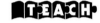

This product comes in print, with a bound-in CD-ROM. Lesson Plans for the *Mastering Medical Coding* are based on chapter-by-chapter learning objectives in 50-minute building blocks, and instructors can customize the Lesson Plans to match their course sequence and add their own content. The Lesson Plans follow chapter content and link all resources of the educational package: PowerPoint slides, the workbook, and class activities. Also included are Background Assessment Questions and Critical Thinking Questions to spur class discussion. Lecture Outlines present the PowerPoint slides with practical talking points and thought-provoking questions to pose to students, intended to spur classroom discussion. Additionally, there is an Evolve component to this manual, providing instructors with access to content from any Web connection.

Medical Coding Practice and Review

A resource for supplemental exercises, *Medical Coding Practice and Review,* provides extra practice with medical record documentation for coding students and practicing coders. Included are more than 350 pieces of medical documentation, all realistic cases for practice with all areas, including Evaluation and Management, Surgery, and Radiology. Educational programs can use this to provide extra coding practice for students, and it is a good resource to prepare students for certification examinations. In addition to coding students, even practicing coders will find it helpful for honing their coding skills, studying for certification, or maintaining their existing certification. All the content has been fully updated to reflect the latest coding information, and the cases have been tailored to the coordinate with the new edition of the textbook.

Coding References and Sources

Although *Mastering Medical Coding* is intended to provide knowledge of concepts for hospital, outpatient, and practice coding, it is not intended to be the resource for third-party carriers in the assignment of codes for services. This book is intended for educational purposes only. The only code books that should be references for third-party justification are the ICD-9-CM and CPT-4.

Coding Updates and Changes

The coding world is constantly changing. Every attempt has been made to ensure that all references to CPT-4, ICD-9-CM, and DRG code assignments are current at the time of publication. Changes that occur after the printing of *Mastering Medical Coding* may affect the assignment of codes. Reference should always be made to the current coding manuals and to any available code books updated to the current year ICD-9-CM and CPT-4. Updates to this text will be made available to instructors through the Evolve companion site when yearly coding updates necessitate change.

ACKNOWLEDGMENTS

Many thanks to the editorial staff at Elsevier who made the publication of this textbook possible.

To Beth LoGiudice, Developmental Editor, for her diligence in reviewing, editing, and critiquing the manuscript. Her insights into the Medical Coding field and her extraordinary vision for this text have been exemplary.

To Susan Cole, Executive Editor, for her foresight in the unique concept of this coding text, compared with other coding textbooks, and the development and design of this textbook. Many thanks for her faith and patience in supporting new ideas and new concepts and thinking outside the "norm."

Thanks also to Jill L. Brown, RN, CPC, CPC-H, MPA, for introducing me to the Elsevier editorial staff, which resulted in the publication of this textbook.

Marsha S. Diamond, CPC, CPC-H

CONTENTS

Section I: Crucial Role of Physician Documentation in the Coding Process

1. Physician Documentation, 2

Section II: ICD-9-CM Diagnostic Coding

2. Determining Physician Diagnosis, 56
3. Using the ICD-9-CM Code Book, 88
4. V Codes and E Codes, 112
5. ICD-9-CM Tables, 128
6. Coding Special Complexities, 146
7. ICD-10-CM, 178

Section III: Physician Procedure Coding

8. Determining Codeable Services, 184
9. Using CPT-4, 188
10. Evaluation and Management Services, 198
11. Anesthesia Services, 248
12. Surgery Services, 260
13. Radiology Services, 300
14. Pathology Services, 314
15. Medicine Services, 322
16. Modifiers, 346
17. HCPCS Codes, 358

Section IV: Hospital Coding and Billing Processes

18. Hospital Coding, 368
19. Hospital/Facility Billing Process, 392

Section V: Putting Together Coding Systems

20. Putting Together CPT-4, ICD-9-CM, and DRG, 410

Section VI: The Reimbursement Perspective

21. Coding from a Reimbursement Perspective, 432

Section VII: Monitoring/Compliance and Certification Review

22. Monitoring and Compliance Process, 448
23. The Certification Process, 466

Appendix A: ICD-9-CM Official Guidelines for Coding and Reporting, 477

Appendix B: Godfrey Regional Practice Information and Forms, 513

Appendix C: Answers, 519

INTRODUCTION

WELCOME to the world of coding! You have chosen your career wisely. The field of medical coding has evolved over the past couple of decades to a profession all its own. From the 1970s and 1980s when coding was only one small facet of the Business Office to a career that demands top pay and is recognized as a distinguished profession, coders today represent the professional expertise that promotes a successful practice or facility.

The real world of coding extends beyond the coders many envision positioned in their cramped cubicles buried in their own little world of code books and medical charts. The coder of today is the key to successful reimbursement for the practice or facility. Having worked in the medical field for well over 30 years, I have seen firsthand that the financial success of the practice/facility always comes back to coding. As a Practice Manager, Billing/Reimbursement Manager, and A/R Manager, I quickly learned that the practice's timely and accurate reimbursement revolved around the CPT-4 and ICD-9-CM coding and the accompanying documentation that supported those codes. Many a practice has come and gone despite the wonderful interpersonal skills of the staff or physicians of the practice.

As a consultant working with practices that had reimbursement issues, I came to understand that if the appropriate coding processes had been followed to support the documentation, there would be no need for any assistance in securing reimbursement. And so, over time, my world eventually revolved around coding.

What Exactly Is Medical Coding?

Medical coding has been defined as the systematic classification of data and assignment of a number system to that service for identification purposes. When these numbers are assigned for diagnoses and procedures, codes are from a predefined classification system, or a grouping together of similar items. In the case of disease classification, the *International Classification of Diseases, Ninth Revision, Clinical Modification (ICD-9-CM)* is used. When procedures are coded, the *Current Procedural Terminology (CPT-4)* is used.

Coding serves a number of purposes, including the retrieval or reporting of information according to diagnosis and procedure. It also plays an integral role in

reimbursement, as previously discussed, because it is the primary tool of communication between the provider of care and the third-party carrier (insurance).

Coding, however, involves much more than just the systematic assignment of codes. Perhaps more complex is extracting the necessary information from the documentation that is required to assign the correct code(s). From the history and physical form, to the surgical operative report, the interpretation of data for coding purposes can often be more involved than the actual code assignment process.

This textbook covers several types of coding. The use of these classifications is based on the location and type of service that is being reported. They are as follows:

Facility/Provider Type	Coding System(s) Used
Facility Inpatient	ICD-9-CM (Diagnosis/Procedures)
Facility Outpatient	ICD-9-CM (Diagnosis/Procedures)
	CPT-4/HCPCS (Procedures)
Physician/Professional	ICD-9-CM (Diagnoses)
	CPT-4/HCPCS (Procedures)

The world of medical coding has become complex. From significantly different guidelines for physicians, inpatient facilities, and outpatient facilities to different coding systems for diagnostic coding and procedural coding, the coder of the twenty-first century is faced with many challenges.

In addition to yearly changes in diagnostic and procedure coding, third-party carriers continue to apply individual caveats on those common guidelines that are available. APCs (Ambulatory Payment Classifications) are relatively new to the scope of coding. Next on the horizon, the coder faces the implementation of ICD-10-CM and possible ICD-10-PCS. Needless to say, the world of the coder is a constant environment of change.

As a result, the successful coder of today needs to remain flexible and informed regarding changes in the coding world. Constant updates, literature, and third-party bulletins make the coder's job a never-ending educational process. For this reason, the national certification organizations require coders to maintain continuing education units (CEUs) each year to make certain that the strive for excellence in coding continues long after the certification process.

The practice or facility coder has a number of responsibilities extending beyond the coding arena. As the "expert" in the practice or facility, the coder also holds the responsibility of educating the entire medical staff on coding issues and the success of the practice or facility through effective coding and monitoring techniques. Although these techniques center on the coder, the office staff (clerical, clinical, and medical) must understand that the practice's success hinges on many individuals in the practice understanding the coding and reimbursement process.

With third-party carriers imposing additional guidelines in their individual contracts with physicians and facilities comes the need for an initial **clean claim,** that insurance claim that is free (clean) of errors. Although this may sound like the job of the billing department, the culmination of this clean claim process begins with the accurate and timely coding for services that you will learn about in this textbook.

Because of the large number of **dirty claims** (not clean), reimbursements are not paid promptly or services are denied. The annual cost for reprocessing claims is well into the billions of dollars. As a result, some state and federal organizations have recommended legislation that some carriers require claims be reviewed by professional certified coders only. Although this has passed in a few states and remains on the agendas of several states and the federal government, the need for certified coders continues to grow.

What about Certification?

As with any profession, an attempt to identify those individuals who have mastered the skill has been made in the field of coding, much like the CPA (Certified Public Accountant) in the business world.

The two main organizations for nationally recognized certification are the American Academy of Professional Coders (AAPC) and the American Health Information Management Association (AHIMA).

The following are the four certification examinations available:

CPC   Certified Professional Coder
CPC-H Certified Professional Coder/Hospital

These two certifications are through the AAPC. The CPC credential is intended for the professional/physician coder, whereas the CPC-H is intended for the coder who performs outpatient facility coding.

CCS   Certified Coding Specialist
CCS-P Certified Coding Specialist/Physician

These two certifications are offered through AHIMA. The CCS-P examination, intended for physician/professional coders, is similar in intent to the CPC offered by AAPC, whereas the CCS offers testing in the mastery of inpatient hospital coding.

Statistics available from these two credentialing organizations indicate that certified coders should expect to

receive an additional 10% to 15% of their salary for their certification expertise.

Testing for all these examinations is available throughout the year at various locations in the United States and in other countries.

Additional information regarding the AAPC and AHIMA and their certification processes are available on their respective Web sites, www.aapc.com and www.ahima.org.

Roles of the Coder in the Twenty-First Century

Coders initially worked within the medical record or health information department of the facility or physician's office performing ICD-9-CM coding, CPT-4 coding, or both. Their jobs seemed rather regimented, and they ranked among the many other staff who prepared for a rather bland, tedious job.

Many physician offices did not even employ full-time coders but instead used a billing office staff to perform both the coding and billing functions. Physicians, too, have now realized the necessity and benefits that a professional coder adds to their organization.

"Traditional" Coder
The traditional role of the coder in the medical practice, outpatient facility, and inpatient facility remains the same in title only. Although the coder continues to perform the functions of ICD-9-CM and CPT-4 coding, the job has developed additional complexities and responsibilities as the years have progressed.

Initially, this position assigned appropriate coding to services performed; however, as coding rules became more complex and individual carriers began to implement coding guidelines specific to individualized contracts, specific guidelines continued to increase, and the specialization of the coder in the traditional sense began to change.

With the rising prominence of managed care contracts came coding restrictions inherent in each individual third-party contract. It is now imperative that the coder be educated on the content of these third-party contracts for effective coding. Most of the answers for nonpayment or denial of claims can be found in the contract.

The traditional coder may assign codes in a myriad of settings. From hospital coders, who perform inpatient facility coding and statistical coding such as tumor registry, to physician coders, who perform coding in the physician practice, MSO, or group practice, the traditional coder performs an array of coding functions in a number of settings. In addition to these settings, many other entities, such as insurance carriers, managed care companies, third-party administrators, and attorneys, are employing coders.

Medical Billing Specialist
Although the medical biller or business office is typically responsible for sending claims, receiving payments/

denials, and working accounts receivable, the successful medical biller should be equipped with the coding knowledge to prepare clean claims and determine coding discrepancies that have created delays or denial of claims.

Most states have some legislation that requires clean claims to be paid within a specified period (sometimes 30 days). This means that when claims are submitted free of errors, the practice should expect payment within a 30- to 60-day period from the date of service. Claims that are missing codes or have incorrect/incomplete information, though, will be delayed by many weeks or months. Thus an accounts receivable that is older than 90 days is created. Statistics reflect that accounts receivable older than 90 days are collected at the rate of 50% or less.

Chart Auditing
A somewhat new field for the medical coder is the area of chart auditing. With the growing problem of fraud and abuse, many facilities find the need for in-house chart auditing or employment of an outside entity to routinely audit charts prospectively for potential fraud and abuse scenarios.

Keep in mind that fraud and abuse may happen even in the best facilities or practices. For instance, when services are billed that are not performed, this may constitute the definition of fraud. This can happen in a practice as a result of the charge document being marked with a service, decision made not to perform the service, perhaps because of time restraints. The oversight is not removing that service from the billing documents, which results in fraudulent billing for services not performed. As fraud and abuse run into billions of dollars a year, the federal government and other third-party carriers are constantly reviewing documentation for medical necessity to make certain that guidelines have been met.

Chart audits performed within the medical practice/facility can ensure that fraud and abuse are not occurring, even by oversight, in the practice. Fraud and abuse as a result of these oversights can be staggering.

For instance, in a practice that incorrectly bills Medicare for two urinalyses per week that are not actually performed, the fines (an average of $5,000 per item) will total $10,000 per week, $40,000 per month, culminating in an annual penalty of approximately $480,000. In the event an audit takes place by a carrier, proof that internal auditing has been performed may eliminate the charge of abuse in that the intent to defraud cannot be proven.

Compliance
The fastest growing field for coders is probably the compliance field. This is the direct result of the continually growing investigation of fraud and abuse. This aspect of medical coding typically requires an experienced coder to be certified. The Compliance Officer, Compliance Coordinator, or coder responsible for compliance must ensure that the identity follows federal, state, and other regulatory guidelines for coding and billing. Compliance staff often formulates a written compliance program and monitors its enforcement. Chart audits at regularly scheduled intervals are a part of the responsibility of the coder in charge of compliance.

The compliance field has also opened up additional opportunities outside the traditional inpatient, outpatient, and physician arena. Many organizations such as insurance carriers have employed compliance individuals to organize and enforce compliance programs for their organizations. In addition, third-party carriers often employ these individuals for monitoring claims for payment.

Educator
The need for coding educators grows with the continuing need for qualified expert coders. Many coders who have experienced the real world of coding have chosen to use their real-world experiences in educating the new coding student.

Conclusion
It should now be obvious that the coder holds a number of responsibilities within the practice, and each facility will expect some or all of these duties from the coder they employ. The facility coder may be responsible for tumor registry, inpatient or outpatient coding, and a number of other coding and management functions within the facility's Health Information Department (previously known as Medical Records). The provider/physician coder often is responsible not only for coding services provided in an outpatient/inpatient setting for the providers within the group, but often for education and training of staff on coding-related issues.

The salary that the coder should expect will obviously be determined by the extent of responsibilities and the individual's credentials and experience.

The role of the coder offers many opportunities to the coding student. Positions such as those outlined can be obtained in a number of facilities such as hospitals, physician offices, insurance carriers, consulting groups, and third-party audit organizations. The opportunities are numerous, diverse, and rewarding. The success of the practice or facility rests in large part with coders and their ability to provide accurate coding assignment and coding education within their organization.

CRUCIAL ROLE OF PHYSICIAN DOCUMENTATION IN THE CODING PROCESS

Most coding texts begin instruction with an introduction of the coding process. This text begins at the beginning—with documentation. As the student will learn, documentation drives the coding process, for without proper documentation, coding cannot be successful.

It is also appropriate that this text ends with the same process that drives coding—documentation. Accurate documentation is maintained throughout the monitoring process, which ensures that documentation is complete and is in compliance with third-party requirements.

In this first section, Crucial Role of Physician Documentation in the Coding Process, the student begins to understand the important role of documentation. It encompasses not only an explanation of the importance of the documentation process, but also a breakdown of the many types of medical chart documentation that drive the coding process. Final discussion focuses on improvement of the documentation process through the use of effective tools and techniques.

The student will have the opportunity to review different medical chart documents and formats and to become familiar with the many types of documents that can be used in the coding and documentation process. The charts contained in this text are real; they range from the incomplete to the complete, from difficult-to-read to the dictated, well-organized record. Such charts represent ones that will be encountered by those who code in the physician's or provider's office or within the hospital setting.

PHYSICIAN DOCUMENTATION

LEARNING OBJECTIVES

Following the completion of this chapter, the student will be able to:

- Comprehend the importance of physician documentation in the coding process.
- Understand that signature requirements are a vital component of the documentation process.
- Identify the various components of the medical chart needed for documentation in both office and hospital settings.
- Identify the various providers of service and locations of service where documentation occurs.
- Realize the importance of identifying documentation deficiencies.
- Understand the need for implementing documentation tools within the practice or facility to overcome documentation deficiencies.
- Develop specific tools and monitoring processes to correct and prevent documentation deficiencies identified in the practice setting.

CODING REFERENCE TOOLS

Tool 1
Dictation Note Guide
Tool 2
History Check-off Guide
Tool 3
Examination Check-off Guide
Tool 4
Emergency Department Chart Documentation Requirements
Tool 5
Emergency Department Record of Treatment
Tool 6
History and Physical Sample Dictation Model
Tool 7
Basic Documentation Do's and Don'ts

KEY TERMS

Assessment, 9
Consultations, 23
Discharge Summary, 23
Examination, 9
Fraud, 3
History, 9
Joint Commission on Accreditation of Healthcare Organizations (JCAHO), 15
Medical Decision Making, 9
Medical Necessity, 4
Medication Record, 9
Objective, 9
Patient History, 9
Pertinent Negative, 9
Plan, 9
Problem List, 9
Qui Tam Action, 4
Signature Lists, 6
SOAP Format, 9
Subjective, 9

DOCUMENTATION DRIVES THE CODING PROCESS

The first and perhaps most important aspect of all coding is the documentation itself. Without appropriate documentation, medical coding is difficult, if not impossible. This chapter deals with physician documentation and its importance and role in both selecting correct coding for reimbursement and establishing medical necessity.

The first and foremost rule of coding and documentation is:

IF IT IS NOT DOCUMENTED, IT DID NOT HAPPEN.

If it did not happen, the provider may not code or collect payment for services. Billing for services that "did not happen" is the basic definition of **fraud,** an attempt to collect for services not furnished or to receive payment for services that would not otherwise be reimbursed. The specific definitions of fraud and abuse are discussed in a later chapter.

In the same regard, **if documentation is not *signed*, it does not exist.** The provider of the service or the provider supervising the delivery of service must indicate that the work was performed or supervised by the provider for documentation to be complete. Carriers and other regulatory agencies differ as to whether this documentation needs to be confirmed with a signature, initials, or some other kind of identifying mark. The use of signature stamps in medical practice should be strongly discouraged because for most third-party carriers the signature stamp does not constitute the physician's authentication of services. Electronic signatures generated by computerized billing or medical records systems are becoming acceptable alternatives to original signatures. These electronic signatures should be verified as acceptable to federal, state, and other regulatory agencies before they are used. It is also prudent to maintain a signature log when more than one provider is represented, so that all staff members are familiar with each provider's signature. This aspect will be discussed later in the chapter.

The following examples may shed some light on the importance of documentation in the coding process.

Real Case Scenario

The gynecological oncologist bills for an abdominal hysterectomy and an appendectomy. Diagnostic codes include malignant neoplasm of the cervix and malignant neoplasm of the appendix. The claim is filed to the insurance carrier who reimburses for both services on the basis of medical necessity of the diagnoses listed.

Later medical review of the chart indicates no documented medical necessity because there was no diagnostic statement regarding malignancy to the appendix. The insurance carrier has reimbursed for services that are not "medically necessary" and thus are not covered.

Problem

Because the physician's documentation did not substantiate the appendectomy as other than incidental, payment was made inappropriately. Should the carrier make a medical chart review, the provider will be liable for refunding the amount reimbursed for the appendectomy (the law now allows for up to three times the amount reimbursed). There may also be fines and penalties, as well as a review of additional charts to identify other potentially fraudulent coding or billing. A representative sampling of similar charts may be made and a percentage of the charges billed in error may be calculated, based on the results of that representative sampling. The percentage of all such procedures billed erroneously will be calculated as the *error percentage,* and that amount will be requested by the carrier for refund as overpayment.

In addition, the provider may be liable for fraud if services were billed and not provided, or if services were deemed not medically necessary because of the lack of medical documentation. Fraud is penalized by the line item; therefore the number of cases calculated to be in error may be charged an average of $5,000 per line item, with additional penalties and interest from the date of billing to the date of discovery by the carrier.

Although the amount reimbursed for the appendectomy represented may be only $400, the penalties will include triple the reimbursement (which equals

$1,200) plus a minimum $5,000 line item fraud charge plus interest. Therefore the single appendectomy refund to the carrier will easily exceed $6,200, plus costs of the investigation into additional billing practices. The average gynecology/oncology office performs many of these services, and the amount assessed could easily run into many thousands of dollars.

In the real world of medical coding and billing, the coder attempts to impress upon the provider and documenter the importance of medical necessity in documentation. The provider may not comprehend such importance from a billing perspective but may fully understand the repercussions from a medical malpractice standpoint.

Until the last couple decades, medical record documentation served solely as the mechanism for tracking patient visits and was used primarily by the physician in the office and the medical staff. The physician or provider could document clearly and concisely, making review of documentation straightforward at the time of a future visit, or could handwrite charts illegibly because no one outside of the office had to deal with the documentation.

More recently, the role of documentation in the coding and billing process has changed dramatically. This has become necessary in light of medical malpractice suits arising from poor documentation of medical care and an increase in fraud and abuse investigation by the federal government and third-party carriers (insurance companies). Increased emphasis on providing only medically necessary services requires that providers pay attention to which services will be paid or denied and submit properly documented claims.

MEDICAL MALPRACTICE/DOCUMENTATION OF MEDICAL CARE

Because of the necessity for supporting documentation, the medical record serves as the best and perhaps the only line of defense against medical malpractice. The best protection from liability is well-documented patient care. Although many physicians may not comprehend the importance of good documentation from a coding and reimbursement perspective, they understand the necessity from a medical and legal standpoint. Take, for example, the following real-life scenario wherein documentation was the determining factor for whether prudent medical care was in fact performed by the physician:

Real Case Scenario

Two years after a patient's death from myocardial infarction (MI), the emergency department (ED) physician is sued for wrongful death. The patient's wife indicates in her suit that the ED physician failed to provide prudent medical care by not reading the electrocardiogram (ECG) performed on her husband during his last ED visit for chest pain before his death. As a result, the physician did not diagnose the MI that caused the patient's death.

The physician's counsel argues that the physician did, indeed, review the ECG, which showed no indication of an impending MI. The plaintiff's attorney asks the physician to present evidence that the ECG was in fact reviewed with no significant findings. The ECG is present in the medical record; there is, unfortunately, no evidence to support the claim that the physician had properly reviewed the ECG at the time of the patient's last visit.

Because of this lack of documentation, the ED physician was held accountable in part for the death of this patient. The outcome was that the plaintiff received a significant monetary award.

MEDICAL NECESSITY

Medical malpractice has not been the only factor that increased the importance of medical documentation. Title XVIII of the Social Security Act of 1966 mandated that the Medicare program (for elderly and disabled Americans) pay only for those services that were deemed "medically necessary." To ensure that the standard of **medical necessity** was being met for all services paid for by the Medicare program, the Health Care Finance Administration (HCFA), now known as the Centers for Medicare and Medicaid Services (CMS), began performing medical reviews. These reviews are performed based on analysis of computerized claims submitted to Medicare, as well as postpayment reviews. Computerized claims submission also allows for physician and practice profiling, including determination of physicians who might be submitting fraudulent claims, claims for procedures deemed not medically necessary, or claims for services either not provided or not documented. This process is responsible for saving the Medicare program billions of dollars annually.

With the implementation of the 1995 Evaluation and Management CPT-4 (Current Procedural Terminology, fourth edition) code specifications, Medicare began conducting random claim audits to verify that the new codes were being used appropriately. To this day, the review of Evaluation and Management services remains a top priority of the federal government and other third-party carriers because the error rate remains significantly high for these services.

The federal government also implemented **qui tam action,** which allows individuals who are aware of potential fraudulent activity to report providers and be awarded a significant amount of the funds recouped from the resulting investigation. Commercial carriers also began to see the cost benefits of implementing claims review processes such as those implemented by Medicare, and they followed suit. Thus the coder needs to be aware that all entities may review charts for potential fraud and abuse, medical necessity, and when appropriate, such entities may request refunds, interest, and perhaps penalties.

During the same time these review processes were being implemented, the cost of health care continued to soar. Third-party carriers recognized that not only did these review processes identify overpayments, they also assisted in containing health care costs. As a result, third-party carriers have invested significant time and resources to identify potential fraud, abuse, and overpayment for undocumented or inappropriately documented services.

REIMBURSEMENT

From the provider's perspective, medical record documentation serves as the means for requesting correct reimbursement for services. The record is the primary source for identifying the appropriate procedures and services performed, as well as the diagnostic documentation to support medical necessity. This information is then reviewed, interpreted, and translated into diagnostic and procedural codes, and then billed for possible reimbursement. This is the primary role of the medical coder.

THE MEDICAL CHART AS A WHOLE

The patient medical record is a compilation of information that is gathered during the patient encounter and recorded to document the care provided. The record contains information regarding the patient's medical, social, and family history, as well as information supplied by the patient with respect to presenting complaints, examination findings by the physician, and medical decisions regarding the patient's care. Because much of the data secured during the patient encounter is recorded in the patient medical record and later used for requesting reimbursement or statistical analysis, the records must contain legible, accurate, and specific information regarding each encounter.

The information contained in the medical record is used to determine whether reimbursement is received for services. In addition, medical records are useful for vital statistics, utilization review, case management, quality assurance, and research.

One of the most common difficulties encountered by the medical biller or coder is the difference between medical terminology used in medical records and the descriptors found in CPT-4 and ICD-9-CM (International Classification-ninth revision-Clinical Modification) references. An understanding of medical terms, abbreviations, and acronyms is imperative in establishing the appropriate diagnostic and procedural codes of the services performed.

The medical record document(s) may be handwritten, dictated, or typed notes, or in the form of preprinted check-off forms.

HANDWRITTEN DOCUMENTATION

Physicians are known for handwriting that is barely legible. Not only does handwritten documentation create ambiguities, it is lengthy and time-consuming to read. The average handwritten chart is one and a half times longer than a dictated report. Dictated reports tend to be more organized, easy to read, and easier to defend in the event of a medical malpractice charge.

DICTATED/TYPED DOCUMENTATION

Dictated notes tend to be more efficient, allowing quicker documentation in a more organized form. Many practices use macros, predesigned blocks of dictation, to streamline the dictation process further.

CHECK-OFF SHEETS AND PREPRINTED FORMS

Although some physicians have abandoned the use of handwritten documentation, dictation may not provide a viable solution for their practices either. The use of a check-off style form may be used for documenting the data gathered during the encounter. Although this mechanism saves time and requires less space than handwritten documentation, it becomes almost too easy for the physician to "check off" items, whether or not they are pertinent. Such a form may discourage documentation of more complete information by limiting space for findings. An alternative format would be a checklist that contains anatomical headings followed by multiple blank lines, thereby providing adequate space for documentation of significant observations.

STANDARD ACRONYMS/ABBREVIATIONS

No matter the format, documentation will almost certainly contain a number of abbreviations and acronyms. Specialty-specific abbreviations and any adopted by the individual physician should be avoided.

A listing of standard abbreviations and acronyms used in a practice is helpful for the new transcriptionist, biller, or coder, as well as during a third-party audit, utilization review, or other review of documentation. Unfortunately, many abbreviations can be interpreted more than one way. The following abbreviations serve as useful examples.

HS (such as HS-bedtime) could be interpreted as:
   at bedtime
   half strength

hamstring
heavy smoker
heel spur
high school
CP (such as chest pain) could be interpreted as:
chest pain
cleft palate
chronic pain
clinical pathway
cor pulmonale
LBP (such as low back pain) could be:
low back pain
low blood pressure

SIGNATURES LIST

When a practice contains multiple providers, the practice should be capable of identifying each individual's signature in both the office setting and the hospital setting. In the event of an audit, office personnel will be relied on to identify signatures that validate whether services coded and billed were documented appropriately. Practices with more than one provider should maintain a physician **signature list** in their files with names and appropriate marks or signatures of each provider for signature authentication purposes.

DOCUMENTATION FORMATS

There are a myriad of forms and formats that may be used in gathering and recording the vital information stored in medical records; a few of the most common forms are reviewed in this chapter. Specific documentation guidelines for each type of service are addressed in more depth in specific chapters.

Because services may be provided in the office, in the outpatient or inpatient setting, or in another facility, a number of documents are generated for record keeping, liability, and reimbursement.

OFFICE PROGRESS NOTE/HISTORY AND PHYSICAL

This document serves as one of the primary source documents for the physician's office. It may be conveyed in many formats and is usually typed or handwritten. Because of the variety of documents used for office notes, the coder must be familiar with a number of formats and possess the ability to decipher both physician's and patient's handwritten notes.

Patient History

In many instances, the documentation process actually begins with the patient. Once the patient has registered, many practices ask the patient to complete a history and physical form that contains a multitude of questions regarding current complaint(s) and medical, family, and social history information. If information from the patient's history form is used to determine the services provided, the physician must indicate that the information has been reviewed by affixing a signature or acceptable authentication, date, and proof in the form of documentation that the information was reviewed. The physician may choose as an alternative to incorporate relevant information from the history form into the patient progress note, in which case the review of the history form would not need to be documented.

In the event the **patient history** form is reviewed in subsequent visits for needed medical data, the physician will need to document each time that information from the form was used in making decisions.

An example of the Patient History and Physical form is illustrated in Figure 1-1. Note the physician designation of "abnormals" and physician authentication by signature, date, and information reviewed on this document as appropriate.

Progress Note/Visit Note

The clinical staff, including nurses or medical assistants, may actually conduct the next part of the documentation process. The patient typically is directed to the clinical area after completion of registration paperwork for "workup" documentation. The following information may be included:

Patient's reason for encounter (chief complaint)
Vital signs
Other pertinent medical data (laboratory results, other services performed that relate to the chief complaint)

These notes made by the clinical staff other than the physician may be incorporated into the diagnostic statement and procedures only if the notes are also mentioned in the provider's report (similar to the patient history described previously). The provider of service must document review of this documentation by signature/authentication and date or by incorporation in the provider's progress note.

Care should be taken that services provided by the clinical staff under the auspices of the health care professional are documented as ordered and performed to the provider's satisfaction. For instance, the patient arrives for an injection by the nurse of vitamin K. An order for that service must exist in the record, as well as the documentation that the service occurred, with review by the provider/billing entity that the provider supervised, reviewed, and approved both the service and its provision in the manner described in the notes.

An example of the staff note is illustrated in Figure 1-2. Note that this information may be incorporated in the physician's encounter documentation as in Figure 1-5, which is discussed shortly.

HISTORY AND PHYSICAL EXAMINATION

Godfrey Regional Hospital History & Physical
Admission: 12/01/00

The patient came from a nursing home and felt weak on the right side. Workers there thought she was alert, but confused. When seen in the ER, she was able to answer questions appropriately and to follow commands but was unable to lift her right leg. She had some motion in her right arm but was unable to squeeze her right hand. When evaluated by the ER physician, she was determined to be confused, and was difficult to understand. CT was obtained, with initial impression of a large, left hemispheric bleed.

Past medical history:

Remarkable for polymyalgia, GERD, hyperthyroid, DJD of the knees. Hospitalizations for pneumonia, gout, situational depression.
CURRENT MEDICATION: Prilosec 20 mg qd, Synthroid .125 mg daily, Propulsid 10 mg bid, Prednisone 20 mg daily, Cardizem CD 120 mg daily.

Family and social history

Unobtainable from patient.

Review of systems:

Unobtainable from patient.

Physical exam

Patient is alert but confused. She is not dysarthric. PERRL. Extraocular movements are normal. Sclera is clear. TMs normal. No skull lacerations noted. Slight right VII nerve weakness. Lungs clear. Abdomen is soft, nontender, without guarding or rebound. Neuro/MS: Full ROM except right arm and leg. Unable to raise her left leg or to move it at all with positive Babinski's on right. Normal labs.

Laboratory/radiology:

X-ray:

Assessment:

Intracranial bleed.

Plan:

GODFREY REGIONAL HOSPITAL
123 Main Street • Aldon, FL 77714 • (407) 555-1234

FIGURE 1-1 Patient History and Physical Form.

STAFF NOTES   Patient name _____

Date	Time	Staff notations

GODFREY MEDICAL ASSOCIATES
1532 Third Avenue, Suite 120 • Aldon, FL 77713 • (407) 555-4000

FIGURE 1-2 Staff/Visit Note.

PROBLEM LIST

Some provider offices will use a **problem list** similar to Figure 1-3 to record each time a patient visits with a new problem. This form serves as a medical summary of problems, medications, illnesses, and injuries for the provider to review at the time of each encounter for consideration in evaluating and managing the current problem. Again, this document must be reviewed and authenticated if information contained in the Problem List will be used to determine diagnostic or procedural services or information incorporated in the physician progress note.

MEDICATION RECORDS

Medications administered may be recorded on a separate document known as a **medication record** contained in the medical records. To be considered part of the diagnostic and procedural information used in the coding and billing process, these records must be documented as reviewed and approved, including orders for the medications and their appropriate administration as ordered by the physician. A minimum of the provider's signature or authentication; the date; and the name, dosage, strength, and administration route of the medication should be recorded. It will become apparent later why all this information is needed for billing and coding purposes. Figure 1-4 is an example of a Medication Record, which may be present in the physician's office or health care provider's facility.

PHYSICIAN OUTPATIENT ENCOUNTER DOCUMENTATION

The provider or physician must document not only the examination of the patient and any relevant findings, but also the "thought process" in evaluating the patient and decision making with respect to possible diagnosis and management options. This documentation should include not only positive findings, but also **pertinent negatives.** By indicating negative findings, the physician documents the thought processes required to arrive at final diagnosis(es) and the procedure(s) or service(s) that should be performed. Thus pertinent negatives, positive findings, and information regarding the history of the patient's chief complaint all play a part in the evaluation and management of the patient's condition.

Physician documentation usually is presented in one of two formats: SOAP or History, Exam, MDM format.

The **SOAP format** has been a nationally recognized method of recording patient visits for decades. The word SOAP is an acronym for (S)ubjective, (O)bjective, (A)ssessment, and (P)lan; however, this format has undergone major changes over the past few years because of documentation necessary for the assignment of Evaluation and Management procedure codes.

The **subjective** portion of the encounter takes into account all the information gathered from the patient, including information regarding the chief complaint, history of the patient, signs and symptoms, and a "patient inventory" of other system signs and symptoms.

The **objective** part of the visit consists of observed objective findings, including any pertinent negatives. For example, such an observation of the patient by the provider might be recorded as "The patient, an elderly 56-year-old female, appears to be in no acute distress." Other objective findings may include observations from the physical examination.

The **assessment** portion consists of the patient's diagnosis or problem, appropriately documented in the chart. It may also consist of differential diagnosis or a list of possible diagnoses considered in the evaluation and management process.

The **plan** portion of the SOAP note is documentation of further workup or planned treatment. A plan for further treatment, workup, and follow-up is usually included in this portion of the record.

With the inception of the 1995 and 1997 Evaluation and Management guidelines came the need for more specific guidelines. In some cases, the SOAP format was simply expanded to include these elements. In other instances, another format that encompassed the needed elements was devised.

As is discussed in Chapter 10 (Evaluation and Management Services), the patient record is composed of documentation regarding history, examination, and medical decision making components of the encounter.

The **history** portion of the record includes the chief complaint and information provided by the patient regarding the reason for the visit, as well as medical, social, and family history that may contribute to the current problem. Such information may include a review of systems gathered by the provider from patient statements or answers to questions.

The **examination** part of the record consists of the provider's findings. As with the history component, pertinent negatives or findings that rule out possible diagnoses are as important to the documentation process as positive findings.

The medical decision making component of the record contains information regarding data, management and diagnostic options, risk, and morbidity or mortality. Clinical information such as x-ray findings, laboratory and other diagnostic tests, previous medical documentation, and discussion of the patient's condition or results with other medical providers is included in the review of data. Management and diagnostic options include whether the problem is new, established, stable, or worsening. The risk of morbidity or mortality refers to the effects the patient may suffer if the condition is not treated appropriately. These components are discussed in greater depth during review of the evaluation and management process in Chapter 10.

Although the actual forms and formats differ significantly from practice to practice, Figures 1-5, 1-6, and 1-7

Text continued on p. 15

Problem list	
Date	Problem

Date	Hospitalizations

Date	Surgeries

Date	Immunizations

Name _____

Phone #: _____

Allergies	

Current medications

Screening tests	Date	Date	Date
Mammogram			
Pap smear			
DRE/PSA			
12 Lead ECG			
ECG stress test			
Colonoscopy			

Last update:

GODFREY MEDICAL ASSOCIATES
1532 Third Avenue, Suite 120 • Aldon, FL 77713 • (407) 555-4000

FIGURE 1-3 Problem List.

MEDICATION FLOW SHEET

Name: _____   Pharmacy: _____

Phone: _____   Phone: _____

Allergies: _____

Medical HX: _____

Medication	Date	Date	Date	Date	Date

GODFREY MEDICAL ASSOCIATES
1532 Third Avenue, Suite 120 • Aldon, FL 77713 • (407) 555-4000

FIGURE 1-4 Medication Flow Sheet.

PROGRESS NOTE

Chief complaint: _____

Date: _____

Vital signs: BP _____ P _____ R _____

History:

Exam:

Diagnosis/assessment:

Patient name: _____

Date of service: _____

GODFREY MEDICAL ASSOCIATES
1532 Third Avenue, Suite 120 • Aldon, FL 77713 • (407) 555-4000

FIGURE 1-5 Physician Progress Note.

PROGRESS NOTE

| Date: 02/05/XX | Vital signs: | T | R |
| Chief complaint: Sore throat, difficulty swallowing | | P | BP |

| 02/05/XX | This is a 7-year-old who has had a sore throat with some difficulty swallowing and a headache for the past two days. Not improving. |

Examination:

She is afebrile. She has retro TM fluid on the left
which is asymptomatic. The right side is normal.
She has considerable amount of oropharyngeal
inflammation, small tender anterior cervical node.
Lungs are clear to auscultation. Heart, sinus without
murmur.

Impression:

Strep tonsillitis

Plan:

She is placed on Amoxil 250 suspension tid for 10 days

Willen Obst MD

Patient name: Anne Novitz
DOB: 2/26/19XX
MR/Chart #: 63223

GODFREY REGIONAL OUTPATIENT CLINIC
3122 Shannon Avenue • Aldon, FL 77712 • (407) 555-7654

FIGURE 1-6 Physician Progress Note.

PROGRESS NOTE

Date: 01/18/XX	Vital signs:	T		R	
Chief complaint: Fever, nasal drainage		P		BP	

01/18/XX	This 9-month-old child with Down's syndrome brought in today by mother with onset of fever and thick greenish drainage from his nose. Also developed a cough again. No history of ear infections and has had a history of pneumonia.

Physical examination:

General appearance of well-developed child in no acute distress

Head: Flat anterior fontanel

Ears: Canals small, cleared of cerumen

Neck: No adenopathy

Lungs: Clear, no wheezing but has noisy inspiratory respiration
        for which he had a recent bronchoscopy

Nose: He does have thick greenish drainage from his nose

Assessment:

Upper respiratory infection with symptoms of pulmonary infection

Plan:

Continue with Ibuprofen and decongestants
Placed on Augmentin 200 mg twice daily

Willen Obst MD

Patient name: Thomas Derringer
DOB: 4/16/20XX
MR/Chart #: 24481

GODFREY REGIONAL OUTPATIENT CLINIC
3122 Shannon Avenue • Aldon, FL 77712 • (407) 555-7654

FIGURE 1-7 Physician Progress Note.

are representative samples of physician progress notes in the provider office setting. Later in the chapter, variations in hospital and facility progress notes are highlighted.

ANCILLARY REPORTS/RECORDS

Ancillary records such as x-ray, laboratory, and other diagnostic tests are typically recorded on separate documents in the medical record. Usually, two physicians are involved with this process: one ordering the procedure and one performing it and interpreting results. When two physicians are involved, only that physician responsible for the final interpretation can bill for the interpretative services. If one physician requires input or collaboration with the other physician (often known as an *overread*), then only the physician ultimately responsible for the interpretation may code and bill for the service. Documentation and billing for these services will differ on the basis of the providers that are involved (see later discussion). These documents may be found in both the physician chart and in the facility chart, depending on where services were performed and which provider is involved in treatment and interpretation.

For illustration, a radiology report (Figure 1-8), laboratory test results (Figure 1-9), a surgical pathology report (Figure 1-10), an ECG (Figure 1-11), respiratory test outcomes (Figure 1-12), and an electromyography report (Figure 1-13) are provided. Specific documentation, signature requirements, and document contents are discussed in detail in the section on Radiology, Laboratory, and Medicine services.

HOSPITAL/FACILITY RECORDS

The hospital record creates another complication in the documentation process. In many instances, either a practice does not have access to the documentation, or access is extremely difficult. In addition, the provider typically does not dictate these hospital visit notes, except perhaps for the Admissions History and Physical. As a result, the documentation is typically short, is sometimes marginally legible, and may not be accessible for every single chart so that level of service for coding and billing purposes may be determined.

In addition, requirements for hospital records often are above and beyond those of office records. The **Joint Commission on Accreditation of Healthcare Organizations (JCAHO),** a national organization that accredits hospitals, has developed additional guidelines for inpatient medical records that include the following:

Patient's medical history
Any known allergies
Medical history completed within the first 24 hours of admission for inpatient
Physical examination completed within the first 24 hours of admission for inpatient

Conclusion drawn from the admitting history and physical examination
Course of action statement planned for the stay
Diagnostic/therapeutic orders
Progress notes by all providers
Consultation reports
Nursing notes
Ancillary procedure reports
Conclusions or discharge summary at the end of the hospital stay

Keep in mind that facility documentation, in the form of nursing notes and notes by other facility employees, may not be considered as part of the provider's record, unless they are documented as reviewed or are incorporated in the provider's medical record.

A number of documents, such as the following, may be included in hospital records:

Admission history and physical
Progress note
Discharge summary
Consultations
Operative/surgical report

Admission History and Physical

A hospital or similar facility requires that a History be taken and a Physical examination be performed on all patients to assess their condition, needs, and plan for treatment. Because this is usually a comprehensive service that takes place during admission, the documentation is typically dictated and includes in-depth information regarding history, present illnesses, examination, and management options. In many facilities, such as hospitals that are governed by JCAHO accreditation standards, this admission history and physical examination, also known as an *H&P,* must be performed within 24 hours of admission. Figure 1-14 is an example of a Hospital History and Physical examination. Although the service may be initially performed by an intern or resident under the governance of the physician, the physician must see and evaluate the patient as well. Legal documentation requirements for residents and providers other than physicians are discussed in later chapters.

Progress Note

The biggest problem with hospital daily visit notes is they are often brief, handwritten, and sometimes illegible, or they may not be present at all. Some of the biggest fraud cases have involved services performed in the hospital setting that were not properly documented. When the provider sees the patient in the hospital, the evaluation of the patient and the provider's assessment and plan should be documented in the daily progress note. Because more than one provider may see the patient

Text continued on p. 23

RADIOLOGY REPORT

MR#:
DOB:
Dr.

Clinical summary:

Abdomen:

Conclusion:

Ddt/mm

D:
T:

_____

, M.D.   Date

GODFREY REGIONAL HOSPITAL
123 Main Street • Aldon, FL 77714 • (407) 555-1234

FIGURE 1-8 Radiology Report.

Patient name: _____	Room #: _____
Age: _____ Sex: _____	Accession #: _____
Collected: _____	Received: _____
Reported: _____	Req. #/Med. Rec. #:_____
Requesting Phys:_____	Pt. ID #: _____

| Test name | Results | | Reference range | TL |
	Out of range	In range		

Testing location (see reverse side)

GODFREY CLINICAL LABORATORIES
465 Dogwood Court • Aldon, FL 77712 • (407) 555-9876

FIGURE 1-9 Laboratory Report.

SURGICAL PATHOLOGY REPORT

Name: _____ Hosp. No.: _____ Path. No.: _____

Date: _____ Room: _____ Age: _____ Sex: _____ Surgeon: _____ M.D.

Operation: _____

Material submitted: _____

Pre-op diagnosis: _____

Post-op diagnosis: _____

Previous material: _____ Pertinent history: _____

Diagnosis:

_____ M.D.
Pathologist

Gross description:

Micro description:

GODFREY CLINICAL LABORATORIES
465 Dogwood Court • Aldon, FL 77712 • (407) 555-9876

FIGURE 1-10 Surgical Pathology Report.

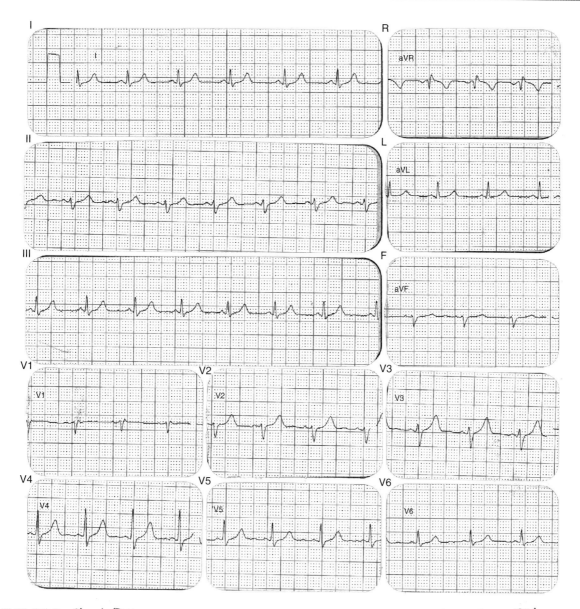

CLIN. DIAG.: Chest Pain

ECG DESCRIPTION: Stat 12 Lead

INTERPRETATION:

PATIENT: Jane Doe

DIG ( ) QUIN. ( ) AGE 29 SEX F B.P. 120/80

ECG REQUEST BY Dr. Hope V. Arewell.....
ATR. RATE ...90..... VENTR. RATE 90......
INTERVALS: P-R..12.. QRS..08.. QTc........
AXIS: Left Axis shift
RHYTHM: Normal Sinus Rhythm

INTERPRETED BY: H. Arewell MD..........
DATE:

FIGURE 1-11 Electrocardiogram. *(From Chester GA: Modern medical assisting, Philadelphia, 1998, WB Saunders.)*

Place top of report No. 3 here

PULMONARY FUNCTION REPORT

Name: _____

ID #: _____

Age: _____ Ht: _____ Wt: _____

Reason for test: _____

Smoker? _____

Dyspnea: _____

Lung surgery: _____

Frequent cough: _____

Pain breathing? _____

Heart disease? _____

Wheeze/asthma? _____

Abnormal X-ray? _____

Test	PRED	ACTL	%PRED
FVC	4.76		81%
FEV1	3.77		88%
FEV1/FVC	81%		107%
FEF 25%–75%	4.64		124%
MMET (sec.)	0.68		49%
FEF max	9.14		127%
FEF 25%	8.43		126%
FEF 50%	6.26		118%
FEF 75%	3.17		56%
ET (sec.)	—		—
Maximal FVC	4.76		81%
Maximal FEV1	3.77		88%
MVV (L/min.)	154.7		100%

BTPS factor: _____ Last cal: _____

Primary normals source: Knudson.

Base: _____

T _____

Operator: _____

Physician: _____

GODFREY CLINICAL LABORATORIES
465 Dogwood Court • Aldon, FL 77712 • (407) 555-9876

FIGURE 1-12 Respiratory Testing Report.

ELECTROMYOGRAPHY LABORATORY REPORT

Nerve conduction studies	Name: _____

NR = No response
M = Motor
S = Sensory
Mx = Mixed
• = no increment after 10 sec. exercise
† = no decrement to 2/sec x3
X = Forearm median to ulnar crossover

Name: _____
Clinic number: _____ Age: _____
Birthdate: _____ Date: _____
Referring physician: _____

Nerve stimulated (Recording site)	Amplitude (Sensory = uV; Meter = mV)					Distal/peak latency (mSec)			Conduction velocity (M/sec)			F-wave latency (mSec)		
	Distal			Proximal										
	Right	Left	Normal	Rt	Lt	Rt	Lt	Normal	Rt	Lt	Normal	Rt	Lt	Normal
Lower right														
Sural (S) Pt.B ankle						NH								
Peroneal (M) knee EDB	3.0					14.8			45					
Peroneal (M) ankle EDB	3.0					4.8								
Posterior tibia (M) knee AH	1.0					14.8			41					
Posterior tibia (M) ankle AH	1.5					4.2								
H-reflex						NR	NR							
Med (s) wrist 1st	9.0					3.6								
Med (m) elbow thenar	2.8					9.6			58					
Med (m) wrist thenar	2.8					4.4								
Ulnar (s) wrist 5th	1440					2.8								

Needle examination:

Summary:

Impression:

_____ , M.D.

GODFREY CLINICAL LABORATORIES
465 Dogwood Court • Aldon, FL 77712 • (407) 555-9876

FIGURE 1-13 Electromyography Report.

HISTORY AND PHYSICAL EXAMINATION

WHITE, Blanche
Admitted: 04/26/XXXX

John Parker, M.D.

Medical record number: 2253546

Patient is an 89-year-old female who presents with abdominal pain, nausea, vomiting and weakness. She has also had a fairly substantial weight loss over the last year or so. Symptoms started getting worse yesterday. She denies fever or chills. Bowels have moved, although not substantially. She says she really has not eaten enough to have a bowel movement at this time. She denied any blood in her emesis. No blood in her stool. The pain seems to be in the epigastric area, although it seems to radiate a little bit to the right side. Denies pain into the back at all. She also denies chest pain or SOB. She had become weak, enough that she has fallen. This had been a problem for her in the past, where she had fallen, but she has not had a fall for quite some time.

Past medical history:

Hypertension, cholelithiasis, depression, osteoarthritis and CHF. She also has cholelithiasis but no cholecystitis. She reports the recent onset of Type II diabetes mellitus. She reports an allergy to Penicillin and Amoxicillin.

Family and social history:

Noncontributory except she does smoke

Review of systems:

Denies dysuria or any difficulty urinating. She denies fever, chills or any swelling in her upper or lower extremities. No difficulties reported in breathing, joint pain, specifically knee pain she has reported in the past.

Physical exam

General:	Alert, oriented, in no obvious distress
Vital signs:	Temperature 98.4, respiration 20, BP 117/43
HEENT:	Negative
Neck:	Supple, no thyromegaly
Chest:	Clear
Heart:	Regular rate and rhythm, normal S1, S2, no gallops, rubs or murmurs
Abdomen:	Soft, epigastric tenderness. No mass or organomegaly. No guarding, rebound or rigidity if noted
Back:	No pain or spinal tenderness is noted on exam
Extremities:	No swelling or edema noted
Neuro:	She appears a little less alert and oriented than she has in the past

Laboratory/radiology:

Lab tests include WBC of 13,200, hemoglobin 11.8, platelet count 220,000. The differential appears within normal range. Panel 20 shows a decreased sodium of 133, Potassium 3.3, BUN and creatinine are 34 and 1.4. Calcium is 8.1, Bilirubin 1.1. Proteins normal, liver functions normal and TSH is 2.2. Urinalysis is normal.

X-ray:

Flat and upright of her abdomen are pending at this time.

Assessment:

Patient with abdominal pain, nausea, and weakness. This would be recurrent cholelithiasis or gastroenteritis.

Plan:

Admit to hospital, and will give her medications for her nausea. IV fluids for rehydration and watch for fever, chills. If things do not improve, will order ultrasound or CT.

GODFREY REGIONAL HOSPITAL
123 Main Street • Aldon, FL 77714 • (407) 555-1234

FIGURE 1-14 Hospital Admission and History.

daily, each document should bear the provider's name, authentication, and date for specific services. Figure 1-15 is an example of a hospital or facility progress note.

Discharge Summary

The **discharge summary** should document the various services provided that prepare the patient for discharge from the inpatient facility. In Chapter 10 (Evaluation and Management Services), it is explained that discharge visits are based on the amount of time required to prepare the patient for discharge, including any services performed on the patient's floor. Services provided; the patient's progress during hospitalization; and discharge instructions, follow-up, and diagnoses are all included in the discharge summary, which is usually dictated because it tends to be lengthy and contains significant data. Figure 1-16 represents a typical discharge note for a hospital or facility. Again, format may differ from one facility to another, but the information contained in this document is typically the same.

Consultations

A **consultation** involves one physician sending the patient to another physician for an expert medical opinion. Documentation must contain a written request and a written report with findings that was sent back to the requesting physician. Consultations are perhaps the most misunderstood medical documents and are often incorrectly coded and billed. For services to remain consultative in nature, the physician rendering an opinion may provide therapy but cannot assume primary care of the patient. Consultations may occur in many settings, including the hospital or facility, physician's office, or any setting where the criteria have been met. Figure 1-17 is an example of a dictated consultation report.

Operative/Procedure Report

A surgical procedure report, regardless of whether the procedure was performed in the hospital or in the office, would be documented in the same manner. The following elements should be included in all such documents:

> Patient identification (Name, Medical Record Number, Date of Birth, Room #)
> Preoperative diagnosis
> Postoperative diagnosis
> Name of procedure
> Surgeon(s)
> Anesthesia/anesthesiologist(s)
> Indications
> Procedure detail
> Findings summary
> Complications/unusual service
> Postoperative condition

One of the most common mistakes made on the interpretation of operative reports is being misled by the word *summary* under "Procedure Performed." Because this summary is abbreviated, it often does not contain all the information necessary to assign diagnostic and procedural codes as appropriate. To code and bill for every service that was provided, the coder must review the entire operative record, sometimes multiple pages, abstract the key elements, and assign codes for all services provided. Chapter 12 (Surgery Services) illustrates how involved this process can be.

An example of an operative report is given in Figure 1-18. In addition, the anesthesiologist would also generate a report of the preanesthesia services, administration of anesthesia, and patient monitoring (Figure 1-19).

HEALTH CARE STAFF NOTES ("NURSING" NOTES)

Notes made by health care staff may be incorporated into the diagnostic statement only if these notes are mentioned in the provider's progress notes. If such documents are to be used in this manner, they must be referenced by the provider's own documentation (date, signature or authentication, and approval of actions taken or treatments provided). These nursing notes are similar to the visit note represented in Figure 1-2, except that the headings will reflect the hospital or facility's information rather than the physician's.

ANCILLARY TEST FINDINGS

Other tests may be considered as part of the history, examination, and medical decision making components used for diagnostic and procedural coding, if the physician provides written interpretation. This interpretation may be recorded on the order slip along with the date and signature or authentication of the provider, or it may be incorporated in the progress note signed and dated by the provider. Reports regarding provider documentation have been previously discussed. Keep in mind that facility tests are performed by employees of the facility or hospital; a qualified provider must perform the interpretations.

For certain ancillary services to be considered for coding, billing, and reimbursement, a minimum amount of information must be provided in the interpretive statement. For example, to consider reimbursement for an ECG, most third-party insurance carriers require a minimum of heart rate, rhythm, and ectopy notation. Should physicians provide various ancillary services, the coder must determine the minimum requirements for reimbursement specified by each carrier, so that requests for reimbursement may be submitted in the proper format.

Text continued on p. 31

PROGRESS NOTE

Date/time

04/27/XX

S:

Patient is feeling a little better, and she is not having as much abdominal pain.
She is still experiencing some trouble with confusion and loose stools. She appears
to have lapsing periods of confusion, and even seeing people that are actually not there.
Otherwise she indicates she feels somewhat better. Denies chest pain, SOB, but reports
she still feels a little weak.

O:

Afebrile, vital signs normal. Chest clear, heart regular rhythm, extremities show no appearance of edema.

A:

Abdominal pain with diarrhea, improved.
Confusion that may be related to infection.

P:

Will get blood cultures and start her on IV medications. If her confusion continues, may determine CT scan
or ultrasound would be appropriate.

John Palermo

Patient ID

WHITE, Blanche
Admit: 04/26/XX
MR# 2253546

PROGRESS NOTES

GODFREY REGIONAL HOSPITAL
123 Main Street • Aldon, FL 77714 • (407) 555-1234

FIGURE 1-15 Hospital Progress Notes.

DISCHARGE SUMMARY

	WHITE, Blanche #2253546
	DOB: 05/17/XX

Admitted: 04/26/XX
Discharged: 04/30/XX

Discharge diagnoses:

1. Diverticulosis
2. Abdominal pain with fever
3. Cholelithiasis
4. Confusion
5. Hypertension
6. Depression
7. Osteoarthritis
8. Congestive heart failure
9. Diabetes mellitus type II

History:

Patient is an 89-year-old female who presented with abdominal pain, nausea, and vomiting. She was also weak. She had lost some weight, mostly I think because of dietary measures to control her newly diagnosed diabetes. She had no fever or chills. Her BMs had been fairly regular although not substantial. I do not feel that she is eating enough because of her recent symptoms to make bowel movements. There was no diarrhea. There has been no blood in the stool. She did have an emesis earlier that had no blood in it. Pain seemed to be over the epigastrium and left side, sometimes would radiate to the right side.

On exam, temperature was 98.4°, respiratory rate 20, blood pressure 117/43. HEENT examination was negative. Chest was clear. Heart had a regular rhythm, normal S1, S2, no gallops, rubs or murmurs. The abdomen was soft, there was epigastric tenderness. No mass or organomegaly. There was no guarding, rebound or rigidity. Extremities had no edema.

Laboratory and radiology studies:

Lab tests include a CBC showing a white count of 15,200, hemoglobin 11.8, platelet count 220,000. Follow-ups remained stable with an improving white count of 7,600. Hemoglobin had dropped to 10.8 with hydration.

On admission her sodium was 133, Potassium 3.3, BUN was elevated at 34, blood sugar 193. Calcium was low at 8.1. Bilirubin was up to 1.1 and her TSH was 2.2. Her sugars were followed in the hospital and they ranged fairly stable with a high being noted at 195, low of 75. Her potassium did respond to supplementation and was 3.9 on discharge. Her sodium also improved to 137 by discharge. BUN was back to normal as was the creatinine. Liver function testing was normal by discharge.

Urinalysis was remarkable for 2–3 WBCs per hpf. Blood cultures were negative.

Flat and upright of abdomen showed degenerative changes and a probable gallstone.

Abdominal ultrasound showed cholelithiasis.

Hospital course:

Patient was admitted to the hospital because of her abdominal symptoms. She was started on Protonix 40 mg IV as well as Demerol for pain. Her pre-hospital medications were continued. Blood cultures were obtained and she was placed on Levaquin 500 mg every 24 hours. Amaryl was also started for her blood sugars, which remained stable except for a low of 56. She was a little symptomatic with this and so sugar was given. Her potassium was supplemented with cocktails in addition to the IV fluids. Over the course of her hospitalization she did feel better with her stomach. She did have some trouble with confusion on occasion, but mostly with the initial episode of her illness and during the time she had a fever. Over the course of her stay however, she was still weak and we needed to watch her blood sugars closely. She was switched to oral Levaquin, told to monitor her blood sugars closely, and continue the Amaryl. She will be started on OT and PT to help in strengthening her gait.

D: 04/30/XX
T: 05/02/XX

GODFREY REGIONAL HOSPITAL
123 Main Street • Aldon, FL 77714 • (407) 555-1234

FIGURE 1-16 Discharge Summary.

CONSULTATIONS

Indication for consultation:

Ventricular tachycardia

History:

54-year-old with known history of cardiac disease who was undergoing outpatient arthroscopy of the knee. Patient's cardiac rhythm was noted to have multiple runs of non-sustained ventricular tachycardia. Patient remained asymptomatic stable.
Status post MI 15 years ago.

FAMILY/SOCIAL HISTORY:
Non-contributory

Exam:

PHYSICAL EXAM:
Head: Normocephalic, atraumatic
Neck: Supple, w/o evidence of JVP, mass or bruit
Chest: Clear to auscultation
Cardiac: Normal carotid upstroke with normal contour
Abdomen: Soft, nontender, no evidence of mass
Extremities: Showed no evidence of clubbing, cyanosis, or edema
Neurologic: Grossly intact, nonfocal
EKG: Ectopic atrial rhythm with delayed precordial transmission

Diagnosis/assessment:

IMPRESSION:
Known history of coronary atherosclerotic heart disease and atrial fibrillation, now presents with run of nonsustained
V tach per report. It would be prudent to continue patient on his current medications and allow him to follow-up with his
primary cardiologist.

We appreciate the opportunity to participate in the overall evaluation and management of this patient.

Patient name: _____

Date of service: _____

GODFREY MEDICAL ASSOCIATES
1532 Third Avenue, Suite 120 • Aldon, FL 77713 • (407) 555-4000

FIGURE 1-17 Dictated Consultation Report.

OPERATIVE REPORT

Patient information:

Patient name:
DOB:
MR#:

Preoperative diagnosis:

Postoperative diagnosis:

Procedure(s) performed:

Anesthesia:

Assistant surgeon:

Description of procedure:

GODFREY REGIONAL HOSPITAL
123 Main Street • Aldon, FL 77714 • (407) 555-1234

FIGURE 1-18 Operative Report.

PRE-ANESTHESIA EVALUATION

Age	Sex ☐ M ☐ F	Height in./cm.	Weight lb./kg.	Pre-procedure vital signs B/P P R T

Proposed procedure

Previous anesthesia/operations *(if none, check here ☐)*	**Current medications** *(if none, check here ☐)*

Family history of anesthesia complications *(if none, check here ☐)*	**Allergies** *(if NKDA, check here ☐)*

Airway/teeth/head and neck	**History from** ☐ Parent/guardian ☐ Poor historian ☐ Chart ☐ Significant other ☐ Patient

System	WNL	Comments	Pertinent study results
Respiratory Asthma Pneumonia Bronchitis Productive cough COPD Recent cold Dyspnea SOB Orthopnea Tuberculosis	☐	Tobacco use: ☐ No ☐ Yes ____ Pack/Day for ____ Years	Chest X-ray Pulmonary studies
Cardiovascular Angina MI Arrhythmia Murmur CHF MVP Exercise tolerance Pacemaker Hypertension Rheumatic fever	☐		EKG
Hepato/gastrointestinal Bowel obstruction Jaundice Cirrhosis N&V Hepatitis Reflux/heartburn Histal hernia Ulcers	☐	Ethanol use: ☐ No ☐ Yes Frequency_____	
Neuro/musculoskeletal Arthritis Paresthesia Back problems Syncope CVA/stroke Seizures DJD TIAs Headaches Weakness Loss of consciousness Neuromuscular disease Paralysis	☐		
Renal/endocrine Diabetes Renal failure/dialysis Thyroid disease Urinary retention Urinary tract infection Weight loss/gain	☐		
Other Anemia Bleeding tendencies Hemophilia Pregnancy Sickle cell trait Transfusion history			

Problem list/diagnoses	ASA PS	**Lab studies** Hgb/HcT/CBC Electrolytes Urinalysis
	1	
	2	
Planned anesthesia/special monitors	3	Other
	4	
	5	
	E	**Post-anesthesia note**

Pre-anesthesia medications ordered	
Signature of evaluator(s)	Signed Date Time

Optional form 517 back

GODFREY REGIONAL HOSPITAL
123 Main Street • Aldon, FL 77714 • (407) 555-1234

FIGURE 1-19 Anesthesia Report.

History from:	☐ Patient	☐ Chart	PRE-ANESTHESIA EVALUATION	☐	See previous anesthesia record dated _____ for information
	☐ Parent/guardian	☐ Poor historian			
	☐ Significant other	☐ Language barrier			

Proposed procedure | **Age** | **Sex** ☐ M ☐ F | **Height** _____ in/cm | **Weight** _____ lb/kg

Pre-procedure vital signs
B/P:　　　　P:　　　　R:　　　T:　　　O₂ SAT %:

Current medications　　☐ None

Previous anesthesia/operations　　☐ None

Airway
☐ MP1　☐ Unrestricted neck ROM　☐ ↓ mouth opening/TMJ　☐ Edentulous
☐ MP2　☐ T-M distance = _____　☐ Hx difficult airway　☐ Facial hair
☐ MP3　☐ Obesity　☐ Teeth poor repair　☐ Short muscular neck
☐ MP4　☐ ↓ neck ROM:　☐ Teeth chipped/loose:

Family HX anes. problems

Allergies　　☐ None

System	Comments	Diagnostic studies
☐ WNL Respiratory	Tobacco use: ☐ Yes ☐ No ☐ Quit _____ Packs/Day for _____ Years	**ECG**
Asthma/RAD　Chronic tonsillitis		
Bronchiolitis　Chronic OM		
COPD　Recent URI		
Emphysema　TB/+PPD		
Bronchitis　Pneumonia		**Chest X-ray**
Respiratory failure　Productive cough		
Pleural effusion　SOB/dyspnea		
Pulmonary embolism　OSA		
Sinusitis/rhinitis　Orthopnea	*Pre-procedure* pulmonary assessment:	**Pulmonary studies**
Environ. allergies　Wheezing		
☐ WNL Cardiovascular		
Hypertension　Abnormal ECG		
Hyperlipoproteinemia　Dysrhythmia		
CAD/cardiomyopathy　Hypovolemia		
Angina　Chronic fatigue		**Laboratory studies**
Stable/unstable　Pacemaker/AICD		
Myocardial infarction　Murmur		
CHF DOE PND　Valvular Dz/MVP		
Peripheral vascular Dz　Rheumatic fever		
Exercise tolerance　Endocarditis		
Excellent/fair/poor　Aneurysm	*Pre-procedure* cardiac assessment:	
☐ WNL Hepato/gastrointestinal	Ethanol use: ☐ Yes ☐ No ☐ Quit Frequency _____ ☐ Hx ETOH abuse	
Obesity　N & V		
Cirrhosis　Diarrhea		
Hepatitis/jaundice　IBS		
Bowel obstruction　Pancreatitis		
Ulcers　Gallbladder Dz		
Hiatal hernia　Diverticulum		PT/PTT/INR:　　T&S/T&C:
GERD　Colon polyps		
☐ WNL Neuro/musculoskeletal		HCG:　　U/A:
Arthritis/DJD　Muscle weakness		LMP:
Back problems (LBP)　Neuromuscular Dz		
CVA/TIA　Paralysis		
Psychiatric disorder　Paresthesia(s)		**Other diagnostic tests**
Headaches　Syncope		
↑ ICP/head injury　Seizures		
Loss of consciousness　Epilepsy		
☐ WNL Renal/endocrine		
Thyroid disease　Prostate		
Cushing's syndrome　BPH/CA		
Renal failure/dialysis　Diabetes mellitus		
Renal insufficiency　Type I/II/Gest.		
Renal stones　UTI		
Adrenocortical insuff.　Pituitary disorder		
☐ WNL Other		
Anemia　Immunosuppressed		
Bleeding disorder　Sickle cell Dz/trait		
Cancer　Recent steroids		
Chemotherapy　Transfusion Hx		
Radiation Tx　Weight loss/gain		
Dehydration　Herbal/OTC drug use		
HIV/AIDS　Illicit drug use		
☐ WNL Pregnancy	☐ AROM　☐ Mg drip	
TIUP　SGA　Multiple gestation	☐ SROM　_____ gm/hr　Weeks gest:	
Pre-eclampsia　LGA　VBAC	☐ Pitocin drip	
HELLP　PROM　IUGR	☐ Induction　G:　P:　EDC:	

Surgical diagnosis/problem list

Post-anesthesia care notes

Location	Time	Controlled medications			
		Medication	Used	Destroyed	Returned
B/P	O₂ Sat ____%				

Physical status: 1 2 3 4 5 E

Pulse	Resp	Temp

Provider　　**Witness**

☐ Awake　☐ Stable　☐ Mask O₂
☐ Somnolent　☐ Unstable　☐ NC O₂
☐ Unarousable　☐ Oral/nasal airway
Intubated - ☐ T-piece ☐ Ventilator
Regional - dermatome level: _____
☐ Continuous epidural analgesia
☐ Direct admit to hospital ward
　(PACU recovery not required)
☐ Recovery recorded on anes. form

☐ No anesthesia related complications noted
☐ Satisfactory post anesthesia/analgesia recovery
☐ See progress notes for anesthesia related concerns

Planned anesthesia/special monitors

Pre-anesthesia medications ordered

Evaluator signature　　**Date**

Provider　　**Date**　　**Time**

GODFREY REGIONAL HOSPITAL
123 Main Street • Aldon, FL 77714 • (407) 555-1234

FIGURE 1-19, cont'd

Continued

ANESTHESIA RECORD

Procedure(s)

	Start	Stop
Anesthesia		
Procedure		
Room time **in**:		**out**:

Date   OR#   Page   of   Surgeon(s)

Pre-procedure

☐ Identified   ☐ ID band   ☐ Questioned
☐ Chart reviewed   ☐ Permit signed
☐ NPO since _____
☐ Patient reassessed prior to anesthesia
   & surgery - Ready to proceed
☐ Peri-operative pain management discussed
   with patient/guardian, plan of care completed
Pre-anesthetic state:
☐ Awake   ☐ Anxious   ☐ Uncooperative
☐ Calm   ☐ Lethargic   ☐ Unresponsive
Other:

Patient safety

☐ Anesthesia machine# _____ checked
☐ Secured with safety belt
☐ Arm(s) secured on armboards: L   R
☐ Arm(s) tucked: L   R   ☐ Axillary roll
☐ Pressure points checked, padded, monitored
☐ Eye care: ☐ Taped closed   ☐ Ointment
              ☐ Saline   ☐ Pads ☐ Goggles
☐ No pressure on orbits when prone

Monitors and equipment

☐ Steth: ☐ Esoph ☐ Precordial ☐ Suprasternal
☐ Non-invasive B/P   ☐ V lead ECG
☐ Continuous ECG   ☐ ST/Dysrhy. analysis
☐ Pulse oximeter   ☐ Nerve stimulator:
☐ End tidal CO_2 ☐ Ulnar ☐ Tibial
☐ Oxygen monitor   ☐ Facial ☐ _____
☐ ET agent analyzer   ☐ Fluid/blood warmer
☐ Temp: _____   ☐ Cell saver   ☐ BIS
☐ Body warmer   ☐ TEE   ☐ ICP
☐ Airway humidifier: ☐ FHT monitor ☐ EEG
                            ☐ Evoked potential:
☐ NG/OG tube   ☐SSEP☐ BAEP☐ MEP
☐ Foley catheter   ☐ Doppler: _____
☐ Arterial line _____
☐ CVP _____
☐ PA line _____
☐ IV(s) _____

Anesthetic technique

GA induction: ☐ Intravenous ☐ Pre-O_2 ☐ RSI
☐ Cricoid pressure   ☐ Inhalation ☐ IM   ☐ PR
GA maintenance: ☐ Inhalation   ☐ Inhalation/IV
☐ GA/regional combination   ☐ TIVA
Regional: Epidural- ☐ Thoracic ☐ Lumbar ☐ Caudal
☐ SAB ☐ Ankle ☐ Femoral ☐ Axillary ☐ Interscalene
☐ CSE ☐ Bier ☐ Continuous spinal ☐ Cervical plexus
☐ Other:
Regional technique: ☐ Position _____
☐ See remarks   ☐ Prep _____
☐ Local _____   ☐ Site _____
☐ Needle _____
☐ LA _____
☐ Narcotic _____
☐ Additive _____
☐ Test dose Rx _____
☐ Attempts x _____   ☐ Level _____
☐ Catheter _____ ☐ Test dose response: +   −
Space _____ cm Skin _____ cm   ☐ Secured
☐ Sedation & analgesia/monitored anesthesia care

Airway management

☐ Oral ETT   ☐ RAE   ☐ L.T.A.   ☐ Magill forceps
☐ Nasal ETT   ☐ LMA # _____
☐ Stylet   ☐ LMA fastrach # _____
☐ DVL   ☐ LMA ProSeal # _____
☐ Tube size:_____   ☐ FOI   ☐ Awake
☐ Blade: _____   ☐ Laser ETT ☐ LIS
☐ Attempts x _____   ☐ EMG ETT ☐ Bougie
☐ Grade: I   II   III   IV ☐ Armored ETT ☐ Blind
☐ Secured at _____ cm   ☐ DLT_____
☐ ET CO_2 present   ☐ Univent _____
☐ Breath sounds = bilateral ☐ _____
☐ Cuffed-min. occ. pres. with:☐ Air ☐ NS ☐ _____
☐ Uncuffed-leaks at _____ cm H_2O
☐ Oral airway   ☐ Nasal airway ☐ Bite block
Circuit: ☐ Circle system   ☐ NRB   ☐ Bain
☐ Mask case   ☐ Via tracheotomy/stoma
☐ Nasal cannula ☐ Simple O_2 mask☐ _____
Nebulizer:
Topicalization:
Nerve block(s):

Time:

Agents

☐ Des ☐ Iso ☐ Sevo ☐ Halo (%)
☐ N_2O ☐ Air   (L/min)
Oxygen (L/min)
(   )
(   )
(   )
(   )
(   )
(   )
(   )
(   )

Totals

Fluids

Urine   (ml)
EBL   (ml)
Gastric   (ml)

Monitors

ECG
% Oxygen inspired (FiO_2)
O_2 saturation (SaO_2)
End Tidal CO_2
Temp: ☐ C ☐ F

PNS/TOF

Peri-op meds

200
180
160
140
120
100
80
60
40
20

(graph values: 150, 120, 100, 80, 50)

Symbols

∨
∧
B/P cuff pressure

⊥
⊤
Arterial line pressure

X
Mean arterial pressure

●
Pulse

○
Spontaneous respiration

Ø
Assisted respiration

⊗
Controlled respiration

T
Tourniquet

Vent

Tidal volume (ml)
Respiratory rate
Peak pressure   (cm H_2O)
☐ PEEP ☐ CPAP   (cm H_2O)
Symbols for remarks
Position

Time of delivery:
Sex: M   F   /
Apgars:

Provider(s)

Patient identification

Remarks:

GODFREY REGIONAL HOSPITAL
123 Main Street • Aldon, FL 77714 • (407) 555-1234

FIGURE 1-19, cont'd

OTHER DOCUMENTATION NEEDS

In addition to the requirements for specific services discussed earlier, other general guidelines exist for documenting services. Certain terms are acceptable in some services but may be disallowed in others. For example, the notation "patient doing well" is not acceptable for complete documentation of a patient visit. As has already been described, a minimum history, physical examination, and medical decision making documentation should be recorded for all such visits. The conclusion or impression of "doing well," however, might be acceptable for an outpatient office visit, with the inclusion of a diagnosis or diagnostic impression. The documentary note "doing well" would NOT be acceptable, however, for a critical care visit, which requires constant attendance to the care of a critically ill or injured unstable patient. In fact, the note "doing well" would be contradictory to the billing of a critical care visit; it would imply that the patient was in fact not critically ill, but rather "doing well." Thus the provider should be careful in the choice of words when recording services.

Descriptors for visits should be chosen carefully. The type of service to be billed should be aligned carefully with the content of the visit documentation. This is described at length in Chapter 10 (Evaluation and Management Services).

Developing Documentation Tools for the Practice

One of the coder's responsibilities is to identify problem areas in the documentation process and educate the staff in rectifying these problems. A number of steps can be taken in this process. The coder must determine effective methods and means for successfully correcting documentation problems within the practice.

Just as the coder enters the coding profession as a career choice, the physician has usually entered the medical profession for the primary purpose of diagnosing and treating patients—not to appropriately document the patient chart for coding and billing. With this in mind, the coder must develop strategies to ensure the collection of proper documentation for coding. Some suggestions for optimizing data collection in patient records are offered in the following paragraphs.

STANDARDIZED DICTATION NOTE GUIDES

Make certain that the physician, provider, or transcriber has available a listing of the elements that must be assessed and noted in the medical documentation during the patient encounter. Develop a guide for such elements presented in a format that is usable by the person responsible for dictating or documenting the record. This may take the form of an outline posted in the dictation area,

or a "pocket card" that can be carried by the provider at all times for reference. A copy of a sample "History and Physical" dictation pocket card is shown in Tool 1.

Other useful tools for making certain that patient records include all the vital elements of documentation are illustrated in Tools 2, 3, and 4.

STANDARDIZED PROGRESS NOTE FORMS

Another way to ensure proper documentation is to incorporate specific guidelines into the practice's standardized forms. For instance, column notations that outline needed documentation such as "social history," "family history," and "differential diagnosis" can be used. Stress to those making documentation the need to record "noncontributory" and "not applicable" when appropriate. Emphasize the importance of following a set format so that third-party carriers and staff can locate specific information at a particular place on the form.

In the event the documenter handwrites the documentation, a standardized form can incorporate time-saving mechanisms such as descriptive words that can be circled when appropriate. Even if the documenter dictates at a later time, the circled information will assist in providing a complete record.

An example of a standardized progress note or record of treatment for the ED setting is illustrated in Tool 5.

In addition, a number of excellent tools are available that allow the documenter to check off normal and abnormal elements without the need for much writing. These serve as excellent alternatives for the physician who uses handwritten progress notes as documentation. Figures 1-20 through 1-26 are excellent representative selections of these documentation tools.

STANDARDIZED "MACROS" FOR DICTATION

If providers dictate documentation, coders can assist them by developing "macros" for specific conditions. Software word-processing packages provide the capability of programming a set paragraph and labeling it as a macro (such as "PHYSICAL"). When the transcriptionist enters the macro command, the body of the text appears, and the health care provider must dictate only the information needed to fill in the blanks. A macro entitled PHYSICAL might appear as follows:

> This ( )-year-old (female, male) presents with the complaint(s) of ( ). Family history and social history are noncontributory to the patient's complaints. Review of systems reveals no significant findings. Vital signs are BP ( ) and pulse ( ); respirations are ( ).

An example of a history and physical template as described is included in Tool 6.

Text continued on p. 49

TOOL 1

DICTATION NOTE GUIDE

ADMISSION HISTORY AND PHYSICAL EXAM	HISTORY AND PHYSICAL PROGRESS NOTE FORMATS
Date Patient's Name Attending **HISTORY** Chief Complaint History of Present Illness Past Medical History Past Surgical History Medications Allergies Social History (ETOH, tobacco) Family History Immunizations Review of Systems	**SOAP FORMAT** **S - SUBJECTIVE** -Major events (ROS, FH, SH, HPI) -Better or worse -Patient's complaints **O - OBJECTIVE** -Vital signs -Physical exam -Labs/ancillaries **A - ASSESSMENT** -Review of data -Diagnosis **P - PLAN** -Treatment -Discharge plan

ADMISSION HISTORY AND PHYSICAL EXAM

Date
Patient's Name
Attending

HISTORY
Chief Complaint
History of Present Illness
Past Medical History
Past Surgical History
Medications
Allergies
Social History (ETOH, tobacco)
Family History
Immunizations
Review of Systems

Constitutional	Musculoskeletal
Eyes	Integumentary
Cardiovasc	Neuro
Respiratory	Psych
GI	Endocrine
GU	Hema/Lymph

Ears, Nose, Mouth, Throat
Allergic/Immunologic

PHYSICAL EXAM
Body Areas:
Gen Appearance (AO, WDWN, NAD)

Head/Face	Chest/Breasts
Neck	Genitalia/Groin/
Abdomen	Buttocks
Back	
Ea Extremity	

Organ Systems:

Eyes	Ears/Nose/Mouth/
Cardiovasc	Throat
Respiratory	Musculoskeletal
GI	Skin
GU	Neurologic
Psych	Hema/Lymph/ Immunologic

MEDICAL DECISION MAKING
Ancillary Services Ordered/Interpret
Differential Diagnoses
Med Data Review
Risks of morbidity/mortality

ASSESSMENT/PLAN
Diagnosis
Treatment Plan
Discharge Instructions

HISTORY AND PHYSICAL PROGRESS NOTE FORMATS

SOAP FORMAT
S - SUBJECTIVE
-Major events
(ROS, FH, SH, HPI)
-Better or worse
-Patient's complaints
O - OBJECTIVE
-Vital signs
-Physical exam
-Labs/ancillaries
A - ASSESSMENT
-Review of data
-Diagnosis
P - PLAN
-Treatment
-Discharge plan

SNOCAMP FORMAT
S - SUBJECTIVE
-Major events
(ROS, FH, SH, HPI)
-Better or worse
-Patient's complaints
**N - NATURE OF PRESENTING
    PROBLEM**
O - OBJECTIVE
-Vital signs
-Physical exam
-Labs/ancillaries
**C - COUNSELING/COORDINATION
    OF CARE**
-Document time
-Document issue(s)
A - ASSESSMENT
-Review of data
-Diagnosis
**M - MEDICAL DECISION
    MAKING**
-Differential dx
-Review of data
-Risk of morbidity/mortality
P - PLAN
-Treatment
-Discharge plan

T O O L   1, cont'd

DICTATION NOTE GUIDE cont'd

OP NOTE	ADMIT/TRANSFER ORDERS/NOTE

OP NOTE

Date
Patient's Name
Medical Record #
Preop Diagnosis
Postop Diagnosis
Operative Procedure(s)
Surgeon
Assistant(s)
Anesthesia
Surgical Procedure in Detail
Findings
Estimated Blood Loss
Drains/Tubes
Pathology, Specimens, Cultures
Complications
Disposition/Condition

ADMIT/TRANSFER ORDERS/NOTE

(ACDAVANDIML)
A - Admit (Floor, ICU, Unit, etc.)
    Attending/Consulting MDs
C - Condition (stable, fair, guarded)
D - Diagnosis
A - Activities (Ad lib, bed rest)
V - Vital Signs Monitoring
    (check BP hourly)
A - Allergies
N - Nursing
    (dressing changes, IV care)
D - Diet (clear liquids, NPO)
 I - IV (access site)
M - Medications
    Preadmission
    Antibiotics
    Pain Meds
L - Labs and Ancillary Services

POSTOP CHECK/NOTE

Subjective
Objective
 - Vital Signs
 - Inputs/Outputs
  Fluids - volume, blood products,
       urine output, drains,
       BM, blood loss
 - Labs
  CBC, SMAC, CXR, ABG
 - Physical Examination - lungs, dressings
          incisions, pulses
Assessment
Plan

DISCHARGE SUMMARY

Patient's Name
Medical Record #
Attending MD
Admit Date/Discharge Date
Primary/Associated Diagnoses
Surgical Procedures
Hospital Course
Consults
Complications
Discharge Condition
Discharge Instructions (Follow-up)
Copies to _____

TOOL 2

HISTORY CHECK-OFF GUIDE

FAMILY HISTORY/SOCIAL HISTORY

FAMILY HISTORY:
- ☐ Marital Status
- Family Hx of:
  - ☐ Parents
  - ☐ Diabetes
  - ☐ Psychiatric Illness
  - ☐ Cancer
  - ☐ Sickle Cell
  - ☐ Hyperlipidemia
  - ☐ CVA
  - ☐ Kidney Dz

Indicate (+) or (-) in applicable boxes
- ☐ Siblings
- ☐ HTN
- ☐ TB
- ☐ Genetic Disease
- ☐ ASHD
- ☐ Arthritis

SOCIAL HISTORY:
- ☐ Smoker
- ☐ PPD
- ☐ Years
- ☐ Cigarettes/Pipe
- ☐ Cigar
- ☐ Alcohol
- ☐ Caffeine
- ☐ Diet
- ☐ Exercise
- ☐ IV Drug Use
- ☐ PCP
- ☐ Crack
- ☐ Cocaine
- ☐ Other:

Sexual Pref:
- ☐ Heterosexual
- ☐ Homosexual
- ☐ Bisexual

Place of Birth: ____
Occupation: ____
Education: ____
Religion: ____

REVIEW OF SYSTEMS

Indicate (+) or (-) in applicable boxes

GENERAL:
- ☐ Weight change
- ☐ Appetite
- ☐ Sleeping habits

HEENT:

Head:
- ☐ Cephalgia
- ☐ Head injury
- ☐ Migraines

Eyes:
- ☐ Blurriness
- ☐ Cataracts
- ☐ Diplopia
- ☐ Photophobia
- ☐ Vision changes

Ears:
- ☐ Discharge
- ☐ Hearing chgs
- ☐ Tinnitus

Nose:
- ☐ Sinusitis
- ☐ Rhinorrhea
- ☐ Epistaxis

Mouth:
- ☐ Tenderness
- ☐ Lesions

Throat:
- ☐ Sore throats
- ☐ Dysphagia
- ☐ Hoarseness

Neck:
- ☐ Injury
- ☐ Masses
- ☐ Pain
- ☐ Stiffness

RESPIRATORY:
- ☐ Asthma
- ☐ Bronchitis
- ☐ COPD
- ☐ Chronic cough
- ☐ Hemoptysis
- ☐ SOB
- ☐ TB
- ☐ Tachypnea

CARDIOVASCULAR:
- ☐ Angina
- ☐ CHF
- ☐ Claudication
- ☐ CVA
- ☐ Cyanosis
- ☐ Dizziness
- ☐ Dyspnea
- ☐ HTN
- ☐ Orthopnea
- ☐ Palpitations
- ☐ Phlebitis
- ☐ Precordial pain
- ☐ TIA

GASTROINTESTINAL:
- ☐ Constipation
- ☐ Diarrhea
- ☐ Dysphagia
- ☐ Gallbladder dz
- ☐ Hematemesis
- ☐ Hematochezia
- ☐ Hemorrhoids
- ☐ Hernia
- ☐ Indigestion
- ☐ Jaundice
- ☐ Melena
- ☐ Nausea/vomit
- ☐ Pancreatitis
- ☐ Rectal bleed

GENITOURINARY:
- ☐ Anuria
- ☐ Dysuria
- ☐ Hematuria
- ☐ Nocturia
- ☐ Discharge
- ☐ Frequency
- ☐ Hesitancy
- ☐ Incontinence
- ☐ Chronic UTI
- ☐ STD
- ☐ Prostatitis

OB/GYN:
- ☐ Pregnancy:
- ☐ Contraceptive use:
- ☐ Discharge

Breasts:
- ☐ Enlargement
- ☐ Tenderness
- ☐ Prior surg
- ☐ + Mammogram

NEUROMUSCULAR:
- ☐ Anesthesias
- ☐ Paresthesias
- ☐ Arthralgias
- ☐ Myalgias
- ☐ Nervousness
- ☐ Syncope
- ☐ Vertigo
- ☐ Weakness

ENDOCRINE:
- ☐ Hot/cold intolerance
- ☐ Paresthesias
- ☐ Excess bruising/ bleeding
- ☐ Polydipsia
- ☐ Polyphagia
- ☐ Thyroid prob
- ☐ Polyuria
- ☐ Anemia

NEURO:
- ☐ Dizziness
- ☐ Syncope
- ☐ Seizures
- ☐ Vertigo
- ☐ Paresthesias
- ☐ Weakness
- ☐ Tremor

RHEUM:
- ☐ Arthritis
- ☐ Joint stiffness/swell
- ☐ Myalgias
- ☐ Gout
- ☐ Lyme
- ☐ Back pain

VASCULAR:
- ☐ Phlebitis
- ☐ Varicose veins
- ☐ Claudication
- ☐ Cramping
- ☐ Raynaud's

HEME:
- ☐ Anemia
- ☐ Easy bruising/bleed
- ☐ Transfusions
- ☐ Blood type
- ☐ Pain
- ☐ Fever
- ☐ Chills
- ☐ Night sweats

DERM:
- ☐ Rashes
- ☐ Moles (recent chgs)
- ☐ Birthmarks
- ☐ Dryness
- ☐ Pruritus
- ☐ Lumps
- ☐ Pigmentation change:

PSYCH:
- ☐ Depression
- ☐ Agitation
- ☐ Panic-anxiety
- ☐ Memory
- ☐ Hallucinations
- ☐ Personality changes

TOOL 3

EXAMINATION CHECK-OFF GUIDE

Indicate (+) or (−) in applicable boxes

PHYSICAL EXAMINATION

GENERAL:
- ☐ Alert
- ☐ Oriented
- ☐ Well developed
- ☐ Nourished
- ☐ NAD
- Race _____   Sex _____

Head/Scalp:
- ☐ Normocephalic
- ☐ Condition scalp

Eyes:
- ☐ PERRLA
- ☐ EOEM
- ☐ Discs
- ☐ Lids
- ☐ Conjunctiva
- ☐ Sclera
- ☐ Visual fields
- ☐ Visual acuity
- ☐ Retinal vessels

Ears:
- ☐ Pinnae
- ☐ Ext auditory canal
- ☐ Ear drum
- ☐ Rinne test
- ☐ Weber's test
- ☐ Acuity

Nose:
- ☐ Mucosa
- ☐ Septum
- ☐ Polyps

Throat/Oral:
- ☐ Lips
- ☐ Buccal mucosa
- ☐ Palate
- ☐ Tongue
- ☐ Tonsils
- ☐ Gingiva
- ☐ Teeth/dentures
- ☐ Gag reflex

Neck:
- ☐ Trachea-larynx
- ☐ Thyroid:
- ☐ Goiter
- ☐ Nodules
- ☐ Bruits
- ☐ Carotid artery:
- ☐ Contour
- ☐ Bruit
- ☐ Jugular venous pressure with waveforms
- ☐ JVD
- ☐ Range of motion

RESPIRATORY:
- ☐ Contour
- ☐ Breath sounds:
- ☐ Wheezes
- ☐ Rales
- ☐ Rhonchi
- ☐ Rub
- ☐ Resonance
- ☐ Diaphragm movement
- ☐ Intercostal muscle retraction

CARDIAC:
- ☐ Heart sounds:
- ☐ S1, S2, S3, S4
- ☐ Systolic click
- ☐ Opening snap
- ☐ Mid-diastolic murmur
- ☐ Murmur:
- ☐ Systolic
- ☐ Diastolic
- ☐ Continuous
- ☐ Radiation
- Location _____
- ☐ Duration _____
- ☐ Loudness
- ☐ Pitch
- ☐ Quality

ABDOMEN:
- ☐ Appearance
- ☐ Bowel sounds
- ☐ Scars
- ☐ Distention
- ☐ Liver
- ☐ Spleen
- ☐ Guarding
- ☐ Rebound
- ☐ Kidneys
- ☐ CVA tenderness
- ☐ Ventral hernia
- ☐ Bladder
- ☐ Masses

GU (MALE):
- ☐ Penis
- ☐ Scrotum
- ☐ Testicles
- ☐ Varicocele
- ☐ Hydrocele
- ☐ Ext genitalia
- ☐ Bartholin gland
- ☐ Urethra

GU (FEMALE):
- ☐ Internal exam:
- ☐ Cervix
- ☐ Uterus
- ☐ Adnexa
- ☐ Rectovaginal area

RECTAL:
- ☐ Ext lesions
- ☐ Hemorrhoids
- ☐ Fissures
- ☐ Sphincter tone
- ☐ Sphincter tenderness
- ☐ Masses
- ☐ Stricture
- ☐ Prostate
- ☐ Occult blood
- ☐ Stool appearance:

MUSCULOSKELETAL:
- ☐ Appearance:
- ☐ Muscle swelling
- ☐ Deformity
- ☐ Tenderness
- ☐ Range of motion
- ☐ Bone
- ☐ Deformity
- ☐ Tenderness
- ☐ Joint swelling
- ☐ Deformity
- ☐ Tenderness
- ☐ Range of motion
- ☐ Hypertrophy
- ☐ Spasm
- ☐ Muscle group atrophy
- ☐ Spinal kyphosis
- ☐ Spinal scoliosis
- ☐ Symmetry
- ☐ Skin changes

BREAST:
- ☐ Tenderness
- ☐ Nipple discharge
- ☐ Retraction
- ☐ Nipple-areola
- ☐ Masses

VASCULAR:
- Arterial pulse contour/bruits:
- ☐ Radial
- ☐ Ulnar
- ☐ Brachial
- ☐ Carotid
- ☐ Abd aorta
- ☐ Femoral
- ☐ Popliteal
- ☐ Post tibial
- ☐ Dorsalis

EXTREMITIES:
- ☐ Clubbing
- ☐ Cyanosis
- ☐ Edema
- ☐ Color
- ☐ Pigmentation
- ☐ Hair
- ☐ Turgor
- ☐ Texture
- ☐ Temperature
- ☐ Lesions
- ☐ Nailbeds

NEURO:
- ☐ Mental status:
- ☐ Orientation
- ☐ Memory
- ☐ Arithmetic
- ☐ Abstract concepts
- ☐ Speech
- ☐ Cortical integration
- ☐ Cranial nerves
- ☐ Motor
- ☐ Sensory
- ☐ Reflexes

TOOL 4

ED CHART DOCUMENTATION REQUIREMENTS

	Chart Documentation Requirements	Chart Content (examples)			Levels of Documentation	
HISTORY **Chief Complaint**	Document in patient's own words	"Pt states"			Req All Levels	
Hx Present Illness	Must be documented by ED phy	Location Timing Assoc S/S	Quality Context Mod Factors	Severity Duration	Brief Extended	1–3 elements >4 elements
Past FH/SH/PMH	May be documented by staff and **confirmed** by ED phy Review pertinent −/+	"Reviewed and agree with nurse/ resident's notes"			Req Levels	4/5
Review of Systems	May be documented by staff and **confirmed** by ED phy "All other systems negative" acceptable after pert problems	*ROS Identified:* Constitutional Musculoskel Eyes Integumen Neuro	Ears,Throat, Nose, Mouth Cardiovasc Psych Endocrine	Gastro Hema/Lymph GU All/Immun	Prob Foc Extend Complete	Prob Pert Only 2–9 rel systems all systems

PHYSICAL EXAM	All abnormal findings of affected areas must be documented
	
	"Negative" or "normal" OK for findings of unaffected areas
	
	Must be able to identify system(s) from negatives listed
		Organ Systems Identified:
		Constitutional
		Eyes
		Ears, Nose,
		  Mouth, throat
		Cardiovasc
			Respiratory
			GI
			GU
			Musculoskel
			Skin
				Neurologic
				Psych
				Hema/
				  Lymph/Imm
					Prob Foc
					Exp Prob Foc
					Detailed
					Complete
						1 element
						2–4 elements
						5–7 elements
						8 or more

		Body Areas Identified: Ea Extremity Neck Abdomen	Genitalia, Groin, Buttocks Chest, incl breasts Head, incl face Back, incl spine			
MED DECISION **Dx/Mgt Options**	Minimal "improving, resolved(ing)" Limited "self-limited" Multiple "inadequately controlled" Extensive "worsening" "failing to respond"	Differential Diagnosis Final Diagnosis Drug Therapy(ies) Procedure(s) Disposition of Patient/Consultations			Minimal Limited Multiple Extensive	1 2 3 4

Amt/Complexity of Data Reviewed	Path/Lab 1>test =1
	Rad 1>test =1
	Dx Test 1>test =1
	Comp Test
	 Results Ea 1 test =2
	Old Records
	Eval Need =1 OR
	Old Records
	Obtain/Review =2
	Discuss with Physician =1
		Physician Documentation of:
		  Medical Necessity of Tests/Orders
		  Test Results
		  Independent Interpretation
		  Eval of Need for Records
		  Eval/Review of Old Records
		  Repeat Procedures
		  Repeat Evaluations/Treatments
					Minimal/None
					Limited
					Moderate
					Extensive
						1
						2
						3
						4 or more

Risk/Morbidity/ Mortality	Presenting Prob Severity
	Diagnostic Proc Ordered
	Management Options Selected
	Discharge Status
	Discharge Instructions
		Mild, moderate, progressive
		X-Rays, Labs, Procedures
		
		Home/Admit/Resolution or Non-Resolution
		  of symptoms
		Rest, Gargle, Bandages
		Non-Rx drugs
		Drug Therapy(ies)
		IV fluids w/ or w/o additives
		Minor procedures
					Straightforward Minimal
					  Self-Lmtd/Minor Problem
					--- 	
					Low
					  >2 Self-Lmtd/Minor
					  1 Stable Chronic Illness
					  Acute Uncompl Illness/Inj
					--- 	
					Moderate
					  >1 chronic ill/mild exac
					  >2 stable chronic ill/inj
					  undiag new problem
					  acute complicated injury
					--- 	
					Extensive
					  >1 chronic ill/severe exac
					  acute/chronic illnesses
					  poses threat life/limb
					  abrupt chg in neuro status	

TOOL 5

EMERGENCY DEPARTMENT RECORD OF TREATMENT

Admit#:		Date:		Time:		Age:		Sex:		Race:

Name:		Address:			

SSN:		DOB:		Phone:

Chief Complaint:	Medications:

Vitals:	Allergies:

HISTORY	**EXAM**	NL if WNL	Noted Exam Abnormalities:
CHIEF COMPLAINT	Constitutional		
HX PRESENT ILLNESS	Skin		
PAST MED HX/FAMILY HX	Eyes		

(P=Pt F=Family)	P	F	Other Hx Information:
HTN/Card/Stroke/Chol			
Cancer/Bleed			
Seizures/Headaches			
Weakness/Coordination			
DM/Kidney/Abdominal			
Surgical Procedures			
Other:			

Ears, Nose, Mouth, Throat		
Neck		
Respiratory		
Cardiovascular		

SOCIAL HX

Occupation/Living Arrangement
Alcohol/Smoking/Drugs

Chest		

REVIEW OF SYSTEMS	NL if WNL	Noted System Abnormalities:	GI		
Constitutional					
Allergic/Immun			GU		
Integumentary					
Eyes			Musculoskeletal		
Ears, Nose, Mouth, Throat					
Cardiovasc			Neurological		
Hematologic					
Endocrine			Lymph/Immun		
Respiratory					
GI			Psych		
GU					
Musculoskeletal			Other Exam		
Neurologic			Abnormalities:		

MEDICAL DECISION MAKING	**FINDINGS:**
Procedures/Treatments/Re-Evaluation:	
	Differential Dx(s):
Prescriptions:	

	NL if WNL	Finding Abnormalities	Final Dx(s):
Lab Results:			
CBC			
UA			
ABG			**DISPOSITION:**
Cultures			Discharge:
ECG			Admit:
Enzymes			Transfer to:
Pulse Ox			CONDITION:
X-Ray: Specify_____			Improved/Stable
Other: _____			Worse/Expired
Other: _____			INSTRUCTIONS:

Consults:	
Resident Signature/Date:	I hereby attest that I have reviewed and concurred with Resident Findings/Treatment:
	Physician Signature/Date:

Name: _____ DoB __/__/__ Cht.# _____ Seen with: ☐ Mth. ☐ Fth. ☐ Other _____

History

Nutrition: ☐ Breast ☐ Formula _____ ☐ WIC

Present _____
_____
_____
_____

Past _____
_____

Family/social _____

Drug allergies? ☐ yes ☐ no _____

Physical Exam   ☒ NI ☒ Abn

Temp _____ Head Cir./% ___/___ Wt %/Ht % ___/___

Constitutional ....☐	Head, fontanels... ☐	Gastrointestinal....☐
Alertness...............☐	Eyes.....................☐	Genitourinary ....☐
Hearing ....☐	ENMT ....☐	Back ....☐
Language.............☐	Lymphatics...........☐	Extremities, hips..☐
Nutrition ....☐	Respiratory ....☐	Muscle tone..........☐
Growth..................☐	Cardiovascular....☐	Skin.......................☐
Motor develop......☐	Femoral pulses....☐	Neuromuscular ....☐

_____
_____
_____

Procedures   ☐ Hep B _____

Immun. current? ☐ yes ☐ no _____

Plan _____
_____

Next visit: _____

Anticipatory Guidance

☐ Immunization (risks/benefits) ☐ Growth ☐ Development ☐ Nutrition (solids) ☐ Fluoride ☐ Sleep (night crying)
☐ Safety (shaking, no walkers, poisons, Ipecac) ☐ Fear of strangers ☐ Educational handouts _____

Provider's sig. ▶

9 mo.	Date/Time	Age	Weight	Height	Assessment:	☐ Referral

FIGURE 1-20 Forms for regularly scheduled interval examinations record the information needed for medical and documentation purposes. *(Courtesy of Piermed, Inc., Lewisville, NC.)*

Name: _____ DoB __/__/__ Cht.# _____ Seen with: ☐ Mth. ☐ Fth. ☐ Other _____

History

Date of injury __/__/__ Time of injury _____ Time of visit _____ Location _____

Description of injury/complications _____
_____
_____

Date of last tetanus: __/__/__

Physical Findings _____
_____
_____

Treatment/Plan _____
_____

Referral? ☐ yes ☐ no   Dr. _____   Findings/recommendations: _____

Anticipatory Guidance ☐ Discussed signs of possible complications and appropriate intervention. _____

Provider's sig. ▶   ☐ Follow up: ☐ phone call _____ ☐ return visit _____

Injury	Date/time	Description:	☐ Referral

FIGURE 1-21 Forms designed to ask injury-specific information are separated from the usual physical examination and illness documentation forms. *(Courtesy of Piermed, Inc., Lewisville, NC.)*

Name: _____	DOB __/__/__	Cht.# _____	Seen with: ☐ Mth. ☐ Fth. ☐ Other _____

Physical Exam   ☒ NI   ☒ Abn   (Circle Abn)

Temp _____ P _____ R_____ BP_____ Peak Fl_____

Constitutional.......... ☐	looks ill 1$^+$, 2$^+$, 3$^+$ Hydration ☐ _____	
Fontanel .... ☐	_____	
Eyes .... ☐	red, drainage (clear, pur.), Fundi ☐ _____	
Ears: . Rtm.............. ☐	red, dull, thick, ↓ mobility, retract., bulging	
	fluid (ser, pur), perf, scarred, tube (in, out)	
Ltm .... ☐	red, dull, thick, ↓ mobility, retract., bulging	
	fluid (ser, pur), perf, scarred, tube (in, out)	
Ext. canal............... ☐	cerumen, swollen, tender, pur. drainage	
Nose .... ☐	drainage (watery, mucoid, pur.), Sinuses ☐	
Mouth/throat .... ☐	ulcers, drainage (mucoid, pur.) inj. _____	
Tonsils .... ☐	enlarged 1$^+$, 2$^+$, 3$^+$, 4$^+$, exudate, petechiae	
Lymphatic .... ☐	_____	
Neck .... ☐	_____	
Cardiovascular....... ☐	_____	
Respiratory .... ☐	rhonchi, wheezes, rales, ↓ br. sounds, retract.	
R ___ L ___	resp. distress 0, 1$^+$, 2$^+$, 3$^+$ _____	

	CPT
Gastrointestinal....... ☐ _____	PF
Genitourinary .... ☐ _____	EPF
Musculoskeletal ...... ☐ _____	D
Skin .... ☐ _____	C
Neurological .... ☐	

History   ☒ Positive ☒ Negative   ☐ Follow-up visit

Chief complaint/duration: _____

restless ☐	fussy ☐	awake at night ☐	↓ appetite ☐

Fever............... ☐	Earache........... ☐	Back pain .... ☐	Vomiting.......... ☐
Congestion ...... ☐	Sw. glands....... ☐	Musc/jnt pain.... ☐	Diarrhea........... ☐
Cough............. ☐	Red eyes......... ☐	Abd. pain......... ☐	Urinary sx. ...... ☐
Sore throat ...... ☐	Headache........ ☐	Constipation ..... ☐	Skin rash.......... ☐

_____

_____

_____   Over ☐

		CPT
Systems reviewed...........☐	Family/Social Hx reviewed............ ☐	PF
Past Hx reviewed............ ☐	Immunizations current? Yes ☐ No ☐	EPF
Current meds: _____		D
Drug allergies? Yes ☐ No ☐		C

Treatment

_____

_____

_____

Provider's sig. ▶	Over ☐

CPT
SF
LC
MC
HC

☐ Report back in 24 hrs.	☐ Call in 48 hrs., prn	☐ Re-examine

Sick	Date/Time	Age	Weight	Height	Diagnosis:	☐ After hrs. ☐ Referral

FIGURE 1-22 Forms designed specifically for "sick" visits record information regarding presenting complaint, history of present illness, physical examination, and medical decision making for both medical and documentation purposes. *(Courtesy of Piermed, Inc., Lewisville, NC.)*

Name: _____ DoB __/__/__ Age _____ Chart No. [_____]

Assessment

Plan

_____ _____
Provider's signature   Return visit

Physical Exam

Ht. _____ Wt. _____ Temp. _____ Resp. _____
B.P. sit. or stand. ____/____ Supine ____/____
Pulse rate and regularity _____

Circle abnormal and pertinent normal findings.
Describe abnormalities above.
☑ Normal   ☒ Abnormal

1. Constitutional
a. ☐ gen. appear., development, body shape, nutrition, deformities, grooming

2. Eyes
a. ☐ conjunctivae, lids
b. ☐ pupils, irises
c. ☐ fundi (optic discs, vessels, exudate, hemorr.)

3. Ears, nose, throat, and mouth
a. ☐ appearance of ears, appearance of nose
b. ☐ auditory canals, tympanic membranes
c. ☐ hearing (whis. voice, finger rub, tun. fork)
d. ☐ nasal mucosa, septum, turbinates
e. ☐ lips, teeth, gums
f. ☐ oropharynx (mucosa, saliv. glands, hard and soft palates, tongue, tonsils, post. pharynx)

4. Neck
a. ☐ appearance, masses, symmetry, tracheal position, crepitus
b. ☐ thyroid (enlargement, tenderness, mass)

5. Respiratory
a. ☐ respiratory effort (intercostal retractions), use of accessory muscles, diaphragm move.
b. ☐ percussion (dullness, flatness, hyper-reson.)
c. ☐ palpation (tactile fremitus)
d. ☐ auscultation (breath sounds, rhonchi, wheezes, rales, rubs)

6. Cardiovascular
a. ☐ palpation (location of p.m.i., size, thrill)
b. ☐ auscultation (abnormal sounds, murmurs)
c. ☐ carotid arteries (pulse amplitude, bruits)
d. ☐ abdominal aorta (size, bruits)
e. ☐ femoral arteries (pulse amplitude, bruits)
f. ☐ pedal pulses (pulse amplitude)
g. ☐ extremities (edema, varicosities)

7. Chest (breasts)
a. ☐ inspection (size, symmetry, nipple discharge)
b. ☐ palpation of breasts and axillae (masses, lumps, tenderness)

8. Gastrointestinal (abdomen)
a. ☐ examination for masses, tenderness
b. ☐ examination of liver, spleen
c. ☐ examination for presence or absence of hernia
d. ☐ examination of (when indicated) anus, perineum, rectum: (sphincter tone, hemorrhoids, masses)
e. ☐ stool for occult blood when indicated

9. Genitourinary
a. ☐ scrotum (hydrocele, spermatocele), tenderness of cord, testicular mass)
b. ☐ examination of penis
c. ☐ digital exam of prostate (size, symmetry, nodularity, tenderness)

10. Lymphatic
a. ☐ palpation of lymph nodes in 2 or more areas:
(Circle: neck, axillae, groin, other)

11. Musculoskeletal
a. ☐ examination of gait and station
b. ☐ inspection and/or palpation of digits and nails (clubbing, cyanosis, inflammatory conditions, petechiae, ischemia, infections, nodes)
c. ☐ assessment of range of motion (pain, crepitation, contracture)
d. ☐ Examination of joint, bone, and muscle of 1 or more of the following 6 areas (circle)
• head/neck
• rt. upper extremities
• spine, ribs, and pelvis
• lt. upper extremities
• rt. lower extremities
• lt. lower extremities
e. ☐ inspection and/or palpation (misalignment, asymmetry, crepitation, defects, tenderness, masses, effusion)
f. ☐ assessment of stability: dislocation (luxation), subluxation or laxity
g. ☐ muscle strength and tone (flaccid, cogwheel, spastic), atrophy or abnormal movement

12. Skin
a. ☐ inspection of skin and sub-Q tissue (rashes, lesion, ulcers)
b. ☐ palpation of skin and sub-Q tissue (induration, sub-Q nodules, tightening)

13. Neurology
a. ☐ test cranial nerves: notation of deficits
b. ☐ examination of DTRs with notation of pathological reflexes (e.g., Babinski)
c. ☐ examination of sensation (touch, pain, vibration, proprioception)

14. Psychiatric
a. ☐ description of patient's judgment and insight
Brief assessment of mental status:
b. ☐ orientation to time, place, and person
c. ☐ recent and remote memory
d. ☐ mood and affect (depression, anxiety, agitation)
e. ☐ other

Procedures and Immunizations

☐ Hearing ☐ Glucose ☐ Cholesterol ☐ CXR
☐ Vision   ☐ PT   ☐ HDL/LDL   ☐ EKG
☐ CBC   ☐ Urine   ☐ TSH

Are immunizations current?
☐ yes ☐ no

☐ dT ☐ Hep B ☐ Influenza

Drug Allergies

Male 19-39 | Date/Time | Summary | ☐ Referral

FIGURE 1-23 Forms designed specifically for complete physical examinations, which are also specific to age and sex, detail the information specific to the particular patient groups. *(Courtesy of Piermed, Inc., Lewisville, NC.)*

Name: _____   Date ____ / ____ / ____

HPI Chief Complaint:

Past/Family History

Current Meds.:

THIS SECTION TO BE COMPLETED BY PATIENT.

Personal/Social History

Are you ...   □ single   □ married
□ live-in partner   □ divorced   □ widowed

Do you have children? □ yes □ no
Age(s) of child(ren) _____
_____

Occupation _____

	YES	NO
a. Are your immunizations up to date?	□	□

Date of last tetanus shot: _____

	YES	NO
b. Do you have any pain or blood on urination?	□	□
c. Do you have lesions, sores or drainage from penis?	□	□
d. Do you have any lumps, swelling, tenderness or pain in groin, scrotum, or testicles?	□	□
e. Are you sexually active now?	□	□

□ same sex   □ opposite sex
□ single partner   □ multiple partners

	YES	NO
Have you had more than 4 lifetime partners?	□	□
f. Do you use condoms?	□	□

	YES	NO
g. Do you have concerns about sexual orientation, sexually transmitted diseases, or exposure to HIV or other sexual concerns?	□	□
h. Do you feel safe/comfortable in your home, with your family, and/or your partner relationship?	□	□
i. Do you smoke or use tobacco products now?	□	□
j. Do you use recreational drugs?	□	□
k. Do you drink alcohol?	□	□

□ daily □ weekly □ rarely

\# of drinks _____

If yes, do you drink: □ beer □ wine □ liquor

Review of Systems

Are you concerned about? (circle concerns)

	YES	NO
1. Recent changes in health status	□	□
2. Eye problems: vision, pain, tearing	□	□
3. Ear, nose, mouth, throat problems	□	□
4. Heart problems: chest pain, blood pressure	□	□
5. Lung problems: coughing, wheezing, infections	□	□

	YES	NO
6. Abdominal pain, stomach, bowel problems	□	□
7. Kidney or bladder problems	□	□
8. Muscle, bone, joint or back problems	□	□
9. Skin, hair or nail problems	□	□
10. Neurologic problems: headaches, dizziness, numbness	□	□
11. Nervousness, anxiety, depression, suicidal thoughts	□	□
12. Excessive thirst and urine output, recent weight changes	□	□
13. Anemia, bruising, blood clots, swollen glands	□	□
14. Food allergies, hay fever, eczema, asthma, decreased immunity	□	□
Do you have any other concerns?	□	□

_____
_____
_____
_____

_____   _____
Patient's signature   Date

Provider Comments:

□ PFSH and ROS have been reviewed.   □ Unresolved problems from previous visit have been addressed.

_____   _____
Provider's signature   Date

Anticipatory Guidance

□ Nutrition   □ Sun exposure   □ Self-exam: testes, skin, oral cavity   □ Auto seat belts
□ Exercise   □ Smoking cessation   □ School/work   □ Smoke detectors
□ Dental care   □ Alcohol/drugs   □ Family   □ Domestic violence
□ Cardiovascular risks   □ Sexual issues   □ Recreation/hobbies   □ Stress
     □ STD prevention   □ Safety/injury/gun safety   □ Educational handouts

FIGURE 1-23, cont'd

New Patient Record (Adults)

Date _____ DoB __/__/__ Chart No. [   ]

Name: _____   Sex ☐ M ☐ F   Referred By _____

Current Medical Problems
List all medical problems and approximate time they began.

Problems   Onset date
_____
_____
_____
_____

Current Medications
List all medications you take (including nonprescription medication).

1 _____   5 _____
2 _____   6 _____
3 _____   7 _____
4 _____   8 _____

Current Allergies or Sensitivities
List anything you are allergic to and describe how it affects you.

_____
_____
_____
_____

Work History

Are you currently employed? ☐ Yes ☐ No
☐ Homemaker ☐ Retired ☐ Disabled
Present type of work _____
In your work are you exposed to:
☐ Harmful toxins   ☐ Extremes in temperatures
☐ Heavy lifting   ☐ Undue stress, pressure
☐ Other _____

Health Care Providers
What other health care providers have cared for you in the past five years?

Year   Doctor/provider   City and state
_____
_____
_____
_____

Do you have other concerns or problems? ☐ Yes ☐ No
_____
_____
_____

Signed _____ Date _____

Family Medical History

Check if you or a member of your family have had the following illnesses or problems.
List which family member.

Health is

Relative	Age(s)	Good	Poor	Deceased
Father	____	☐	☐	☐
Mother	____	☐	☐	☐
Brothers	____	☐	☐	☐
Sisters	____	☐	☐	☐
Spouse	____	☐	☐	☐
Children	____	☐	☐	☐

Illness(es) _____
_____

Cause(s) of Death _____
_____

☐ Allergies _____
☐ Asthma _____
☐ Eczema, rashes _____
☐ Eye problems _____
☐ Thyroid problems _____
☐ Lung problems _____
☐ Heart diseases _____
☐ Cholesterol problems _____
☐ High blood pressure _____
☐ Phlebitis _____
☐ Stomach or intestinal
   problems _____
☐ Liver diseases _____
☐ Kidney problems _____

☐ Diabetes _____
☐ Hereditary diseases _____
☐ Cancer _____
☐ Anemia or blood diseases _____
☐ Epilepsy _____
☐ Nervous breakdown or
   mental illnesses _____
☐ Depression _____
☐ Suicide attempt _____
☐ Alcohol or drug problem _____
☐ Other _____

History updated (date)

500-50

FIGURE 1-24 New patient records should include specific medical information for new patients so that all the pertinent history and medical information is included both for the physician and for documentation purposes. *(Courtesy of Piermed, Inc., Lewisville, NC.)*

Name: _____ DoB __/__/__ Age _____ Chart No. [ ]

Assessment

Plan

_____ _____
Provider's signature   Return visit

Physical Exam

Ht. ____ Wt. ____ Temp. ____ Resp. _____
B.P. sit. or stand.____/____ Supine ____/____
Pulse rate and regularity _____

Circle abnormal and pertinent normal findings.
Describe abnormalities.
☑ Normal   ☒ Abnormal

1. Constitutional
a. ☐ gen. appear. (e.g., development, nutrition, body habitus, deformities, attention to grooming)

2. Head and face

3. Eyes
a. ☐ inspection of conjunctivae and lids (e.g., xanthelasma)

4. Ears, nose, throat and mouth
a. ☐ inspection of teeth, gums and palate
b. ☐ inspection of oral mucosa with notation of presence of pallor or cyanosis

5. Neck
a. ☐ examination jugular veins (e.g., distention; a, v or cannon a waves)
b. ☐ examination of thyroid (e.g., enlargement, tenderness, mass)

6. Respiratory
a. ☐ assessment of respiratory effort (e.g., intercostal retractions, use of accessory muscles, diaphragmatic movement)
b. ☐ auscultation of lungs (e.g., breath sounds, adventitious sounds, rubs)

Comments:

7. Cardiovascular
a. ☐ palpation of heart (e.g., location, size and forcefulness of the point of maximal impact; thrills; lifts; palpable S3 or S4)
b. ☐ auscultation of heart, including normal sounds, abnormal sounds and murmurs
c. ☐ measurement of blood pressure in two or more extremities when indicated (e.g., aortic dissection, coarctation)

Examination of:

d. ☐ carotid arteries (e.g., waveform, pulse amplitude, bruits, apical-carotid delay)
e. ☐ abdominal aorta (e.g., size, bruits)
f. ☐ femoral arteries (e.g., pulse, amplitude, bruits)
g. ☐ pedal pulses (e.g., pulse, amplitude)
h. ☐ extremities for peripheral edema and/or varicosities

8. Chest (breasts)

9. Gastrointestinal (abdomen)
a. ☐ examination of abdomen with notation of presence of masses or tenderness
b. ☐ examination of liver and spleen
c. ☐ obtain stool sample for occult blood from patients who are being considered for thrombolytic or anticoagulant therapy

10. Genitourinary (abdomen)

11. Lymphatic

12. Musculoskeletal
a. ☐ examination of the back with notation of kyphosis or scoliosis
b. ☐ examination of gait with notation of ability to undergo exercise testing and/or participation in exercise program
c. ☐ assessment of muscle strength and tone (e.g., flaccid, cogwheel, spastic) with notation of any atrophy and abnormal movements

13. Extremities
a. ☐ inspection and palpation of digits and nails (e.g., clubbing, cyanosis, inflammation, petechiae, ischemia, infections, Osler's nodes)

14. Skin
a. ☐ inspection and/or palpation of skin and subcutaneous tissue (e.g., stasis dermatitis, ulcers, scars, xanthomas)

15. Neurological/psychiatric
Brief assessment of mental status:
a. ☐ orientation to time, place, and person
b. ☐ mood and affect (e.g., depression, anxiety, agitation)

Procedures

☐ CBC
☐ Urine
☐ Glucose
☐ BUN
☐ Creatinine
☐ Electrolytes
☐ Liver funct. tests
☐ Cholesterol
☐ HDL/LDL
☐ Triglycerides
☐ Serum enzymes
☐ PT time
☐ Digitalis level
☐ CXR
☐ ECG
☐ Ambulatory ECG
☐ Echocardiogram
☐ Stress test
☐ Other

Drug Allergies:

Cardiology	Date/Time	Summary	☐ Referral ☐ Consultation

FIGURE 1-25 Patient records that are specialty specific detail the information needed for evaluating, treating, and managing specific-specialty problems, such as those in cardiology. *(Courtesy of Piermed, Inc., Lewisville, NC.)*

Continued

| Name: _____ | Date ___ / ___ / ___ |

HPI Chief Complaint:

Current Meds.:

Past, Family/Social History

THIS SECTION TO BE COMPLETED BY PATIENT.

Review of Systems

Are you concerned about? (circle concerns)

YES NO

1. Have you had recent health concerns (circle): changes in the way you feel, weight loss or gain, ↓ appetite, ↓ energy, ↑ tiredness or weakness, problems with sleep? ☐ ☐

2. Eye problems: vision, pain, tearing ☐ ☐

3. Ear, nose, mouth, throat problems ☐ ☐

4. Heart problems:

   a. Have you had any heart problems? ☐ ☐

   b. Have you ever had high blood pressure? ☐ ☐

   c. Do you take any heart, blood pressure, or cholesterol medications? ☐ ☐

   d. Do you have any chest pain? If yes, (circle) does it occur with rest, after exercise, after eating, during stress or emotional strain, associated with shortness of breath, nausea or vomiting? ☐ ☐

   e. Do you have any shortness of breath? ☐ ☐

YES NO

f. Do you sleep on more than one pillow? ☐ ☐

g. Have you noticed any fluttering, skipped beats, pounding or heart irregularity? If yes, is this worse after drinking tea, coffee or colas? ☐ ☐

h. Have you had any fainting or passing out episodes? ☐ ☐

i. Have you been tiring more easily? ☐ ☐

j. Have you noticed ankle or leg swelling? If yes, does the swelling decrease after resting and elevation of legs? ☐ ☐

k. Do you have pain in the calves of your legs after walking? ☐ ☐

l. Have you been coughing up blood? ☐ ☐

m. Have you noticed any bluish discoloration or paleness to your skin? ☐ ☐

n. Do you smoke? ☐ ☐

o. Do you drink alcoholic beverages? ☐ ☐

YES NO

5. Lung problems: coughing, wheezing, infections ☐ ☐

6. Abdominal pain, stomach or bowel problems ☐ ☐

7. Kidney or bladder problems ☐ ☐

8. Muscle, bone, joint or back problems ☐ ☐

9. Skin, hair or nail problems ☐ ☐

10. Neurologic problems: headaches, dizziness, numbness ☐ ☐

11. Nervousness, anxiety, depression, suicidal thoughts ☐ ☐

12. Excessive thirst and urine output, recent weight changes ☐ ☐

13. Anemia, bruising, blood clots, swollen glands ☐ ☐

14. Food allergies, hay fever, eczema, asthma, decreased immunity ☐ ☐

Do you have any other concerns?

_____

_____

_____

| Patient's signature | Date |

Provider Comments:

☐ PFSH and ROS have been reviewed. ☐ Unresolved problems from previous visit have been addressed.

| Provider's signature | Date |

Anticipatory Guidance

☐ Nutrition
☐ Low-salt diet
☐ Weight reduction
☐ Exercise

☐ Aspirin
☐ Smoking cessation
☐ Caffeine
☐ Alcohol

☐ Work
☐ Stress
☐ Oral contraceptive risks
☐ Postmenopausal hormones

FIGURE 1-25, cont'd

Name: _____ DoB __/__/__ Age _____ Chart No. [   ]

Assessment

Plan

_____   _____
Provider's signature   Return visit

Physical Exam

Ht. ____ Wt. ____ Temp. ____ Resp. _____
B.P. sit. or stand.____/____ Supine ____/____
Pulse rate and regularity _____

Circle abnormal and pertinent normal findings.
Describe abnormalities.
☑ Normal   ☒ Abnormal

1. Constitutional
a. ☐ gen. appear., development, body habitus, nutrition, deformities, grooming

2. Head and face

3. Eyes

4. Ears, nose, throat and mouth

5. Neck
a. ☐ appearance, masses, symmetry, tracheal position, crepitus
b. ☐ thyroid (enlargement, tenderness, mass)

6. Respiratory
a. ☐ respiratory effort (intercostal retractions) use of accessory muscles, diaphragm move
b. ☐ auscultation (breath sounds, rhonchi, wheezes, rales, rubs)

7. Cardiovascular
a. ☐ femoral arteries (pulse amplitude, bruits)
b. ☐ pedal pulses (pulse amplitude)
c. ☐ extremities (edema, varicosities)

8. Chest (breasts)
a. ☐ inspection and palpation of breasts (e.g., masses or lumps, tenderness, symmetry, nipple discharge)

9. Gastrointestinal (abdomen)
a. ☐ examination for masses, tenderness
b. ☐ examination of liver and spleen
c. ☐ examination for presence or absence of hernia
d. ☐ stool for occult blood when indicated
e. ☐ digital rectal examination including sphincter tone, presence of hemorrhoids, rectal masses

10. Genitourinary
Pelvic exam. (with or without specimen collection for smears or cultures), including:
a. ☐ external genitalia (e.g., gen. appearance, hair distribution, lesions)
b. ☐ urethral meatus (e.g., size, location, lesions, prolapse)
c. ☐ urethra (e.g., masses, tenderness, scarring)
d. ☐ bladder (e.g., fullness, masses, tenderness)
e. ☐ vagina (e.g., gen. appearance, estrogen effect, discharge, lesions, pelvic support, cystocele, rectocele)
f. ☐ cervix (e.g., gen. appearance, lesions, discharge)
g. ☐ uterus (e.g., size, contour, position, mobility, tenderness, consistency, descent or support)
h. ☐ adnexa/parametria (e.g., masses, tenderness, organomegaly, nodularity)
i. ☐ anus and perineum

11. Lymphatic
a. ☐ palpation of lymph nodes in neck, axillae, groin, other locations _____

12. Musculoskeletal

13. Extremities

14. Skin
a. ☐ inspection and/or palpation of skin and sub-Q tissue (e.g., rashes, lesions, ulcers)

15. Neurological/psychiatric
Brief assessment of mental status:
a. ☐ orientation to time, place, and person
b. ☐ mood and affect (depression, anxiety, agitation)

Comments:

Procedures and Immunizations

Are immunizations current? ☐ yes ☐ no

☐ CBC
☐ Glucose
☐ TSH
☐ Urine

☐ Cholesterol
☐ HDL/LDL
☐ FSH
☐ Prolactin
☐ Estradiol
☐ VDRL

☐ PAP test
☐ Mammogram
☐ Stool guaiac
☐ Chlamydia screen
☐ Rubella screen
☐ GC screen

☐ Other
☐ dT
☐ Hep B
☐ Influenza
☐ Rubella

Drug Allergies:

GYN	Date/Time	Summary	☐ Referral

FIGURE 1-26 Another example of a specialty-specific history, examination, and medical decision making form that aids the physician in properly documenting patient information for charting purposes and fulfilling documentation requirements. *(Courtesy of Piermed, Inc., Lewisville, NC.)*

Continued

Name: _____ Date ___/___/___

HPI Chief Complaint:

Current Meds.:

Past/Family History

THIS SECTION TO BE COMPLETED BY PATIENT.

Personal/Social History

Are you ... ☐ single ☐ married
☐ live-in partner ☐ divorced ☐ widowed

Do you have children? ☐ yes ☐ no
Age(s) of child(ren) _____
No. of pregnancies _____ Miscarriages _____
Occupation _____

YES NO

a. Do you have concerns about your breasts? (circle): changes in size or shape, changes in skin color, lumps, tenderness, ulcerations, discharge or blood from nipple, inverted nipple ☐ ☐

b. Do you have concerns about your menstruation (circle): frequency of periods, amount of flow, cramping, premenstrual tension, menopausal symptoms, postmenopausal bleeding? ☐ ☐

c. Do you take hormones (estrogen)? ☐ ☐

d. Do you have concerns about (circle): vaginal itching, dryness or discharge; pain or bleeding with intercourse; fertility problems; lack of enjoyment of sex? ☐ ☐

e. Concerns about lesions, lumps or swelling on your vulva or vagina? ☐ ☐

f. Do you have (circle) pain on urination, blood in urine, repeated urinary infections, awakening at night to urinate, urine leakage or incontinence? ☐ ☐

YES NO

g. Do you have concerns about abdominal pain or swelling, constipation or diarrhea, laxative or antacid use, rectal pain or bleeding, hemorrhoids? ☐ ☐

h. Approximate date of last menstruation _____

i. Approximate date of last pelvic exam _____

j. Approximate date of last Pap test _____

k. Approximate date of last mammogram _____

l. Are you sexually active now? ☐ ☐
  ☐ same sex   ☐ opposite sex
  ☐ single partner ☐ multiple partners

  Have you had more than 4 lifetime partners? ☐ ☐

m. Birth control method _____

n. Do you have concerns about sexual orientation, sexually transmitted diseases, exposure to AIDS or other sexual concerns? ☐ ☐

o. Do you feel safe/comfortable in your home, with your family, and/or your partner relationship? ☐ ☐

p. Do you smoke or use tobacco products now? ☐ ☐

q. Do you use recreational drugs? ☐ ☐
                                  ☐ ☐

r. Do you drink alcohol? ☐ ☐
  ☐ daily ☐ weekly ☐ rarely
  # of drinks _____
  If yes, do you drink: ☐ beer
  ☐ wine ☐ liquor

Review of Systems
Are you concerned about? (circle concerns)

YES NO

1. Recent changes in health status ☐ ☐
2. Eye problems: vision, pain, tearing ☐ ☐
3. Ear, nose, mouth, throat problems ☐ ☐
4. Heart problems: chest pain, blood pressure ☐ ☐
5. Lung problems: coughing, wheezing, infections ☐ ☐
6. Abdominal pain, stomach or bowel problems ☐ ☐
7. Kidney or bladder problems ☐ ☐
8. Muscle, bone, joint or back problems ☐ ☐
9. Skin, hair or nail problems ☐ ☐
10. Neurologic problems: headaches, dizziness, numbness ☐ ☐
11. Nervousness, anxiety, depression, suicidal thoughts ☐ ☐
12. Excessive thirst and urine output, recent weight changes ☐ ☐
13. Anemia, bruising, blood clots, swollen glands ☐ ☐
14. Food allergies, hay fever, eczema, asthma, decreased immunity ☐ ☐

Do you have any other concerns? ☐ ☐

_____

_____

_____
Patient's signature   Date

Provider Comments:

☐ PFSH and ROS have been reviewed.   ☐ Unresolved problems from previous visit have been addressed.

_____
Provider's signature   Date

Anticipatory Guidance

☐ Nutrition
☐ Exercise
☐ Calcium
☐ Multivit. with folate

☐ Cardiovascular risks
☐ Osteoporosis risks
☐ Estrogen
☐ Sun exposure
☐ Smoking cessation
☐ Alcohol/drugs

☐ Sexual issues
☐ Family planning/contraception
☐ STD prevention
☐ Menopause
☐ Self-exam: breasts, skin, oral cavity
☐ Family

☐ Recreation/hobbies
☐ Safety/injury/gun safety
☐ Auto seat belts
☐ Domestic violence
☐ Stress
☐ Educational handouts

FIGURE 1-26, cont'd

T O O L   6

HISTORY AND PHYSICAL SAMPLE DICTATION MODEL

Patient:	If Applicable:
Age:	Attending Physician:
Gender:	Date of Admission:
Date of Physical:	Room #:

Chief Complaint:
As Related to Provider by Patient
Character, Location, Onset, Radiation, Intensity, Duration, Intermittency, Events associated with, Palliative, Provocative Factors

Past Medical History:
Patient denies/positive for:

-Arthritis	-Diabetes	-Hepatitis	-Rheumatic Fever
-Asthma	-Emphysema	-Heart Disease	-Seizure
-Blood Disease	-Epilepsy	-Hypertension	-Thyroid Disease
-Bronchitis	-Flu	-Liver Disease	-TB
-Cancer	-Gout	-Pneumonia	-Ulcers
			-UTI

Past Surgical History:

Injuries:

Chronic Diseases/Disabilities:

Family History:

Social History:
Patient presently lives with:
Occupation:
Patient denies/positive for history of:
- Cigarettes/Smoking (# years/ppd)
- ETOH (frequency, # years)
-Substance Abuse (# years/substance)

Medications:

Allergies:

Review of Systems:

General -	Recent change in weight, appetite, sleeping habits
HEENT:	Head: Cephalgia, head injury, migraines Eyes: Blurring, cataracts, diplopia, photophobia, vision changes Ears: Discharge, hearing changes, tinnitus Nose: Chronic sinusitis, decreased smell, rhinorrhea, epistaxis, nasal fractures Mouth/Throat: Tenderness/lesions oral cavity, frequent sore throats, dysphagia, persistent hoarseness Neck: History of injury, masses, pain, stiffness
Respiratory:	Asthma, bronchitis, COPD, chronic cough, hemoptysis, SOB, TB, tachypnea
Cardiovascular:	Angina, CHF, claudication, CVA, cyanosis, dizziness, exertional dyspnea, hypertension, orthopnea, palpitations, phlebitis, precordial pain, TIA

Continued

T O O L 6, cont'd

HISTORY AND PHYSICAL SAMPLE DICTATION MODEL
(continued)

Gastro:	Constipation, diarrhea, dysphagia, gallbladder disease, hematemesis, hematochezia, hemorrhoids, hepatitis, hernia, indigestion, jaundice, melena, nausea, vomiting, pancreatitis, rectal bleeding
GU:	Dysuria, hematuria, nocturia, discharge, frequency, hesitancy, incontinence, chronic UTI, STD, prostatitis
Ob/Gyn:	Pregnancy history, last Pap/breast exam, contraceptive use, menstrual history
Breasts:	Discharge, enlargement, pain, tenderness, prior surgery/biopsy, +mammogram
Neuromuscular:	Anesthesias, paresthesias, arthralgias, myalgias, nervousness, syncope, vertigo, weakness
Endocrine:	Hot/cold intolerance, paresthesias, polydipsia, polyphagia, polyuria, anemia, excessive bruising/bleeding, diabetes, thyroid enlargement/problems

Physical Examination:

Vital Signs:	BP____ P____ T____ R____
General:	This is a ___ year old ____ who appears well hydrated and properly nourished and whose appearance is appropriate with the stated age. The patient is alert, cooperative, and in no acute distress at this time.
Skin:	Skin texture, turgor and pigmentation appear normal. No rashes, cyanosis. Normal hair pattern for sex and age.
Head:	Atraumatic, normocephalic, symmetrical and without deformities
	Eyes: PERRLA EOMI bilaterally. No conjunctival injection, ptosis or sclera icterus. Fundoscopic exam reveals no AV nicking, retinal hemorrhages or retinopathy seen.
	Ears: External ear exam reveals no abnormalities seen. External ear canals are patent, TM intact with normal light reflex and without injection.
	Nose: No deviated septum, turbinates normal appearing. Moist mucosa without discharge noted.
	Mouth: Pink gums without bleeding. Mucosa moist. Teeth appear in good condition.
	Throat: Trachea midline and mobile. No JVD, thyroid not palpable, nor enlarged. No cervical lymphadenopathy or rigidity present.
Lungs/Thorax:	Lungs clear to auscultation, no rales, rhonchi or wheezes. Breath sounds normal without prolonged expiratory phase. Respirations normal with good chest motion. No lymphadenopathy noted.
Heart:	Regular rate and rhythm without murmurs; no clicks, gallups, rubs, or extra heart sounds.
Abdomen:	Reveals soft, nontender abdomen. No masses, organomegaly, rebound tenderness or scars noted. Active bowel sounds noted in all quadrants. No pulsations, bruits or flank pain.
Extremities:	No clubbing, cyanosis, edema or varicosities noted. Pulses equal and adequate.
Neurological:	Patient oriented X 3. DTRs equal and adequate in upper and lower extremities. Good grip strength noted bilaterally. Sensation intact.

"GOOD WORDS/BAD WORDS" LIST

Provide a list of descriptive words considered acceptable in certain medical documentation, and a list of other terms that are not. Post it prominently wherever dictation or documentation is performed. These terms will vary by specialty. "Doing well" may be acceptable documentation (although not preferred) in a family physician's chart, but it would not be appropriate for documenting service provided to a critical care patient.

DOCUMENTATION DO'S AND DON'TS LIST

After a thorough review of the habits and practices of dictating or documenting information, develop a list of words and phrases that should be included and a list of those that should be excluded in documentation, as illustrated in Tool 7.

PROCEDURE FOR REVIEWING SIGNATURE REQUIREMENTS

Documentation is crucial to the practice from a reimbursement standpoint, as well as from a legal one. When appropriate signature requirements are not met, the documentation is of no value with respect to reimbursement and may leave the practice vulnerable to legal difficulties.

Records are often filed after a visit and subsequent dictation have been concluded. Develop a procedure for reviewing each medical record to ensure that signatures have been provided. Put into writing whether such a procedure is to be implemented just before the next visit or the next time the chart is pulled. As part of the office policy, this procedure should be clearly outlined and distributed to all employees. In addition to the established procedures for optimizing documentation, a monitoring process **must** also be included. The components of a successful compliance and monitoring program for a medical practice are discussed in Chapter 22.

A MONITORING PROCEDURE FOR DOCUMENTATION SUCCESS

After providing input and devising tools for effective documentation, monitor their implementation and success. If documenters still are not providing acceptable documentation, continue to educate and to identify alternatives tools and techniques that may be more successful. In a large practice, monitoring techniques must be incorporated into the company compliance program as well.

After the coder has developed effective tools and techniques to optimize the documentation process, the first skill to be developed for successful diagnostic and procedural coding is selecting appropriate information from the medical documentation. Some primary rules exist for this selection process and are specific to physi-cian coding for services. In a later chapter, the differences in physician and hospital coding, and the rationale for those differences are discussed.

GODFREY REGIONAL HOSPITAL PROVIDERS AND FACILITIES

As already discussed, a number of forms and formats may be used for record keeping and reimbursement purposes. These forms and formats may also occur in different locations. As mentioned in the Preface, this text has adapted a real-life-scenario approach to help students understand the coding process. Toward this end, the following providers from various locations are represented throughout the textbook and its ancillaries. Some charts are dictated and typed, whereas others are handwritten, sometimes bordering on illegible. A list of these providers and facilities is included in Table 1-1. For easy reference, a copy of Table 1-1 is included in Appendix B.

Providers and locations have been established so that students may practice the multitudinous skills required in medical coding. A signature log is required so that office personnel may identify signatures of individual physicians providing the various services. Table 1-2 contains the signature log for the medical groups.

Keep in mind that physicians may provide services in a number of facilities at different locations. As an exercise, put together one medical chart and review the documents that are contained in that chart. Typically, the physician chart will be tabbed on the basis of like services and like locations, such as the following:

Office visit/progress notes
Laboratory/x-ray tests
Other ancillaries
Hospital services
Correspondence/patient records

Typically, the following would be included in the record, starting from front to back:

Tab 1: Office Visits/Progress Notes (chronological order, current first)
Figure 1-3   Problem list
Figure 1-4   Medication flow sheet
Figure 1-2   Staff/visit note (chronological order, current first)
Figure 1-5   Progress note (most current)
Figure 1-5   Progress note (oldest)
Tab 2: Lab/X-Ray
Figure 1-18   Radiology report (chronological order, current first)
Figure 1-19   Laboratory report (chronological order, current first)
Tab 3: Other Ancillaries
Figure 1-11   Respiratory report (chronological order, current first)
Figure 1-13   Electromyography report (chronological order, current first)
Tab 4: Hospital Services
Figure 1-16   Discharge summary (chronological order, current first)

T O O L   7

BASIC DOCUMENTATION DO'S AND DON'TS

	Do	Don't
HISTORY Present	Vital sign review Duration/severity symptoms	Allow other personnel to document hx present illness
Past	Pertinent negative hx Pertinent positive hx	
Systems Review	Document all systems hx review incl "WNL" notations	
Family/Social	Include notations such as: Not available/noncontributory Unable to obtain due to_____	
PHYSICAL EXAM	Include: Body areas/organ systems Abnormal findings notated Pertinent negatives notated	
MEDICAL DECISION MAKING Diagnostic Tests	Document orders Document interpretations INTERPRETATIONS NOT DOCUMENTED CANNOT BE CHARGED	Document dx interpretations as "WNL" or "Abn"—document specifics that make them normal/abnormal
Clinical Impression	Record primary/2nd diagnoses Record contributory dx which may have resulted in increased level of care Include differential diagnoses	Use "rule out," "probable," "suspect," as part of the diagnostic statement
Treatment Plan	Record all medications/orders & sign Record all discharge instructions including preprinted handouts Resolution/nonresolution of symptoms Documentation of risks	Allow nurse documentation of meds unless signed off by the physician
SIGNATURE REQUIREMENTS	Sign all charts Countersign all academic residents Include notation "examined and concur" CHARTS NOT SIGNED ARE CONSIDERED NOT DOCUMENTED — NO CHARGE	Allow signature stamps Allow "dictated but not read"
SPECIAL NOTATIONS:	Document addtl time spent for: Excessive data review/counseling due to: Lengthy past med history Lengthy review of records Patient inability to comprehend Procedures documented separately	Forget to document time for these elements

TABLE 1-1   Godfrey Regional Health Facilities and Providers

Facility Names and Addresses

Godfrey Regional Outpatient Clinic	3122 Shannon Avenue Aldon, FL 77712 (407) 555-7654
Godfrey Regional Hospital	123 Main Street Aldon, FL 77714 (407) 555-1234
Godfrey Clinical Laboratories	465 Dogwood Court Aldon, FL 77712 (407) 555-9876
Godfrey Medical Associates	1532 Third Avenue, Suite 120 Aldon, FL 77713 (407) 555-4000

Provider Names

Provider	Specialty	Location(s) of Service
Maurice Doates, MD	Internal Medicine	Godfrey Regional Hospital Godfrey Regional Outpatient Clinic Godfrey Medical Associates
Robert Rais, MD	Emergency Department	Godfrey Regional Hospital
Stanley Krosette, MD	Internal Medicine	Godfrey Regional Hospital Godfrey Regional Outpatient Clinic Godfrey Medical Associates
William Obert, MD	Family Medicine	Godfrey Regional Hospital Godfrey Medical Associates
Felix Washington, MD	Family Medicine	Godfrey Regional Hospital Godfrey Medical Associates
Jay Corman, MD	Internal Medicine	Godfrey Regional Hospital Godfrey Medical Associates
Nancy Connelly, MD	Emergency Department	Godfrey Regional Hospital
Adam Westgate, MD	Surgeon/General	Godfrey Regional Hospital Godfrey Regional Outpatient Clinic Godfrey Medical Associates
Patrick Chung, MD	Surgeon/Orthopedics	Godfrey Regional Hospital Godfrey Regional Outpatient Clinic Godfrey Medical Associates
Rachel Perez, MD	Surgeon/General	Godfrey Regional Hospital Godfrey Regional Outpatient Clinic Godfrey Medical Associates
Lisa Valhas, MD	Radiologist	Godfrey Regional Hospital Godfrey Regional Outpatient Clinic
John Parker, MD	Internal Medicine	Godfrey Regional Hospital Godfrey Regional Outpatient Clinic Godfrey Medical Associates
Nathan Brady, MD	Internal Medicine Cardiology	Godfrey Regional Hospital Godfrey Regional Outpatient Clinic Godfrey Medical Associates
Luis Perez, MD	Anesthesiologist	Godfrey Regional Hospital Godfrey Regional Outpatient Clinic
Steven Speller, MD	Pathologist	Godfrey Clinical Laboratories
Maria Callaway, MD	Surg Pathologist	Godfrey Regional Hospital Godfrey Regional Outpatient Clinic
Patrick Adams, MD	Gastroenterologist	Godfrey Regional Hospital Godfrey Medical Associates
James Ellicott, MD	Otolaryngologist	Godfrey Regional Hospital Godfrey Regional Outpatient Clinic
Linda Patrick, MD	Ophthalmologist	Godfrey Regional Hospital Godfrey Medical Associates
Vincent DiMarco, MD	Neurologist	Godfrey Regional Outpatient Clinic Godfrey Regional Hospital

Figure 1-15   Hospital progress note (chronological order, current first)

Figure 1-14   Admission and history (chronological order, current first)

Figure 1-18   Operative report (chronological order, current first)

Figure 1-19   Anesthesia report

Tab 5: Correspondence/Patient Records

Figure 1-17   Consultation report (chronological order, current first)

Figure 1-1   Patient history

TABLE 1-2 Godfrey Regional Medical Signature Log

Provider	Signature
Maurice Doates, MD	
Robert Rais, MD	
Stanley Krosette, MD	
William Obert, MD	
Felix Washington, MD	
Jay Corman, MD	
Nancy Connelly, MD	
Adam Westgate, MD	
Patrick Chung, MD	
Rachel Perez, MD	
Lisa Valhas, MD	
John Parker, MD	
Nathan Brady, MD	
Luis Perez, MD	
Steven Speller, MD	
Maria Callaway, MD	
Patrick Adams, MD	
James Ellicott, MD	
Linda Patrick, MD	
Vincent DiMarco, MD	

CHAPTER IN REVIEW

CERTIFICATION REVIEW

At this point, it is assumed that the student of coding has not completed his or her studies and is not prepared to actually take the certification examination. Therefore certification exercises are included in the chapters on coding that occur later in the text.

Coding Concepts

- The cardinal rule of coding is: If it is not documented, it did not happen.
- All documentation used for coding must be appropriately signed to be considered complete.
- Documentation is important from both coding and medical liability standpoints.
- Key components of all medical documentation used in medical coding are history, physical examination, and medical decision making.
- Elements constituting history include chief complaint, history of present illness, medical history, family history, social history, and review of systems.
- Information included in the review of systems is used to identify the patient problem, assist in the arrival at a diagnosis, identify differential diagnoses, and determine the testing necessary to attain a definitive diagnosis.
- Elements of the physical examination component may be classified by specific body area or by organ system.
- Medical decision making is composed of review of information from tests and data; diagnosis and management options; and risks of morbidity, mortality, and complications.
- Complete ancillary records include medication records, health care staff notes, operative notes, and laboratory and other ancillary test results.
- Documentation requirements for hospital records include history and physical, admission records, hospital progress notes, and consultations.
- Documentation tools can help in the development of adequate medical documentation for medical coding and compliance.

STUDENT STUDY GUIDE

- Study Chapter 1.
- Review the Learning Objectives for Chapter 1.
- Review the Certification Review for Chapter 1.
- Complete the Chapter Review exercise to reinforce the concepts learned in this chapter.

CHAPTER REVIEW EXERCISE

Identify where the following services might be performed and on the basis of that location, identify the appropriate form(s) that would be used:

			Location	Type of Form(s)
1.	Patient visit	Godfrey Regional Hospital	*Hospital*	*H+P progress note*
2.	Patient visit	Godfrey Medical Associates	*office*	*office progress note*
3.	Patient visit	Godfrey Regional Outpatient Clinic	*outpatient clinic*	*office progress note physician outpt encounter documentation*
4.	Patient visit	Emergency department/ Godfrey Regional Hospital	*Hospital*	*emergency department note*
5.	Laboratory report		*office/Hosp*	*lab report ancillary report*
6.	Radiology report		*office/Hosp*	*radiology report*
7.	Admission history and physical		*Hospital*	*History + Physical H+P*
8.	Staff documentation of office visit		*office*	*Staff visit note*
9.	Patient history		*office*	*patient history form*
10.	Patient problem list		*office*	*Problem list*
11.	Anesthesia record		*hospital*	*Anestology rep*
12.	Operative report		*Hospital*	*operative report*
13.	Discharge summary		*Hospital*	*DC summary*
14.	Consultation		*office/ hosp.*	*consultation report*

II

ICD-9-CM DIAGNOSTIC CODING

In Section I of this text, many documents and techniques used in the documentation process were identified. This section contains diagnostic coding guidelines applicable to physicians and providers and provides an explanation of how to apply these rules to actual physician documents. The format of the ICD-9-CM diagnostic code book and its use for correct diagnostic code assignment are covered. Hospital and facility diagnostic coding are discussed in depth later in this text.

A brief review of the first building block in the process of correctly identifying and coding diagnostic components of the medical documentation, or WHY services were performed, follows. This outline is intended to provide a simple approach to the complicated process covered in depth by this part of the text.

Many think that diagnostic coding involves only the selection of the correct numerical ICD-9-CM diagnostic code; however, the process also involves many rules and considerations. As mentioned in Chapter 1, documentation plays a key role in determining which diagnostic statements are the correct ones to use. The steps for identifying correct diagnostic codes include the following:

Step 1. Identify key elements and words for possible use in the diagnosis.
Step 2. Determine which diagnostic statements are necessary for proper diagnosis.
Step 3. Determine the appropriate diagnostic code order.
Step 4. Assign diagnostic codes to diagnoses selected from the ICD-9-CM code book.

After reading the discussion of each step thoroughly, use the Diagnostic Documentation Worksheet to evaluate the information contained in the coding example. This form is included in Appendix B.

2

DETERMINING PHYSICIAN DIAGNOSIS

LEARNING OBJECTIVES

Following the completion of this chapter, the student will be able to:

- Identify key elements and words in physician documentation.
- Identify which key elements and words should be used for coding and documentation purposes.
- Recognize the differences between signs, symptoms, and diagnoses.
- Determine correct diagnostic code order.

CODING REFERENCE TOOLS

Tool 8
Rules for Selecting Appropriate Diagnoses (for Physician Coding)
Tool 9
Signs and Symptoms Rules
Tool 10
Diagnosis Do's and Don'ts
Tool 11
Diagnostic Order Rules

ICD-9-CM PHYSICIAN DIAGNOSTIC CODING

Step 1

Identify Key Elements and Words for Possible Use in the Diagnosis

Some primary rules exist for selecting appropriate diagnoses from medical documentation. These rules are specific to physician coding for services. The differences between physician and hospital coding, and the rationale for those differences are described later in the chapter. Keep in mind when reviewing the medical documentation, one must identify WHY the services are being provided. While only interested in assigning diagnoses at this point, the student must also identify services for the purpose of making certain all services have an appropriate diagnosis assigned.

Using the basic coding documentation rules found in Tool 8, look at the progress note in Figure 2-1 and identify items that would or would not be selected as **key elements** or **phrases.**

In the example, identify those components that might be used for diagnostic and procedural coding. Look for elements that identify **WHY** (diagnosis, signs, or symptoms) the encounter took place, as well as **WHAT** (procedures, services) was provided to help the patient. Later chapters on ICD-9-CM diagnostic coding and CPT-4 procedural coding examine which elements should be retained for coding purposes. Because all documentation will not be the same, it is important to keep in mind that the medical record should be reviewed for more than "Impression." In some instances, additional information is contained in the body of the documentation. A complete review will be necessary to select the correct diagnostic statements for coding purposes.

Look at the keywords identified in the sample documentation that are needed for diagnostic and procedural coding purposes.

WHAT (Service Elements)	WHY (Diagnostic Elements)
Physician office visit	Cough, fever, cold symptoms
	Upper respiratory infection
	Urinary frequency, urinary tract infection
Chest x-ray	Cough, fever, cold symptoms
	Upper respiratory infection
CBC	Cough, fever, cold symptoms
	Upper respiratory infection
Urinalysis	Urinary frequency, urinary tract infection

TOOL 8

RULES FOR SELECTING APPROPRIATE DIAGNOSES
(For Physician Coding)

1. **If it is not documented, it did not happen.**

2. The condition, problem, or other circumstance chiefly responsible for the health encounter/visit/problem is reported. This will be referred to as **Chief Reason for Encounter.**

3. Unconfirmed diagnoses described as "possible," "probable," "questionable," "rule out," "ruled out," "suspect(ed)," CANNOT be utilized for physician diagnoses or physician coding.

4. Code the condition to the **highest level of specificity.**
   In some cases, this may be the sign, symptom, abnormal test, or reason for visit/encounter.

5. If the physician does not identify a definite condition or problem at the conclusion of the patient visit/encounter, the coder should select the documented chief complaint or chief reason for the encounter.

6. Never code a diagnosis not listed by the physician.
   In the event the coder feels the physician has not listed an appropriate diagnosis, the coder must check with the physician.

   If the physician believes the information has been omitted in error, the provider may add an addendum to the original medical record, and, at that time, the coder may code accordingly.

PROGRESS NOTE

Date:	Vital signs:	T	R
Chief complaint:		P	BP

This is a 65-year-old female who presents due to ongoing problem with cough, fever, and cold symptoms.

Examination:

Chest x-ray and CBC are ordered, which indicate the presence of an upper respiratory infection. Patient also complains of urinary frequency; therefore, a urinalysis is performed that confirms the diagnosis of urinary tract infection.

Impression:

Upper respiratory infection
Urinary tract infection

Plan:

The patient will be treated with antibiotics and should follow-up in approximately 7–10 days.

Patient name:

DOB:

MR/Chart #:

GODFREY REGIONAL OUTPATIENT CLINIC
3122 Shannon Avenue • Aldon, FL 77712 • (407) 555-7654

FIGURE 2-1 Progress Note.

Note the necessity of matching **WHAT** service was provided with **WHY** that particular service was necessary. Refer to Figure 2-2 for completing Step 1 (identifying key elements for possible use in coding) of the Diagnostic Documentation Worksheet.

STOP AND PRACTICE

Review the following diagnostic information and identify the key words that would be appropriate for determining diagnostic statements that may be considered for diagnostic purposes.

	Utilize for Diagnostic Purposes?	
	Yes	No
1. Rule out pneumonia		✓
Cough		
2. Dysuria		✓
Probably urinary tract infection		
3. Leg pain		
Tibia fracture	✓	
4. Femur fracture		
Closed femur fracture	✓	
5. Tonsillitis		
Strep tonsillitis	✓	
6. Bronchitis		
Acute bronchitis	✓	
7. Abdominal pain	✓	
Rule Out (R/O) appendicitis		✓
8. Shortness of breath		
Asthma	✓	
Asthma, status asthmaticus	✓	
9. Abdominal pain	✓	
Right upper quadrant (RUQ)		
Abdominal pain	✓	
Possible cholecystitis		
10. Upper respiratory illness (URI)		
Upper respiratory infection	✓	

Step 2

Determine Which Diagnostic Statements Are Necessary for Proper Diagnosis Coding Purposes

Step 2 involves determining which of the elements selected will be used for diagnostic coding. This requires elimination of unneeded signs and symptoms and determination of those that are necessary for coding. In an actual medical document, a number of statements can be found regarding why the patient is being seen, or why the services are being performed. Some of these statements are diagnoses—statements about the patient's condition after evaluation has taken place. Signs and symptoms are information gathered throughout the course of the evaluation. In some instances, the physician may be unable to make a final diagnosis, in which case, the final diagnostic statement may be nothing more than signs and symptoms. The physician may make a final diagnostic statement after the conclusion of the encounter. Therefore these statements may not be used for that encounter.

For instance, the patient has symptoms of cough and fever. At the conclusion of the encounter, the physician orders a chest x-ray and makes a diagnosis of cough, ruling out pneumonia. The final diagnostic statement encompassing "rule out" cannot be used; the cough and fever may be coded as signs and symptoms because the pneumonia diagnosis has not be definitively established at the conclusion of the encounter.

When the patient arrives at the radiology center to undergo a chest x-ray, and the diagnosis of pneumonia is determined before the conclusion of the chest x-ray visit, however, pneumonia may be used as a diagnosis for the chest x-ray services, but not the physician office visit.

In the event that it is necessary to use signs, symptoms, or other conditions that do not qualify as a true diagnosis, the additional rules found in Tool 9 also apply.

DIAGNOSTIC DOCUMENTATION WORKSHEET

Chart#/Patient Name:

WHAT (Service/Procedure)	WHY (MEDICAL NECESSITY) (Diagnostic Information)			
Step 1 Select all words for possible use as diagnosis/diagnostic statement from the document	Office Visit — Cough, Fever, Cold Symptoms, Upper Respiratory Infection Urinary Frequency, Urinary Tract Infection Chest X-Ray — Cough, Fever, Cold Symptoms, Upper Respiratory Infection CBC — Cough, Fever, Cold Symptoms, Upper Respiratory Infection Urinalysis — Urinary Frequency, Urinary Tract Infection			
Step 2 Determine which words are appropriate for inclusion: (Carry these forward) Diagnosis vs. signs/symptoms				
Step 3 Based on each service performed, determine the appropriate order of diagnosis for each service performed				
Step 4 Look up/assign the proper dx codes				

FIGURE 2-2 Step 1 of the diagnostic coding process. (Courtesy of MD Consultative Services, Orlando, Florida. All rights reserved.)

T O O L   9

SIGNS AND SYMPTOMS RULES

Signs and symptoms should be used **ONLY** when:

1 Principal diagnosis has not been established at the conclusion of the visit or encounter.

2 No more specific diagnoses for the specific condition can be made at the end of the encounter/visit.

3 Presenting signs/symptoms are transient and no definitive diagnosis is made.

4 The symptom is treated in an outpatient setting without the additional workup necessary to arrive at a more definitive diagnosis at the conclusion of the encounter.

Signs and symptoms need NOT be used when they are an integral part of the underlying diagnosis or condition already coded.

STOP AND PRACTICE

Look at the following diagnostic statements. Identify whether the statements are "signs and/or symptoms" (SS) or "diagnosis" (D).

	(SS)	(D)
1. Upper respiratory infection		✓
2. Nausea	✓	
3. Vomiting	✓	
4. Headache	✓	
5. Angina	⊘	✓
6. Abdominal pain	✓	
7. Ovarian cyst		✓
8. Shoulder strain		✓
9. Ankle fracture		✓
10. Shortness of breath	✓	
11. High blood pressure	⊘	✓
12. Ankle contusion		✓
13. Viral illness		✓
14. Nasal congestion	✓	
15. Fatigue	✓	
16. Sore throat	✓	

In 17 to 26, try to eliminate (cross out) those diagnoses, signs, or symptoms that are an integral part of the final diagnosis for each case. This will leave only those statements that should be used for coding purposes.

In accordance with the rules, the signs and symptoms that are an integral part of the diagnostic statement can be eliminated in the sample. The procedure (service) elements are addressed in the CPT-4 procedural section of the textbook.

17. Upper respiratory infection
    Cough
    Acute bronchitis ✓
18. Nausea
    Vomiting
    Gastroenteritis ✓
19. Shortness of breath
    Chronic obstructive pulmonary disease (COPD) ✓
20. Angina
    Coronary artery disease ✓   *code both*
    Status post (S/P) bypass graft ✓
21. Otitis media ✓ *ear pain*
    Acute bronchitis ✓
    Diaper rash ✓
    Cough
22. Urinary retention
    Urinary frequency
    Urinary tract infection ✓
23. Urinary tract infection ✓
    Kidney stone ✓
24. Abdominal pain
    Appendicitis ✓
25. Fever
    Influenza ✓
26. Fever
    Urinary tract infection ✓

WHY (Diagnostic Elements)
Cough, fever, cold symptoms
Upper respiratory infection
Urinary frequency, urinary tract infection

The key elements and phrases listed on the previous page were previously identified in the sample chart as diagnostic elements to be considered for diagnosis coding. In accordance with the rules, the following can be eliminated:

Cough, Fever, Cold Symptoms   These are signs and symptoms that are part of the actual diagnosis of upper respiratory infection. This is referred to as "coding to the highest level of specificity." Be as specific as possible. Obviously, an upper respiratory infection has the symptoms of cough, fever, and cold as an integral part of the upper respiratory infection diagnosis. Therefore the diagnosis of upper respiratory infection is coded to the highest specific level possible.

As long as the coder is confident that the signs and symptoms listed are integral to that disease or diagnostic process, they need not be coded.

Urinary Frequency   This is considered a sign or symptom of the more specific diagnosis of urinary tract infection. Because urinary frequency signs and symptoms are an integral part of the urinary tract infection diagnosis, it is not necessary to code this sign or symptom.

Refer to Figure 2-3 for completion of Step 2 in determining the diagnostic statements to eliminate or include in this coding exercise, and then proceed to the "Stop and Practice" section.

Key elements have been identified for diagnostic statements; signs and symptoms not necessary to list and code have been determined. Next are additional diagnostic statements that may be found in the documentation.

ADDITIONAL DIAGNOSTIC DO'S AND DON'TS

Physician documentation frequently includes statements regarding previous conditions, chronic conditions, and abnormal findings. Tool 10 provides additional rules entitled **Diagnosis Do's and Don'ts** for determining which of the diagnoses selected thus far should be coded.

T O O L   10

DIAGNOSIS DO'S AND DON'TS

1. For previous conditions stated as diagnosis
   when previous condition has no bearing on current visit — **DO NOT CODE**
   Coder may utilize a "V" code (history of) if significant

2. Chronic conditions not the thrust of treatment — **DO CODE**
   Certain diseases such as hypertension, Parkinson's disease, diabetes, COPD are examples of systemic diseases that require continued clinical evaluation and monitoring during each visit.
   If visit does not involve evaluation of condition — **DO NOT CODE**

3. Conditions that ARE an integral part of the disease — **DO NOT CODE**
   Example: Patient with nausea and vomiting due to infectious gastroenteritis. Nausea and vomiting are common symptoms of this disease process and need not be coded.

   Conditions that are NOT an integral part of the disease — **DO CODE**
   Example: 5-year-old with 104° fever associated with pneumonia, also experienced convulsions. Pneumonia is coded (fever usually associated with pneumonia need not be coded), convulsions is coded (not always associated with pneumonia/fever).

4. Diagnosis not listed in final diagnostic statement — **CHECK WITH PHYSICIAN**
   If integral to correct coding, ask the physician to incorporate this information into the final diagnostic statement.

5. Abnormal findings — **CODE WHEN NECESSARY**
   Should be assigned only when physician is unable to arrive at a diagnosis prior to the conclusion of the encounter. If abnormal findings is the only diagnostic information available, the coder should check with the physician to make certain a codeable diagnosis is not available.

DIAGNOSTIC DOCUMENTATION WORKSHEET

Chart#/Patient Name:

	WHAT (Service/Procedure)	WHY (MEDICAL NECESSITY) (Diagnostic Information)
Step 1 Select all words for possible use as diagnosis/diagnostic statement from the document	Office Visit	Cough, Fever, Cold Symptoms, Upper Respiratory Infection
		Urinary Frequency, Urinary Tract Infection
	Chest X-Ray	Cough, Fever, Cold Symptoms, Upper Respiratory Infection
	CBC	Cough, Fever, Cold Symptoms, Upper Respiratory Infection
	Urinalysis	Urinary Frequency, Urinary Tract Infection
Step 2 Determine which words are appropriate for inclusion: (Carry these forward) Diagnosis vs. signs/symptoms	Office Visit	Upper Respiratory Infection
		Urinary Tract Infection
	Chest X-Ray	Upper Respiratory Infection
	CBC	Upper Respiratory Infection
	Urinalysis	Urinary Tract Infection
Step 3 Based on each service performed, determine the appropriate order of diagnosis for each service performed		
Step 4 Look up/assign the proper dx codes		

FIGURE 2-3 Step 2 of the diagnostic coding process. *(Courtesy of MD Consultative Services, Orlando, Florida. All rights reserved.)*

Differentiating signs and symptoms used as the diagnosis from those that are an integral part of a stated disease or condition is a cornerstone of the basic guidelines for reviewing documentation and identifying key elements.

Reevaluate the choice of diagnostic statements presented in Figure 2-3 to make certain these diagnostic statements are still appropriate based on the coding guidelines discussed thus far. All the key elements can be identified by circling, marking, or highlighting the information within the physician documentation. Then those elements that are not necessary for coding purposes can be eliminated.

Step 3

Determine the Appropriate Diagnostic Code Order
Order is significant in coding and reimbursement. Keep in mind that some third-party carriers allow for only one diagnostic code per service billed. In those instances, the first diagnosis for each service billed is the ONLY diagnosis code considered. Also, it is assumed that the most acute or severe diagnoses typically would be the **chief reason for the encounter.** Each service billed should include the appropriate "matching" reason WHY that service was medically necessary. Although the diagnosis code is indicative of the medical necessity for the service, it will justify only those services billed in the correct combination. Additional rules for diagnostic order are found in Tool 11.

Take another look at the medical chart in Figure 2-1. Each listed service should specifically include the primary reason that the service was provided (medical necessity), followed by any contributing diagnoses that support the intensity or complexity of that particular service. For instance, a patient in the physician's office with multiple complaints typically would have multiple diagnoses for the office visit. These additional diagnoses add to the complexity of the physician's office visit. In the case of laboratory services, blood specimens or urine specimens, for example, would include specific diagnostic statements for results identified from these tests.

Revisit the previous example and look at the order of diagnosis for each of the services identified.

WHAT (Service Elements)	**WHY (Diagnostic Elements)**
Physician office visit	Upper respiratory infection
	Urinary tract infection
Chest x-ray	Upper respiratory infection
CBC	Upper respiratory infection
Urinalysis	Urinary tract infection

Physician Office Visit

On the basis of the rules already discussed, several of the elements identified as signs or symptoms of a stated condition or disease have been eliminated. Therefore the remaining diagnostic statements for the physician office visit are the following:

TOOL 11

DIAGNOSTIC ORDER RULES

1. Signs and symptoms are assigned only after diagnoses, and only when NOT an integral part of the diagnostic statement.

2. Acute conditions are coded as the primary diagnosis in most instances as it is assumed they are the primary reason for encounter. The exception would be the case of a significantly more serious condition.

   EXCEPTION: Myocardial Infarction not listed as Acute Otitis Media.

   Note that many serious conditions are "automatically" assumed as acute.

3. Chronic conditions (when coded by previous rules) are coded secondary to any acute conditions or primary reasons for encounter. Make sure to use chronic codes when applicable.

4. Physician diagnosis allows for only four (4) diagnoses per service (line item) billed on the physician claim form. Choose them wisely, keeping in mind that some insurance carriers consider only the first diagnosis per service in determining medical necessity for the service and whether reimbursement is made.

   Select more than four (4) diagnoses in total for all services if necessary; however, only four (4) may be utilized per each service.

Urinary tract infection
Upper respiratory infection

Several factors would be considered in determining which diagnosis would best justify the medical necessity of the office visit. Because neither condition listed is acute or chronic, those considerations are not involved. Certainly, the fact that the patient reports ongoing problems with the signs and symptoms now diagnosed as upper respiratory infection (probably prompting the visit to the physician in the first place) would be a consideration.

The other consideration would be the complexity of each diagnosis. The upper respiratory infection necessitated both a chest x-ray and a complete blood cell count (CBC), both more significant than the urinalysis ordered for the urinary tract infection. Thus the upper respiratory infection would be coded as the primary diagnosis for the physician visit. This does NOT mean it will necessarily be the primary diagnosis for each of the other services provided.

Certainly, a urinalysis would not be required for the primary diagnosis of upper respiratory infection, nor would the urinalysis be justified from a medical necessity standpoint.

Chest X-Ray

This radiological test allowed the provider to render unequivocally the diagnosis of upper respiratory infection. Symptoms of cough, fever, and cold were eliminated as integral parts of the upper respiratory infection diagnosis. The urinary tract infection has no bearing on a radiological test; therefore it is not used at all to justify this service.

Complete Blood Cell Count

The CBC would not be considered medically necessary for the diagnosis of urinary tract infection. This test was performed only for the medical necessity of establishing the diagnosis of upper respiratory infection.

Urinalysis

Urinalysis is performed on a specimen for the symptom of urinary frequency, diagnosed to the higher level of specificity of urinary tract infection. The other diagnosis of upper respiratory infection has no bearing on the medical necessity of a urinalysis; therefore it is not used to justify this service.

The following is a recap of the services, the appropriate diagnoses, and the order of the diagnostic statements for these services.

Service/Encounter (WHAT)	Diagnosis (WHY)
Physician office visit	Upper respiratory infection
	Urinary tract infection
Chest x-ray	Upper respiratory infection
CBC	Upper respiratory infection
Urinalysis	Urinary tract infection

Note that each encounter or service may include a different diagnosis. Some encounters or services may have more than one diagnosis. Figure 2-4 is the correct diagnostic code order for this sample chart. Use this same technique in coding Step 3 in the Stop and Practice section.

STOP AND PRACTICE

Review the following diagnostic statements, signs, and symptoms. Eliminate unnecessary statements and place the remaining diagnostic statements in appropriate order for an office encounter. Place a numerical assignment next to each remaining statement.

1. Upper respiratory infection
   R/O pneumonia
   Acute bronchitis
2. Cholecystitis
   Cholecystitis with cholelithiasis
3. Cough
   Fever
   Bronchitis

4. Seizures
   Epilepsy ruled out
5. Shortness of breath (SOB), cause undetermined
6. 2-year-old child with fever, rhinorrhea
   Diagnosis: acute sinusitis and acute otitis media
7. Bronchitis with cough
8. Chronic heart failure (CHF) with SOB
9. Headache
   Probably migraine
10. Abdominal mass with jaundice
    Consider hepatitis

Because all the required steps have been completed before the assignment of the proper ICD-9-CM code, coding of the selected diagnosis can now proceed. These steps may seem of little consequence for the simple physician charts discussed here, but the same guidelines are used to determine the assignment of diagnostic codes in even the most complex situations.

So far, the steps discussed have helped to accomplish the following:

- Identify the key elements and phrases used in diagnostic coding
- Distinguish signs or symptoms from actual diagnoses and determine when their use is appropriate

DIAGNOSTIC DOCUMENTATION WORKSHEET

Chart#/Patient Name:

	WHAT (Service/Procedure)	WHY (MEDICAL NECESSITY) (Diagnostic Information)
Step 1 Select all words for possible use as diagnosis/diagnostic statement from the document	Office Visit	Cough, Fever, Cold Symptoms, Upper Respiratory Infection
		Urinary Frequency, Urinary Tract Infection
	Chest X-Ray	Cough, Fever, Cold Symptoms, Upper Respiratory Infection
	CBC	Cough, Fever, Cold Symptoms, Upper Respiratory Infection
	Urinalysis	Urinary Frequency, Urinary Tract Infection
Step 2 Determine which words are appropriate for inclusion: (Carry these forward) Diagnosis vs. signs/symptoms	Office Visit	Upper Respiratory Infection
		Urinary Tract Infection
	Chest X-Ray	Upper Respiratory Infection
	CBC	Upper Respiratory Infection
	Urinalysis	Urinary Tract Infection
Step 3 Based on each service performed, determine the appropriate order of diagnosis for each service performed	Office Visit	1) Upper Respiratory Infection (addtl services performed)
		2) Urinary Tract Infection (1 addtl service performed)
	Chest X-Ray	1) Upper Respiratory Infection
	CBC	1) Upper Respiratory Infection
	Urinalysis	1) Urinary Tract Infection
Step 4 Look up/assign the proper dx codes		

FIGURE 2-4 Step 3 of the diagnostic coding process. (Courtesy of MD Consultative Services, Orlando, Florida. All rights reserved.)

- Identify the rules for coding
- Determine the appropriate order of diagnosis for services rendered

The last step of the diagnostic coding process is to open the ICD-9-CM coding books and begin assigning appropriate codes.

Step 4

Assign Diagnostic Codes to Diagnoses Selected from the ICD-9-CM Code Book

Keep in mind that the universal insurance claim form (CMS-1500) or inpatient billing form (UB-92) that is used for coding, billing, and reimbursement to insurance carriers affords the coder the opportunity to assign code numbers only to **WHAT** services are rendered (CPT-4 procedural codes) and **WHY** those services are medically necessary (ICD-9-CM diagnostic codes). There is insufficient room to display descriptions or to further describe services and diagnoses. In addition, most health insurance claim forms are now read by optical scanners that are unable to decipher descriptors other than code numbers. Therefore a justification exists for **ICD-9-CM,** a standardized coding method for reporting diagnosis information with numerical codes only.

CHAPTER IN REVIEW

CERTIFICATION REVIEW

- Always code the chief reason for encounter/service as the primary diagnosis.
- Always code to the highest level of specificity.
- Always select appropriate diagnoses that "tie" to the services performed.
- Every chart should have a **WHY** (diagnostic code) and **WHAT** (CPT-4 code) in completely describing the services performed and the medical necessity for those services.
- Keywords such as *rule out, probable,* and *possible* may NOT be used for physician diagnostic coding.
- Acute conditions or those with the word *acute* included in the diagnostic statement should be coded as primary because they are assumed to be the chief reason for the encounter.
- Chronic systemic conditions should be coded in addition to the primary reason(s) for encounter when such conditions influence the physician's decision making and final diagnostic statement.
- Signs and symptoms may be used for diagnostic statements; however, they should be used only when a more specific diagnosis is not available.

STUDENT STUDY GUIDE

- Study Chapter 2.
- Review the Learning Objectives for Chapter 2.
- Review the Certification Review for Chapter 2.
- Complete the Stop and Practice exercises contained in Chapter 2
- Complete the Chapter Review exercise to reinforce concepts learned in this chapter.

CHAPTER REVIEW EXERCISE

Determine which of the following diagnoses would be used in the final diagnostic statement, as well as the appropriate order for the diagnoses selected.

	Diagnostic Statement(s) Selected in Appropriate Order
1. Otitis media	1
Dehydration	2
Nausea/vomiting	3
2. Strep throat	2
Acute pharyngitis	1
Sore throat	
3. Unstable angina	2
Hypertension (previously diagnosed)	3
Coronary artery disease (CAD) (previously diagnosed)	1
4. Gastroenteritis, ~~probably~~ ~~viral~~	~~X~~ 1
Nausea and vomiting	X NO
5. Chickenpox	1
Dehydration	
6. Acute sinusitis	1
Bronchitis	2
7. Viral hepatitis	1
Viral illness	
8. Abdominal pain RUQ due to pancreatitis or cholecystitis	Abdominal pain
9. Chest pain, probably angina	chest pain
10. Syncope with a fever in a 6-year-old child R/O meningitis	Syncope

PRACTICAL APPLICATION

Using the concepts presented in Chapter 2, identify the key elements or statements used for diagnostic purposes and place them in appropriate diagnostic order in the following charts. The Diagnostic Coding Worksheet for assigning diagnoses that is found in Appendix B may continue to be used.

1. Borderline Hypercholesterolemia

PROGRESS NOTE

Chief complaint: _____

Date: _____

Vital signs: BP____   __P__   ___R___

History:

This 45-year-old patient came to the physician for evaluation of her borderline hypercholesterolemia for which she takes niacin in doses of 1500 mg daily. Her cholesterol initially was 345, and it has now dropped to 252. She has a history of hypoglycemia, which has improved with diet and supplements. She also has an approximately 6-month history of insomnia. Allergy to codeine. Has had some bloating after meals and extremely cold extremities for which she wears gloves in the house during the winter months. Family history—mother with valvular heart disease, father with heart attack.

SOCIAL/FAMILY HISTORY:
Drinks coffee and rarely alcohol.

Exam:

Diagnosis/assessment:

Borderline hypercholesterolemia
Hypoglycemia
Insomnia
Cold extremities/intolerance to cold

Stany Krault MD

Patient name: _____

Date of service: _____

GODFREY MEDICAL ASSOCIATES
1532 Third Avenue, Suite 120 • Aldon, FL 77713 • (407) 555-4000

Service Provided: Office Visit Only

Diagnostic Statement #1: _____

Diagnostic Statement #2: _____

Diagnostic Statement #3: _____

2. Shortness of Breath versus Angina

PROGRESS NOTE

| Date: | Vital signs: | T | R |
| Chief complaint: | | P | BP |

This 58-year-old female noted a sensation of shortness of breath in the high substernal region of her chest. She also describes a feeling of heaviness or pressure. I believe that this sensation is more consistent with angina than true air hunger. This sensation reportedly lasted about 20 minutes. There was no radiation with discomfort and no associated symptoms.

Physical examination:

EXAM: Neck supple without masses. Thyroid gland not enlarged. Carotid arterial pulses equal and full. Prominent normal jugular venous pulsations with patient in supine position. Chest is symmetrical with equal respiratory sounds. No thoracic deformity or tenderness. Breast normal, free of masses or tenderness. No visible or palpable precordial activity. There is a grade III/VI systolic ejection murmur. Lungs clear to auscultation and percussion. Extremities free of cyanosis, clubbing, and peripheral edema. Femoral and distal pulses are present and normal. EKG reveals T-wave inversions that are symmetrical in leads V1 and V3; lead V4 reveals very flat T wave, consistent with anterior myocardial ischemia.

Assessment:

Angina

Plan:

Will order stress test and possible cardiac catheterization as EKG already shows ischemic heart disease.

Maurice Doaters, MD

	Patient name:
	DOB:
	MR/Chart #:

GODFREY REGIONAL OUTPATIENT CLINIC
3122 Shannon Avenue • Aldon, FL 77712 • (407) 555-7654

SERVICE PROVIDED: _____   SERVICE PROVIDED: _____
Diagnostic Statement #1: _____   Diagnostic Statement #1: _____
Diagnostic Statement #2: _____   Diagnostic Statement #2: _____
Diagnostic Statement #3: _____   Diagnostic Statement #3: _____

3. Pain in Chest

PROGRESS NOTE

Chief complaint: _____

Date: _____

Vital signs: <u>BP</u>___   <u>P</u>___   <u>R</u>___

History:

This 40-year-old gentleman presents to this office because of pain in the chest that has been noted for some time. The pain is radiating in nature, and the patient has become concerned.

Medical history reveals no diabetes or history of rheumatic fever. Social history is one-pack-a-day cigarette smoker, no ETOH intake. Family—both parents died as the result of strokes.

Exam:

Neck is supple, no carotid bruit. Lungs clear to percussion and auscultation. Heart reveals regular rate and rhythm with no gallop, rub, or murmur. EKG is within normal limits. Treadmill stress test using the Bruce protocol was normal; no abnormalities were noted.

Diagnosis/assessment:

Chest pain, noncardiac in nature; probably musculoskeletal in nature

John Palermo

Patient name: _____

Date of service: _____

GODFREY MEDICAL ASSOCIATES
1532 Third Avenue, Suite 120 • Aldon, FL 77713 • (407) 555-4000

SERVICE PROVIDED: _____   SERVICE PROVIDED: _____
Diagnostic Statement #1: _____   Diagnostic Statement #1: _____
Diagnostic Statement #2: _____   Diagnostic Statement #2: _____
Diagnostic Statement #3: _____   Diagnostic Statement #3: _____

4. Slow Heart Beat

EMERGENCY ROOM RECORD

Name:		Age:	ER physician:
		DOB:	

Allergies/type of reaction:	Usual medications/dosages:

Triage/presenting complaint:	This 65-year-old patient presents to the emergency room complaining of an irregular heart beat and shortness of breath. The patient has a history of COPD.

Initial assessment:	

Time	T	P	R	BP	Other:					
Medication orders:										

Lab work:	

X-Ray:	

Physician's report:

Following the administration of O_2, ABG, EKG, and chest x-ray, the final diagnosis is bradycardia and severe exacerbation of COPD. The patient will be admitted for further study and treatment.

Diagnosis:	Physician sign/date
	Nancy Caulley MD

Discharge	Transfer	Admit	Good	Satisfactory	Other:

GODFREY REGIONAL HOSPITAL
123 Main Street • Aldon, FL 77714 • (407) 555-1234

SERVICE PROVIDED: _____   SERVICE PROVIDED: _____
Diagnostic Statement #1: _____   Diagnostic Statement #1: _____
Diagnostic Statement #2: _____   Diagnostic Statement #2: _____
SERVICE PROVIDED: _____   SERVICE PROVIDED: _____
Diagnostic Statement #1: _____   Diagnostic Statement #1: _____
Diagnostic Statement #2: _____   Diagnostic Statement #2: _____

5. Motor Vehicle Accident

EMERGENCY ROOM RECORD

Name:		Age:	ER physician:
		DOB:	

Allergies/type of reaction: | **Usual medications/dosages:**

Triage/presenting complaint: | This 46-year-old male presents to the emergency room via ambulance following a motor vehicle accident where he lost control of his car and hit a tree off the side of the road. Upon presentation, the patient complains of pain to the lower right extremity, especially when the leg is moved. It appears to have obvious deformity.

Initial assessment:

Time	T	P	R	BP	Other:					

Medication orders:

Lab work:

X-Ray:

Physician's report:

An x-ray of the femur and hip reveal a right comminuted intertrochanteric fracture as well as a distal transverse femur fracture. The patient also complains of abdominal pain, and bruising and contusions appear throughout the abdominal area. Urinalysis reveals frank hematuria. The patient's lower extremity is splinted for mobility and the patient is transferred for evaluation of the above-listed problems.

Diagnosis: | **Physician sign/date**

Robert Rai MD

Discharge	Transfer	Admit	Good	Satisfactory	Other:

GODFREY REGIONAL HOSPITAL
123 Main Street • Aldon, FL 77714 • (407) 555-1234

SERVICE PROVIDED: _____
Diagnostic Statement #1: _____
Diagnostic Statement #2: _____
SERVICE PROVIDED: _____
Diagnostic Statement #1: _____
Diagnostic Statement #2: _____

SERVICE PROVIDED: _____
Diagnostic Statement #1: _____
Diagnostic Statement #2: _____
SERVICE PROVIDED: _____
Diagnostic Statement #1: _____
Diagnostic Statement #2: _____

6. Chest Pain in Elderly Patient

PROGRESS NOTE

Date:	Vital signs:	T	R
Chief complaint:		P	BP

A 92-year-old female presents with recurrent chest pain along with dizziness and weakness. The patient has been in the office on numerous occasions with similar complaints.

Examination:

Following examination, a chest x-ray, EKG, and cardiac enzymes are performed.

Impression:

The patient is diagnosed with chest pain, probably anxiety-related.

Plan:

Willem Obot MD

Patient name:

DOB:

MR/Chart #:

GODFREY REGIONAL OUTPATIENT CLINIC
3122 Shannon Avenue • Aldon, FL 77712 • (407) 555-7654

SERVICE PROVIDED: _____
Diagnostic Statement #1: _____
Diagnostic Statement #2: _____
SERVICE PROVIDED: _____
Diagnostic Statement #1: _____
Diagnostic Statement #2: _____

SERVICE PROVIDED: _____
Diagnostic Statement #1: _____
Diagnostic Statement #2: _____
SERVICE PROVIDED: _____
Diagnostic Statement #1: _____
Diagnostic Statement #2: _____

7. Upper Abdominal Pain

EMERGENCY ROOM RECORD

Name:		Age:	ER physician:
		DOB:	

Allergies/type of reaction:		Usual medications/dosages:

Triage/presenting complaint:	This 47-year-old male presents to the emergency room with abdominal pain, especially in the right upper abdomen. The patient has had these symptoms for the past 4–5 days, more at night while sleeping. Nothing has improved the symptoms, and they have steadily increased over the last 24 hours.

Initial assessment:

Time	T	P	R	BP	Other:				

Medication orders:

Lab work:

X-Ray:

Physician's report:

Exam of the abdomen, chest, HEENT, and labs (liver enzymes) are performed. Liver enzymes are significantly elevated. The patient will be watched for probable cholelithiasis in the observation unit.

Diagnosis:	Physician sign/date
	Nancy Caulby MD

Discharge	Transfer	Admit	Good	Satisfactory	Other:

GODFREY REGIONAL HOSPITAL
123 Main Street • Aldon, FL 77714 • (407) 555-1234

SERVICE PROVIDED: _____
Diagnostic Statement #1: _____
Diagnostic Statement #2: _____
SERVICE PROVIDED: _____
Diagnostic Statement #1: _____
Diagnostic Statement #2: _____

SERVICE PROVIDED: _____
Diagnostic Statement #1: _____
Diagnostic Statement #2: _____
SERVICE PROVIDED: _____
Diagnostic Statement #1: _____
Diagnostic Statement #2: _____

8. Severe Headache

PROGRESS NOTE	
Date:	Vital signs: T R
Chief complaint:	P BP

This 7-year-old presents with a 2–3 hour history of severe headaches, including intermittent nausea and vomiting. The patient refused vehemently any diagnostic testing including labs, CT scans, etc.

Physical examination:

Assessment:

Plan:

The patient will be seen by the pediatric neurologist and admitted to rule out seizures and migraine headaches.

Felix Wander M

Patient name:

DOB:

MR/Chart #:

GODFREY REGIONAL OUTPATIENT CLINIC
3122 Shannon Avenue • Aldon, FL 77712 • (407) 555-7654

SERVICE PROVIDED: _____

Diagnostic Statement #1: _____

Diagnostic Statement #2: _____

SERVICE PROVIDED: _____

Diagnostic Statement #1: _____

Diagnostic Statement #2: _____

9. Finger Laceration

PROGRESS NOTE				
Date:		**Vital signs:**	T	R
Chief complaint:			P	BP

A 25-year-old male presents with a laceration of finger which resulted from a knife cut while working at the bakery where he is currently employed.

Examination:

Laceration appears deep, almost down to the bone. It is examined for vessel and tendon involvement, which appears to be negative. An x-ray of the finger reveals no other damage other than the laceration. The wound is irrigated and sutured appropriately.

Impression:

Plan:

Jay Corim MD

Patient name:

DOB:

MR/Chart #:

GODFREY REGIONAL OUTPATIENT CLINIC
3122 Shannon Avenue • Aldon, FL 77712 • (407) 555-7654

SERVICE PROVIDED: _____   SERVICE PROVIDED: _____
Diagnostic Statement #1: _____   Diagnostic Statement #1: _____
Diagnostic Statement #2: _____   Diagnostic Statement #2: _____

10. Shortness of Breath

EMERGENCY ROOM RECORD

Name:		Age:	ER physician:
		DOB:	

Allergies/type of reaction:	Usual medications/dosages:

Triage/presenting complaint:	A patient is brought in with shortness of breath and history of COPD. The patient appears diaphoretic, in obvious distress.

Initial assessment:

Time	T	P	R	BP	Other:					
Medication orders:										

Lab work:

X-Ray:

Physician's report:

A chest x-ray and ABG are performed. The patient will be admitted for acute exacerbation of COPD, with impending ARDS.

Diagnosis:	Physician sign/date
	Robert Rai MD

Discharge	Transfer	Admit	Good	Satisfactory	Other:

GODFREY REGIONAL HOSPITAL
123 Main Street • Aldon, FL 77714 • (407) 555-1234

SERVICE PROVIDED: _____
Diagnostic Statement #1: _____
Diagnostic Statement #2: _____
SERVICE PROVIDED: _____
Diagnostic Statement #1: _____
Diagnostic Statement #2: _____

SERVICE PROVIDED: _____
Diagnostic Statement #1: _____
Diagnostic Statement #2: _____

11. Chest Discomfort

PROGRESS NOTE

Date:	Vital signs:	T	R
Chief complaint:		P	BP

A 26-year-old patient presents to the office with complaints of chest discomfort. He presents with history that he fell while taking out the trash approximately two weeks ago, and experienced some chest discomfort following the fall. Today, he fell while walking down the steps to his home and the pain afterward appeared to become worse.

Examination:

A chest x-ray and rib x-ray were performed which revealed multiple rib fractures, probably the 5th and 6th ribs.

Impression:

Plan:

He was advised on the treatment for this injury and tape was applied to the rib cage.

Willen Obt MD

Patient name:

DOB:

MR/Chart #:

GODFREY REGIONAL OUTPATIENT CLINIC
3122 Shannon Avenue • Aldon, FL 77712 • (407) 555-7654

SERVICE PROVIDED: _____   SERVICE PROVIDED: _____
Diagnostic Statement #1: _____   Diagnostic Statement #1: _____
Diagnostic Statement #2: _____   Diagnostic Statement #2: _____
SERVICE PROVIDED: _____
Diagnostic Statement #1: _____
Diagnostic Statement #2: _____

12. Injury Trauma

EMERGENCY ROOM RECORD

Name:	Age:	ER physician:
	DOB:	

Allergies/type of reaction:	Usual medications/dosages:

Triage/presenting complaint:	This 28-year-old male presents with complaints of pain to the lower back area following an accident where he lost control of his car, hitting a nearby tree.

Initial assessment:	

Time	T	P	R	BP	Other:					

Medication orders:

Lab work:

X-Ray:

Physician's report:

Back x-rays were performed which were negative. However, a urinalysis revealed hematuria and kidney trauma is suspected. A kidney ultrasound was also negative. The patient will be admitted for further evaluation and treatment.

Diagnosis:	Physician sign/date
	Nancy Cauley MD

Discharge	Transfer	Admit	Good	Satisfactory	Other:

GODFREY REGIONAL HOSPITAL
123 Main Street • Aldon, FL 77714 • (407) 555-1234

SERVICE PROVIDED: _____
Diagnostic Statement #1: _____
Diagnostic Statement #2: _____
SERVICE PROVIDED: _____
Diagnostic Statement #1: _____
Diagnostic Statement #2: _____

SERVICE PROVIDED: _____
Diagnostic Statement #1: _____
Diagnostic Statement #2: _____

13. History of Bipolar Disorder

PROGRESS NOTE

Date:	Vital signs:	T	R
Chief complaint:		P	BP

This 42-year-old male presents with shortness of breath and history of bipolar disorder.

Examination:

Upon the patient's insistence, an EKG, chest x-ray, and cardiac enzymes were ordered, all of which were negative.

Impression:

Plan:

The patient was discharged with a diagnosis of shortness-of-breath episode due to anxiety.

Robert Rai MD

Patient name:

DOB:

MR/Chart #:

GODFREY REGIONAL OUTPATIENT CLINIC
3122 Shannon Avenue • Aldon, FL 77712 • (407) 555-7654

SERVICE PROVIDED: _____
Diagnostic Statement #1: _____
Diagnostic Statement #2: _____
SERVICE PROVIDED: _____
Diagnostic Statement #1: _____
Diagnostic Statement #2: _____

SERVICE PROVIDED: _____
Diagnostic Statement #1: _____
Diagnostic Statement #2: _____

14. Admitted Patient with Chills

PROGRESS NOTE
Date/time
04/27/XX

S:

Pt states she feels tired, no more chills, denies cough denies N/V/D
C/o dysuria

O:

Lungs, clear, T 10z, Abdomen, positive bowel sounds, soft unttender
WBC:16.7, 85.8% segs

A:

Fever of unknown origin, cultures pending

P:

Continue IVF and antibiotics. Will repeat UA for symptoms

Maurice Doater, MD

PROGRESS NOTES

GODFREY REGIONAL HOSPITAL
123 Main Street • Aldon, FL 77714 • (407) 555-1234

SERVICE PROVIDED: _____
Diagnostic Statement #1: _____
Diagnostic Statement #2: _____
SERVICE PROVIDED: _____
Diagnostic Statement #1: _____
Diagnostic Statement #2: _____

SERVICE PROVIDED: _____
Diagnostic Statement #1: _____
Diagnostic Statement #2: _____

15. Shortness of Breath This Evening–Emergency Department (ED) Visit

EMERGENCY ROOM RECORD

| Name: | Age: | ER physician: |
| | DOB: | |

| Allergies/type of reaction: | Usual medications/dosages: |
| None | |

Triage/presenting complaint:

Initial assessment:

| Time | T | P | R | BP | Other: | | | | | |

Medication orders:

Lab work:

X-Ray:

Physician's report:

Check-off form completed.

Diagnosis:	Physician sign/date
	Nancy Cauley MD
	11/24/XX

| Discharge | Transfer | Admit | Good | Satisfactory | Other: |

GODFREY REGIONAL HOSPITAL
123 Main Street • Aldon, FL 77714 • (407) 555-1234

SERVICE PROVIDED: _____
Diagnostic Statement #1: _____
Diagnostic Statement #2: _____
SERVICE PROVIDED: _____
Diagnostic Statement #1: _____
Diagnostic Statement #2: _____

SERVICE PROVIDED: _____
Diagnostic Statement #1: _____
Diagnostic Statement #2: _____

16. Episode of Dyspnea

HISTORY AND PHYSICAL EXAMINATION

Stanley Krosette, MD

This 67-year-old female noticed trembling and restlessness in her left leg, eventually had shortness of breath and presented to the ER. Her chest x-ray, EKG and basic labs were normal. Her venous Doppler study of the LLE revealed no evidence of deep vein thrombosis. She will be admitted for possible DVT.

Past medical history:

Recently hospitalized for perforated appendix. Patient has had multiple admissions for other health problems.
CURRENT MEDICATIONS:
These include Synthroid 0.3 mg 4 X weekly, Digoxin 0.25 daily, Reglan 10 mg qid and prn Tylenol.

Family and social history

The patient and her spouse have been able to maintain with the help of family members. The patient does not drink or smoke.

Review of systems:

Musculoskeletal, patient has had numerous and gradually increasing musculoskeletal symptoms of reports many years of trembling or restless leg syndrome.

Physical exam

General: Patient's temperature was 98.6, pulse 54 and regular, respiratory rate of 18
             Patient's BP 127/51, patient is very hard of hearing
HEENT: Pupils equal and reactive to light and accommodation. EOM in tact
CHEST: Mild degree of kyphosis and breath sounds relatively distant. No dullness to Percussion of the thorax. No rales.
CV: Normal first and second heart sounds, no jugular venous distention
ABDOMEN: Soft, flat, nontender. Well healed surgical scars present on the central abdomen.

Laboratory/radiology:

X-ray:

CXR and Doppler normal

Assessment:

Episode of Dyspnea, LLE Restlessness, Severe hearing loss, Recent perforated appendix with peritonitis

Plan:

Stanley Krosette, MD

GODFREY REGIONAL HOSPITAL
123 Main Street • Aldon, FL 77714 • (407) 555-1234

SERVICE PROVIDED: _____
Diagnostic Statement #1: _____
Diagnostic Statement #2: _____
SERVICE PROVIDED: _____
Diagnostic Statement #1: _____
Diagnostic Statement #2: _____

SERVICE PROVIDED: _____
Diagnostic Statement #1: _____
Diagnostic Statement #2: _____

17. Radiology Report–Venous Doppler Ultrasound

RADIOLOGY REPORT

MR#:
DOB:
Ordered by: Dr. Stanley Krosette, MD

Clinical summary:

Shortness of breath

Abdomen:

CHEST BEDSIDE:
Single frontal view of the chest was obtained and compared with last chest x-ray performed 02/28/xxxx. The heart is normal in size, lungs clear. Diaphragm slightly flat raising the possibility of chronic obstructive pulmonary disease. Otherwise negative.

Conclusion:

IMPRESSION:
Hyperinflation of the lungs with possible COPD

Ddt/mm

D:

T:

_____
, M.D.   Date

GODFREY REGIONAL HOSPITAL
123 Main Street • Aldon, FL 77714 • (407) 555-1234

SERVICE PROVIDED: _____
Diagnostic Statement #1: _____
Diagnostic Statement #2: _____
SERVICE PROVIDED: _____
Diagnostic Statement #1: _____
Diagnostic Statement #2: _____

SERVICE PROVIDED: _____
Diagnostic Statement #1: _____
Diagnostic Statement #2: _____

18. Note

PROGRESS NOTE
_____

Date/time
_____
03/01/xxxx

S:

"My leg has trembled off and on for years"

O:

Alert, great loss of hearing, lungs, clear, no dyspnea

A:

Restless leg syndrome
Dyspnea

P:

Chronic and progressive health problems
Will almost certainly need full nursing home care

Stony Kratt, MD

PROGRESS NOTES

GODFREY REGIONAL HOSPITAL
123 Main Street • Aldon, FL 77714 • (407) 555-1234

SERVICE PROVIDED: _____
Diagnostic Statement #1: _____
Diagnostic Statement #2: _____
SERVICE PROVIDED: _____
Diagnostic Statement #1: _____
Diagnostic Statement #2: _____

SERVICE PROVIDED: _____
Diagnostic Statement #1: _____
Diagnostic Statement #2: _____

19. Fever of Unknown Origin

RADIOLOGY REPORT

MR#:
DOB:
Ordered by: Dr. Stanley Krosette, MD

Clinical summary:

Fever of unknown origin

Abdomen:

PA and lateral chest:
Pulmonary markings are prominent with definite infiltrate identified. No change. Heart size is normal.

Conclusion:

Normal chest

Ddt/mm

D:
T:

_____
, M.D.   Date

GODFREY REGIONAL HOSPITAL
123 Main Street • Aldon, FL 77714 • (407) 555-1234

SERVICE PROVIDED: _____   SERVICE PROVIDED: _____
Diagnostic Statement #1: _____   Diagnostic Statement #1: _____
Diagnostic Statement #2: _____   Diagnostic Statement #2: _____
SERVICE PROVIDED: _____
Diagnostic Statement #1: _____
Diagnostic Statement #2: _____

20. Bilateral Pedal Edema

PROGRESS NOTE

Date:		Vital signs:	T	R
Chief complaint:			P	BP

56-year-old male presents with bilateral pedal edema increasingly getting worse. Patient states he has a prior history of heart failure and recently discontinued all of his medications on his own accord.

PAST MEDICAL HISTORY: No known allergies, discontinued all meds on his own
Bilateral hernia repair, gallbladder removal 1995. CHF, cirrhosis of liver, COPD, ETOH. Abuse.

Examination:

Patient does not appear to be in discomfort. Vital Signs: T98.3, P 92, R22, BP 180/72. Chest normal, heart irregularity. Irregular rhythm, regular rate, no murmurs, rubs. Abdomen, flat, positive bowel sounds
MS: Good range of motions of all joints. No erythema, tenderness or swelling. Pedal edema 2+ bilaterally in lower extremities. Radial and dorsalis pedal pulses +2 out of 4 bilaterally.

Impression:

Pedal Edema
CHF

Plan:

Restart meds

Jay Corsm mo

Patient name:

DOB:

MR/Chart #:

GODFREY REGIONAL OUTPATIENT CLINIC
3122 Shannon Avenue • Aldon, FL 77712 • (407) 555-7654

SERVICE PROVIDED: _____   SERVICE PROVIDED: _____
Diagnostic Statement #1: _____   Diagnostic Statement #1: _____
Diagnostic Statement #2: _____   Diagnostic Statement #2: _____
SERVICE PROVIDED: _____
Diagnostic Statement #1: _____
Diagnostic Statement #2: _____

3

USING THE ICD-9-CM CODE BOOK

LEARNING OBJECTIVES

Following the completion of this chapter, the student will be able to:

- Comprehend the reasons for the establishment of a uniform coding system.
- Use the ICD-9-CM code book conventions and format.
- Correctly locate diagnoses in the ICD-9-CM code book.
- Understand the use of the tabular and alphabetical sections of the ICD-9-CM code book.
- Know the terminology unique to ICD-9-CM.
- Recognize the signs and symbols unique to ICD-9-CM and their application in the diagnostic coding process.

CODING REFERENCE TOOLS

Tool 12
Helpful Hints in Locating Diagnoses in ICD-9-CM
Tool 13
10 Steps to Accurate Coding from the ICD-9-CM Book
Tool 14
CMS Guidelines for ICD-9-CM Coding
Tool 15
Index to ICD-9-CM Tabular List (by Disease Process)

INTRODUCTION TO ICD-9-CM

ICD

Two versions of the ICD (International Classification of Diseases) are available. The original version, known only as **ICD,** was developed by the World Health Organization (WHO) to facilitate standardized reporting of diseases throughout the world. It is still used today by that same organization. The medical profession in the United States has created an adaptation of this widely used reference book.

ICD-9-CM CODE BOOK

All ICD reference books use the version or edition number following the name *ICD.* Thus ICD-9 represents the ninth edition of the reference book. Medical professionals have adapted the ICD version developed by WHO for use in statistical reporting and medical services billing in the United States. This clinical modification is identified as **ICD-9-CM** for **I**nternational **C**lassification of **D**iseases, **9**th edition, **C**linical **M**odifications.

ICD-10

WHO has already released the tenth revision of ICD; however, the ICD-10-CM version is not expected to be available until sometime after 2006. Proposed changes in ICD-10-CM are discussed in Chapter 7. The ICD-9-CM serves as a standardized means of reporting medical diagnostic information for the health care industry in the United States. Hospitals, physicians, and medical facilities, as well as the nation's health care insurance industry, all accept ICD-9-CM as the standard for reporting diagnostic information regarding services, medical necessity, and WHY services are performed.

USES OF ICD-9-CM

Hospitals use ICD-9-CM when billing for services, as well as for maintaining a statistical database of admitting diagnosis, principal diagnosis, days of hospital stay, and required government statistics, such as tumor registries and medical indices. Although hospitals report statistical data for billing and reimbursement on a different form than physicians do, they use the standard coding found in ICD-9-CM for reporting both medical necessity and the chief reason(s) for the encounter.

Physicians also use ICD-9-CM for reporting medical necessity for services performed, and for including this information in statistical databanks. This same information is used for grant and research projects, and for the determination of specific diagnostic protocols referred to as *standards of care.* Because the ICD-9-CM code is the only means of communicating medical necessity for services provided, the health care provider must ensure that coding is performed accurately to attain maximum reimbursement.

Third-party carriers, or insurance companies, use these diagnostic codes to evaluate the medical necessity for services billed by physicians, hospitals, and other health care entities. They also store these data for reference purposes in determining such matters as preexisting conditions. In addition, this statistical evidence is used to examine the incidences of certain diagnoses and to classify data according to age group, sex, and other categories. For example, statistical evidence that breast cancer is the number one disease in women ages 30 to 45 is the result of coding from ICD-9 and ICD-9-CM.

Because these data are of considerable magnitude in the health care field, the importance of accurate coding and the negative impact of incorrect coding on reimbursement, statistics, and insurance rates can be understood. Following are a few real case scenarios that demonstrate the importance of correct (or incorrect) diagnosis coding.

Real Case Scenario #1

A 4-year-old female was seen by the hematologist/oncologist for a suspicious cyst on her face. The cyst, which proved to be benign, was removed. Coding, however, indicated "malignant neoplasm of the brain." Several years later, when the child is an adult who has not maintained insurance coverage over the previous few years, her application for life insurance is denied because of "preexisting conditions."

Problem

Several years after the cyst was removed, the patient was faced with attempting to determine who coded the service incorrectly, contacting that physician's office, having the error corrected, and making certain all sources were informed of the correction after needed changes were made. This process can take an excessive amount of time. In some instances, the individual may never be able to determine at exactly what time and place the error occurred.

Real Case Scenario #2

A 34-year-old male presents to the physician's office with a laceration to the left hand following an accident. Health insurance claim forms filed to the carrier are denied, indicating "previous amputation of left hand in 1999," and a physician audit takes place because of the possibility of fraudulent billing.

Problem

The patient had a traumatic amputation of the RIGHT hand in 1999—not the left— as indicated at the time of amputation. Therefore claims for injuries would not be considered until the correction on the 1999 amputation claim was made.

Real Case Scenario #3

A 45-year-old female is involved in an automobile accident in which she is a *passenger* in a vehicle driven by another individual. Injuries are significant; the patient is seen in the emergency department and is subsequently admitted. Hospital charges are reported to the patient's auto insurance carrier. Charges are denied on the basis of "no accident report for this insured" because they are filed to *her* insurance carrier.

Problem

The patient was the *passenger* in the vehicle, and the claim should be filed first to the driver's automobile insurance, where an accident report has been made. The diagnosis coded for the injuries, however, was "Motor Vehicle Accident, *Driver,*" which led the insurance carrier to believe incorrectly that the patient was indeed the driver of the accident vehicle.

Real Case Scenario #4

According to the statistical data coded from several area hospitals in the Southeast, the average hospital stay for an appendectomy with perforation has dropped from 6 to 3 days. The Centers for Medicare and Medicaid Services (CMS) in the Southeast office computes these data and attains a new average stay of 4 days for this hospital procedure in the Southeast CMS region. Reimbursement for these hospital diagnosis-related groups (DRGs) is adjusted accordingly, and all hospitals in the Southeast have their reimbursements lowered.

Problem

After complaints from several hospitals in the Southeast, the data were investigated. It appeared that several hospitals were coding inappropriately. What had been coded as an appendectomy with perforation was, in fact, a simple appendectomy without perforation, for which the correct average stay is 3 days. Resubmission of corrected claims and reanalysis of statistical data were necessary at all hospitals involved, as well as with the CMS data. The hospitals that had coded these data incorrectly were audited for the possibility of fraudulent billing practices because they did not perform the services as reported.

The previous examples demonstrate only a few of the many situations that can be created as the result of incorrect diagnostic coding and its effect on reimbursement, patients, and statistical data.

ICD-9-CM AND MEDICAL NECESSITY

The data integrity of ICD-9-CM depends on both coding to the highest level of specificity and correct coding

compliance. Medical necessity has become a hot topic with the federal government, specifically with claims filed to the Medicare and Medicaid programs. Fraud and abuse occur daily in the United States, and millions of dollars in reimbursement are lost because of inadequate documentation for medical necessity. In addition to lost revenue, fraud and abuse fines are frequently charged. If found guilty, the provider is responsible for repayment of overpaid claims at three times the original payment amount, along with fines that vary from $2,000 to $10,000 per service billed.

The medical record often does not accompany the medical claim for services, so the ICD-9-CM code is the only effective means of communicating medical necessity for services. In the event that the insurance carrier needs additional information regarding medical necessity, the medical chart documentation must substantiate the ICD-9-CM diagnostic codes used. The coder then not only must code for accurate reimbursement purposes, but must act as statistician as well.

DIFFERENCES IN HOSPITAL AND PHYSICIAN DIAGNOSTIC CODING

It is important to understand the basic principles underlying the diagnostic coding differences for inpatient and physician coding. Hospitals are reimbursed for services performed. Global capitations under managed care contracts are billed as DRGs. The theory behind this reimbursement method is that the hospital provides certain services to a patient as a result of procedures and workups for conditions or suspected conditions. Therefore the hospital has the ability to incorporate diagnosis codes with descriptions such as "rule out," "suspect," and "probable." An example of this can be seen in two patients entering the hospital with an admitting diagnosis of "chest pain, rule out MI" (myocardial infarction). Although MI was subsequently diagnosed in one patient, the other was later discharged with a diagnosis of "chest pain, rule out MI." The DRG might remain the same for both patients because their workups included such services as electrocardiograms (ECGs), chest x-rays, laboratory tests, and hospital days. Both received services and workups for a possible MI.

Physicians would be reimbursed only on the services performed and documented at the time of the encounter. The emergency department physician in the situation described previously would be paid for the documented history, physical examination, and medical decision making performed for chest pain. Therefore the physician's diagnostic statement based on the chief reason for the encounter would probably be "chest pain."

In the outpatient setting, hospitals code for facility charges associated with a procedure performed by a provider or physician. They use procedural coding from CPT-4, as well as ICD-9-CM coding from Volume 3–Procedural Coding, to indicate the procedure performed rather than the medical necessity for that facility charge.

Hospital and outpatient coding are discussed in detail in Chapters 18 and 19. The rules discussed thus far are specific to physician or provider coding.

Before ICD-9-CM codes can be properly assigned, the correct use of the ICD-9-CM coding book must be learned.

ICD-9-CM CONVENTIONS AND FORMATS

GENERAL FORMAT

First, a look at the format, abbreviations, and symbols used in the ICD-9-CM would be appropriate. The ICD-9-CM coding book is divided into several sections. The three primary areas include the following:

1. Numerical (Tabular Listing of Diseases–Volume 1)
2. Alphabetical (Alphabetical Index to Diseases–Volume 2)
3. Procedural (Index to Procedures–Volume 3), if applicable

The coder must understand that many ICD-9-CM books incorporate multiple volumes in one book. Thus physician coders typically purchase only Volumes 1 and 2 together in one book because they do not need Volume 3. Hospital coders, however, must have all three volumes, usually purchased in one book. Despite the differences in selecting the correct key elements, diagnosis, signs, or symptoms for coding purposes, the methods for using the ICD-9-CM are universal across all types of coding—physician, hospital, and outpatient surgery alike.

A look at the ICD-9-CM book reveals that main terms are located flush with the left margin. Indentations indicate further information regarding the diagnosis listed. These indented terms are referred to as *subterms*. An example of this follows:

Blepharitis (Eyelid) 373.00
Angularis 373.01
Ciliaris 373.00
With Ulcer 373.01
Marginal 373.00
With Ulcer 373.01
Simple Blepharitis of the Eyelid, not otherwise specified, 373.00
Angularis Blepharitis 373.01
Ciliaris Blepharitis With Ulcer 373.01

One of the most common errors made in selecting the correct ICD-9-CM code from the key elements, diagnosis, signs, and symptoms is selecting a code without reviewing all available choices. Make certain, after locating the correct terms, to review all indented codes for possible

higher specificity, which would include more diagnostic information than the key element alone.

ABBREVIATIONS

NOS   Not Otherwise Specified

The designation of *not otherwise specified* (NOS) indicates a lack of sufficient detail to permit assignment to a more specific subdivision. This abbreviation is used when the physician, provider, or documenter does not further specify the condition.

Physician documents "Otitis media"

Code 382.9 otitis media

A number of other otitis media codes that are more specific are listed in ICD-9-CM; however, the physician has not provided further information to allow coding to a higher level of specificity.

Note: These codes may not be reimbursed by some insurance carriers. In the case of specialists, insurance carriers expect a higher level of specificity.

NEC   Not Elsewhere Classified (Other Specified)

The abbreviation of *not elsewhere classified* (NEC) indicates that the physician has further classified the diagnosis to a higher level of specificity; however, ICD-9-CM does not contain a code to the same level of specificity stated. For example, consider the following diagnosis:

Physician documents "Viral Rickettsiosis Fever"

Diagnosis given by the physician is more specific than the diagnoses listed in ICD-9-CM. Rickettsiosis is coded as 083 with the additional fourth digit of "8" for other specified, or NEC. Therefore the correct ICD-9-CM code is 083.8 Other Specified Rickettsiosis.

PUNCTUATION

( )   Parentheses

Parentheses enclose supplementary words that may be present or absent in a statement of diagnosis. PARENTHESES DO NOT AFFECT THE CODE NUMBER ASSIGNED. Information in parentheses is provided to aid in selection of an ICD-9-CM code that is as close to the information provided by the physician as possible.

Physician documents "Subacute bacterial endocarditis"

Code 421.0 Acute and Subacute Bacterial Endocarditis

Endocarditis (Acute) (Chronic) (Subacute)

Note: The information contained in ICD-9-CM in this example indicates that the words in parentheses may or may not be part of the physician's diagnostic statement.

[ ] Brackets

Brackets are used to enclose synonyms, alternate words, or explanatory phrases. Many physicians use a variety of phrases or abbreviations to describe one diagnosis or condition.

> Physician documents "SBE"
>
> Code 421.0 Acute and Subacute Bacterial Endocarditis [SBE]

: Colon

A colon is used after an incomplete term that requires one or more modifiers.

> Bronchitis: (need additional modifiers)
>   Asthmatic
>   Chronic

{ } Braces

Braces are used to connect a series of terms to a common stem.

> Endocarditis
>
> Myoendocarditis} Acute/Subacute
>   Periendocarditis

TYPEFACES

Bold   All codes and titles in a Tabular List are in bold.
Italic   All exclusion notes are in italics.

RELATED TERMS

AND   Interpreted for ICD-9-CM as "and/or."
WITH   Both parts of the title must be present in the diagnostic statement.

SYMBOLS

Several symbols are used in ICD-9-CM to provide instructional notes regarding the proper use of specific codes. Although the symbols vary from one code book to another, the concepts they represent remain the same. Reviewing the specific color and shape representation for each of these concepts in its respective ICD-9-CM code book may be helpful.

Differing Code Symbol	Indicates that a code and its description are not the same in ICD-9-CM and ICD-9.
New Code Symbol	Indicates that a code is new to this revision.
Text Revision Symbol	Denotes a revision of an existing code in text or notes.
Additional Digit Symbol	Indicates that additional digits are required.
Symbol	Indicates that additional digits are required.

Nonspecific Code Symbol	Denotes a nonspecific code; a more specific code should be used if possible. These codes may not be reimbursed by some carriers.
Unspecified Code Symbol	Denotes an unspecified code; a more specific code should be used if possible. These codes may not be reimbursed by some carriers.
Manifestation Code Symbol	Indicates an unacceptable principal diagnosis, meaning that a given diagnosis is a manifestation of another disease process. The other primary diagnosis should be coded first (the code typically references the primary diagnosis needed).

INSTRUCTIONAL NOTATIONS

Includes	Indicates separate terms, modifying adjectives, sites, or conditions entered under a subdivision, such as category. Used to further define or give examples of content of category.
Excludes	Enclosed in a box and printed in italics to draw attention to presence. In other words, all terms following the word *Excludes* are coded elsewhere. ICD-9-CM usually refers the coder to the correct codes.
Notes	Used to define terms and to give coding instructions.
See	Acts as a cross-reference and directs the coder elsewhere. Often found when the referenced term is not the appropriate medical term for the condition (e.g., Headache, See Cephalgia).
See Category	Refers the coder to a specific category for assigning a correct code.
See Also	Refers the coder to a reference elsewhere if the main term or subterms alone are not sufficient for coding.
Code Also	Used when more than one code is required to fully describe a stated condition or diagnosis. Notation requires that the underlying disease be coded first, and the particular manifestation coded second.
Use Additional Code	The coder may wish to add further information by using an additional code to give a more complete description of the diagnosis or the medical necessity.

NUMERICAL AND ALPHABETICAL INDEX (VOLUMES 1 AND 2)

The ICD-9-CM book is NOT intended to be used with the numerical or the alphabetical section alone. These two indices are intended to complement each other.

Codes should be located in the alphabetical volume, identified to the highest level of specificity, and cross-referenced in the numerical volume. Additional notes, such as fifth-digit classification information, "includes," "excludes," and other instructional notes, are included ONLY in the numerical volume when cross-referencing occurs. Take extreme caution to ALWAYS cross-reference these codes. Most coding errors can be avoided if coders make certain to perform this "cross-check" every time they select a code.

Take time to look at some entries in the ICD-9-CM code book and to become familiar with the format, lookup, and abbreviations so that key elements, signs and symptoms, and diagnoses identified for coding purposes will be correctly coded. Complete the following exercises to develop those skills.

STOP AND PRACTICE

Take each diagnostic statement and indicate where the diagnosis will be located in the ICD-9-CM code book.

Diagnosis	Location (Where to Look Up)
Ex: Upper respiratory infection	INFECTION, Respiratory, Upper
Ex: Headache	CEPHALGIA
1. Acute myocardial infarction	_____
2. Finger laceration	_____
3. Otitis media	_____
4. Gastrointestinal hemorrhage	_____
5. Abdominal pain	_____
6. Fractured femur	_____
7. Bacterial pneumonia	_____
8. Senile cataract	_____
9. Incarcerated inguinal hernia	_____
10. Sepsis	_____
11. Renal insufficiency	_____
12. Congestive heart failure (CHF)	_____
13. Upper respiratory infection (URI), possible pneumonia	_____
14. Chronic obstructive pulmonary disease (COPD), with acute bronchitis	_____
15. Ingrown toenail	_____
16. Acute bronchitis with URI	_____
17. Femur fracture, closed	_____
18. Cough, normal chest	_____
19. Chronic pulmonary edema	_____
20. Acute URI due to pneumococcus	_____

ADDITIONAL GUIDELINES

With now being more familiar with the specific format, standardized abbreviations, and symbols of the ICD-9-CM code book, use Tool 12 to gather additional hints for locating codes. These helpful hints will assist in locating the correct term or word for proper coding of diagnoses the **first** time. Correct coding is important; however, time is also valuable. Many facilities require a specified correct coding rate and a minimum chart load per day, per coder. Because time is an important element in successful coding, coders must make certain that they quickly identify the key elements and locate the correct codes in ICD-9-CM. In the following exercises, practice a few more diagnostic terms and determine how they will be identified for lookup in the ICD-9-CM book.

STOP AND PRACTICE

Take each diagnostic statement and indicate where the diagnosis will be located in the ICD-9-CM code book.

Diagnosis	Location (Where to Look Up)
Ex: Abdominal pain	PAIN, Abdominal
1. Chronic obstructive pulmonary disease	_____
2. Closed wrist fracture	_____
3. Laceration repair, thumb (This is **what** service was provided; think about **why** laceration repair was necessary for the correct selection of diagnosis)	_____
4. Abscess of right great toe	_____
5. Infectious gastroenteritis	_____
6. Streptococcal infection	_____
7. Fibrocystic breast disease	_____
8. Fracture of tibia/fibula	_____
9. Coronary artery disease	_____
10. Bilateral pedal edema	_____
11. Postoperative wound infection	_____
12. Right upper quadrant (RUQ), left lower quadrant (LLQ) abdominal pain	_____
13. Dupuytren's contracture	_____
14. Rupture, head of biceps Chronic shoulder pain	_____
15. Acute respiratory distress syndrome (ARDS) with shortness of breath (SOB)	_____
16. Abdominal pain Abdominal mass Rule out (R/O) liver metastases (mets)	_____
17. Obstructive sleep apnea with adenotonsillar hyperplasia	_____
18. Acute appendicitis Appendicitis with peritonitis	_____
19. Cholelithiasis with acute cholecystitis	_____
20. R/O endometriosis and uterine anomaly lesions, right utero ligament	_____

T O O L   12

HELPFUL HINTS IN LOCATING DIAGNOSES IN ICD-9-CM

1. **Cross-reference codes in alphabetic/numeric indices**
   Always look up the code in the alphabetical section and cross-verify with the tabular section for correct code selection as well as highest level of specificity.

2. **Code to highest level of specificity**
   Make certain you have gathered all modifying words to the selected key elements, such as acute, chronic, open, closed.

3. **Do not assume chronic or acute unless specified by physician**
   If diagnosis requires presence of chronic or acute in order to utilize code selected, make certain the physician has indicated such. Remember that most acute conditions are identified as the chief reason for the encounter.

4. **Determine the "root word" that all other words modify to look up code correctly the first time**
   EXAMPLE: Diagnosis As Stated:
           Stress Fracture, Tibia
   ICD-9-CM: **Fracture, pathologic, tibia – 733.16**
   TIP: Think of identifying the proper "term" much like diagramming sentences in junior high school. Identify the subject, the noun, and all other words and descriptive modifiers. In this way, those diagnoses that appear to be complex are, in fact, just as simple as the one- or two-word diagnostic statements.
   EXAMPLE: Cystic Breast Disease
           Main Subject – Disease
           Modifying Factor – Breast = Disease, Breast
           Additional Modifying Factor – Cystic
           Look - up will be as follows:
           Disease, breast, cystic — ICD-9-CM: 610.1

5. **Make sure to convert nonmedical terminology to medical terms**
   If the documentation does not utilize a medical term, the coder may need to convert these nonmedical terms for coding purposes:
   EXAMPLES: Headache   = Cephalgia
             Heart Attack = Infarction, Myocardial

Take the time to identify key elements and choose the correct lookup **before** locating the diagnosis in the ICD-9-CM; both are essential time-saving steps. A summary of the steps for accurate coding from ICD-9-CM is found in Tool 13.

The CMS, formerly known as the Health Care Finance Administration (HCFA), has also provided additional guidelines for coding standardization. These are shown in Tool 14.

The first exercise is to identify the diagnosis needed to code and to select the correct code from the ICD-9-CM book. Give the following examples a try and remember to locate the MAIN term first before attempting to locate the correct codes.

	Diagnostic Term to Reference	ICD-9-CM Code
1. Acute bronchitis	Bronchitis, Acute	_____
2. Cough	_____	_____
Fever	_____	_____
Upper respiratory infection	_____	_____

Hints:

1. Acute bronchitis
   "Bronchitis" is the key term, with "Acute" as a modifier (adjective) to the description. Therefore BRONCHITIS, Acute, would be looked up.

2. Cough
   Fever
   Upper respiratory infection

T O O L   13

10 STEPS TO ACCURATE CODING FROM THE ICD-9-CM BOOK

1. Locate the main term within the diagnostic statement.

2. Locate the main term in the Alphabetic Index (Volume 2).
   Keep in mind that:
   —Primary arrangement for main terms is by condition
   —Main terms can be referred to in ill-defined lay terms

3. Refer to all notes under the main term. Check instructions in any notes appearing in a box immediately after the main term.

4. Examine any modifications appearing in parentheses next to the main term.
   Check if any of these apply to the qualifying terms used in the diagnostic statement.

5. Note the subterms indented beneath the main term.

6. Follow any cross-reference instructions (terms such as "see" or "see also" must be followed to ensure correct codes).

7. Confirm your code selection in the Tabular List (Volume 1).

8. Follow instructional terms in the Tabular List (Volume 1). Watch for exclusion notes as well as fourth/fifth-digit requirements. Be sure to check all the way back to the original heading for that section as the instructional information may be located on one or more pages preceding the actual page where the code is located.

9. Assign the code number you have determined correct. Repeat these steps for each diagnostic code selected, making certain those integral to another diagnosis are not coded.

10. Place the diagnostic code(s) for each service in the appropriate order.

Fever and cough are both signs and symptoms of a URI. Therefore neither of these must be coded. The only diagnosis for this chart is Upper Respiratory Infection. The main term here is "Infection," modified by "respiratory," which is further modified by "upper." This diagnosis can be located under INFECTION, Respiratory, Upper.

STOP AND PRACTICE

Select the diagnoses that should be coded and locate the correct diagnosis codes. See Figure 3-1 to review the coding selection process.

	Diagnostic Term to Reference	ICD-9-CM Code
1. Incomplete miscarriage		
2. URI		
3. Acute bronchitis with cough		
4. Virus, varicella		
5. Viral syndrome		
6. Psychogenic ulcerative colitis		
7. Diabetes mellitus		
8. Benign hypertension		
9. Acute lymphocytic leukemia		
10. Blood loss anemia		
11. Acute serous otitis media		
12. Streptococcal pneumonia		
13. Irritable bowel syndrome		
14. Gastrointestinal bleed		
15. COPD with bronchitis		
16. Hepatitis C		
17. Cholelithiasis with cholecystitis		
18. Asthmatic dyspnea		
19. URI with cough		
20. Fever, cough, pneumonia		

T O O L   14

CMS GUIDELINES FOR ICD-9-CM CODING

1. Identify each service, procedure, or supply with an ICD-9-CM code from 002.0 through V82.9 to describe the **diagnosis, symptom, complaint, condition, or problem.**

2. Identify services or visits for circumstances other than disease or injury, such as follow-up care for chemotherapy, with **V codes.**

3. **Code the principal diagnosis first,** followed by the secondary code, and so on. Code any coexisting conditions that may affect the treatment or outcome of treatment of the patient for that service as supplementary information.

4. **Do not code a diagnosis that is no longer applicable.**

5. **Code to the highest level of specificity.** Carry the numerical code to the appropriate 4th/5th digit. There are only approximately 100 codes with three digits; therefore, most of the codes should be 4th/5th digits in length.

6. **Code chronic diseases when applicable** to the patient's treatment or service for that encounter.

7. When **ancillary services** are provided, **list the appropriate V code first** and the problem second. This follows the rule that the primary diagnosis should be the chief reason for the encounter or service being billed.

8. **For surgical procedures, code the procedure that is most applicable to the principal diagnosis.**

HELPFUL CODING HINTS

To prevent selection of an incorrect code, consider the following in your selection of correct ICD-9-CM codes.

1. Always check the anatomical or system area selected. All the codes can never be memorized; however, if the breakdowns within ICD-9-CM become familiar enough, confirmation that a selection is at least in the correct category is possible.
Diabetes mellitus
Code erroneously selected was 350.00. Because the 300 series of ICD-9-CM codes are psychiatric in nature, the code selected cannot be correct. The correct code series for diabetes is 250.XX.
CODING TIP: Develop an INDEX for the Tabular Section of ICD-9-CM to crosscheck selections easily. An example is shown in Tool 15. This may be incorporated directly into the ICD-9-CM book as a reference.

2. Always check fourth and fifth digits carefully. Only the third or fourth digit may have been selected correctly. Necessary additional digits may not have been selected, or incorrect additional digits may have been selected.
Diabetes mellitus
Code selected was 250.0.
The coder selected the correct first four digits; however, a fifth digit is necessary. Omitted additional digits result in denial from insurance carriers.

3. Make certain to read all notes regarding "excludes," "includes," and so forth. The correct code may seem to have been selected; however, there may be an exclusion listed for the specific condition or diagnosis coded. The ICD-9-CM book will direct the coder to the appropriate code.
Congenital dentofacial deformities
Code selected was 754.0 Congenital Skull, Face, Jaw Deformities
This code **excludes** dentofacial anomalies. ICD-9-CM directs the coder to codes 524.0-524.9.

4. Remember to cross-reference all codes from the alphabetical to the numerical sections, reading all information from one indentation to the next, to ensure correct coding.

DIAGNOSTIC DOCUMENTATION WORKSHEET

Chart#/Patient Name:

	WHAT (Service/Procedure)	WHY (MEDICAL NECESSITY) (Diagnostic Information)
Step 1 Select all words for possible use as diagnosis/diagnostic statement from the document	Office Visit	Cough, Fever, Cold Symptoms, Upper Respiratory Infection
		Urinary Frequency, Urinary Tract Infection
	Chest X-Ray	Cough, Fever, Cold Symptoms, Upper Respiratory Infection
	CBC	Cough, Fever, Cold Symptoms, Upper Respiratory Infection
	Urinalysis	Urinary Frequency, Urinary Tract Infection
Step 2 Determine which words are appropriate for inclusion: (Carry these forward) Diagnosis vs. signs/symptoms	Office Visit	Upper Respiratory Infection
		Urinary Tract Infection
	Chest X-Ray	Upper Respiratory Infection
	CBC	Upper Respiratory Infection
	Urinalysis	Urinary Tract Infection
Step 3 Based on each service performed, determine the appropriate order of diagnosis for each service performed	Office Visit	1) Upper Respiratory Infection (addtl services performed)
		2) Urinary Tract Infection (1 addtl service performed)
	Chest X-Ray	1) Upper Respiratory Infection
	CBC	1) Upper Respiratory Infection
	Urinalysis	1) Urinary Tract Infection
Step 4 Look up/assign the proper dx codes	Office Visit	Upper Respiratory Infection = Infection, Respiratory, Upper 465.9
		Urinary Tract Infection = Infection, Urinary Tract 599.0
	Chest X-Ray	Upper Respiratory Infection = Infection, Respiratory, Upper 465.9
	CBC	Upper Respiratory Infection = Infection, Respiratory, Upper 465.9
	Urinalysis	Urinary Tract Infection = Infection, Urinary Tract 599.0

FIGURE 3-1 Step 4 of the diagnostic coding process. (Courtesy of MD Consultative Services, Orlando, Florida. All rights reserved.)

TOOL   15

INDEX TO ICD-9-CM TABULAR LIST
By Disease Process

Infectious and Parasitic Diseases	001-139
Neoplasms	140-239
Endocrine, Nutritional and Metabolic Diseases, Immunity Disorders	240-279
Diseases of Blood/Blood-Forming Organs	280-289
Mental Disorders	290-319
Inflammatory Diseases of Central Nervous System	320-326
Hereditary/Degenerative Diseases of Central Nervous System	330-337
Other Diseases Central Nervous System	340-349
Disorders of Peripheral Nervous System	350-359
Disorders of Eye and Adnexa	360-379
Diseases of Ear and Mastoid Process	380-389
Diseases of Circulatory System	390-459
Diseases of Respiratory System	460-519
Diseases of Digestive System	520-579
Diseases of Genitourinary System	580-629
Complications of Pregnancy, Childbirth, and Puerperium	630-677
Diseases of Skin and Subcutaneous Tissue	680-709
Diseases of Musculoskeletal System and Connective Tissue	710-739
Congenital Anomalies	740-759
Certain Conditions Originating in the Perinatal Period	760-779
Symptoms, Signs, and Ill-Defined Conditions	780-799
Injury and Poisoning	800-999

CHAPTER IN REVIEW

CERTIFICATION REVIEW

- The ICD-9-CM code book is an offshoot of the "ICD" book published by the World Health Organization (WHO).
- The ICD-9-CM codebook comprises three sections:
  1. Numerical (Tabular—Volume 1)
  2. Alphabetical (Volume 2)
  3. Procedural (Volume 3)
- Volume 3 (Procedures) is used primarily for coding hospital services.
- When using the ICD-9-CM code book, the coder should always cross-reference the selection in the numerical section of the code book.
- ICD-9-CM signifies the use of an incomplete code number with the use of a specific symbol.

- NEC (not elsewhere classified) defines diagnostic statements in which the physician has classified the diagnosis to a higher level than what is available in the ICD-9-CM code book.
- NOS (not otherwise specified) pertains to diagnostic statements in which the physician has not classified the diagnosis to the highest level available in ICD-9-CM.
- The term AND is interpreted as "and/or" for the purpose of the ICD-9-CM code book.

STUDENT STUDY GUIDE

- Study Chapter 3.
- Review the Learning Objectives for Chapter 3.
- Review the Certification Review for Chapter 3.

- Complete the Stop and Practice exercises contained in Chapter 3
- Complete the Chapter Review exercise to reinforce concepts learned in this chapter.

CHAPTER REVIEW EXERCISE

Assign diagnostic codes as appropriate for the following:

Diagnosis Code(s)

1. Osteomyelitis _____
2. Rheumatoid arthritis, hand _____
3. Infectious otitis media _____
4. Pelvic mass, R/O cervical neoplasm _____
5. Nonunion of fracture, tibia _____
6. Laceration of hand _____
7. Angina _____
8. Pendred's syndrome _____
9. Nontraumatic perforation of bowel _____
10. *Klebsiella* pneumonia _____
11. Abdominal distress _____
12. Athlete's foot _____
13. Epileptic attack _____
14. Low back pain _____
15. Barrett's syndrome _____
16. Bell's disease _____
17. Bell's palsy _____
18. Bennett's fracture _____
19. Premature infant birth _____
20. Birthmark _____
21. Centipede bite _____
22. Fever blister _____
23. Bright's disease _____
24. Bradycardia _____
25. Bronchospasm with acute bronchiolitis _____
26. Burkitt's tumor _____
27. Acquired limb deformity _____
28. Degenerative spinal cord _____
29. Single episodic depression _____
30. Allergic eyelid dermatitis _____
31. Bacterial diarrhea _____
32. Capsulitis, hip _____
33. Cervicalgia _____
34. Cervicitis during pregnancy _____
35. Acute cholecystitis _____
36. Ear canal cholesteatoma _____
37. Alcoholic cirrhosis _____
38. Charcot's cirrhosis _____
39. Eating compulsion _____
40. Abdominal cramps _____
41. Fatty cirrhosis _____
42. Forearm contusion _____
43. Epigastric pain _____
44. Liver contusion _____
45. Smoker's cough _____
46. Muscle cramps _____
47. Congenital spine curvature _____
48. Baker's cyst _____
49. Ovarian cyst _____
50. High-frequency hearing loss _____
51. Amino acid deficiency _____
52. Clotting deficiency _____
53. Elbow dislocation _____
54. Difficulty breast-feeding _____
55. Rubber dermatitis _____
56. Mitral valve deficiency _____
57. Arterial dilatation _____
58. Bouillaud's disease _____
59. Heart disease with acute pulmonary edema _____
60. Acute gastric dilatation _____
61. Congenital heart disease _____
62. Osteofibrocystic disease _____
63. Paget's disease _____
64. Adult polycystic kidney disease _____
65. Dislocation anterior hip _____
66. Stress disorder _____
67. Dislocation, humerus, proximal end _____
68. Sympathetic reflux dystrophy _____
69. Elevated SGOT (serum glutamate oxaloacetate transaminase) _____
70. Distal end ulnar dislocation _____
71. Petit mal epilepsy _____
72. Exposure to cold _____
73. Parrot fever _____
74. Abnormal heart sounds _____
75. Rocky Mountain spotted fever _____
76. Anal fissure _____
77. Abnormal thyroid function _____
78. Ureterosigmoidoabdominal fistula _____
79. Foreign body, anus _____
80. Toxic goiter _____
81. Liver hematoma _____
82. Traumatic liver hematoma _____
83. Hemophilia A _____
84. Obstructed Richter's hernia _____
85. Postoperative hematoma _____
86. Adrenal hypoplasia _____
87. Idiopathic hypotension _____
88. Hormonal imbalance _____
89. Eye infection _____
90. Bartholin's gland inflammation _____
91. Breast inflammation _____
92. Irritable bowel _____

93. Cold intolerance _____
94. Postpartum breast inflammation _____
95. Inflammation, lumbar disc _____
96. Intelligence quotient (IQ) under 20 _____
97. Krukenberg's tumor _____
98. Spinal cord lesion _____
99. Infective mastitis _____
100. Myocarditis with rheumatic fever _____
101. Breast mass _____
102. Nursemaid's elbow _____
103. Nystagmus _____
104. Phase of life problem _____
105. Vasomotor phenomenon _____
106. Food aspiration pneumonia _____
107. Positive stool culture _____
108. Premature ventricular contractions _____
109. Premature labor _____
110. Rales _____
111. Diaper rash _____
112. Rasmussen's aneurysm _____
113. Radiculitis, arm _____
114. Rapid respirations _____
115. Fluid retention _____
116. Granulomatous rhinitis _____
117. Leg scar _____
118. Allergic reaction _____
119. Burning sensation _____
120. Seborrheic wart _____
121. Abnormal heart rhythm _____
122. Sleeping sickness _____
123. Sleep disorder _____
124. Convulsions _____
125. Splenic flexure syndrome _____
126. Spina bifida with hydrocephalus _____

127. Fertility testing _____
128. Hemoptysis _____
129. Sternoclavicular sprain _____
130. Cardiac bypass graft status _____
131. Suture abscess _____
132. Thyroid storm _____
133. Rectal stricture due to chemical burn _____
134. Drug-induced delusional syndrome _____
135. Shaken infant syndrome _____
136. Jet lag syndrome _____
137. Parkinsonism _____
138. Central nervous system syphilis _____
139. Congenital syphilis _____
140. Tay-Sachs disease _____
141. Articular cartilage tear _____
142. Grinding teeth _____
143. Child temper tantrum _____
144. Saphenous vein thrombosis _____
145. Thrombocytopenia _____
146. Omental torsion _____
147. SOB _____
148. CHF with mild pedal edema _____
149. Abnormal ECG _____
150. Cough, normal chest _____

PRACTICAL APPLICATION

Now that all four steps of the ICD-9-CM diagnostic coding guidelines have been completed, take the following charts and use these steps for assigning diagnostic codes, placing them in the correct order, and assigning the appropriate ICD-9-CM diagnostic code(s). Also, assign diagnostic codes and place in the appropriate order for the following charts.

1. Acute Onset of Left-Side Chest Pain

PROGRESS NOTE

Date:	Vital signs:	T	R
Chief complaint:		P	BP

This 21-year-old presents with acute onset of left-sided-only chest pain. His EKG performed in the office today is entirely within normal limits, and is not suggestive of pericarditis.

Examination:

Examination shows no rub, gallop, or pathological heart sounds. I suspect he has no organic heart disease.

Impression:

Chest pain, musculoskeletal in nature.

Plan:

I recommended he take the rest of the week off work, rest, take analgesics for pain, and return to work after that time, if he is pain free.

Willen Obrt MD

Patient name:
DOB:
MR/Chart #:

GODFREY REGIONAL OUTPATIENT CLINIC
3122 Shannon Avenue • Aldon, FL 77712 • (407) 555-7654

Diagnostic Statement #1: _____
ICD-9-CM Code: _____

Diagnostic Statement #2: _____
ICD-9-CM Code: _____

2. Postpartum with Multiple Complaints

PROGRESS NOTE

Date:	Vital signs:	T	R
Chief complaint:		P	BP

This is a 32-year-old female who presents today with a cough of 2 weeks' duration, now producing yellow-colored mucus. She presents today because of these symptoms, as well as hemorrhoidal bleeding, which has increased over the past 2 to 3 days, and diarrhea, which began yesterday. Of note, the patient is 6 weeks postpartum vaginal delivery.

Examination:

Circumferential external hemorrhoids noted, nonthrombosed, very indurated, and tender. HEENT unremarkable except for slight nasal drainage. Chest—perhaps some faint wheezing present, consistent with bronchial involvement process.

Impression:

Diarrhea, acute bronchitis, external hemorrhoids

Plan:

Will treat with amoxicillin 500 mg bid x 10 days for acute bronchitis. Patient instructed on care of external hemorrhoids and given diet instructions for complaints of diarrhea, which is not considered to be severe at this time.

Jay Corم MD

	Patient name:
	DOB:
	MR/Chart #:

GODFREY REGIONAL OUTPATIENT CLINIC
3122 Shannon Avenue • Aldon, FL 77712 • (407) 555-7654

Diagnostic Statement #1: _____
ICD-9-CM Code: _____
Diagnostic Statement #2: _____
ICD-9-CM Code: _____

Diagnostic Statement #3: _____
ICD-9-CM Code: _____

3. Leg Pain/Bacterial Infection

PROGRESS NOTE

Date:	Vital signs:	T	R
Chief complaint:		P	BP

This is a 66-year-old female who comes to the physician's office complaining that she has a bacterial infection in her legs. She has already been treated for this infection but states she is having severe pain and is unable to buy the bandages for dressing changes. Patient denies diabetes. Has had history of hypertension and myocardial infarction in 1993. Medications are Monoket, Cotrim, Lasix, and Altace. Family and social history are noncontributory. Patient is having no chest pain, no shortness of breath, and no abdominal pain, but feels nauseated.

Physical examination:

Vital signs are normal; patient is alert. HEENT is unremarkable. Abdomen–obese, soft, and nontender. She has marked edema of the lower extremities. She has erythema from the knees to the feet. Has a necrotic ulceration on the left tibial aspect of her left lower leg. She has marked oozing, crusting, and drainage from both legs consistent with venous stasis and cellulitis. Peripheral pulses are intact, and she has good capillary refill.

Assessment:

DIAGNOSIS: Venous stasis with cellulitis of lower extremities

Plan:

There is no way she can care for herself at home; therefore, we will admit her for care to include whirlpool treatments, dressing changes, and antibiotic therapy.

Maurice Doater, MD

| Patient name: |
| DOB: |
| MR/Chart #: |

GODFREY REGIONAL OUTPATIENT CLINIC
3122 Shannon Avenue • Aldon, FL 77712 • (407) 555-7654

Diagnostic Statement #1: _____
ICD-9-CM Code: _____
Diagnostic Statement #2: _____
ICD-9-CM Code: _____

Diagnostic Statement #3: _____
ICD-9-CM Code: _____

4. Abdominal Pain

PROGRESS NOTE
Date/time

S:

Patient is feeling better and not having the same level of abdominal pain. She is still experiencing dysuria and incontinence. Otherwise she indicates she feels somewhat better. Denies chest pain, SOB, reports she still feels a little weak.

O:

Afebrile, vital signs normal. Chest clear. Extremities normal, Abdomen normal

A:

Abdominal pain, possible UTI

P:

Treat with IV medications

[signature] MD

PROGRESS NOTES

GODFREY REGIONAL HOSPITAL
123 Main Street • Aldon, FL 77714 • (407) 555-1234

Diagnostic Statement #1: _____
ICD-9-CM Code: _____
Diagnostic Statement #2: _____
ICD-9-CM Code: _____

Diagnostic Statement #3: _____
ICD-9-CM Code: _____

5. Possible Hypertension

PROGRESS NOTE

Date:	Vital signs:	T	R
Chief complaint:		P	BP

This is a 56-year-old male who presents with headaches and possible high blood pressure.

Examination:

Chest clear, Vital signs normal, Abdomen, soft, nontender. Repeated BP were all within normal range.

Impression:

Headaches with possible HTN

Plan:

Follow with BP History for next 30 days.

Willen Obrt MD

Patient name:
DOB:
MR/Chart #:

GODFREY REGIONAL OUTPATIENT CLINIC
3122 Shannon Avenue • Aldon, FL 77712 • (407) 555-7654

Diagnostic Statement #1: _____   Diagnostic Statement #3: _____
ICD-9-CM Code: _____   ICD-9-CM Code: _____
Diagnostic Statement #2: _____
ICD-9-CM Code: _____

6. Severe Epigastric Cramping

EMERGENCY ROOM RECORD

Name:	Age:	ER physician:
	DOB:	

Allergies/type of reaction:	Usual medications/dosages:

Triage/presenting complaint: 60-year-old male presents with severe epigastric cramping. He states that the pain started after eating dinner tonight. He has had continual cramping and severe abdominal discomfort. The patient has taken some Lorazepam and had 2 episodes of emesis but no fever and does not feel nauseated at the present time.

Initial assessment: Severe epigastric cramping

| Time | T 98 | P 70 | R 16 | BP 182/98 | Other: | | | | | |

Medication orders:

Lab work:

X-Ray: Labs show WBC 4.5, Hgb 12, platelets 86, sodium 41, potassium 3.9, BUN 21. Reglan 10 mg IV given.

Physician's report:

Patient unable to lie on bed, walking back and forth with distress. Lungs clear, heart regular, abdomen minimally distended but soft. He has hyperactive but non-tympanitic bowel symptoms.

Diagnosis: Abdominal pain unclear etiology / Anxiety

Physician sign/date Nancy Cauly MD

Discharge   Transfer   Admit   Good   Satisfactory   Other:

GODFREY REGIONAL HOSPITAL
123 Main Street • Aldon, FL 77714 • (407) 555-1234

Diagnostic Statement #1: _____
ICD-9-CM Code: _____
Diagnostic Statement #2: _____
ICD-9-CM Code: _____

Diagnostic Statement #3: _____
ICD-9-CM Code: _____

7. Radiology Report, Abdominal Pain

RADIOLOGY REPORT

MR#:
DOB:
Ordered by: Maurice Doates, MD

Clinical summary:

Abdominal pain since 11 AM

Abdomen:

ABDOMEN, 1 VIEW:
One view of the abdomen was obtained. Non-obstructive bowel gas pattern. No calcification overlying kidneys or ureters.

Conclusion:

IMPRESSION:
No abnormality on one view of abdomen

Ddt/mm

D:
T:

_____
                        , M.D.   Date

GODFREY REGIONAL HOSPITAL
123 Main Street • Aldon, FL 77714 • (407) 555-1234

Diagnostic Statement #1: _____
ICD-9-CM Code: _____
Diagnostic Statement #2: _____
ICD-9-CM Code: _____

Diagnostic Statement #3: _____
ICD-9-CM Code: _____

8. Garbled Speech, Gait Instability

HISTORY AND PHYSICAL EXAMINATION

William Obert, MD

82-year-old with episode of shortness of breath, some vague chest pain. Said he got confused, had some slurred speech and could not walk. His wife indicates they were coming home and she noticed he was more mixed up and confused and having some garbled speech. She says that he has had two previous episodes of this in the past. Denies any cough, fever, chills, nausea or vomiting. Evidence of some COPD, is an ex-smoker. No history of CAD.

Past medical history:

Systolic hypertension, DJD, hyperlipidemia, COPD, has had left cataract extraction.

Family and social history

Review of systems:

Denies any weight changes, appetite changes, fever or chills. Denies any problems with tinnitus, hearing loss. Denies sore throat, dysphagia. No history of CAD, Denies cough or hemoptysis. Lot of arthritis, denies dysuria, urgency, frequency. Denies any anemia.

Physical exam

General:	Alert, oriented male resting comfortably. No acute distress.
VITAL SIGNS:	BP 132/78, Pulse 97, Respirations 20
HEENT:	Normocephalic and atraumatic
NECK:	Supple without adenopathy
CARDIAC:	Regular rate and rhythm
LUNGS:	Decreased lung exchange throughout with some fine crackles
NEUROLOGICAL:	Alert, oriented to person, place and time. Somewhat vague in his history. Finger-to-toe able to complete.

Laboratory/radiology:

CBC shows WBC 14,000, Hgb 12.4, 84 neutrophils, 4 bands. BMP sodium 137, potassium 3.8, chloride 106. Troponin 0.1. EKG shows normal sinus rhythm. Chest x-ray is normal.

X-ray:

Assessment:

Plan:

Episode of garbled speech with gait instability, possible cerebrovascular accident versus transient ischemic attached. We will check neuros and vital signs every two hours. Repeat his EKG and enzymes in four hours. Needs a CT scan of his head.

William Obert MD

GODFREY REGIONAL HOSPITAL
123 Main Street • Aldon, FL 77714 • (407) 555-1234

Diagnostic Statement #1: _____
ICD-9-CM Code: _____
Diagnostic Statement #2: _____
ICD-9-CM Code: _____

Diagnostic Statement #3: _____
ICD-9-CM Code: _____

9. Consultation

CONSULTATIONS

Indication for consultation:

Ventricular tachycardia

History:

54-year-old with known history of cardiac disease who was undergoing outpatient arthroscopy of the knee. Patient's cardiac rhythm was noted to have multiple runs of non-sustained ventricular tachycardia. Patient remained asymptomatic stable.
Status post MI 15 years ago.

FAMILY/SOCIAL HISTORY:
Non-contributory

Exam:

PHYSICAL EXAM:
Head: Normocephalic, atraumatic
Neck: Supple, w/o evidence of JVP, mass or bruit
Chest: Clear to auscultation
Cardiac: Normal carotid upstroke with normal contour
Abdomen: Soft, nontender, no evidence of mass
Extremities: Showed no evidence of clubbing, cyanosis, or edema
Neurologic: Grossly intact, nonfocal
EKG: Ectopic atrial rhythm with delayed precordial transmission

Diagnosis/assessment:

IMPRESSION:
Known history of coronary atherosclerotic heart disease and atrial fibrillation, now presents with run of nonsustained V tach per report. It would be prudent to continue patient on his current medications and allow him to follow-up with his primary cardiologist.

We appreciate the opportunity to participate in the overall evaluation and management of this patient.

Ruth Brady M

Patient name: _____

Date of service: _____

GODFREY MEDICAL ASSOCIATES
1532 Third Avenue, Suite 120 • Aldon, FL 77713 • (407) 555-4000

Diagnostic Statement #1: _____
ICD-9-CM Code: _____
Diagnostic Statement #2: _____
ICD-9-CM Code: _____

Diagnostic Statement #3: _____
ICD-9-CM Code: _____

10. Knee Arthroscopy

OPERATIVE REPORT

Patient information:

Patient name:
DOB:
MR#:

Preoperative diagnosis:

Torn medial meniscus, left knee

Postoperative diagnosis:

Torn medial meniscus, left knee

Procedure(s) performed:

Arthroscopy of left knee with partial medial Meniscectomy, medial femoral condyle chondroplasty

Anesthesia:

General

Assistant surgeon:

Description of procedure:

Patient placed supine on table and satisfactory general anesthetic was given. Left leg was prepped and draped in the usual sterile fashion. Arthroscope cannula was introduced via anterolateral port at the joint line. Knee was distended with normal saline, there was no pathology or loose body in the suprapatellar area. The medial plica showed no evidence of pathology or damage. The cartilaginous surface of the medial femoral condyle showed extensive changes of chondromalacia. The posterior horn of the medial meniscus was torn of its free edge. A combination of hand-held cutters and rotary shavers were used to trim back to the tear of the posterior horn of the medial meniscus.

The knee was irrigated throughout the procedure via normal saline delivered by the arthroscopy pump. All instruments were removed.

Patrick Chung, MD

GODFREY REGIONAL HOSPITAL
123 Main Street • Aldon, FL 77714 • (407) 555-1234

Diagnostic Statement #1: _____
ICD-9-CM Code: _____
Diagnostic Statement #2: _____
ICD-9-CM Code: _____

Diagnostic Statement #3: _____
ICD-9-CM Code: _____

4

V CODES AND E CODES

LEARNING OBJECTIVES

Following the completion of this chapter, the student will be able to:

- Understand the proper use of V codes.
- Understand the proper use of E codes.
- Understand that primary guidelines for assigning the chief reason for encounter apply, even with the assignment of V codes as primary when appropriate.
- Use an index for E code and V code sections of the ICD-9-CM code book for inclusion as tools with the coding book.

CODING REFERENCE TOOLS

Tool 16
V Code Index
Tool 17
E Code Index

KEY TERMS

Clean Claims, 117
E Codes, 116
External Causes, 116
V Codes, 113

In addition to the numerical codes used for diagnostic coding, ICD-9-CM has a series of special codes that are applied in specific circumstances. For the most part, these codes are NOT used as primary diagnostic codes; however, there are always exceptions to the rules.

V CODES

APPROPRIATE USAGE

This section of the ICD-9-CM book deals with those instances when events other than disease or injury classifiable to the numerical section are recorded as the diagnosis, problem, condition, or chief reason for encounter. A section on V codes ("Supplementary Classification of Factors Influencing Health Status and Contact with Health Services") covers codes V01 through V82. V codes are typically used for the following reasons:

- Patient does not present with a problem or condition, yet a physician encounter takes place for a specific purpose, such as organ donor or vaccination. In most instances, these events probably would not occur in the hospital setting, but in the outpatient or physician office setting.
- Patient with a specific disease or problem has an encounter for the purpose of specific treatment of that disease or problem (e.g., chemotherapy for malignancy). Remember that under the basic rules for **coding the chief reason for an encounter or service,** the primary diagnosis in the previous instance would require a V code for chemotherapy, followed by the supplemental malignancy diagnosis.
- Patient with a circumstance or problem that influences health status but currently is not an illness or injury (e.g., exposure of a pregnant patient to a communicable disease).

Identify the subsection within the V code section in which the appropriate code is located. This saves time in the coding process because the coder avoids thumbing through the entire V code section, and it helps in cross-checking whether the code selected is from the correct chapter.

V CODE INDEX

V codes are indexed in the alphabetical index of ICD-9-CM, along with the other diseases, signs, and symptoms. Unlike other ICD-9-CM descriptors that are located under the condition, illness, injury, sign, or symptom, V codes are located under the terms that describe the

reason for the encounter or visit. The following terms categorize services that have assigned V Codes:

Admission	Newborn
Aftercare	Observation
Attention (to)	Outcome of delivery
Care	Pregnancy
Carrier (suspected)	Problem
Contact	Prophylactic
Contraception, contraceptive	Replacement artificial/
Convalescence	mechanical device
Counseling	Resistance, resistant
Dependence	Screening
Dialysis	Status
Donor	Supervision
Examination	Test
Exposure	Therapy
Fitting (of)	Transplant
Follow-up	Unavailability of medical
Health	facilities
History (personal)	Vaccination
Maintenance	

Most ICD-9-CM code books do not include a general classification range of V codes. Tool 16 is provided as a valuable tool that can be included in the coder's ICD-9-CM code book.

V01-V06   Persons with Potential Health Hazards Related to Communicable Diseases

These codes are used for encounters with patients who are exposed to, who are in contact with, or who need prophylactic treatment for a disease. Codes from this subsection are identified by the following key word(s):

Contact
Exposure
Prophylactic
Vaccination

EXAMPLES: V01.6 Contact/exposure to venereal disease

V02.1 Carrier or suspected carrier of typhoid

V03.7 Need for prophylactic vaccination tetanus toxoid

V06.4 Need for prophylactic multiple vaccination, mumps, measles, rubella (MMR)

V07-V09   Persons with Need for Isolation, Other Potential Health Hazards, and Prophylactic Measures

Codes from this category are typically used when medical documentation indicates resistance to specific medications or health hazards or potential health hazards. Codes

---

V CODE INDEX

Persons with Potential Health Hazards Related to Communicable Disease(s)	V01-V06
Persons with Need for Isolation, Other Potential Health Hazards and Prophylactic Measures	V07-V09
Persons with Potential Health Hazards Related to Personal and Family History	V10-V19
Persons Encountering Health Services in Circumstances Related to Reproduction and Development	V20-V28
Observation and Evaluation of Newborns and Infants for Suspected Conditions Not Found	V29
Liveborn Infants According to Type of Birth	V30-V39
Persons with a Condition Influencing Their Health Status	V40-V49
Persons Encountering Health Services for Specific Procedures and Aftercare	V50-V59
Persons Encountering Health Services in Other Circumstances	V60-V69
Persons Without Reported Diagnosis Encountered During Examination and Investigation of Individuals and Populations	V70-V82

---

from this subsection are identified by the following key words:

Resistance (resistant)
Replacement

EXAMPLES: V07.4 Postmenopausal hormone replacement therapy
V09.0 Infection with microorganisms resistant to penicillin

V10-V19 Persons with Potential Health Hazards Related to Personal and Family History

When personal history or family history of certain diseases influences the health status of patient or is a pertinent contribution to the health status of the patient, a code from this section will be used. Care should be taken to differentiate between family history and personal history by assigning codes from the following categories:

V10-V15 **Personal History**
V16-V19 **Family History**

Codes from this section are located under the following alphabetical heading:

History

EXAMPLES: V10.3 Personal history, malignant breast neoplasm

V16.3 Family history, malignant breast neoplasm
V10.11 Personal history, malignant lung neoplasm
V16.1 Family history, malignant lung neoplasm

V20-V29 Persons Encountering Health Services in Circumstances Related to Reproduction and Development

Codes from this range are used to describe supervision of pregnancy, care of infant, postpartum care, contraceptive management, sterilization, outcome of delivery, and antenatal screening. Codes from the V22 category are usually used in the outpatient setting because the supervision of a normal pregnancy most often does not require inpatient services. Code V22.2 is assigned either to indicate the primary reason for the encounter or to indicate a pregnant patient who is seen for an unrelated condition that is not complicated or related to the pregnancy. Codes from the V24 series are indicative of uncomplicated follow-up during the postpartum period. V27 codes are used as an additional diagnostic code on the mother's medical record to indicate the outcome of delivery. Codes from this category will be identified with the following key word(s):

Pregnancy
Observation
Postpartum

Contraception
Outcome of delivery

EXAMPLES: V20.2 Routine child health care
V22.2 Supervision of first normal pregnancy
V23.0 Pregnancy with history of infertility
V24.2 Routine postpartum follow-up
V25.2 Sterilization
V27.0 Single liveborn
V28.0 Screening for chromosomal anomalies by amniocentesis
V29.2 Observation for suspected respiratory condition

V30-V39 Liveborn Infants According to Type of Birth

Recorded as the first diagnosis on the newborn hospital record, codes from the V30 range describe the number of live and stillborn births, as well as the location of birth and type of delivery (e.g., cesarean). Fourth (and in some instances fifth) digits are required for this section as follows:

Fourth digit identifies location of birth:
.0 Born in hospital (also requires fifth digit)
.1 Born before hospital admission
.2 Born outside hospital and not hospitalized

Fifth digit (required when fourth digit equal to "0"):
0 Delivered without mention of cesarean delivery
1 Delivered by cesarean delivery

EXAMPLES: V30.00 Single liveborn, born in hospital without mention of cesarean delivery
V32.01 Twin, mate stillborn, born in a hospital, delivered by cesarean delivery

V40-V49 Persons with Conditions Influencing Health Status

This subcategory of codes is used for conditions that influence the patient's health and increase the complexity of the patient's chief reason for the encounter. Conditions including transplant status, the presence of an artificial opening such as a tracheostomy, and S/P (status postoperative) conditions such as S/P coronary artery bypass grafting (CABG) are all included in this category. Key words for this category are the following:

Status
Dependence

EXAMPLES: V42.1 Transplant, heart, S/P
V44.0 Tracheostomy

V50-V59 Persons Encountering Health Services for Specific Procedures and Aftercare

This range of codes covers encounters that take place for the purpose of dealing with residual states or to prevent recurrence of diseases or injuries that are no longer present. These codes may be assigned for fitting and adjustment of prosthetic devices, orthopedic aftercare (such as removal of an internal fixation device), attention needed to artificial openings, encounters for dialysis, physical therapy, speech therapy, and other therapies. Key words for this subcategory would include the following:

Admission
Aftercare
Attention to

EXAMPLES: V54.81 Aftercare following joint replacement
V58.1 Encounter for chemotherapy

V60-V69 Persons Encountering Health Services in Other Circumstances

When encounters are for purposes other than disease, illness, injury, signs or symptoms, codes from this category would be appropriate. Examples would be convalescent and palliative care, and visit for the purpose of follow-up examinations. Key words for this category would be the following:

Admission
Follow-up

EXAMPLES: V67.00 Postoperative examination unspecified
V68.2 Request expert evidence

V70-V72 Persons without Reported Diagnosis Encountered during Examination and Investigation of Individuals and Populations

General medical examinations, observation for suspected conditions that are not found, and special examinations are included in this category. There are a number of medical examinations, and they are subcategorized within this section as follows:

V70.0 Routine general medical examination
V70.1 General psychiatric examination, requested by authority
V70.2 General psychiatric examination, other/unspecified
V70.3 Other examinations for administrative purposes
V70.4 Examinations for medicolegal reasons
V70.5 Examinations for defined population
V70.6 Examinations for population surveys
V70.7 Examinations for clinical trial participant
V70.8 Other specified medical examinations
V70.9 Unspecified medical examinations

Key words would include such terms as the following:

Admission
Observation

EXAMPLES: V70.0 Routine general medical
examination
V71.4 Observation following accident

V73-V83   Screening Examinations for Specified Conditions

When patient encounters are screening examinations for conditions that are currently inactive, codes from this

subcategory would be appropriate. Key words to identify services from within this section are the following:

Screening

EXAMPLES: V76.1 Screening for malignant
neoplasm
V79.2 Screening for mental retardation

STOP AND PRACTICE

Assign the appropriate V codes to the following:

	Section Where Located	V Code			
1. Pregnancy examination			11. Removal of surgical rods		
2. Preoperative examination			12. Dressing changes		
3. Exposure to rubella			13. Peritoneal dialysis		
4. Visit for tetanus immunization			14. Chemotherapy administration		
5. Donation of bone marrow			15. Physical therapy		
6. Personal history of malignant liver neoplasm			16. Single liveborn birth		
7. Visit for normal pregnancy			17. Supervision of high-risk pregnancy, multiple births		
8. Visit for routine child care			18. Family history of malignant neoplasm of gastrointestinal (GI) tract		
9. Contraceptive counseling			19. Observation following automobile accident		
10. General medical examination			20. Visits to the laboratory for routine blood work		

E CODES

APPROPRIATE USAGE

The **External Causes (E code)** section of the ICD-9-CM coding book is included to provide a mechanism for coding "external" causes of injury and poisoning. This section is used to code environmental events, circumstances, and conditions that cause injury, poisoning, or other adverse effects.

The E code is NEVER used as the primary diagnostic code for services because this event typically is not the chief reason for the encounter or service. The illness, injury, poisoning, or condition resulting from the external cause is usually the primary diagnosis and the primary reason for the encounter.

The E code is important from a reimbursement perspective. This code typically clarifies how, where, and why an accident happened. It therefore is used to help assign liability and responsibility of the appropriate insurance carrier.

Open wound of the arm
Occurred during a worksite fire

The appropriate numerical code for the chief reason for encounter, "Wound, Open, Arm," should be assigned. The E code for "Worksite Fire" should also be coded, however, because this indicates that workers' compensation should be billed rather than private health insurance.

Omission of appropriate E codes culminates in either inappropriate or delayed payment until this information is provided on request from the carrier. Requests from the carrier for information typically result in a much longer time for payment than required if the information is provided initially. The health insurance carrier typically has an average of 30 days to process a claim. After processing the claim and determining the need for additional information about an injury, the carrier sends a request letter to the provider. The average response time for the provider adds another 7 to 10 days to the process. The additional claim information is now mailed to the carrier, adding 7 to 10 more days for mailing and receipt.

Unlike the laws passed by most states that specify a certain amount of time that insurance carriers have to initially process a claim, there typically are no rules as to how quickly they must respond when additional information is needed. This process takes several weeks or months before reimbursement is made for services rendered, as opposed to the 30-day rule for a "clean claim."

A **clean claim** is a claim that does not require additional information, correction, or research for processing. Coding must be complete so that payment may be demanded and received within a reasonable period of time.

Some general coding guidelines for the assignment of E codes are the following:

- E codes may be used in conjunction with codes from the 001-V83 range to indicate an injury, illness, or adverse effect due to an external cause.
- E codes should be assigned for all initial treatments of injuries, illness, or adverse effects; however, if the encounter is not for the initial treatment, it would not be appropriate to assign an E code.
- As many E codes as necessary should be assigned to fully explain how, why, and where the injury occurred.
- E codes can never be used as primary diagnosis.

E CODE INDEX

The alphabetical index to External Causes is a separate index in ICD-9-CM. It is located in different locations according to the publisher and edition of ICD-9-CM used in the practice. It is organized by main terms that identify an accident, event or specific cause of injury, or adverse effect. In some instances, these external causes are environmental, such as an earthquake, or are caused by other sources such as dog bites or broken glass. In addition to providing information regarding how the accident or injury occurred, an additional E code assignment may be made for the Place of Occurrence or the location where the injury or accident occurred. As with the V codes, most ICD-9-CM books do not include a general index for the E code section, so such an index has been included in Tool 17.

This section is a break from some of the more difficult exercises completed thus far. Remember, the chief encounter for each service is the primary diagnosis; therefore E codes are NOT primary. Identifying where the code is located in the E code section prevents the coder from looking through the entire E code section.

T O O L   17

E CODE INDEX

Railway Accidents	E800-E807
Motor Vehicle Traffic Accidents	E810-E819
Motor Vehicle Nontraffic Accidents	E820-E825
Other Road Vehicle Accidents	E826-E829
Water Transport Accidents	E830-E838
Air and Space Accidents	E840-E845
Vehicle Accidents Not Classified Elsewhere	E846-E848
Place of Occurrence	E849
Accidental Poisoning by Drugs, Medicinal Substances, Biologicals	E850-E858
Accidental Poisoning by Other Solid and Liquid Substances, Gases, Vapors	E860-E869
Misadventure to Patients During Surgical/Medical Care	E870-E876
Surgical/Medical Procedures Cause of Abnormal Reaction of Patient or Later Complication, Without Mention of Misadventure at Time of Procedure	E878-E879
Accidental Falls	E880-E888
Accidents by Fire and Flames	E890-E898
Accidents Due to Natural/Environmental Factors	E900-E909
Accidents Caused by Submersion, Suffocation and Foreign Bodies	E910-E915
Other Accidents	E916-E928
Late Effects of Accidental Injury	E929
Drugs, Medicinal and Biological Substances Causing Adverse Effects in Therapeutic Use	E930-E949
Suicide and Self-Inflicted Injury	E950-E959
Homicide and Injury Purposely Inflicted by Other Persons	E960-E969
Legal Intervention	E970-E978
Injury Undetermined Whether Accidentally or Purposely Inflicted	E980-E989
Injury Resulting from Operations of War	E990-E999

STOP AND PRACTICE

Assign the appropriate E codes to the following:

	Section Where Located	E Code
Example: Boiling water	Other Accidents	E924.0

1. Cut from electric can opener _____ _____
2. Auto accident, driver _____ _____
3. Burns from fire, warehouse _____ _____
4. Scuba diving accident _____ _____
5. Contusion from fall _____ _____
6. Struck by fellow soccer player _____ _____

7. Rape _____ _____
8. Stabbing _____ _____
9. Gunshot wound _____ _____
10. Tripped and fell on stairs _____ _____
11. Fell from bed _____ _____
12. Cut finger with piece of glass _____ _____
13. Scuba accident _____ _____
14. Accidental drowning _____ _____
15. Accident due to farm cultivator _____ _____
16. Struck by furniture _____ _____
17. Fell into well _____ _____
18. Fall from ladder _____ _____
19. Lightning exposure _____ _____
20. Dog bite _____ _____

CHAPTER IN REVIEW

CERTIFICATION REVIEW

- V codes constitute the "Supplemental Classification of Factors Influencing Health Status and Contact with Health Services" in the ICD-9-CM code book.
- V codes are used when a patient does not present with any diagnoses, signs, or symptoms, yet an encounter takes place.
- V codes may be the primary diagnosis when the chief reason for encounter is best described by the use of a V code (encounter for chemotherapy).
- E codes are NOT applied for primary diagnoses because they provide additional information for coding the cause of the injury or poisoning.
- E codes are important from a reimbursement perspective because they assign liability and the appropriate insurance carrier responsibility.
- Clean claims are those received and processed without the need for additional information, correction, or research.
- Clean claims ensure prompt payment because they are processed on the initial submission.
- Many states have laws specifying time limits within which carriers must adjudicate (provide payment or response for) clean claims submitted.

STUDENT STUDY GUIDE

- Study Chapter 4.
- Review the Learning Objectives for Chapter 4.
- Complete the Certification Review for Chapter 4.
- Complete the Stop and Practice exercises contained in Chapter 4.

- Complete the Chapter Review exercise to reinforce concepts learned in this chapter.

CHAPTER REVIEW EXERCISE

Assign V codes, E codes, and ICD-9-CM codes as appropriate.

	E Code/V Code/Other
1. Exposure to HIV	_____
2. History of hypertension	_____
3. Malignant neoplasm of cervix, treated successfully 10 years ago	_____
4. Fracture of tibia, removal of screws and pins	_____
5. Dialysis treatment for end-stage renal disease (ESRD)	_____
6. CABG status	_____
7. Pregnancy	_____
8. Well-child examination	_____
9. Worried well (examination for which there is no diagnosis)	_____
10. Viral illness with exposure to strep throat	_____
11. Family history ovarian cancer	_____
12. Exposure to sexually transmitted disease (STD)	_____
13. History of colon carcinoma	_____
14. Single delivery, liveborn	_____

15. S/P tracheostomy _____
16. HIV counseling _____
17. Postmenopausal state _____
18. History of malaria _____
19. History of alcoholism _____
20. Removal of orthopedic pin _____
21. Substance abuse counseling _____
22. Family history of mental illness _____
23. S/P percutaneous transluminal coronary angioplasty (PTCA) _____
24. Newborn, suspicion of brain damage _____
25. Supervision of first pregnancy _____
26. Infant, single liveborn _____
27. Screening sickle cell _____
28. Adjustment of arm prosthetic _____
29. Evaluation following rape _____
30. Glaucoma screening _____
31. History renal stones _____
32. History of myocardial infarction _____
33. Insertion of intrauterine device (IUD) _____
34. Sterilization _____
35. Supervision of high risk pregnancy _____
36. S/P pacemaker _____
37. S/P heart transplant _____
38. S/P aortic valve replacement _____
39. Amniocentesis screening chromosome abnormalities _____
40. History of allergy to penicillin _____
41. History colon polyps _____
42. History of malignant melanoma _____
43. History of cigarette smoking _____
44. Family history of mental retardation _____
45. Need for DTP (diphtheria-tetanus-pertussis) immunization _____
46. Renal dialysis status _____
47. Breast augmentation _____
48. Screening mammogram _____
49. Preemployment physical _____
50. Replacement gastrostomy tube _____

51. High risk screening mammogram _____
52. Human immunodeficiency virus (HIV) positive status _____
53. Fall on steps of bus _____
54. Bicycle accident _____
55. Fall off steps of airplane, passenger _____
56. Traffic accident _____
57. Auto accident involving tree _____
58. Fall from ladder on boat _____
59. Injury in private driveway _____
60. Accidental fall _____
61. Fall from bed _____
62. Injury on football field _____
63. Injury at beach _____
64. Lead poisoning, lead-based paint at home _____
65. Barbiturate poisoning, accidental _____
66. Fall into storm drain _____
67. Fall on stairs _____
68. Fall out of tree _____
69. Drowning/submersion in bathtub _____
70. Injury from colliding with another person _____
71. Fall on pitchfork _____
72. Adverse reaction, chlorine fumes _____
73. Crushed by crowd _____
74. Injury caused by foreign body, ear _____
75. Suicide by hanging _____
76. Suicide by jumping from window of home _____
77. Adverse reaction to bee sting venom _____
78. Injury from lifting heavy objects _____
79. Injury from can opener _____
80. Accidental overdose, acetaminophen _____
81. Inhalation of asbestos _____
82. Family history of congenital defects _____
83. Need for flu vaccine _____
84. Need for rabies immunization _____
85. Fall on escalator _____
86. Fall from tripping _____
87. Sprain/strains from strenuous activity _____
88. Injury occurring at industrial site _____

89. Adverse effects, digoxin taken correctly _____

90. Adverse effects, hormones taken correctly _____

91. Injury from electric can opener _____

92. Intentional self-inflicted knife wound _____

93. Gunshot wound, homicide attempt _____

94. Injured by object dropped on patient _____

95. Fall in bathtub _____

96. School physical _____

97. Sports physical _____

98. Car versus car highway accident _____

99. Family history of breast cancer _____

100. S/P loss of limb, below knee _____

PRACTICAL APPLICATION

Review the following case scenarios and assign ICD-9-CM codes as appropriate. Assign both numerical and V codes and E codes as appropriate, listing them in the correct order for each service.

Scenario #1

PROGRESS NOTE

Chief complaint: _____

Date: _____

Vital signs: BP_____   P_____   R____

History:

Patient arrives for visit relating her brother recently underwent colon resection for colon cancer and would like to discuss need for colonoscopy screening.

The patient is a 48-year-old female who presents with no symptoms, no dysuria, no change in bowel habits, no recent weight loss, concerned about the history of colon cancer in her family.

She relates that her brother was recently diagnosed with colon cancer, and in 2002, her mother was diagnosed with colon cancer as well as two other siblings in the past ten years.

She is on no medications, no chronic problems, past surgical history is cesarean section times two with two normal healthy children, now age 28, and 26. She indicates she does not smoke or drink, and is currently unemployed.

Exam:

On exam, the patient is alert and oriented. HEENT exam reveals PERRLA, EOM. Neck supply, no carotid bruits, no thyroidmegaly noted. Heart sounds are regular, no murmurs, rubs or gallops. Lungs clear to auscultation. Neurologically intact.

Diagnosis/assessment:

Discussed with patient the need for screening colonoscopy for over age 40 adults as well as with her significant family history of colon cancer. We will get her scheduled for a screening colonoscopy in the near future. She presents with no signs or symptoms indicative of colon disease; however, would recommend screening colonoscopy due to age and family history.

Steny Knott, MD
Godfrey Regional Outpatient Clinic

Patient name: _____
Date of service: _____

GODFREY MEDICAL ASSOCIATES
1532 Third Avenue, Suite 120 • Aldon, FL 77713 • (407) 555-4000

Codes: _____

Scenario #2

PROGRESS NOTE

| Date: | | Vital signs: | T | | R | |
| Chief complaint: | | | P | | BP | |

2-year-old returns for MMR and Oral Polio immunization series. At her last visit, she was diagnosed with otitis media. Due to the fact she was running a low grade fever, we opted to hold off on her immunizations.

Examination:

Vital signs, including temperature are normal.

Impression:

Plan:

We will proceed with her MMR immunization and Oral Polio today.

Mom understands the benefits and risks of these immunizations, and warning signs, and wishes to proceed.

William Obst MD

Patient name:

DOB:

MR/Chart #:

GODFREY MEDICAL ASSOCIATES
1532 Third Avenue, Suite 120 • Aldon, FL 77713 • (407) 555-4000

Codes: _____

Scenario #3

PROGRESS NOTE

Chief complaint: _____

Date: _____

Vital signs: BP_____   P_____   R_____

History:

22-year-old patient presents today with complaints of abdominal pain, and amenorrhea for approximately 6–8 weeks. She is currently not on any birth control, married, and suspects she may be pregnant.

Exam:

On exam, the patient presents as a normal, healthy 22-year-old female who wishes to determine whether she is pregnant. Patient is alert and oriented, HEENT is normal, neck supple, abdomen, soft, no masses, heart normal rate and rhythm.

Diagnosis/assessment:

Laboratory pregnancy test was performed which was positive. We will refer patient to an Ob/Gyn for care during her pregnancy, and she will return to our office for any non-pregnancy related problems.

Julie Wander M
Godfrey Regional Hospital

Patient name: _____

Date of service: _____

GODFREY MEDICAL ASSOCIATES
1532 Third Avenue, Suite 120 • Aldon, FL 77713 • (407) 555-4000

Codes: _____

Scenario #4

PROGRESS NOTE

Date:	Vital signs:	T	R
Chief complaint:		P	BP

SUBJECTIVE:
22-year-old complains that she fell and injured her right ankle in the parking lot of her office building yesterday. Of note, the patient is approximately 22 weeks pregnant, G1 P1 A 0. She is being followed by Dr. Smith for her pregnancy.

PAST MEDICAL HISTORY:
Allergies, None
Medications, None

Physical examination:

OBJECTIVE:
Alert, oriented pregnant female. BP 120/80, respirations 20, pulse 70. She appears in no distress. She has moderate swelling of the right ankle, tender over the lateral malleolar area. Good range of motion, good pulses. We will not x-ray at this time due to her pregnancy.

Assessment:

Right ankle sprain, elevate the leg, immobilze with Swede-O splint.

Plan:

Take Tylenol only (no narcotics) on a PRN basis. Avoid walking any more than is necessary during the next 2–3 days.

Jay Corm MD

Patient name:

DOB:

MR/Chart #:

GODFREY REGIONAL OUTPATIENT CLINIC
3122 Shannon Avenue • Aldon, FL 77712 • (407) 555-7654

Codes: _____

Scenario #5

PROGRESS NOTE

Date:	Vital signs:	T	R
Chief complaint:		P	BP

Patient presents for follow-up exam for breast cancer. She was seen approximately one year ago, following mastectomy, chemotherapy and radiation therapy for infiltrating ductal carcinoma of the left breast. She has had no recurrence, and was instructed to follow-up on a yearly basis.

Examination:

Alert, female, in no acute distress. Weight 170, pulse 90, temperature 98.6. Examination of the breasts reveals no masses, no abnormalities. Left breast reveals well healed surgical scar. She indicates she is doing well, without complaints. Has continued to perform monthly breast self exams and has felt no lumps or masses. There is no lymphadenopathy. Neck is supple, no thyroidmegaly.

Impression:

Plan:

We will order a mammogram and CA-125 and await the test results, however, appears to be a resolved infiltrating ductal carcinoma without reoccurrence.

Adm Westg MD

Patient name:

DOB:

MR/Chart #:

GODFREY REGIONAL OUTPATIENT CLINIC
3122 Shannon Avenue • Aldon, FL 77712 • (407) 555-7654

Codes: _____

Scenario #6

PROGRESS NOTE

Date:	Vital signs:	T	R
Chief complaint:		P	BP

Patient presents having been injured at home while walking across the lawn. He apparently was pushing a lawnmower, tripped and hit his head on the curb along the sidewalk. Complains of headache, nausea and nasal pain caused by impact. Also complaints of skin laceration to nose.
No previous hospitalizations, surgeries or major illnesses. He is up-to-date on his immunizations, including tetanus toxoid.

Examination:

25-year-old male who was working in his yard on this date and apparently tripped, hit his head and presents with a 2.0 cm laceration of the nose. Examination reveals a 2.0 cm gaping laceration along the septal edge, and apparently a deviated septum which resulted from his fall. He indicates the septal defect was not present prior to the accident. This may need reconstructive surgery in the future. He reports no loss of consciousness or other symptoms other than some nausea and headache from the impact. Head, normal assemetry, no motor or sensory deficits noted. Normal gait. He reports no dizziness or light-headedness. Eyes, PERRLA, EOM, neck supple, full ROM without any limitation. Lungs clear to ausculation, heart regular rate and rhythm, abdomen, nondistended, non-tender. Back and extremities appear normal, no contusions, abrasions, lacerations, full ROM.

Impression:

Laceration to the nose was approximated and closed with 2 sutures, bandaged and taped.

Plan:

Patient to return in 7–10 days for suture removal and re-evaluation of septal defect. Patient should clean wound daily with hydrogen peroxide and water, change bandage as needed and avoid extensive nose blowing for the next 24 hours.

John Palermo

	Patient name:
	DOB:
	MR/Chart #:

GODFREY REGIONAL OUTPATIENT CLINIC
3122 Shannon Avenue • Aldon, FL 77712 • (407) 555-7654

Codes: _____

Scenario #7

PROGRESS NOTE

Date:	Vital signs:	T	R
Chief complaint:		P	BP

19-year-old male was playing soccer and was accidentally kicked by another player instead of the soccer ball. Patient experiencing pain in the calf area and unable to bear full weight on right leg.

Examination:

X-ray was negative for fracture or other injury.

Impression:

Leg pain from leg contusion due to kick

Plan:

Will treat conservatively with NSAIDS and Tylenol for pain.

Patient name:

DOB:

MR/Chart #:

GODFREY REGIONAL OUTPATIENT CLINIC
3122 Shannon Avenue • Aldon, FL 77712 • (407) 555-7654

Codes: _____

5

ICD-9-CM TABLES

LEARNING OBJECTIVES

Following the completion of this chapter, the student will be able to:

- Understand the proper use of the Drugs and Chemicals Table located in the ICD-9-CM code book.
- Understand the proper use of the decision tree (Tool 18) for determining the appropriate ICD-9-CM codes for assigning the adverse effects of drugs or poisonings.
- Make the determination whether ingestion of drugs and chemicals is the result of:
  Accidental poisoning
  Therapeutic use of drugs
  Suicide or assault
  Undetermined causes
- Properly use the Hypertension Table located in the ICD-9-CM code book.
- Comprehend the relationship of other medical conditions that complicate hypertension with assumptions that are made in coding these conditions.
- Understand the proper rules and guidelines for assigning codes to neoplasms.
- Identify the differences among the categories of neoplasms identified in ICD-9-CM.
- Know the proper use of the neoplasm table contained in the ICD-9-CM code book.
- Know the correct assignment order of primary and secondary neoplasms.
- Perceive the proper use of V codes for neoplastic diagnoses.

CODING REFERENCE TOOLS

Tool 18
Adverse Effects of Drugs/Poisonings (Several tables are included in the ICD-9-CM book as well.)
Tool 19
Neoplastic Diagnostic Coding Rules

KEY TERMS

Accidental Overdose, 130
Assault, 130
Benign, 132
Carcinoma in Situ, 134
Malignant, 132
Metastatic From, 132
Metastatic To, 132
Neoplasm, 132
Poisoning, 129
Primary, 134
Secondary, 134
Suicide Attempt, 130
Therapeutic Use, 130
Uncertain Behavior, 134
Unspecified Behavior, 134

In the alphabetical section of ICD-9-CM are diagnoses that are so extensive that the codes are arranged in a table format. For these tables to be used correctly, there are specific guidelines for coding and for selecting the appropriate code(s). The hypertension and neoplasm tables are contained in the alphabetical section, whereas the Table of Drugs and Chemicals is frequently independent of the alphabetical section.

TABLE OF DRUGS AND CHEMICALS

APPROPRIATE USAGE

The Table of Drugs and Chemicals found in the ICD-9-CM book provides a concise guide to **poisoning** and external causes for adverse effects of drugs and other chemical substances. Each of the listed drugs or chemical substances is assigned a code on the basis of the diagnostic statement as to whether the cause is the result of the following:

- Poisoning
- Overdose
- Wrong substance given or taken
- Intoxication

Codes from the Drugs and Chemical Table are used only when the chief reason for the encounter is the result of exposure to a drug or chemical. Codes in the Table of Drugs and Chemicals are arranged by the drug or chemical name in alphabetical order.

The categories in the Drugs and Chemicals Table are as follows (Figure 5-1):

- Poisoning
- Accident

Substance	Poisoning	External Case (E-Code)				
		Accident	Therapeutic Use	Suicide Attempt	Assault	Undetermined
Adalin (acteyl)	967.3	E852.2	E937.3	E950.2	E962.0	E980.2
Adenosine (phosphate)	977.8	E858.8	E947.8	E950.4	E962.0	E980.4
Adhesives	989.89	E866.8	—	E950.9	E962.1	E980.9
ADH	962.5	E858.0	E932.5	E950.4	E962.0	E980.4
Adicillin	960.0	E856	E930.0	E950.4	E962.0	E980.4
Adiphenine	975.1	E855.6	E945.1	E950.4	E962.0	E980.4
Adjunct, pharmaceutical	977.4	E858.8	E947.4	E950.4	E962.0	E980.4
Adrenal (extract, cortex, or medulla) (glucocorticoids) (hormones) (mineralocorticoids)	962.0	E858.0	E932.0	E950.4	E962.0	E980.4
ENT agent	976.6	E858.7	E946.6	E950.4	E962.0	E980.4
ophthalmic preparation	976.5	E858.7	E946.5	E950.4	E962.0	E980.4
topical NEC	976.0	E858.7	E946.0	E950.4	E962.0	E980.4

FIGURE 5-1 Excerpt from Table of Drugs and Chemicals. *(From the U.S. Department of Health and Human Services, Centers for Medicare and Medicaid Services.)*

- **Therapeutic Use**
- **Suicide Attempt**
- **Assault**
- Undetermined

Poisoning (960-979)

Codes from this category are ONLY used when the substance involved was not taken according to physician instructions. This means the substance has to be prescribed and taken exactly as intended. Examples of the appropriate use of the poisoning codes would include such scenarios as the following:

- Wrong dosage of medication given in error
- Medication given to wrong person
- Medication taken by wrong person
- Patient takes wrong medication
- Intoxication (other than that resulting from cumulative ingestion)
- Overdose
- The combination of medications with other substances (such as other medications, alcohol, over-the-counter medications), which creates an adverse effect

In addition to the assignment of a poisoning code when appropriate, the external cause for the condition should also be assigned an appropriate external code (E code).

Accident (E850-E869)

These codes include **accidental overdose** of drug, wrong substance, drug taken in error, accidents in the use of drugs or biologicals during medical or surgical procedures, and external causes of poisoning classifiable to 980-989.

Therapeutic Use (E930-E949)

These codes take in the correct substance administered properly and as prescribed in therapeutic or prophylactic dosage.

Suicide Attempt (E950-E952)

Self-inflicted injuries or poisonings are involved. Make certain that the diagnostic statement confirms that injuries or poisonings are self-inflicted. Many times, the physician or provider is unable or unwilling to make the diagnosis of suicide attempt because he or she may be unable to ascertain, especially in the case of drug overdose, whether the injury or poisoning was intentional or accidental.

Assault (E961-E962)

These codes indicate injury or poisoning that has been inflicted by another person, with the intent to do bodily harm, injure, or kill. This information must be documented and included in the diagnostic information used for coding.

Undetermined (E980-E981)

Undetermined codes are used when the intent of the poisoning or injury is similar to that mentioned in the suicide attempt or assault section, and the provider cannot or will not make a definite diagnostic statement as to whether the injury was accidental or intended.

DOCUMENTATION REQUIREMENTS

As with all the other ICD-9-CM diagnoses codes that have been discussed so far, the drug and chemical codes are dependent on documentation. In some instances, documentation will be unclear about the circumstances under which the drug or chemical was ingested. Consider the following example:

A 30-year-old female presents to the emergency department by way of ambulance because of seizures from an overdose of acetaminophen (Tylenol). Physician documentation does not specify whether the overdose was intentional, for the purpose of suicide, or accidental.

In this instance, the coder must assign an undetermined external cause code. Even when intent seems apparent and is likely the cause of the adverse effect, caution must be taken to make certain the information is documented appropriately. See the following example:

A 35-year-old male presents to the emergency department for abdominal bleeding due to a gunshot wound.

Without further information, the coder cannot assume that the gunshot wound is the result of an attempted assault. The wound could have been accidental (self-inflicted or inflicted accidentally by another individual) or self-inflicted in a suicide attempt. Take extreme caution to consider all possibilities before assigning the E code for drug and chemical codes. The undetermined code will often be assigned because of insufficient or unclear documentation. In some cases, the physician may be unable to determine the cause, as in the example of the patient who ingested acetaminophen.

DRUGS/CHEMICALS FLOWCHART

The most complex part of coding arises from the inability to determine from the documentation provided whether

T O O L   18

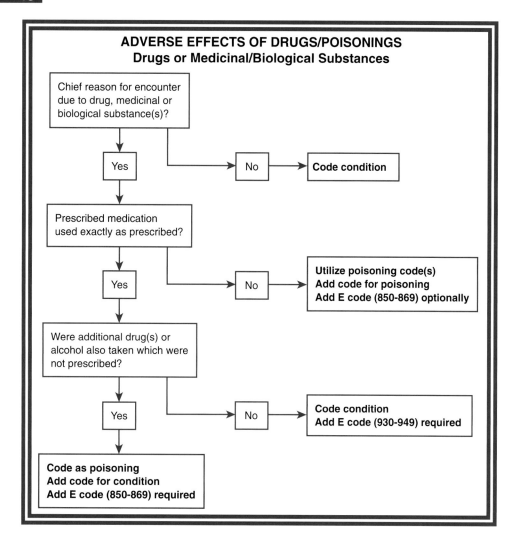

poisoning is the result of an accident, proper therapeutic use, a suicide attempt, or assault. Because of the complexity of this decision-making process, a diagnosis flowchart can be helpful in this determination (Tool 18). Keep in mind that code assignment will typically require a minimum of two codes for any scenario. In some situations, three codes will be assigned to code these appropriately.

As discussed in the introductory chapters on ICD-9-CM coding, the condition would be assigned as the chief reason for the encounter, followed by the external codes or poisoning codes or both. In most instances, this would be the presenting condition, such as coma, seizures, or abdominal pain caused by the drugs and other substance, followed by the cause of the adverse effect.

STOP AND PRACTICE

Identify the external cause category for each of the following. Assign the appropriate E code.

	External Cause Category	E Code

(poisoning, accident, therapeutic, suicide, assault, undetermined)

1. Overdose of fluoxetine _____ _____
2. Digoxin toxicity _____ _____
3. Accidental ingestion of diphenhydramine _____ _____
4. Suicidal ingestion of acetaminophen _____ _____
5. Ingestion of antifreeze _____ _____
6. Rattlesnake bite _____ _____
7. Intentional poisoning of another individual, rat poison _____ _____
8. Ingestion of smelter fumes _____ _____
9. Ingestion of poisonous plant, not classified _____ _____
10. Vitamin B_{12} toxicity _____ _____

NEOPLASMS

Neoplasms are listed in table format in the alphabetical section of ICD-9-CM. These codes are arranged in alphabetical order according to the anatomical site of the neoplasms. Before consideration of the neoplasm table, however, some review of the terminology associated with neoplasm would be appropriate.

DEFINITIONS

A **neoplasm** is *any new and abnormal growth*. That growth may be **malignant** or **benign** or as yet undetermined. Additional definitions and rules for coding neoplastic diagnoses are necessary to assist with correct coding.

Metastatic from	Spread to a distant site of the solid primary neoplasm with a new center of malignancy.
Metastatic to	Indicates the site mentioned is secondary or metastatic.
Metastatic from	Site mentioned is the primary site.
Metastatic (unqualified)	Code as unspecified site for that type.
Codes 199.0-199.1	Malignant neoplasms without specification as to whether the site used is primary or secondary. These codes should be used when no further information is documented.
	199.0 Disseminated malignant neoplasm, without specification of site.
	199.1 Other malignant neoplasm, without specification of site.

In addition to the ICD-9-CM codes discussed in this chapter, the ICD-9-CM code book includes Morphology Codes, which are prefixed by an *M*. Hospital coders specifically use these codes, usually for the purpose of identifying tumor locations for tumor registries. Although these are used solely by the inpatient/outpatient facility coder, an understanding of the code breakdown is necessary. The first four digits identify the type of neoplasm, whereas the fifth digit identifies the behavior, as in the following example:

/0 Benign
/1 Uncertain or borderline malignancy
/2 Carcinoma in situ
 Intraepithelial
 Noninfiltrating
 Noninvasive
/3 Malignant, primary site
/6 Malignant, metastatic site
 Secondary site
/9 Malignant, uncertain whether primary or secondary

GUIDELINES FOR USAGE

In addition to the guidelines already discussed, those found in Tool 19 should be used for the coding of neoplastic diseases. Although they are used to cover specific coding complexities, many of the rules are simply delineations of the rules already learned. For instance, because the primary diagnosis for each encounter or service will always be the chief reason for that encounter or service, most of the specific neoplasm guidelines are no different than those guidelines already presented.

DOCUMENTATION GUIDELINES

As with the other service codes in the ICD-9-CM book, appropriate neoplastic diagnostic codes rely on good documentation. Basic coding guidelines apply to neoplasm codes as well. When the neoplasm is not specified as primary or secondary malignancy, it will be assigned as primary. As with the other ICD-9-CM codes, the chief

T O O L 19

NEOPLASTIC DIAGNOSTIC CODING RULES

1. When treatment is directed at the primary site, the malignancy is designated as the principal site. (Chief reason for encounter still applies.)

2. When treatment is directed at the secondary or metastatic site, the secondary site would be designated as the principal diagnosis, followed by the primary site listed as a secondary diagnosis.

   (Again, the chief reason for this encounter is the secondary site; therefore, the chief reason for the encounter rule applies here as well.)

3. Care for ancillary services such as chemotherapy/radiotherapy—Chief reason for these encounters would be coded with V58.0–V58.1 as these are the chief reasons for this service/encounter. The neoplastic disease being treated with the radiotherapy/chemotherapy may be listed as additional diagnosis(es).

4. When the primary neoplasm is no longer under treatment, it is not appropriate to code the encounter with a neoplasm code. The V codes, personal history, would be utilized as this, again, as the chief reason for encounter. An example of the use of the personal history V codes would be patients who return annually for a re-examination to their hematologist/oncologist who is not being and has not been treated for the disease for some time as the neoplasm is no longer present.

5. Admissions for complications associated with a malignant neoplasm would be coded with that complication listed first. Again, the chief reason for this encounter/service would be the chief complaint/condition rather than the malignant neoplasm. The primary/secondary diagnosis could be the primary and/or secondary neoplasm, whichever is still present.

---

reason for the encounter is assigned as the primary diagnostic code. Consider the following example:

A 42-year-old woman presents for chemotherapy for metastatic cervical cancer originating in the breast. The breast cancer was treated approximately 5 years ago and is no longer present.

The primary code is assigned to the encounter for chemotherapy, the second code is given to the secondary neoplasm of the uterus, and a V code is added for history of breast carcinoma as the third code.

V58.1   Encounter for Chemotherapy
198.82   Secondary Malignant Neoplasm, Uterus
V10.3   Personal History of Breast Carcinoma

In those instances in which neoplasms are not specified as benign or malignant, codes from the uncertain or unspecified behavior categories are applied.

CATEGORIZATION OF NEOPLASMS

The following are the primary categories for the neoplasm table.

Malignant Neoplasms (Codes 140-208)

Malignant or cancerous neoplasms are further defined as tumor cells that extend or attach themselves to an adjacent structure and spread to distant sites. Two types of malignant neoplasms are coded as the following:

Solid Malignant Neoplasms (Codes 140-199)	Single localized point of origin. These neoplasms tend to metastasize to adjacent or remote sites.
Hematopoietic/ Lymphatic Neoplasms (Codes 200-208)	Reticuloendothelial and lymphatic system and blood-forming tissue neoplasms: Primary neoplasms of lymph nodes or glands (Codes 200-202)

Lymphoma—can be malignant or
benign
Hodgkin's disease
Multiple myeloma/leukemia (Codes
203-208)

Malignant neoplasms are further subdivided in the neoplasm table as **primary,** the site where the neoplasm originated, and **secondary,** the site where the neoplasm has spread. When a malignant neoplasm is not specified as primary or secondary, it is assumed to be primary in nature.

Carcinoma in Situ (Codes 230-234)

These codes refer to malignant neoplasms that are undergoing malignant changes; however, they remain confined at the point of origin without any invasion of surrounding normal tissue.

Benign (Codes 210-229)

When neoplasms, or new growths, do not invade or spread and are noncancerous, they are designated benign neoplasms. Use codes from the benign column of the neoplasm table. These neoplasms are not invasive; they do not spread to other sites.

Uncertain Behavior (Codes 235-238)

When neoplasms have the behavior of both benign and malignant neoplasms and the pathologist has been unable to determine the specific nature, they will be coded to this category. These codes might also be used for an initial visit to the physician when a neoplasm is identified during an examination. The behavior of the neoplasm is unknown and cannot be ascertained until a biopsy or an excision is performed.

Unspecified Behavior (Code 239)

In some instances, the nature of the neoplasm has not been specified in the medical documentation. A code would be used from this column of the neoplasm table. This designation should not be confused with behavior that cannot be determined. In the case of **unspecified behavior,** the diagnostic information has not specified the nature of behavior that may be known.

A look at the layout of the Neoplasm Table shows how these codes are further divided (Figure 5-2).

	Malignant					
	Primary	Secondary	Ca in situ	Benign	Uncertain Behavior	Unspecified
Neoplasm *(continued)*						
bone (periosteum)	170.9	198.5	—	213.9	238.0	239.2
Note—Carcinomas and adenocarcinomas, of any type other than intraosseous or odontogenic, of the sites listed under "Neoplasm, bone," should be considered as constituting metastatic spread from an unspecified primary site and coded to 198.5 for morbidity coding and to 199.1 for underlying cause of death coding.						
acetabulum	170.6	198.5	—	213.6	238.0	239.2
acromion (process)	170.4	198.5	—	213.4	238.0	239.2
ankle	170.8	198.5	—	213.8	238.0	239.2
arm NEC	170.4	198.5	—	213.4	238.0	239.2
astragalus	170.8	198.5	—	213.8	238.0	239.2
atlas	170.2	198.5	—	213.2	238.0	239.2
axis	170.2	198.5	—	213.2	238.0	239.2
back NEC	170.2	198.5	—	213.2	238.0	239.2
calcaneus	170.8	198.5	—	213.8	238.0	239.2

FIGURE 5-2 Excerpt from Table of Neoplasms. *(From the U.S. Department of Health and Human Services, Centers for Medicare and Medicaid Services.)*

STOP AND PRACTICE

Take a look at the following neoplasms and determine which coding category the neoplasm occupies. The categories are Malignant (Primary, Secondary, In Situ), Benign, Uncertain Behavior, and Unspecified Behavior.

	Neoplasm Behavior/Category
1. Metastatic neoplasm of the spine	_____
2. Breast cancer	_____
3. Breast cancer, in situ	_____
4. Breast neoplasm	_____
5. Breast lipoma	_____
6. Adenocarcinoma of the thyroid	_____
7. Adrenal adenoma	_____
8. Acute myeloid leukemia	_____
9. Carcinoma of the brain from the lung	_____
10. Acute lymphatic leukemia	_____

TABLE 5-1	Neoplasm Coding Order Guidelines

Reason for Encounter	Code(s) to Assign
Primary neoplasm	Primary neoplasm
Chemotherapy/radiation	V code chemotherapy V code radiation Malignant site being treated Other site(s) if appropriate
Complications from chemotherapy/treatment	Complications V code for treatment modality Malignant site being treated Other site(s) if appropriate
Admission for removal of malignancy with treatment during admission	Primary neoplasm V code for treatment modality
Malignant neoplasm with signs/symptoms	Malignant neoplasm only
Encounter for follow-up for malignancy previously	History of code only
Encounter for condition related to malignancy	Condition Malignant neoplasm

Table 5-1 delineates the proper assignment of ICD-9-CM diagnostic code(s) based on the reason for encounter.

Medical terminology is important in the proper assignment of diagnostic codes. Here are a few additional terms related to neoplasms:

Mass	not regarded as a neoplasm, not determined to be a new growth
Carcinoma	cancerous tumor
Sarcoma	malignant neoplasm of connective tissue
Lymphosarcoma	form of non-Hodgkin's lymphoma
Burkitt's tumor	form of non-Hodgkin's lymphoma
Dysplasia	precursor condition to carcinoma

Assign the appropriate ICD-9-CM diagnostic code(s) in the correct order to the following conditions.

	ICD-9-CM Code(s)
1. Right renal mass	_____
2. Severe dysplasia, cervix; chronic cervicitis	_____
3. Bronchial adenoma	_____
4. Neurofibromatosis, Type 2	_____

5. Carcinoma in situ, skin of anus	_____
6. Metastatic carcinoma from lung	_____
7. Metastatic carcinoma to brain	_____
8. Metastatic carcinoma of brain	_____
9. Acute myeloblastic leukemia	_____
10. Benign lymphoma of axillary nodes	_____

HYPERTENSION

APPROPRIATE USAGE

Hypertension is coded from the table in the alphabetical index of ICD-9-CM. All hypertensive disorders and diseases, and those associated with hypertension, are listed in the hypertensive table. There are four columns in the table, which are outlined as follows:

Column 1	Hypertensive condition (e.g., antepartum, cardiovascular)
Column 2	Malignant hypertension Accelerated severe form of hypertension. Symptoms may include headaches, blurred vision, dyspnea, or uremia.
Column 3	Benign hypertension Relatively stable hypertension (usually mild, continuous blood pressure elevation) that with proper treatment does not threaten the life span of the patient. It is considered a risk factor for heart disease and cerebrovascular disease.
Column 4	Unspecified hypertension Hypertensive heart disease refers to secondary effects of prolonged hypertension on the heart. Hypertensive disorders should be coded as in Figure 5-3.
Hypertension, hypertension, essential, or NOS	Hypertension defined as essential, primary, systemic, or not otherwise specified would be coded as category 401. Do not use malignant or benign hypertension designations unless the documentation supports this diagnosis.
Hypertension, controlled	This category of codes 401 through 405 is usually assigned to hypertension that is controlled with therapy.
Hypertension, uncontrolled	This designation refers to either untreated hypertension or hypertension

	Malignant	Benign	Unspecified
Hypertension, hypertensive (arterial) (arteriolar) (disease) (essential) (fluctuating) (idiopathic) (intermittent) (labile) (low rennin) (orthostatic) (paroxysmal) (primary) (systemic) (uncontrolled) (vascular)	401.0	401.1	401.9
with			
heart involvement (conditions classifiable to 428, 429.0-429.3, 429.8, 429.9 due to hypertension) (*see also* Hypertension, heart)	402.00	402.10	401.90
with kidney involvement – *see* Hypertension, cardiorenal			
renal involvement (only conditions classifiable to 585, 586, 587) (excludes conditions classifiable as 584) (*see also* Hypertension, kidney)	403.00	403.10	403.90
with heart involvement – *see* Hypertension, cardiorenal			
failure (and sclerosis) (*see also* Hypertension, kidney)	403.01	403.11	403.91
sclerosis without failure (*see also* Hypertension, kidney)	403.00	403.10	403.90
accelerated (*see also* Hypertension, by type, malignant)	401.0	—	—
antepartum – *see* Hypertension, complicating pregnancy, childbirth, or the puerperium			

FIGURE 5-3 Excerpt from Hypertension Table. *(From the U.S. Department of Health and Human Services, Centers for Medicare and Medicaid Services.)*

Hypertension, transient
that is not responding to medical treatment or therapy. Codes 401 through 405 are used for coding this type of hypertension.
When elevated blood pressure is documented without a diagnosis of hypertension (code 796.2), transient hypertension should be assigned, unless there is a documented, established diagnosis of hypertension for the patient.

HYPERTENSION DOCUMENTATION GUIDELINES

Often the documentation of hypertension lacks specificity. As a result, the diagnosis code 401.9 (hypertension, unspecified) must be assigned when documentation lacks information regarding the nature of the hypertension (benign compared with malignant). Other descriptive words may accompany the diagnosis of hypertension, including hypertensive crisis, orthostatic hypertension, uncontrolled hypertension, essential hypertension, intermittent hypertension, primary hypertension, or systemic hypertension. These terms do not specify the nature of the hypertension, though. Therefore these diagnostic statements will also be assigned a diagnosis code of 401.9, hypertension, unspecified. The use of malignant or benign hypertension codes is not appropriate without supporting medical documentation.

OTHER CODING GUIDELINES

When another condition complicates the treatment of hypertension, typically both conditions are coded. The primary reason for the encounter, which may be the complicating condition, is coded as the primary diagnosis and the hypertension is coded as the secondary diagnosis. Complicating conditions of hypertension include the following.

Hypertension in Pregnancy

As indicated in Chapter 6 (Coding Special Complexities) complications that arise during or after pregnancy are assigned codes from the 600 series of ICD-9-CM. This guideline also applies to hypertension in pregnancy. Regardless of whether the condition occurred during pregnancy or was present before pregnancy, a code from the 600 series would be assigned. Should the condition of hypertension still exist following the postpartum period, a diagnostic code from the 400 series would again be assigned.

Hypertension with Heart Disease

Certain heart conditions (Codes 425.8, 428, and 429) are assigned a code from category 402 when the stated condition is due to hypertension or the statement implies that such is the case (use of the word "hypertensive" in the documentation). The coder must use only the code from category 402 in these instances. When this relationship is not stated, each condition is coded separately.

Hypertensive Renal Disease with Chronic Renal Failure

When conditions that are coded in categories 585 through 587 occur with hypertension, codes from category 403 are appropriate. ICD-9-CM assumes a relationship between chronic renal failure and hypertension. Acute renal failure is not included in this assumption.

Hypertensive Heart and Renal Disease

Combination codes from category 404 are used for coding these two diseases. The coder may assign a relationship between hypertension and renal disease when both are stated in the diagnosis, whether they are connected or not.

Other Associated Complications of Hypertension Requiring Two Codes

Hypertensive cerebrovascular disease
Hypertensive retinopathy
Secondary hypertension

These complications of hypertension must be assigned two diagnostic codes for the conditions stated. One code is assigned for the underlying condition and the other for the hypertension.

Hypertension Coding as a Chronic Condition

Because many patients will have hypertension in addition to other illnesses, injuries, signs, and symptoms, it is important to keep in mind that only those conditions chiefly responsible for the encounter would be appropriate. If the patient presents for the evaluation and treatment of hypertension or if the condition of hypertension is involved in evaluation and management during the encounter, the assignment of hypertension is appropriate. Only when the chief reason for the encounter is hypertension would this condition be listed first. When hypertension is a contributing illness, it is listed as a secondary diagnostic code. Keep in mind that the coding guidelines are relative to physician coding, and that facility coders may use the hypertension diagnosis in other circumstances that are discussed in the brief overview of hospital/facility coding.

STOP AND PRACTICE

Code the following hypertension exercises.

ICD-9-CM Code(s)

1. Hypertension _____
2. Postoperative hypertension _____
3. Elevated blood pressure _____
4. Postpartum hypertension _____
5. Pulmonary hypertension _____

6. Myocarditis due to hypertension _____
7. Hypertension with chronic renal failure _____
8. Hypertension due to brain tumor _____
9. Gestational hypertension _____
10. Hypertension, possibly malignant _____

CHAPTER IN REVIEW

CERTIFICATION REVIEW

- The Table of Drugs and Chemicals located in ICD-9-CM is intended to simplify the assignment of adverse effects.
- Each drug or chemical is assigned a code based on the diagnostic statement as to whether the injury is the result of poisoning, overdose, wrong substance given or taken, or intoxication.
- Some adverse effects require two ICD-9-CM codes: one for the poisoning and an additional E code for the external cause.
- When the cause of adverse effects is not stated by the physician, the coder must use the Undetermined category. This is particularly important in potential suicide cases in which the physician does not or will not state that the adverse effects were intentionally inflicted.
- Adverse effects from therapeutic use occur only when the correct substance is administered correctly as prescribed.
- Accidental poisoning codes are used only when accidental overdose of a drug, wrong substance, drug taken in error, or accidents in the use of drugs or biologicals are identified.
- Drugs and chemicals listed in the Table of Drugs and Chemicals in the ICD-9-CM codebook are listed alphabetically; generic names are used for prescription drugs.
- A neoplasm is defined as any new and abnormal growth. That growth may be malignant, benign, or undetermined.
- Masses are not coded or classified as neoplasms unless the physician states "neoplasm" or "neoplastic" in the diagnostic statement.
- When secondary or metastatic neoplasms are coded, the primary site should always be coded. If the site is known, use the appropriate code. If the site is not known but is known to exist, use 199.0 or 199.1. If the site no longer exists, use history of malignant neoplasm codes.
- Carcinoma in situ refers to malignant neoplasms that stay confined to the point of origin without invading surrounding areas.

STUDENT STUDY GUIDE

- Study Chapter 5.
- Review the Learning Objectives for Chapter 5.
- Complete the Stop and Practice exercises.
- Complete the Certification Review for Chapter 5.
- Complete the Chapter Review exercise to reinforce concepts learned in this chapter.

CHAPTER REVIEW EXERCISE

Code the following:

Code Assigned

1. Essential hypertension _____
2. Suicide attempt by cocaine _____
3. Open wound of abdomen due to shotgun blast to abdomen _____
4. Overdose of phenobarbital, prescribed by physician, taken as directed _____
5. Hypertensive heart and renal disease _____
6. Attempted homicide by rat poison _____
7. Hypertension in pregnancy, antepartum _____
8. Secondary hypertension due to pulmonary edema _____
9. Allergic reaction to spider bite _____
10. Asbestos poisoning _____
11. Secondary hypertension _____
12. Pulmonary hypertension _____
13. Transient hypertension of pregnancy _____
14. Accidental overdose, doxycycline _____
15. Accidental ingestion, gas fumes/vapors _____
16. Benign hypertension _____
17. Preexisting hypertension in pregnancy with preeclampsia _____
18. Adverse effects of bupivacaine hydrochloride (Marcaine), administered subcutaneously _____
19. Renovascular hypertension _____
20. Suicide attempt by ingestion of gas _____
21. Overdose of diazepam, accidental _____
22. Adverse effects, topical neomycin sulfate (Neosporin) _____
23. Adverse effects, laxatives, therapeutic _____
24. Lithium, taken as directed _____
25. Adverse effects, bee sting _____
26. Elevated blood pressure reading _____
27. Hypertensive renal disease _____
28. Secondary hypertension due to Cushing's disease _____
29. Hypertension due to polycystic kidney disease _____
30. Intraocular hypertension _____
31. Squamous cell carcinoma in situ, floor of mouth _____

32. Metastatic malignant melanoma
    from left lateral chest wall to
    axillary lymph node   _____

33. Carcinoma, rectosigmoid junction
    and prostate   _____

34. Adenocarcinoma, right upper
    lobe, lung, with metastases to
    mediastinal lymph nodes   _____

35. Breast mass   _____

PRACTICAL APPLICATION

1.

PROGRESS NOTE

Date:	Vital signs:	T	R
Chief complaint:		P	BP

63-year-old female who has taken Norvasc for approximately the past five years for hypertension presents for evaluation and urinary tract symptoms and nausea. She is on no other medications, and has had hypertension for approximately the past two decades.

Social History/Past Medical History:
Non-smoker, non-drinker. Past surgeries include three cesarean sections, a hysterectomy in 1999, cholecystectomy in 2001.

Physical examination:

She is afebrile. Vital signs are stable. Color normal, she is not diaphoretic. Neck is supple, carotids are normal. Chest is clear, with good air movement. Abdomen, soft and nontender. Pulses are normal.

LABS:
CBC and Comprehensive Metabolic Panel revealed patient in renal failure.

Assessment:

IMPRESSION:
Hypertension, acute renal failure

Plan:

Arrangements will be made for the patient to begin dialysis ASAP.
Continue hypertension medications and we will consider additional medications after dialysis has improved her renal function somewhat.

Maurice Doater, MD

	Patient name:
	DOB:
	MR/Chart #:

GODFREY REGIONAL OUTPATIENT CLINIC
3122 Shannon Avenue • Aldon, FL 77712 • (407) 555-7654

Codes: _____

2.

PROGRESS NOTE

Date:	Vital signs:	T	R
Chief complaint:		P	BP

A 68-year-old male presents for evaluation of increasing shortness of breath over the past several weeks. He has experienced no other symptoms other than feeling a bit run down and lethargic over the past several days. Feels effort must be taken to complete daily tasks and feels exhausted when he returns from work.
Past Medical History: History of smoking 2 packs per day/20 years. Ceased smoking in 1998 following a scare with a lung mass that was thought to be malignant, however, repeat x-rays revealed poor x-ray technique and no mass could be appreciated after multiple repeated x-rays.
Patient works in the sales field, traveling from city to city, and a great deal of driving is involved.

Examination:

This gentleman appears short winded and a bit anxious. Color is good, P 84, R 12, BP 120/80. Chest: Lungs bilaterally clear to auscultation. Heart: Regular rate and rhythm. Abdomen: Postive bowel sounds, soft and nontender. Extremities: normal strength and sensation with no cyanosis and a minimal pitting edema around the ankles. He reports that he has some edema as the result of sitting and driving for many hours a day. This has been present for years.

Chest x-ray was performed, which revealed a mass in the left lower lobe of the lung. We will schedule for additional testing to include a CT Scan as well as an MRI to determine primary site and any other possible involvement.

Impression:

Lung mass, suspicious for malignant neoplasm

Plan:

Stony Kralt, MD

Patient name:
DOB:
MR/Chart #:

GODFREY MEDICAL ASSOCIATES
1532 Third Avenue, Suite 120 • Aldon, FL 77713 • (407) 555-4000

Codes: _____

3.

PROGRESS NOTE

Chief complaint: _____

Date: _____

Vital signs: BP_____ P_____ R_____

History:

SUBJECTIVE:
68-year-old male returns following initial evaluation for shortness of breath which revealed a suspicious lesion in the left lower lobe of the lung. CT Scan and MRI were ordered to determine primary site and any other possible involvement. MRI of the bone was performed that was positive for metastases to the bone. CT of the lung confirmed a malignant oat cell carcinoma of the left lower lobe. MRI of the brain also revealed metastatic involvement in the brain as well.

Exam:

OBJECTIVE:
68-year-old male who appears anxious for his test results.
He is informed that the diagnosis is guarded, with primary oat cell carcinoma of the left lower lobe with metastatic changes in the brain and bone.

Diagnosis/assessment:

ASSESSMENT:
Primary oat cell carcinoma
Metastatic to brain and bone

PLAN:
Will refer to Oncologist for intervention probably to include both chemotherapy and radiation therapy. Offer reassurance, however, explained that the prognosis was guarded until oncologist has ability to evaluate.

Jay Corson MD
Godfrey Medical Associates

Patient name: _____
Date of service: _____

GODFREY MEDICAL ASSOCIATES
1532 Third Avenue, Suite 120 • Aldon, FL 77713 • (407) 555-4000

Codes: _____

4.

PROGRESS NOTE

Date:	Vital signs:	T		R	
Chief complaint:		P		BP	

Patient is a 12-month-old active female who presents with a rash over the trunk and lower extremities. She was in approximately 1 week ago with complaints of sore throat, fever and cough and was diagnosed with an upper respiratory infection. She was prescribed penicillin for her URI at that time.

Allergies: None reported

Examination:

She appears to be an active, normal healthy 12-month-old female in no acute distress. She does continue to cough and her upper respiratory infection is not resolved. Lungs, congested. HEENT: Normal. Heart, normal rate and rhythm. Abdomen: soft and non-tender. Coarse rash over the lower trunk and lower extremities that seems to have spread diffusely. Mom indicates no new foods, detergents or lotions have been introduced in the past couple weeks.

Impression:

Non-resolved URI
Allergic reaction to Penicillin

Plan:

Will switch to Keflex for 10 day course

Felix Warden MD

| Patient name: |
| DOB: |
| MR/Chart #: |

GODFREY REGIONAL OUTPATIENT CLINIC
3122 Shannon Avenue • Aldon, FL 77712 • (407) 555-7654

Codes: _____

5.

PROGRESS NOTE

Date:	Vital signs:	T	R
Chief complaint:		P	BP

34-year-old female presents for extremely anxious feelings. Reports that she takes Solumedrol for her asthma and accidentally took twice the normal dosage recommended and prescribed. She has had asthma since the age of 8 and uses Solumedrol and inhaler therapy to keep her asthma under control.

Examination:

Anxious appearing 34-year-old female who appears in no acute distress. Her breathing is rapid, however, her lungs are clear and her asthma appears to be well-controlled at this time. HEENT normal. Vital signs are stable. PERRLA, neck, soft. Abdomen, soft and nontender. Heart, regular rate and rhythm.

Impression:

Accidental overdose of Solumedrol
Asthma, under control

Plan:

Patient is cautioned about adhering to the correct dosages for her medications and not to overdose even when her asthma is not well-controlled. She should seek medical attention when her medications are not controlling her asthma rather than taking additional dosages.

Stony Knutt, MD

	Patient name:
	DOB:
	MR/Chart #:

GODFREY REGIONAL OUTPATIENT CLINIC
3122 Shannon Avenue • Aldon, FL 77712 • (407) 555-7654

Codes: _____

6.

EMERGENCY ROOM RECORD

Name:		Age:	ER physician:
		DOB:	

Allergies/type of reaction:	Usual medications/dosages:

Triage/presenting complaint:	24-year-old male presents to the ER via ambulance in a non-responsive state. He is accompanied by friends who indicate he had been drinking this evening, several beers and a few mixed drinks. He returned home, and was unable to sleep, so he took some prescribed Valium to sleep.

Initial assessment:

Time	T	P	R	BP	Other:					

Medication orders:

Lab work:

X-Ray:

Physician's report:

24-year-old male who presents in a non-arousable state after ingesting alcohol and prescription sleeping medications. Pulse is rapid and irregular, BP 80/60. Patient is intubated and his stomach contents lavaged. Following treatment, the patient became arousable, began to improve and his pulse became regular, his BP stabilized to 120/80 over a period of approximately 4 hours in the ER.

Diagnosis:	Physician sign/date
ASSESSMENT: Adverse reaction to alcohol and prescription sleeping aids PLAN: Patient will be discharged with follow-up to an outpatient alcohol treatment facility as he indicates he is binge drinking on a fairly regular basis, at least 2–3 times weekly.	*Nancy Caulley* MD

Discharge	Transfer	Admit	Good	Satisfactory	Other:

GODFREY REGIONAL HOSPITAL
123 Main Street • Aldon, FL 77714 • (407) 555-1234

Codes: _____

6

CODING SPECIAL COMPLEXITIES

CODING REFERENCE TOOLS

Tool 20
Pregnancy/Postpartum Coding Guidelines
Tool 21
Guidelines for Coding Trauma/Injuries
Tool 22
Injury/Trauma/Burn Index
Tool 23
Injury/Trauma Coding Matrix

KEY TERMS

Alcohol Abuse, 151
Alcohol Dependence, 151
Closed Fracture, 163
Compression Fracture, 163

First-Degree Burn, 166
IDDM, 148
Myocardial Infarction, 153
NIDDM, 148
Normal Delivery, 158
Open Fracture, 163
Rule of Nines, 166
Second-Degree Burn, 166
Third-Degree Burn, 166
Type I Diabetes, 148
Type II Diabetes, 148

There are several areas of diagnostic coding that require special attention because they are complex. Because special circumstances surround each of these areas, each is addressed individually. Some of these areas, such as drugs and chemicals, hypertension, and neoplasms, are presented in table format in the ICD-9-CM book and are discussed in Chapter 5. This chapter deals with other ICD-9-CM diagnostic coding complexities, which are presented by system in the order they appear in the ICD-9-CM code book.

DOCUMENTATION GUIDELINES FOR CODING COMPLEXITIES

Guidelines for coding medical complexities vary from one section to another within the ICD-9-CM code book. Documentation drives the coding process and specific diagnoses can only be used when supporting documentation is present in the medical record. In many instances, when specific documentation does not exist, it is necessary to use an unspecified code.

The coder should keep in mind that, as mentioned at the beginning of ICD-9-CM coding, part of her or his responsibility is to educate. It is important that the coder not simply assign the unspecified code, but educate the provider on the appropriate information needed to code the diagnosis to the highest level of specificity.

INFECTIOUS AND PARASITIC DISEASES (CODES 001-139)

When codes are assigned for infectious and parasitic diseases, the medical record must be reviewed for body site, severity of disease (acute compared with chronic), the specific organism involved (unspecified if unknown), cause of the infection (if known), and any associated signs and symptoms.

In Chapter 1 of the ICD-9-CM book (Infectious and Parasitic Diseases), many conditions are covered by one combination code that identifies both the condition and the specific organism. Consider the following examples:

034.0	Streptococcal sore throat
038.2	Pneumococcal septicemia

Many conditions in this section, however, require two codes: one to describe the condition and the other to describe the organism.

599.0	Urinary tract infection
041.4	*E coli*

In Chapter 1 (Infectious and Parasitic Diseases), the following conditions can be located:

Infectious Gastroenteritis (003-008). Inflammation of the gastrointestinal (GI) tract caused by different organisms such as bacteria, viruses, or parasites.

Tuberculosis (010-018). Acute or chronic infection resulting from *Mycobacterium tuberculosis*. The fifth digit for tuberculosis (TB) is determined by the method used for confirming this disease as in the following examples:

0	unknown
1	bacteriological/histological examination

Codes from the Nonspecific Abnormal Findings section of ICD-9-CM are used when the condition is only reported as an abnormal finding rather than confirmation of the TB bacteria.

795.5	Positive PPD Test, without Diagnosis of TB

Streptococcal Sore Throat (034). Infection from beta hemolytic *Streptococci* organism; the following conditions are assigned codes from the 034 series of the Infectious/Parasitic Disease category:

Streptococcal pharyngitis
Streptococcal laryngitis
Streptococcal tonsillitis
Septic sore throat

Septicemia (038). Defined as the entrance of bacterial into the bloodsteam; extreme caution should be taken in the assignment of these codes. Infection alone does not constitute septicemia, and these codes should only be used when the record indicates clinical evidence of this condition.

Meningitis (036). This code is for meningitis caused by bacterial infections. Codes from the 321 series, meningitis due to other organisms, should be assigned if the causal agent is other than bacteria.

HIV (042). Care should be taken in the assignment of the Human Immunodeficiency Virus code. Category 042 includes the following:

Human immunodeficiency virus
AIDS-related complex
Symptomatic HIV infection

V codes (V08) should be used for asymptomatic HIV virus infection and in patients with HIV infection without any HIV-related illness.

Childhood Communicable Disease (052-056). Examples include the following:

052   Varicella, commonly known as chickenpox
055   Measles
056   Rubella, commonly known as German measles

Herpes (053-054). Herpes zoster (053), known as shingles, is caused by the varicella zoster virus. Herpes simplex (054) is a recurrent viral infection resulting from the herpes virus hominis.

Viral Hepatitis (070). There are five forms of hepatitis in this category:

Type A (HAC)
Type B (HBV)
Type C (HCV)
Type D (HDV-delta)
Type E (HEV)

Sexually Transmitted Diseases (090-099). Diseases from this section are also known as venereal diseases and are usually spread through sexual intercourse or genital contact. Some examples are the following:

Syphilis
Gonorrhea
Chlamydia

SPECIFIC DOCUMENTATION ISSUES

Caution should be taken in the assignment of infectious and parasitic disease codes to observe the appropriate order for code assignment. The coder must keep in mind the primary guideline discussed in general ICD-9-CM coding guidelines—assign the chief reason for the encounter. If the infectious or parasitic disease is not the chief reason for the encounter, it would not be coded first. Consider the following examples:

Patient presents 24 weeks pregnant with complaints of sore throat, fever, and chills.

Laboratory tests reveal streptococcal sore throat.

Coding would be as follows:

647.61   Other viral/parasitic disease in pregnancy complicating pregnancy
034.0   Streptococcal sore throat

Patient with AIDS seen by physician for acute lower abdominal pain.

Studies reveal acute cholecystitis.

Coding would be as follows:

575.0   Acute cholecystitis
042   AIDS

STOP AND PRACTICE

Assign ICD-9-CM code(s) as appropriate for the following exercises:

                                     ICD-9-CM Code(s)

1. Poliomyelitis   _____
2. Acute streptococcal pharyngitis _____
3. Viral hepatitis, Type C   _____
4. Gastroenteritis due to *Salmonella* infection _____
5. Gastroenteritis, probably viral _____
6. Varicella _____
7. Pneumonia due to *E. coli* _____
8. Encephalitis due to malaria _____
9. Bacterial meningitis _____
10. Asymptomatic HIV infection _____

NEOPLASMS (CODES 140-239)

Neoplasms are discussed in Chapter 5 because these codes are presented in ICD-9-CM in a table format.

ENDOCRINE, NUTRITIONAL, AND METABOLIC DISEASES, AND IMMUNITY DISORDERS (CODES 240-279)

The most common and perhaps complicated diagnostic coding from this section involves the correct assignment of codes for diabetes mellitus. Diabetes is classified by a fifth digit that indicates the type of diabetes and whether the current status of diabetes is controlled or uncontrolled. The fifth digits for diabetes are as follows:

0   **Type II (Non–Insulin-Dependent) NIDDM, Adult-Onset Type, or Unspecified type, not stated as uncontrolled**
1   **Type I (Insulin-Dependent) IDDM, Juvenile Type, not stated as Uncontrolled**
2   **Type II (Non–Insulin-Dependent) NIDDM, Adult-Onset Type, or Unspecified type, uncontrolled**
3   **Type I (Insulin-Dependent) IDDM, Juvenile Type, uncontrolled**

When patients with diabetes receive insulin during hospitalization, it should NOT be assumed that the patient is insulin dependent. It is not unusual for patients with Type II diabetes to require short-term administration of insulin for regulation of diabetes.

Many complications occur as sequelae of diabetes mellitus. Acute metabolic changes arise but do not require assignment of an additional code. When conditions occur in other body areas or organ systems as the result of diabetes, two codes are required: one for the diabetic complication and one for the manifestation. Subcategories for these conditions are as follows:

250.1x   Diabetes with ketoacidosis
250.2x   Diabetes with hyperosmolarity
250.3x   Diabetes with other coma
250.4x   Diabetes with renal manifestations
250.5x   Diabetes with ophthalmic manifestations
250.6x   Diabetes with neurological manifestations
250.7x   Diabetes with peripheral circulatory disorders
250.8x   Diabetes with other specified manifestations
250.9x   Diabetes with unspecified complications

Further explanation of some of the most common complications follows. Fifth digits are required.

DIABETES WITH KETOACIDOSIS (250.1x)

Diabetic ketoacidosis occurs because of lack of insulin. Most often, this condition occurs in patients with insulin-dependent diabetes. For that reason, code 250.11 should be assigned unless the medical documentation specifically states NIDDM (non–insulin-dependent diabetes mellitus).

DIABETES WITH RENAL MANIFESTATIONS (250.4x)

Conditions related to the kidneys are coded with 250.4x, as well as a manifestation code of 583.81 (nephritis and nephropathy, not specified as acute or chronic, in diseases classified elsewhere). When the renal condition has progressed to reported chronic renal failure (CRF), codes 585.9 (chronic renal failure) and 250.4x would be assigned. It is not necessary to assign the additional code of 583.81.

DIABETES WITH OPHTHALMIC MANIFESTATIONS (250.5)

Another manifestation of diabetes is the development of diabetic cataract, also referred to as a *snowflake cataract*. Senile cataracts occur frequently in patients with diabetes but are not a result of the diabetic condition. Therefore a regular diabetes code, 250.0x, and a regular ICD-9-CM code for the cataract, such as 366.10, would be assigned.

DIABETIC FOOT ULCERS

Foot complications, most commonly foot ulcers, are a common complaint with diabetes. In many instances, these foot ulcers result from peripheral vascular disease. When documentation supports that the ulcer results from existing peripheral vascular disease, codes from 250.6 and 250.7 series are used. If documentation does not specify whether the ulcer is due to peripheral vascular disease, a code from the 250.8 series, other specified manifestations, is appropriate.

DIABETES AND PREGNANCY

Codes from the 600 series are assigned for conditions that arise or require treatment during pregnancy. Therefore the 250.0x codes would not apply during the antepartum and postpartum periods.

OTHER CONDITIONS

Hyperthyroidism and hypothyroidism are conditions listed in this section. Hypothyroidism is coded to category 244, whereas hyperthyroidism is categorized to 242. The most common form of hyperthyroidism is known as Graves' disease, characterized by goiter, weight loss, sweating, diarrhea, tremor, palpitations, and heat intolerance.

STOP AND PRACTICE

Assign ICD-9-CM code(s) as appropriate to the following exercises:

ICD-9-CM code(s)

1. Diabetes, NIDDM   _____
2. Diabetes, IDDM   _____
3. Hypothyroidism   _____
4. Hyperthyroidism   _____
5. Diabetes mellitus with hypoglycemic coma   _____

6. Iatrogenic hypothyroidism   _____
7. Hyperlipidemia   _____
8. Diabetic ophthalmic neuropathy _____
9. Diabetic nephritic syndrome   _____
10. Cystic fibrosis with pulmonary exacerbation _____

BLOOD, BLOOD-FORMING ORGANS (CODES 280-289)

Chapter 4 of ICD-9-CM contains codes related to blood and the blood-forming organs such as anemias, coagula-

tion defects, and other disorders associated with hemorrhage. The most common condition in this chapter is anemia, which has multiple causes. Anemia is defined as a decrease in red blood cell numbers, or the quantity of hemoglobin, or the volume of red cells contained in the blood.

Types of anemias contained in Chapter 4 include the following:

280-281	Deficiency Anemia
282-283	Hemolytic Anemia

284	Aplastic Anemia
285	Unspecified Anemia

STOP AND PRACTICE

Assign ICD-9-CM code(s) to the following exercises:

ICD-9-CM Code(s)

1. Iron deficiency anemia   _____
2. Iron deficiency anemia due to blood loss   _____
3. Sickle cell anemia   _____
4. Sickle cell anemia in crisis   _____

5. Screening for iron deficiency anemia   _____
6. Acquired aplastic anemia   _____
7. Atypical anemia   _____
8. Nutritional anemia   _____
9. Eosinophilia   _____
10. Chronic lymphadenitis   _____

MENTAL DISORDERS (CODES 290-319)

The types of mental disorders classified in this section are categorized in the following sections.

ORGANIC BRAIN SYNDROME

Organic brain syndrome (OBS) may be psychotic or nonpsychotic, depending on the level of distortion of reality. The symptoms associated with OBS are related to impaired cerebral function. Levels of OBS range from acute and reversible to chronic and irreversible and are considered when this disorder is coded. Keep in mind the same rules already learned for diagnostic coding. Only the documentation listed may be used for diagnostic coding purposes. If the provider does not document the specific type of OBS, a nonspecific code may be required.

Remember that caution should be used in assigning nonspecific codes because of their effect on reimbursement. As mentioned previously, unspecified or nonspecific codes may be reimbursed in some instances; however, insurance carriers are less likely to reimburse nonspecific diagnostic statements made by the specialist. For instance, should the family practitioner make the initial diagnosis of OBS, he or she quite possibly could be reimbursed for this diagnostic statement. In contrast, the psychiatrist, psychologist, and other professional specializing in the field of psychiatry would be expected to specify the level of this disorder.

When a provider in the psychiatry field does not specify this information, the coder should compile a list of diagnoses or diagnostic statements that will be acceptable for coding, billing, and reimbursement.

ALZHEIMER'S DISEASE

Alzheimer's disease is coded as 331.0. This disease is a progressive atrophic process that involves the degenera-tion of nerve cells. As the disease progresses, mental changes occur that range from mild or moderate intellectual deterioration to full-blown dementia.

Keep in mind that the patient with Alzheimer's disease is usually elderly and may be receiving treatment for several diseases. Alzheimer's disease must be documented as the confirmed disease process when this condition is coded. If the diagnosis has not been made, only signs, symptoms, or conditions such as dementia can be coded. Should the patient with Alzheimer's seek medical care for a laceration or illness, the chief reason for the encounter—not Alzheimer's disease—would be coded. In this case, Alzheimer's disease would be coded as a secondary diagnosis only if the condition is involved in the encounter.

METABOLIC ENCEPHALOPATHY

Metabolic encephalopathy is an altered state of consciousness. This disease process is often associated with delirium and may involve treatment by professionals other than psychiatrists, such as critical care specialists.

TRANSIENT GLOBAL AMNESIA

The diagnosis of transient global amnesia is not considered psychiatric and is therefore not coded as such. Code 437.7 is used for this condition, which may be the result of trauma, accident, or injury and usually only lasts for a few hours. Because this code is not considered psychiatric, the reimbursement guidelines followed by third-party carriers are the usual reimbursement guidelines rather than those subject to the limitations that a psychiatric diagnosis might have.

SCHIZOPHRENIC DISORDERS

Schizophrenic disorders are coded to category 295. The fourth and fifth digits for schizophrenic disorders delineate the type of schizophrenia and the level of the condition. Fifth digits for schizophrenic disorders are defined as follows:

0 unspecified
1 subchronic
2 chronic
3 subchronic with acute exacerbation
4 chronic with acute exacerbation
5 in remission

Most psychiatrists are aware of the specific level of coding necessary for psychiatric diagnoses. If the psychiatric providers do not use fifth digits other than unspecified, consider developing a tool for guidance. The coder may not be able to determine the level of the condition on the basis of review of the documentation. The provider should include this information in the diagnostic statement.

AFFECTIVE DISORDERS

Coded to category 296, affective disorders are characterized by mood changes that recur on a cyclical basis. The patient experiences "highs and lows" that vary from periods of deep depression to periods of elation.

Affective disorders are diagnosed when mood disorders are beyond the usual range of mood swings. If in addition to this cyclical mood disorder, the patient experiences manic and depressive periods, the disorder would be further diagnosed as circular or bipolar. The fifth digit for this category determines the level of the condition:

0 unspecified
1 mild
2 moderate
3 severe, without mention of psychotic behavior
4 severe, specified as with psychotic behavior
5 in partial or unspecified remission
6 in full remission

PSYCHOPHYSIOLOGICAL DISORDERS

This type of disorder arises from mental factors such as hyperventilation or paralysis and manifests itself with physiological malfunctions. Psychophysiological disorders are assigned code 306.

REACTIONS TO STRESS

Only acute and adjustment reactions to stress are categorized for this disorder. The psychiatric specialist must categorize the levels of reaction to stress. Code 308 is used for acute reactions to stress, and code 309 is used for adjustment reactions.

SUBSTANCE ABUSE DISORDERS

Probably the most common coding error made in this category is the coding of alcoholism, or **alcohol depen-**

dence, compared with alcohol abuse. In most cases, the confusion is the result of inadequate or incomplete documentation.

Alcoholism, or alcohol dependence, is seen in the patient who is dependent on alcohol and is unable to control the drinking process. As with all diagnostic codes, the physician or provider must place the patient within this category. The most common codes for this category are the following:

303.0 Alcohol Dependence Syndrome
303.0 Alcohol Dependence Syndrome, Acute Alcoholic Intoxication
303.0 Patient presents for care in an intoxicated state; specified by the provider or physician
303.9 Other and unspecified alcoholism

The other disorder, **alcohol abuse,** is defined as problem drinking that has not been documented as physical dependence. In many cases, the patient may, in fact, be alcohol dependent; however, the treating provider does not have sufficient history or documentation to state this diagnostically. Code 305.0 is used for alcohol abuse with the following fifth digit:

0 unspecified
1 continuous
2 episodic
3 in remission

As with the alcohol diagnostic codes, there is differentiation between drug dependence and drug abuse. Drug dependence is seen in those patients who are dependent on drugs and are unable to stop using drugs, as diagnostically stated by the physician. Drug abuse is coded for those patients who have a drug problem but in whom drug dependence has not been and cannot be diagnosed at the time of the specific encounter.

SUBSTANCE-RELATED PSYCHOSIS

Many patients in whom substance and alcohol abuse or dependence is diagnosed will have additional physical conditions or problems that include psychotic symptoms. Alcohol-related psychosis is coded to category 291; drug-related psychosis is coded to 292.

SPECIFIC DOCUMENTATION ISSUES

Care should be used in assigning diagnostic codes for psychiatric conditions. Keep in mind that the chief reason for the encounter or service should always be the primary diagnosis for each procedure or service provided.

When using diagnostic codes from the mental illness section (290-319) the coder must realize that the attachment of a mental disorder diagnosis will trigger third-party attention. Third-party reimbursement for mental disorders may be limited under many health insurance contracts. All services reported with a mental disorder diagnosis will be attached to the maximum amount per calendar year or contract period.

For example, when a patient presents with a problem of upper respiratory infection (URI) and mentions that he or she is depressed, unless the physician incorporates the depressive disorder diagnosis in the diagnostic statement, the depression should not be coded. In those instances when the physician actually treats the depression (e.g., by prescription or hospital orders) and includes this information in the diagnostic statement, the coder should include the appropriate mental disorder codes. The codes must be placed in the correct order. Remember that if the patient presents with URI and indicates depression, the chief reason for the encounter is the URI, with a secondary diagnosis of depression.

Keep the basic ICD-9-CM coding rules in mind; always code the chief reason for the encounter as primary. Mental disorder codes are treated no differently than other diagnostic codes.

The mere mention by the patient of a "depressed" feeling or state does not require coding for "depressive disorder" unless documented by the physician or provider. When the chief reason for the encounter is an injury that was inflicted because of a mental disorder, the chief reason for the encounter is the injury, followed by the mental disorder.

Psychiatric coding is a specialty all its own. In addition to the ICD-9-CM coding book, psychiatric practices typically use the DSM-IV book for diagnostic purposes.

The primary rules of coding apply to the patient with a psychiatric disorder: all encounters must be coded with the chief reason for that encounter, admission, or visit. In some instances, the visit will be for the evaluation and treatment of the mental disorder. In other instances, the patient will present for another problem, unassociated or perhaps associated, with the mental disorder and the problem would be coded as the principal diagnosis. The mental disorder or associated problem would be coded as a secondary or contributory diagnosis only if that disorder is also treated or is part of the clinical consideration for the presenting problem.

STOP AND PRACTICE

Code the following ICD-9-CM exercises for mental disorders:

	ICD-9-CM Code(s)
1. Severe manic disorder, recurrent	_____
2. Bipolar disorder, manic phase, mild	_____
3. Bipolar disorder, atypical	_____
4. Psychogenic paralysis	_____
5. Schizophrenia, subchronic	_____
6. Depression with anxiety, dependent personality	_____
7. Anxiety reaction	_____
8. Anxiety reaction manifested by tachycardia	_____
9. Psychotic depression reaction	_____
10. Aggressive personality, adjustment reaction	_____

NERVOUS SYSTEM AND SENSE ORGANS (CODES 320-389)

Codes from these chapters deal with diseases of the nervous system and sense organs. Subcategories for Chapter 6 of the ICD-9-CM code book include the following:

320-326	Inflammatory Diseases of the Central Nervous System
330-337	Hereditary and Degenerative Diseases of the Central Nervous System
340-349	Other Disorders of the Central Nervous System
350-359	Disorders of the Peripheral Nervous System
360-379	Diseases of the Eye and Adnexa
380-389	Diseases of the Ear and Mastoid Process

NERVOUS SYSTEM

The nervous system, which is composed of the central (brain and spinal cord) and peripheral nervous systems, is covered in Chapter 6 of ICD-9-CM. One of the most common conditions in this section would probably be epilepsy, defined as any disorder or condition characterized by recurrent seizures. The assignment of code(s) for epilepsy would include one of the following fifth digit categories:

0   without mention of intractable epilepsy
1   with intractable epilepsy

Obviously, the statement of intractable epilepsy would need to be documented in the medical order for the fifth digit of "1" to be assigned.

SPECIFIC DOCUMENTATION ISSUES

Several types of epilepsy may be assigned codes such as grand mal and petit mal. None of the specific types of epilepsy may be assigned without the appropriate medical documentation.

Physicians may document terms such as "recurrent seizure" or "seizure disorder." It should not be assumed that either of these statements is intended to be coded as epilepsy unless documented by the physician.

SENSE ORGANS

The eyes and ears are categorized as sense organs and are included in Chapter 6 of ICD-9-CM. One of the most common disorders is cataract, an opacity of the lens of the eye or its capsule. Congenital cataracts are not included with other cataracts but are assigned codes from the 743 series because they are congenital anomalies. When specific documentation is not present as to the nature of the cataract, it is coded as 366.9, cataract, unspecified.

The ear is also considered a sensory organ and is also included in Chapter 6. Otitis media and otitis externa are both common conditions of the ear. Otitis media, or inflammation of the middle ear, is often categorized further as follows:

381.00	Acute nonsuppurative otitis media, unspecified
381.01	Chronic serous otitis media
381.10	Chronic serous otitis media, simple/unspecified
381.3	Other/unspecified chronic nonsuppurative otitis media
381.4	Nonsuppurative otitis media, not specified as acute/chronic
382.00	Acute suppurative otitis media w/out spontaneous rupture eardrum
382.01	Acute suppurative otitis media w/spontaneous rupture eardrum
382.3	Unspecified chronic suppurative otitis media
382.4	Unspecified suppurative otitis media
382.9	Unspecified otitis media

STOP AND PRACTICE

Assign the appropriate ICD-9-CM code(s) to the following exercises:

ICD-9-CM Code(s)

1. Otitis media, NOS _____
2. Chronic suppurative otitis media _____
3. Senile cataract _____
4. Cataract, NOS _____
5. Migraine headache _____
6. Trigeminal neuralgia _____
7. Parkinson's disease _____
8. Bell's palsy _____
9. Congenital hereditary muscular dystrophy _____
10. Reflex sympathetic dystrophy _____

CIRCULATORY SYSTEM (CODES 390-459)

Chapter 7 includes codes for the cardiovascular or circulatory system. Subcategories for this section include the following:

390-392	Acute Rheumatic Fever
393-398	Chronic Rheumatic Heart Disease
401-405	Hypertensive Disease
410-414	Ischemic Heart Disease
415-417	Diseases of Pulmonary Circulation
420-429	Other Forms of Heart Disease
430-438	Cerebrovascular Diseases
440-448	Diseases of Arteries, Arterioles, Capillaries
451-459	Diseases of Veins, Lymphatics, Other Diseases of Circulatory System

Hypertension is included in diseases of the circulatory system. Because the codes are provided in table format in the ICD-9-CM book, coding of this disorder is discussed in Chapter 5 of this book.

Rheumatic fever typically occurs after a streptococcal infection such as a sore throat. It is included in the circulatory system section because of the possibility for collateral heart damage. Rheumatic fever can recur, so categories are included for acute rheumatic fever and chronic rheumatic heart disease.

Ischemic heart disease, also known as *arteriosclerotic heart disease* or *coronary artery disease,* is also included in Chapter 7. Three forms of heart disease are classified under ischemic heart disease: angina, chronic ischemic heart disease, and **myocardial infarction** (MI).

MI is the sudden inadequate flow of blood to the heart. Code 410 is assigned for the diagnosis of MI with a fourth digit describing the specific location as follows:

0   anterolateral wall
1   other anterior wall
2   inferolateral wall
3   inferoposterior wall
4   other inferior wall
5   other lateral wall
6   true posterior wall
7   subendocardial infarction
8   other specific site(s)
9   unspecified site(s)

Fifth digits are assigned based on the episode of care as follows:

0   episode of care unspecified
1   initial episode of care—newly diagnosed MI without regard to the number of times the patient is seen/transferred
2   subsequent episode of care—following the initial episode of care that patient is seen or admitted

for additional care or observation for the previously diagnosed MI within an 8-week period

CHRONIC ISCHEMIC HEART DISEASE

Both arteriosclerosis and atherosclerosis are the narrowing of the arterial wall by the deposit of plaque. This condition is the major cause of ischemia and is reported as 414.0 with the following fifth digit(s):

0   unspecified type of vessel
1   native coronary artery
2   autologous vein bypass graft
3   nonautologous biological bypass graft
4   artery bypass graft
5   unspecified type of graft

If medical documentation does not reflect that the disease presents in a native vessel or graft, the fifth digit "0" should be assigned.

CARDIAC DYSRHYTHMIAS

Cardiac dysrhythmias are defined as disturbances in the electrical activity of the heart muscle. When additional information regarding the nature of the disturbance is not available, code 427.9 would be assigned. Specific cardiac dysrhythmias include the following:

427.31   Atrial fibrillation
427.32   Atrial flutter
427.41   Ventricular fibrillation
427.0   Paroxysmal supraventricular tachycardia
427.81   Sick sinus syndrome
426.11   First-degree heart block
426.12   Second-degree heart block, Type I
426.13   Second-degree heart block, Type II
426.0   Third-degree heart block

CEREBROVASCULAR DISEASE

Any condition that pertains to the blood vessels or blood flow to the brain is classified in the cerebrovascular disease section. The 430 series of ICD-9-CM covers codes for cerebrovascular diseases and identifies specific conditions. Subcategories are as follows:

430   Subarachnoid hemorrhage
431   Intracerebral hemorrhage
432   Other/unspecific intracranial hemorrhage
433   Occlusion/stenosis of precerebral arteries
434   Occlusion, cerebral arteries
435   Transient cerebral ischemia
436   Acute, ill-defined, cerebrovascular disease
437   Other, ill-defined, cerebrovascular disease
438   Late effects of cerebrovascular disease

Make certain that when fourth and fifth digits are necessary, for instance with codes 433 and 434, that the additional digits are assigned appropriately.

PHLEBITIS AND THROMBOPHLEBITIS

Phlebitis, or inflammation of the vessels, leads to thrombophlebitis or thrombus formation in the deep or superficial veins. Category 451 is assigned for these conditions, with additional digits to classify the specific vessel(s) or site(s) involved.

SPECIFIC DOCUMENTATION ISSUES

Documentation issues associated with hypertension are discussed in Chapter 5. Those codes are presented in table format.

MI should always be coded with a five-digit ICD-9-CM diagnostic code that identifies both the site and the episode of care. In the outpatient setting, the fifth digit will typically be assigned as "2."

STOP AND PRACTICE

Assign the appropriate ICD-9-CM diagnostic code(s) to the following exercises:

		ICD-9-CM Code(s)
1.	Mitral valve stenosis	_____
2.	Old MI	_____
3.	Myocardial infarction NOS	_____
4.	Congestive heart failure	_____
5.	Thrombophlebitis, deep femoral vein	_____
6.	CVA	_____
7.	Arteriosclerosis	_____
8.	Unstable angina	_____
9.	Cardiomegaly	_____
10.	Atrioventricular block, first degree	_____

DISEASES OF THE RESPIRATORY SYSTEM

Chapter 8 covers infections and other diseases associated with the respiratory system. A brief review of the codes is provided here.

BRONCHITIS

Bronchitis, or inflammation of the bronchi, can be classified as either acute or chronic. Acute bronchitis, coded to 455.0, includes the following:

- Acute tracheobronchitis
- Viral bronchitis

- Pneumococcal bronchitis
- Membranous bronchitis
- Septic bronchitis

CHRONIC OBSTRUCTIVE PULMONARY DISEASE

Coded to 496 when no further specification is available, chronic obstructive pulmonary disease (COPD) associated with other respiratory conditions is assigned codes as follows:

491.20	Obstructive chronic bronchitis without acute exacerbation
	Chronic asthmatic bronchitis
	Emphysema with chronic bronchitis
491.21	Chronic obstructive bronchitis with acute exacerbation
	Acute exacerbation of COPD
	Acute bronchitis with COPD
	Acute and chronic obstructive bronchitis
	Chronic asthmatic bronchitis with acute exacerbation
	Emphysema with acute and chronic bronchitis
492.8	COPD with emphysema
493.2x	COPD with asthma

PNEUMONIA

Specific codes for pneumonia, or inflammation of the lung, are assigned according to the underlying cause (e.g., bacterial or viral).

Viral pneumonia (category 480) is further divided based on the identity of the virus.

Pneumococcal pneumonia (category 481) is used when pneumonia results from pneumococcal bacteria. Category 482 is used for other bacterial infections that cause pneumonia. When pneumonia is a secondary diagnosis to an infectious disease process, the underlying disease code and a code from category 484 are assigned. When the record lacks identification of a specific organism, 485, pneumonia, organism unspecified would be assigned.

ASTHMA

When the condition *reactive airway disease* is documented, the diagnosis of asthma would be appropriate. Specific types of asthma are assigned a fourth digit as follows:

0	Extrinsic asthma
1	Intrinsic asthma
2	Chronic obstructive asthma
3	Unspecified

A required fifth digit classification, indicating whether the patient was in status asthmaticus, would be assigned as follows:

0	without mention of status asthmaticus
1	with mention of status asthmaticus
2	with acute exacerbation

STOP AND PRACTICE

Assign ICD-9-CM diagnostic code(s) as appropriate to the following exercises:

ICD-9-CM Code(s)

1. Tonsil hypertrophy _____
2. Pneumonia, NOS _____
3. Viral pneumonia _____
4. Chronic respiratory failure _____
5. Asthma _____
6. ARDS _____
7. COPD with bronchitis _____
8. URI _____
9. Lower respiratory infection _____
10. Sinusitis _____

DISEASES OF THE DIGESTIVE SYSTEM

The category of digestive diseases is subdivided as follows:

520-529	Diseases of the Oral Cavity, Salivary Glands, Jaws
530-537	Diseases of the Esophagus, Stomach, and Duodenum
540-543	Appendicitis
550-553	Hernia of the Abdominal Cavity
555-558	Noninfectious Enteritis and Colitis
450-569	Other Diseases of the Intestine and Peritoneum
570-579	Other Digestive Diseases

The following diseases are classified within the digestive disease section.

GASTROINTESTINAL ULCERS

Ulcers are further classified as inflammatory or necrotic. The specific location of the ulcers, (e.g., gastric, duodenal, peptic, or gastrojejunal) should also be given.

HERNIAS

There are numerous types of hernias assigned codes from the digestive disease section of ICD-9-CM. The appropriate codes are assigned based on the following:

- Location of hernia (e.g., inguinal, umbilical, hiatal)
- Severity (unspecified, strangulated, incarcerated)

GASTROENTERITIS

Gastroenteritis, or inflammation of the stomach, small intestine, and colon, may be caused by a number of factors. Codes are based on the nature of the inflammation as follows:

003.0   Due to *Salmonella* infections
005.9   Food poisoning
008.8   Viral gastroenteritis NEC

009.0   Infectious gastroenteritis
556.9   Ulcerative colitis
558.3   Allergic gastroenteritis and colitis
558.9   Other/unspecified noninfectious gastroenteritis

CHOLECYSTITIS AND CHOLELITHIASIS

Cholecystitis, or inflammation of the gall bladder, is assigned codes from the 575 series of ICD-9-CM. When stones are also involved, codes from the 574 series are assigned as a combination code for this disorder.

APPENDICITIS

Inflammation of the appendix, or appendicitis, is classified to the 540 series of ICD-9-CM. Additional digits are assigned for complications such as perforation, abscess, and peritonitis.

STOP AND PRACTICE

Assign ICD-9-CM diagnostic code(s) as appropriate for the following exercises:

ICD-9-CM Code(s)

1. Inguinal hernia   _____
2. Gastroenteritis, probably viral   _____
3. Nausea and vomiting with
   gastroenteritis   _____
4. Recurrent inguinal hernia, with
   strangulation   _____

5. Reflux esophagitis   _____
6. Acute pancreatitis   _____
7. Acute cholecystitis with
   cholelithiasis   _____
8. Hematemesis   _____
9. GI hemorrhage   _____
10. Anal fistula   _____

DISEASES OF THE GENITOURINARY SYSTEM

Diseases of the genitourinary system include the following:

580-589   Nephritis, Nephrotic Syndrome, and Other Kidney Diseases
590-599   Diseases of the Urinary System
600-608   Diseases of the Male Genital Organs
610-611   Breast Disorders
614-616   Female Pelvic Organ Inflammatory Diseases
617-629   Other Disorders of the Female Genital Tract

Listings in this section of ICD-9-CM include diseases and disorders of the urinary, female, and male systems. Some of the diseases included in this section are listed in the following paragraphs.

CHRONIC RENAL FAILURE

Usually the result of progressive loss of renal function, CRF is assigned code 585.9. This is one of the few codes

in ICD-9-CM that does not require five digits. Additional ICD-9-CM codes may be required for additional complications or manifestations that often occur with CRF.

Care should be taken to assign CRF only when appropriate. Acute (series 584) should be assigned when documentation does not support the use of CRF.

URINARY TRACT DISORDERS

Disorders of the urinary tract can include pyelonephritis (590.xx series), cystitis (595.xx series), calculus of the urinary system (592.x-594.x series), and urinary tract infection (599.x). Pyelonephritis usually involves an infection that moves from the lower urinary tract into the kidneys. Cystitis involves infection or inflammation of the urinary bladder and ureters. The fourth digit assigned for cystitis identifies the type, severity, and location of the infection:

0   Acute
1   Chronic interstitial
2   Other chronic
3   Trigonitis
4   Cystitis in diseases classified elsewhere

8   Other specified types
9   Unspecified

When a specific organism is identified, code(s) from the Infectious and Parasitic Disease section should also be assigned. Consider the following example:

UTI due to *E. coli*
Urinary tract infection   599.0
E. coli   041.4

Calculi are stones that form in the kidney, ureter, or bladder. Fourth digits are assigned based on the location as follows:

592.0   Kidney
592.1   Ureter
592.9   Urinary calculus, unspecified
594.0   Diverticulum of bladder
594.1   Other calculus of bladder
594.2   Urethra
594.8   Other lower urinary tract
594.9   Lower urinary tract, unspecified

SYMPTOMS OF THE URINARY TRACT

In many instances, signs and symptoms of the urinary tract are often reported when a specified diagnosis has not been determined at the conclusion of the encounter. Consider the following examples:

599.7   Hematuria
788.20-788.29   Urinary retention
788.1   Urinary dysuria
788.3   Urinary incontinence
788.41   Urinary frequency
788.42   Polyuria
788.43   Nocturia
788.5   Oliguria

HYPERPLASIA OF THE PROSTATE

Code 600, hyperplasia of the prostate, includes a number of forms of prostatic enlargement such as the following:

600.0   Benign hypertrophy
600.1   Nodular prostate
600.2   Benign localized hyperplasia
600.3   Cyst
600.9   Unspecified hyperplasia

BREAST DISORDERS

Those breast disorders that are not defined as neoplasms are listed in categories 610 and 611 of the genitourinary system. Examples would include the following:

- Inflammatory diseases of the breast
- Hypertrophy of the breast
- Lump/mass in breast
- Fibroadenosis
- Fibrosclerosis
- Mastodynia

INFLAMMATORY DISEASE OF THE FEMALE PELVIC ORGANS

Codes from 614 through 616 are assigned for inflammatory diseases of the female pelvic organs. An additional code is assigned when the organism causing the inflammation is identified. Consider the following example:

Acute inflammatory uterine infection due to streptococcal infection

615.0   Acute inflammatory uterine infection
041.00   Unspecified streptococcal infection

GYNECOLOGICAL DISORDERS NOT RELATED TO REPRODUCTION

Codes from 616 through 626 are assigned for gynecological disorders not related to reproduction. Examples from this section would include the following:

617.x   Endometriosis
616.0   Cervicitis
618.x   Genital prolapse
622.1   Cervical dysplasia
620.x   Ovarian cyst
626.x   Disorders of menstruation/abnormal bleeding

STOP AND PRACTICE

Assign ICD-9-CM diagnostic code(s) to the following exercises:

ICD-9-CM Code(s)

1. Hematuria   _____
2. Acute renal failure   _____
3. Amenorrhea   _____
4. Polycystic kidney disease

5. Interstitial cystitis   _____
6. Endometriosis, ovaries   _____
7. Breast mass   _____
8. Acute prostatitis   _____
9. Benign hypertrophy of the
   prostate   _____
10. Ureter calculus   _____

COMPLICATIONS OF PREGNANCY, CHILDBIRTH, AND THE PUERPERIUM

Conditions usually classified elsewhere that complicate the obstetrical condition are listed in Chapter 11 of ICD-9-CM. Conditions that occur during pregnancy are assumed to arise as the result or as a complication of pregnancy unless otherwise specified by the provider. This guideline differs from instances other than pregnancy because in those cases, the coder will assign the least significant service or diagnosis codes when documentation does not clarify otherwise.

When the provider indicates that the obstetrical condition is coincidental, the diagnosis code of V22.2, pregnancy state, incidental, will be used after the primary diagnoses are coded.

Codes from Chapter 11 of the ICD-9-CM book take priority over codes from other sections. Codes from other chapters may be listed as additional codes only when necessary or when they add to the diagnostic statement for the encounter.

Codes from Chapter 11 of the coding book are subdivided into the following categories:

640-648	Complications Related Mainly to Pregnancy
650-659	Normal Delivery; Other Indications for Care in Pregnancy, Labor, and Delivery
660-669	Complications Occurring Mainly During the Course of Pregnancy
670-677	Complications of Puerperium

These codes are used for the period that begins with conception and ends 6 weeks after delivery.

Fourth digits for this section typically provide additional information regarding complications that have occurred during the specified pregnancy period. The fifth digit contains information specific to the episode of care, as indicated in the following list:

1 delivered, with or without mention of antepartum condition

2 delivered, with mention of postpartum complication

3 antepartum condition or complication, not delivered

4 postpartum condition or complication, delivery occurred during previous episode of care

Make certain that the fifth digit chosen for the pregnancy condition is allowed for the diagnosis selected. Some diagnostic codes in this section typically take place during a specific period only, such as postpartum hemorrhage.

Tool 20 provides a decision tree for determining the appropriate diagnosis to be used in pregnancy and postpartum coding. This tool, which will assist the coder in assignment of numerical as well as V codes, will prove invaluable for the specialty coder in Ob/Gyn.

OTHER MATERNITY CODING ISSUES

Normal Delivery

Code 650 is used for coding an admission and the subsequent delivery of a baby. This code is used only when the entire delivery is normal and yields a single liveborn outcome. Code 650 cannot be used with any other code from the categories 630 through 677; these codes indicate other than completely normal deliveries.

Conditions that existed during the pregnancy but are not present during the delivery admission would not be coded. Code 650, **normal delivery,** could still be used as long as there were no other complications.

For code 650 to be used, all the following conditions must be met:

- Presentation must be head/occipital.
- Abnormalities during labor and/or delivery cannot exist.
- Complications of the antepartum period cannot be present at the time of the delivery admission.
- Single live birth can be the only delivery. Multiple births or stillbirth cannot be coded as 650.
- No obstetrical procedures can be performed other than episiotomy, amniotomy, manually assisted delivery, fetal monitoring, or sterilization.

Fetal Abnormality Affecting Management of the Mother

Codes from the 655 section may be used only when the condition of the fetus is responsible for affecting the usual obstetrical care of the mother. If no change is made in the mother's care, the codes from this section should not be used.

When conditions in other sections of ICD-9-CM complicate pregnancy, childbirth, or puerperium, they are coded from Chapter 11.

Preexisting hypertension is considered a complication of pregnancy, childbirth, and puerperium. Coding is changed from the 400 series hypertension codes to category 642 as follows:

642.00-642.04	Benign essential hypertension
642.10-642.14	Hypertension secondary to renal disease
642.20-642.24	Other preexisting hypertension

Other complications of hypertension may develop during pregnancy such as eclampsia or preeclampsia. When this condition arises, it is coded based on the preexistence of hypertension before the pregnancy.

642.4-642.6	Without preexisting hypertension
642.7x	With preexisting hypertension

As with the coding of hypertension in the nonpregnant patient, hypertension in the pregnant patient may be coded only when the diagnosis has been made.

T O O L   20

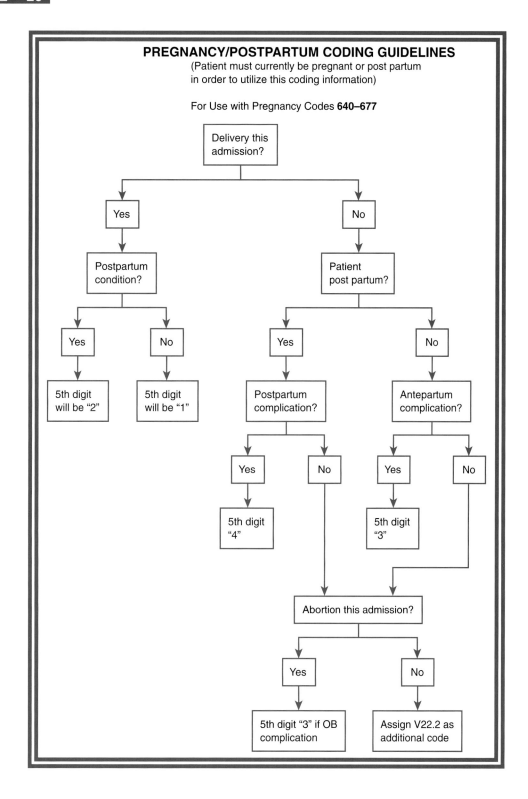

PREGNANCY/POSTPARTUM CODING GUIDELINES
(Patient must currently be pregnant or post partum
in order to utilize this coding information)

For Use with Pregnancy Codes **640–677**

Elevated blood pressure or abnormal findings alone do not constitute justification for coding hypertension in the pregnant or nonpregnant patient.

Postpartum Conditions and Complications

Postpartum conditions and complications are defined as problems arising during the 6-week postpartum period. Should the condition occur during the delivery admission, the fifth digit "2" is assigned. Fifth-digit "4" identifies those complications occurring after discharge and during the postpartum period.

Outcome of Delivery

V27 codes should be assigned to designate the delivery consequences (e.g., single liveborn) and therefore would be coded only to the mother's diagnostic statement.

Sterilization

Typically, the coder tries to avoid the use of a V code as a primary diagnostic code; however, when sterilization is coded, category V25 is appropriate. Although the service for the delivery may indicate the code 650, normal delivery, and V27.0, single liveborn, the service for sterilization has a different primary diagnosis. This series of V25 codes may be used as primary or secondary diagnoses when appropriate. The hospital will code the previous case as follows:

650   Primary Diagnosis for Admission
V27.0   Single Liveborn
V25.2   Sterilization

STOP AND PRACTICE

Code the following maternity cases:

ICD-9-CM Code(s)

1. Hypertension in pregnancy _____
2. Preeclampsia, delivered _____
3. Cephalopelvic disproportion _____
4. Fetal distress, delivered _____
5. Uterine fibroids, pregnant _____
6. Poor fetal growth _____
7. Post dates, delivered _____
8. Premature rupture of membranes, not delivered _____
9. Retention of placenta, postpartum _____
10. False labor, not delivered _____

DISEASES OF THE SKIN AND SUBCUTANEOUS TISSUE

Chapter 12 of the ICD-9-CM book describes conditions of the skin, hair, and nails, all components of the integumentary system. Inflammation is perhaps the most common problem with the skin and subcutaneous tissue. This may take the form of cellulitis, an acute localized inflammation of superficial tissue, or dermatitis, an inflammation of the skin. Codes for cellulitis are assigned on the basis of the location of the infection (e.g., arm [682.3], breast [611.0], cervix [616.0], eyelid [373.13], neck [682.1]). When a specific organism is involved, an additional code(s) should be assigned to identify the causal pathogen as well.

Chronic ulcers of the skin are assigned codes from the 707 category. Decubitus ulcers, or ulcerations due to prolonged pressure such as a bedsore, are assigned to code 707.0 without regard to the site involved.

STOP AND PRACTICE

Assign ICD-9-CM diagnostic code(s) to the following exercises:

ICD-9-CM Code(s)

1. Cellulitis, arm _____
2. Allergic urticaria _____
3. Ingrown toenail _____
4. Decubitus ulcer _____
5. Contact dermatitis due to perfume _____
6. Abscess of the arm _____
7. Impetigo _____
8. Pilonidal cyst _____
9. Psoriasis _____
10. Keloid scar _____

DISEASES OF THE MUSCULOSKELETAL SYSTEM

Chapter 13 of the ICD-9-CM covers diseases of the musculoskeletal system. Injuries to the musculoskeletal system, including fractures, open wounds (lacerations), contusions, abrasions, sprains, and dislocations, are covered in Chapter 17 (Injuries, Poisonings, and Adverse Effects). Musculoskeletal injuries are covered later.

Subsections for Chapter 13 include the following:

710-719   Arthropathies and Related Disorders
720-724   Dorsopathies

725-729   Rheumatism, Excluding the Back
730-739   Osteopathies, Chondropathies, Acquired Musculoskeletal Deformities

Diseases and conditions of the musculoskeletal system are discussed in the following sections.

SYSTEMIC LUPUS ERYTHEMATOSUS

Systemic lupus erythematosus (SLE) is assigned to code 717.0. Because this disease is systemic, additional code(s) may be necessary for additional manifestations.

ARTHRITIS

The various types of arthritis are classified to the following codes:

711   Arthropathy associated with infections
712   Crystal arthropathies
713   Arthropathies associated with disorders classified elsewhere
714   Rheumatoid arthritis
715   Osteoarthrosis and associated disorders
716   Other/unspecified arthropathies

STOP AND PRACTICE

Assign appropriate ICD-9-CM diagnostic code(s) to the following:

                                    ICD-9-CM Code(s)

1. Dupuytren's contracture   _____
2. Acute osteomyelitis   _____
3. SLE   _____
4. Rheumatoid arthritis, hand   _____
5. Osteoarthritis, knee   _____
6. Pain, knee   _____
7. Fracture, vertebra, pathological _____
8. History of arthritis   _____
9. Nonunion of femur fracture   _____
10. Chondromalacia, knee   _____

CONGENITAL ANOMALIES AND CERTAIN CONDITIONS ORIGINATING IN THE PERINATAL PERIOD

The perinatal period begins at birth and lasts through the twenty-eighth day following birth. Congenital abnormalities are present at, and exist from, the time of birth. An appropriate code from the 740-759 series of ICD-9-CM should be assigned for each of these conditions. When the condition presents itself during the admission when the child is born, the congenital anomaly code(s) would be assigned in addition to the primary diagnosis of V30-V39, Liveborn Infants categorization.

Liveborn female infant born with spina bifida at the hospital

V30.00   Liveborn infant born at hospital
741.0   Unspecified spina bifida

Specific conditions contained in this section include the following.

OTHER JOINT DISORDERS

Category 719 covers other or unspecified joint disorders such as:

719.0   Effusion of the joint
719.1   Hemarthrosis
719.2   Villonodular synovitis
719.3   Palindromic rheumatism
719.4   Pain in joint
719.5   Stiffness in joint
719.6   Symptoms referable to joint
719.7   Difficulty walking

ACQUIRED MUSCULOSKELETAL DEFORMITIES

Bone deformities acquired from fractures caused by disease, or from nonunion or malunion of a fracture are coded from this section.

Pathological fractures (733.1x) result from an existing disease process or occur spontaneously. Malunions, classified to 733.81, arise when fragments or ends of a fractured bone are not aligned and thereby heal improperly. Nonunion, the failure of fractured bone fragments or ends to unite is classified to 733.82.

SPINA BIFIDA

Spina bifida is defined as a defective or incomplete closure of the vertebral column. With the exception of spina bifida occulta, spina bifida is assigned as 741. Further digits describe the presence or absence of hydrocephalus and the site of the spina bifida. Other conditions, such as hydrocephalus, are commonly associated with spina bifida and are assigned additional codes accordingly.

CARDIAC DEFECTS/ABNORMALITIES

Congenital heart defects are categorized according to anomalies of the cardiac septal closure and of the heart. Category 745, cardiac septal closure anomalies, includes such common congenital disorders as the following:

745.1x   Transposition of great vessels
745.2   Tetralogy of Fallot
745.3   Ventricular septal defect

CLEFT LIP/CLEFT PALATE

Cleft lip and cleft palate are the two most common congenital anomalies of the upper body. Cleft palate is categorized to 749.0x; cleft lip is categorized to 749.1x. A combination code, 749.2x, is used for cleft lip and palate occurring together.

MATERNAL CAUSES OF PERINATAL MORBIDITY AND MORTALITY

When a medical condition or complication of pregnancy, labor, or delivery results in conditions that affect the newborn, codes from this section (760-763) should be assigned. If the condition does not cause adverse affects in the newborn, it is not necessary to assign codes. Consider the following example:

Mother consumes alcohol during pregnancy but child does not have any adverse effects.

Code only the liveborn infant code V30.00

For codes from these categories to be assigned, the condition(s) must develop at birth or within 28 days of birth. If a condition develops after this time, codes from the usual ICD-9-CM chapters would be used. Consider the following example:

3-month-old female has strep throat

034.0 Streptococcal sore throat

Note that no codes from this section (760-763) would be assigned because the condition did not develop within 28 days after birth.

SIGNS, SYMPTOMS, AND ILL-DEFINED CONDITIONS

When a specific diagnosis is not available at the conclusion of the encounter, code(s) from the signs, symptoms, and ill-defined conditions would be appropriate. Codes from this section are assigned in the following instances:

- No further diagnosis can be made at the conclusion of the encounter
- Signs/symptoms are transient and cannot be determined at the time of the encounter
- Patient is referred for further treatment/evaluation
- Signs/symptoms did not have the workup necessary to establish a definitive diagnosis at the conclusion of the encounter

The use of signs and symptoms is discussed in Chapter 2 (Determining Physician Diagnoses).

Codes from categories 790-796 (Nonspecific Abnormal Findings) are required for findings on laboratory, x-ray, and other diagnostic tests when the results are inconclusive and a definitive diagnosis cannot be made at the conclusion of the encounter. These codes should only be used when a diagnosis is not possible. In many cases, codes from this section are necessary to justify additional testing necessary to either rule out or diagnose a condition.

Codes from 797-799 (Ill-Defined and Unknown Causes of Morbidity and Mortality) are assigned when additional information is not available in the medical record. Consider the following examples:

799.1 Asphyxia
799.2 Respiratory Arrest
799.4 Cachexia

Codes from the Common Signs and Symptoms category are assigned to signs and symptoms that do not have a definitive diagnosis, and they do not represent a significant finding over and above the underlying cause or disease.

Examples of Common Signs and Symptoms would be the following:

780.2	Syncope
780.31-780.39	Convulsions/seizures
780.4	Dizziness and giddiness
782.0	Disturbance of skin sensation
784.7	Epistaxis
785.1	Palpitations
786.01	Hyperventilation
786.05	Shortness of breath
786.07	Wheezing
786.2	Cough
786.50	Chest pain, unspecified
787.0x	Nausea and vomiting
787.1	Heartburn
787.2	Dysphagia
787.91	Diarrhea
789.0x	Abdominal pain

STOP AND PRACTICE

Assign ICD-9-CM diagnostic code(s) to the following exercises:

	ICD-9-CM Code(s)
1. RUQ pain	______
2. Abdominal pain, NOS	______
3. Abnormal chest x-ray	______
4. Cough	______
5. Abnormal Pap smear	______
6. Dyspnea	______
7. Hemoptysis	______
8. Respiratory arrest	______
9. Seizures	______
10. Urinary incontinence	______

INJURIES, POISONINGS, AND ADVERSE EFFECTS

Perhaps the most difficult part of coding injuries and trauma is the identification of the type of injury. As mentioned in the musculoskeletal chapter discussion, diagnoses that occur as the result of an injury such as fractures, intracranial injuries, open wounds, and dislocations are located in Chapter 17 of the ICD-9-CM book. Of course, most of the codes assigned from this section will necessitate the addition of an E code to describe the external or environmental cause of the injuries. Some examples of conditions included in this section are listed in the following paragraphs.

FRACTURES

Different types of fractures are specified by the following definitions:

Open—A wound permitting direct contact of the bone and tissues with the environment. Typical descriptors for open fractures include the following terminology:

- compound
- infected
- puncture

Closed—The integrity of the overlying muscle and skin has not been breached. Any fracture not specified as open is classified as closed. Typical descriptors for closed fractures include the following terminology:

- comminuted
- depressed
- greenstick
- simple
- spiral

Pathological—Bones weakened by disease
Compression—Due to disease or trauma
Vertebral—Involves spinal cord injury
Skull—Fifth digit–specified level of consciousness

Fractures that are due to birth injuries are classifiable elsewhere. Fractures that are not classified as open or closed are always coded as closed. The coder always assumes the lowest, least complex service or encounter and the least complicated diagnosis when specific information is not available.

INTRACRANIAL INJURIES

Intracranial injuries include the following conditions and diagnoses:

- concussion
- cerebral laceration or contusion
- intracranial hemorrhage

Code 850 is used for concussions, with the fifth digit used for coding the level of consciousness associated with the injury.

INTERNAL INJURIES

Codes from this category include injury to internal organs such as:

- heart
- lung
- liver
- kidney
- pelvic organs

Internal injuries constitute a variety of wounds such as lacerations, tears, traumatic rupture, penetrating wounds, blunt trauma, and other open wounds. The fourth digit for internal injuries specifies whether there is an associated open wound.

OPEN WOUNDS

This classification includes all open wounds other than those due to internal injury. Included are injuries or wounds to the skin, tendon, or muscle. They may be caused by laceration, puncture, trauma, or avulsion. Open wounds may be classified as complicated or uncomplicated. For open wound injuries to be classified as complicated, medical documentation and the diagnostic statement must specify delayed healing or treatment, the presence of a foreign body, or infection. The fourth digit indicates whether the wound is simple or complicated, or if there is tendon involvement.

BLOOD VESSEL/NERVE INJURIES

These codes are used when a primary injury results in minor damage to peripheral nerves or blood vessels. Injuries to nerves or the spinal cord are coded with codes 950 through 957. Blood vessel injuries are coded with codes 900 through 904.

SUPERFICIAL INJURIES

These codes include injuries that involve blisters, abrasions, and friction burns.

CONTUSIONS

Contusions include bruises and hematoma without a fracture or open wound. If a fracture or open wound occurs at the same time, the coder should code whichever is the most significant injury to that site—the fracture or the open wound.

CRUSH INJURY

Crush injuries include those injuries not complicated by concussion, fracture, injury to internal organs, or intracranial injury.

DISLOCATION

This injury includes subluxation or displacement. As with fractures, dislocations may be open or closed. If not specified, the dislocation should be coded to the least specific level of closed.

SPRAIN/STRAIN

Sprain or strain injuries can occur to joint capsules, ligaments, muscles, and tendons. The rules listed in Tool 21 for coding injuries and trauma may assist in the correct assignment of ICD-9-CM codes for these cases. In addition, Tool 22 is an index for locating the proper injury, trauma, and burn codes. The type of injury has been defined so that the coder may select the proper category for coding the injury. Additional information regarding the injury involves the location and complications.

The coder may wish to develop an "Injury/Trauma Coding Matrix" such as Tool 23. Keep in mind that the coder should develop this matrix on the basis of the diagnoses most commonly used in the practice. Also remember that this matrix, as well as others that have been developed, serves as a reference tool and should be updated with each new edition of ICD-9-CM and CPT-4 books. As with any coding matrix that has been developed, the codes should be cross-referenced in the alphabetical and numerical indexes of ICD-9-CM until each and every code has been verified. The coder may wish to mark codes in the ICD-9-CM code book after they have been cross-referenced. After completion of cross-reference verification, the coder will want to document the verification of this information and keep a copy of this information on file.

STOP AND PRACTICE

Assign the appropriate ICD-9-CM codes to these injury and trauma cases.

ICD-9-CM Code(s)

1. Paralysis of right wrist   _____
2. Nonunion of fracture, neck of femur   _____
3. Fracture, pelvis, right femur, right foot _____
4. Contusions, right cheek/right forearm/
   right hand   _____
5. Open wound, right thigh and knee   _____
6. Fracture, left hip   _____
7. Compound fracture, left tibia/fibula _____
8. Fracture, left pelvic   _____
9. Pneumothorax trauma w/o mention
   of open wound   _____
10. Stab wound of abdominal wall,
    infected   _____

BURNS

All burns (except friction burns and sunburn, which are not considered burns) are classified to categories 940 through 949. Friction burns are classified as superficial injuries. Sunburn is coded to 692.71, Inflammatory Conditions of Skin and Subcutaneous Tissues.

T O O L   21

GUIDELINES FOR CODING TRAUMA/INJURIES

1 Primary axis indicates the type of injury (e.g., fracture).

2 Injuries classifiable to more than one subcategory should be coded separately unless a combination code is available.

3 Always code the most severe injury as primary diagnosis.

4 Late effect injury codes are always coded after the residual condition.

5 Assign V codes for aftercare required for wires, pins, plates, external fixation devices.

6 Assign E codes for accidents.

T O O L   22

INJURY/TRAUMA/BURN INDEX

Fractures	820 – 829
Dislocations	830 – 839
Sprains/Strains	840 – 848
Intracranial Injuries	850 – 854
Internal Injuries	860 – 869
Open Wounds	870 – 897
Blood Vessel Injuries	900 – 904
Late Effects of Injuries	905 – 909
Superficial Injuries	910 – 919
Contusions	920 – 924
Crushing Injuries	925 – 929
Foreign Body Entering Through Orifice	930 – 939
Burns	940 – 949
Nerve/Spinal Cord Injuries	950 – 957
Complications of Trauma and Unspecified Injuries	958 – 959

T O O L 23

INJURY/TRAUMA CODING MATRIX

Site	Contusion	Superficial Injury*	Wound, Open		Sprain/ Strain	Fracture		Dislocation		Burns		
			Uncomp	Comp		Closed	Open	Closed	Open	1st deg	2nd deg	3rd deg
Abdomen	922.2	911	879.2	879.3	848.8	N/A	N/A	N/A	N/A	942.13	942.23	942.33
Ankle	924.21	916	891.0	891.1	845.00	824.8	824.9	837.0	837.1	945.13	945.23	945.33
Arm	923.9	913	884.0	884.1	840.9	818.0	818.1	839.8	839.9	943.10	943.20	943.30
Shoulder												
Humerus												
Elbow												
Forearm												
Wrist												
Finger(s)												
Back	922.31	911	876.0	876.1	847.9	805.80	805.90	839.8	839.9	942.14	942.24	942.34
Cervical	922.31	911	876.0	876.1	847.0	805.00	805.10	839.00	839.10	942.14	942.24	942.34
Coccyx	922.32	911	876.0	876.1	847.4	805.60	805.70	839.41	839.51	942.14	942.24	942.34
Dorsal	922.31	911	876.0	876.1	847.1	805.20	805.30	839.21	839.31	942.14	942.24	942.34
Lumbar	922.31	911	876.0	876.1	847.2	805.40	805.50	839.20	839.30	942.14	942.24	942.34
Leg												
Femur												
Knee												
Tibia												
Fibula												

* Superficial injuries require 4th digit for 910-917, 919:

0 = Abrasion/Friction Burn, No Infection
1 = Abrasion/Friction Burn, With Infection
2 = Blister, No Infection
3 = Blister, With Infection
4 = Insect Bite, Nonvenomous, No Infection
5 = Insect Bite, Nonvenomous, Infection
6 = Superficial Foreign Body, No Infection
7 = Superficial Foreign Body, Infection

NOTE: Always develop any coding matrix tools directly from your CURRENT ICD-9-CM MANUAL.
Keep in mind these codes should be used ONLY when no additional coding documentation to code to a higher level of specificity is available.

(Courtesy of MD Consultative Services, Orlando, Florida. All rights reserved.)

Categorization of Burns

When coding burns, remember the following information regarding the degree of burn:

First-degree burn—Erythema
Second-degree burn—Blistering
Third-degree burn—Full-thickness involvement

In burn codes, the numbers identify and code the following:

First axis—identifies the anatomical site
Fourth digit—identifies the depth of the burn
Fifth digit—provides more specified site information

In the event of burns of more than one site, code the most severe burn first. When the body service area codes are used, the **Rule of Nines** applies.

Each arm—9%
Each leg—18%
Anterior trunk—18%
Posterior trunk—18%
Genitalia—9%

When third-degree burns are coded, it is necessary to code the body surface area involved. Code 958.3 should be used for posttraumatic wound infection that is not elsewhere classified.

STOP AND PRACTICE

Complete these ICD-9-CM burn exercises. Remember to use E codes when appropriate.

ICD-9-CM Code(s)

1. First-degree and second-degree burns, thumbs and two fingers, from kitchen fire _____
2. Second-degree burns in factory fire, determined to be arson _____
3. Burns 30% of body—10% third degree, 20% second degree, firefighter in forest fire _____
4. Severe sunburn of face, neck, shoulders _____
5. Third-degree burns, shoulder, upper arm, elbow, garage fire _____
6. First-degree burn of left foot, second-degree burn of toes, bonfire _____
7. Burn of trachea due to accidental ingestion of caustic substance _____
8. Allergic dermatitis, face _____
9. First- and second-degree burns of arm _____
10. Second- and third-degree burns of lower leg, house fire _____

CHAPTER IN REVIEW

CERTIFICATION REVIEW

- Normal delivery diagnostic codes are used when the entire delivery process is normal, there are no additional diagnostic problems, and the delivery results in a single liveborn only.
- All deliveries should include the outcome of delivery code.
- Fractures are classified into two main areas, open and closed. The coder should code the least significant (closed) injury when diagnostic information does not state the category.
- Lacerations are defined in ICD-9-CM as open wounds; therefore, they are located under the category "wound, open (site)."

- Burns are classified into three categories: first (erythema), second (blisters), and third (full-thickness involvement) degree.
- Alcohol or drug dependence is defined as the inability to cease the intake of alcohol or drugs; this must be so designated by physician documentation for coding purposes.
- Alcohol or drug abuse is defined as problem drinking and drug use that has not been given the diagnosis of dependence in the physician diagnostic statement.
- Fifth digits for substance abuse codes define the period of the abuse, such as continuous, episodic, or in remission. These must be stated as such by the physician diagnosis statement.

- Codes for specific diagnoses by body area and organ system are defined by the guidelines for the specific chapter in which they are found.

STUDENT STUDY GUIDE

- Study Chapter 6.
- Review the Learning Objectives for Chapter 6.
- Complete the Stop and Practice exercises.
- Complete the Certification Review for Chapter 6.
- Complete the Chapter Review exercise to reinforce concepts learned in this chapter.

CHAPTER REVIEW EXERCISE

Complete the following:

ICD-9-CM Code(s)

1. Maternal venereal disease, not delivered _____
2. Twin pregnancy _____
3. Threatened abortion _____
4. Breech presentation, delivered _____
5. Mild concussion following accidental fall down steps, no LOC _____
6. Head injury _____
7. Laceration to hand _____
8. Contusions to left elbow _____
9. Sprained ankle _____
10. Burns to left cheek from stove _____
11. First-degree burns, 10% body surface, arm _____
12. Obsessive-compulsive disorder _____
13. Depressive disorder _____
14. Hyperventilation syndrome _____
15. Failed attempted abortion _____
16. Fetal disproportion _____
17. Rh incompatibility _____
18. Four (4) rib fractures _____
19. Burns to left lower extremity, hand _____
20. Sternoclavicular joint sprain _____
21. Shoulder laceration _____
22. Corneal foreign body _____
23. Depression _____
24. Antisocial personality _____
25. Paranoid reaction _____
26. Separation anxiety _____
27. Abdominal mass _____
28. Cervical cancer _____
29. Uterine ca, squamocolumnar junction _____
30. Maternal venereal disease _____
31. Varicose veins/legs in pregnancy _____
32. Umbilical cord around neck with compression _____
33. Concussion with less than 1 hour LOC _____
34. Knee laceration _____
35. Dislocation, metacarpophalangeal joint _____
36. Chemical burns of eyelids _____
37. Sander's disease _____
38. Schizophrenia _____
39. Juvenile delinquency _____
40. Multiple personality disorder _____
41. Spontaneous abortion _____
42. Insect bite, leg _____
43. Traumatic pneumothorax _____
44. Elbow dislocation, lateral _____
45. Bimalleolar fracture _____
46. Coin in nostril _____
47. Mental retardation _____
48. Drug addiction _____
49. Psychogenic asthenia _____
50. Arthritis, ankle _____
51. IDDM Diabetes _____
52. Hyperthyroidism _____
53. Nonvenomous insect bite, elbow, infected _____
54. Gestational diabetes _____
55. Acute pyelonephritis due to *E. coli* _____
56. Fibroadenosis of breast _____
57. Anorexia nervosa _____
58. Simple greenstick fracture, radius _____
59. Laceration of wrist with tendon involvement _____
60. Compound fracture, proximal end of ulna _____
61. Traumatic laceration of kidney _____
62. Aortic stenosis _____
63. Ventricular septal defect _____
64. Diverticulosis of colon _____
65. Maternal drug dependency _____
66. Fetal distress _____
67. Postpartum cardiomyopathy _____
68. Abrasion, finger _____
69. Skull base fracture _____
70. Open C1 fracture _____
71. Infected insect bite, finger _____
72. Acid burns to cornea _____
73. Brief depressive reaction _____
74. Developmental dyslexia _____
75. Cocaine dependency _____
76. Hysterical paralysis _____
77. Hiatal hernia _____
78. Alcohol liver cirrhosis _____
79. Aortic valve insufficiency _____
80. Hypoglycemia _____
81. Triplet pregnancy _____
82. Third-degree perineal laceration _____
83. Traumatic amputation of leg, below knee _____
84. Lung contusion _____
85. Attention deficit disorder _____
86. Aggressive personality _____

87. Viral hepatitis _____
88. Bacterial meningitis _____
89. Hepatitis B _____
90. Placenta previa _____
91. Antepartum hemorrhage _____
92. Gestational hypertension _____
93. Anxiety reaction _____
94. Septicemia due to streptococcus _____
95. Right lower extremity paralysis _____
96. Gouty arthritis _____

97. Acute alcoholic intoxication _____
98. Chronic alcohol abuse _____
99. Barbiturate abuse, episodic _____
100. Separation anxiety disorder _____

PRACTICAL APPLICATION

Review the following medical charts. Determine the appropriate ICD-9-CM diagnostic code(s) and arrange them in the appropriate order.

1.

PROGRESS NOTE

Chief complaint: _____

Date: _____

Vital signs: BP_____ P_____ R_____

History:

SUBJECTIVE:
35-year-old with known history of asthma presents with shortness of breath, feeling of tightness and inability to move air. She has experienced these symptoms in the past when her asthma has not been under good control.

Exam:

OBJECTIVE:
35-year-old female in slight distress, obviously anxious. BP 120/80, pulse 70, R20 and shallow. Heart, normal rate and rhythm, HEENT, normal, PERRLA, normal, neck, soft and supple. Lungs have coarse rhonchi which cleared with bronchodilator treatments X 2.

Diagnosis/assessment:

ASSESSMENT:
Acute exacerbation of asthma

PLAN:
Treated with two bronchodilator treatments, prescribed antibiotics and IV steroids.

Jay Corman MD

Godfrey Medical Associates

Patient name: _____
Date of service: _____

GODFREY MEDICAL ASSOCIATES
1532 Third Avenue, Suite 120 • Aldon, FL 77713 • (407) 555-4000

Codes: _____

2.

PROGRESS NOTE

Date:	Vital signs:	T	R
Chief complaint:		P	BP

58-year-old male presents with complaints of abdominal pain for the past 24–48 hours. States somewhat nauseated, however, no vomiting. No fever, chills or other symptoms. No unusual foods during the past 24–48 hour period.

Past history: History of Cholelithiasis

Examination:

58-year-old in no acute distress. BP 128/82, Pulse 71, Temperature 98.2. Color is good, HEENT normal. Abdomen, guarded but soft and tender. Heart, normal rate and rhythm. Lungs are clear to auscultation. Labs indicated elevated liver function is a patient with known cholelithiasis.

Impression:

Abnormal Liver Function, possibly due to cholelithiasis

Plan:

John Palermo

Patient name:

DOB:

MR/Chart #:

GODFREY REGIONAL OUTPATIENT CLINIC
3122 Shannon Avenue • Aldon, FL 77712 • (407) 555-7654

Codes: _____

3.

PROGRESS NOTE

Date:	Vital signs:	T	R
Chief complaint:		P	BP

SUBJECTIVE:
Patient presents with history of 3–4 weeks of headaches, fever and chills. Was prescribed antibiotics for an apparent viral infection, however, little or no improvement over the past few weeks. He has finished the antibiotic regimen, and still experiences fever and headaches, nonchanged from his original complaint(s) 3–4 weeks ago. No history of hypertension, diabetes, infections, cardiac problems. Has been apparently in good health until this incident 3–4 weeks ago.

Physical examination:

OBJECTIVE:
Patient exam reveals a 37-year-old male in slight distress, probably from anxiety but appearing worn from his recent illness period. Vital signs are stable, HEENT normal, abdomen soft and nontender, heart regular rate and rhythm.

Labs show WBC 12.3, hemoglobin 13.2, Hepatitis B panel is positive. Chest x-ray was returned as normal.

Assessment:

Hepatitis B

Plan:

Will admit for inpatient treatment to stabilize his condition with IV antibiotics and IV fluids.

Willen Obst MD

	Patient name:
	DOB:
	MR/Chart #:

GODFREY REGIONAL OUTPATIENT CLINIC
3122 Shannon Avenue • Aldon, FL 77712 • (407) 555-7654

Codes: _____

4.

PROGRESS NOTE

Chief complaint: _____

Date: _____

Vital signs: BP_____ P_____ R_____

History:

SUBJECTIVE:
Patient is known-diabetic who presents with nausea and vomiting over the past week. No shortness of breath, no palpitations, however reports nausea and vomiting as well as increased urination over the past 24–48 hours.

Exam:

OBJECTIVE:
Pleasant appearing 39-year-old female who appears in no acute distress. Vital signs are normal. Appears pale, with multiple episodes of vomiting while in the office. Lungs are clear to ausculation, neck soft and supple. HEENT normal. PERRLA. Neurologically intact. Abdomen is tender from multiple episodes of vomiting, positive for bowel sounds, soft and tender apparently only from the vomiting.

Labs indicated blood sugar over 600 is a patient with known Type I diabetes mellitus.

Diagnosis/assessment:

Diabetes Type I
Diabetic Ketoacidosis

Maurice Doater, MD
Godfrey Regional Outpatient Clinic

Patient name: _____
Date of service: _____

GODFREY MEDICAL ASSOCIATES
1532 Third Avenue, Suite 120 • Aldon, FL 77713 • (407) 555-4000

Codes: _____

5.

PROGRESS NOTE

Chief complaint: _____

Date: _____

Vital signs: BP_____ P_____ R_____

History:

SUBJECTIVE:
Patient presents with fever and chills 3 days prior to presenting to office. She has experienced nausea, vomiting, fever and chills for several days with shortness of breath over the past 24 hours.

PAST MEDICAL HISTORY:
She is a known hypertensive, with unstable blood pressure readings in the past. She also had a myocardial infarction approximately 4 weeks ago and is continuing to be followed.

Exam:

OBJECTIVE:
Upon examination, she appears ill, with shortness of breath noted. Her vital signs are stable, except for her blood pressure reading which was 190/117; however, as mentioned, her BP readings have been unstable in the past. She is not experiencing chest pain, however, has had anxiety problems in the past, and appears anxious. Heart, normal rate and rhythm. HEENT normal, neck soft and supple. Abdomen, soft and non-tender. Her lungs had bilateral crackles upon ausculation.

Chest x-ray revealed bilateral lower lobe pneumonia.

Diagnosis/assessment:

Bilateral lower lobe pneumonia, old myocardial infarction, hypertension, anxiety state

Stong Knatt, MD
Godfrey Medical Associates

Patient name: _____
Date of service: _____

GODFREY MEDICAL ASSOCIATES
1532 Third Avenue, Suite 120 • Aldon, FL 77713 • (407) 555-4000

Codes: _____

6.

PROGRESS NOTE

Date:	Vital signs:	T		R
Chief complaint:		P		BP

79-year-old female presents with 3 days history of severe epigastric pain associated with considerable nausea, minimal vomiting. Patient has no history of food reactions, or consumption of any unusual foods over the past few days. Denied melena, shortness of breath, diarrhea, constipation, or fever.

Medications: The patient takes hypertensive medication however does not remember the name of the medication.

Examination:

Normal appearing 79-year-old female who appears pale in color and anxious. Vital signs are stable, HEENT normal, PERRLA. Abdomen is non-tender with normal bowel sounds. The pain appears to be high in the abdominal area rather than in the actual abdominal area. Extremities are normal with no clubbing or cyanosis. Heart and lungs are normal.

Impression:

Will order gall bladder ultrasound to rule out possible cholecystitis and upper GI for possible stomach ulcer.

Plan:

Patient will have tests performed at the hospital on an outpatient basis and return as soon as tests are completed for further evaluation and treatment.

Stony Knott, MD

	Patient name:
	DOB:
	MR/Chart #:

GODFREY REGIONAL OUTPATIENT CLINIC
3122 Shannon Avenue • Aldon, FL 77712 • (407) 555-7654

Codes: _____

7.

PROGRESS NOTE

Chief complaint: _____

Date: _____

Vital signs: BP_____ P_____ R_____

History:

SUBJECTIVE:
25-year-old patient presents for routine prenatal visit with complaints of hyperemesis. This is her first pregnancy and 24 weeks and she continues to have intermittent nausea and vomiting throughout her pregnancy. On her last visit, she was informed that she was anemic and should carefully watch her intake of food and vitamins.

Exam:

OBJECTIVE:
25-year-old female who appears in no distress. 24-week gestation with normal development. Fetal heart tones appear normal. CBC indicates that the patient continues to be anemic, and we will supplement her vitamins with additional medications as she appears unable to hold down food on a regular basis. She will also report to the OB Unit at the hospital for IV hydration at which time a Fetal Non-Stress test will also be performed.

Diagnosis/assessment:

Anemia
Hyperemesis Gravidarum

Felix Wanler M
Godfrey Medical Associates

Patient name: _____
Date of service: _____

GODFREY MEDICAL ASSOCIATES
1532 Third Avenue, Suite 120 • Aldon, FL 77713 • (407) 555-4000

Codes: _____

8.

PROGRESS NOTE

Date:	Vital signs:	T	R
Chief complaint:		P	BP

23-year-old patient presents 4 days postoperative for cesarean section at 39 weeks for fetal distress. She delivered a healthy 6 pound 14 ounce female, with apgars of 6 and 8 and both the mother and child are doing fine.

Examination:

Her temperature is normal, vital signs are stable. The wound shows no signs of infection and is healing nicely. She is encouraged to apply lotion to the area and warned of lifting anything heavy for the next several weeks. Staples are removed and she is to return at 6 weeks for her postpartum re-check and discharge.

Impression:

Normal postpartum check and suture removal

Plan:

Return at six weeks postpartum for re-check and discharge.

Adm Westg MD

Patient name:

DOB:

MR/Chart #:

GODFREY MEDICAL ASSOCIATES
1532 Third Avenue, Suite 120 • Aldon, FL 77713 • (407) 555-4000

Codes: _____

9.

EMERGENCY ROOM RECORD

Name:	Age:	ER physician:
	DOB:	

Allergies/type of reaction: | **Usual medications/dosages:**

Triage/presenting complaint: | Patient presents to the Emergency Room having been involved in a minor automobile accident. He went to his family physician complaining of left leg pain and the physician noted the left lateral leg to be swollen, pain to touch and sent the patient to the Emergency Room for further evaluation and x-ray.

Initial assessment:

Time	T	P	R	BP	Other:					

Medication orders:

Lab work:

X-Ray:

Physician's report:

The patient appears in no acute distress. Vital signs are normal. Leg appears swollen, painful to touch and an x-ray is ordered that reveals a small fracture of the proximal tibia. Splint is placed and the patient is instructed to non-weight bear for approximately 7 days and then partial weight-bearing for approximately 3–4 weeks. Patient should return to his physician for further follow-up.

Diagnosis:	Physician sign/date
ASSESSMENT: Proximal Tibia Fracture PLAN: Follow up with physician in approximately 6 weeks for further evaluation and treatment.	Robert Rai MD
Discharge Transfer Admit Good Satisfactory Other:	

GODFREY REGIONAL HOSPITAL
123 Main Street • Aldon, FL 77714 • (407) 555-1234

Codes: _____

10.

PROGRESS NOTE

Date:	Vital signs:	T	R
Chief complaint:		P	BP

SUBJECTIVE:
14-year-old presents to the physician's office for evaluation and treatment following an altercation with his brother at home. He complains of multiple injuries consisting of bruises, cuts and scrapes and his mother requests evaluation and appropriate treatment. He denies any loss of consciousness, double vision or any other symptoms. Apparently the altercation was more of a wrestling match and neither party appeared to have been injured significantly.

Physical examination:

OBJECTIVE:
14-year-old in no acute distress who presents with multiple cuts and scrapes on his upper extremities. Head is atraumatic, neck soft and supple, PERRLA. His left upper extremity has multiple contusions on the anterior surface, with a minimal laceration to the lower part of his upper extremity which does not require suturing or treatment. His right upper extremity has an area of swelling with discoloration but not open wounds or concerns.

Assessment:

Abrasions to upper extremities
Contusion to R upper extremity
Open wound to arm
Resulting from altercation

Plan:

Willen Obt MD

Patient name:
DOB:
MR/Chart #:

GODFREY REGIONAL OUTPATIENT CLINIC
3122 Shannon Avenue • Aldon, FL 77712 • (407) 555-7654

Codes: _____

7

ICD-10-CM

LEARNING OBJECTIVES

Following the completion of this chapter, the student will be able to:

- Grasp the changes that will be effective with the introduction of ICD-10-CM.
- Comprehend the basic layout of ICD-10-CM.
- Understand the concepts of code families and service categories with the implementation of ICD-10-CM.

INTRODUCTION TO ICD-10-CM

EXPECTED DATE

An update to ICD-9-CM is expected sometime late in 2007. The information contained herein regarding ICD-10-CM may change in some respects. Make certain to check the final information in ICD-10-CM when it is published.

It appears that the rules and guidelines currently used for coding purposes will not change significantly. Significant content and format changes will be noted in ICD-10-CM. These changes are presented in some detail later in the chapter.

LAYOUT AND CONVENTIONS

The ICD-10-CM is scheduled to be divided into chapters:

Chapter 1 Tabular List
Chapter 2 Instruction Manual (may not be included in ICD-10-CM)
Chapter 3 Alphabetical Index (by diagnosis)

ICD-10-CM coding will begin with A00 and will end with Z99. Codes are scheduled to include a maximum of six digits (those currently used in ICD-9-CM include no more than five digits). Therefore many facilities will need to reformat their computerized billing and coding systems to accommodate the increased number of digits. Each diagnosis code will be composed of the following:

1 alphabetical character + 2 numerical characters + up to 3 additional digits (e.g., X22.444)

The place of each character in the code will convey a specific meaning. The first character will denote **service category:**

0   Medical and Surgical Services
1   Obstetrics
2   Placement
3   Administration
4   Measurement and Monitoring
5   Imaging
6   Nuclear Medicine
7   Radiation Oncology
8   Osteopathic Services
9   Rehabilitation and Diagnostic Audiology
B   Extracorporeal Assistance and Performance
C   Extracorporeal Therapies
D   Laboratory Services
F   Mental Health Services
G   Chiropractic Services
H   Miscellaneous

The second character will indicate the **body system** affected:

0   Central Nervous System
1   Peripheral Nervous System
2   Heart and Great Vessels
3   Upper Arteries
4   Lower Arteries
5   Upper Veins
6   Lower Veins
7   Lymphatic and Hematologic Systems
8   Eye
9   Ear, Nose, Sinus
B   Respiratory System
C   Mouth and Throat
D   Gastrointestinal System
F   Hepatobiliary System/Pancreas
G   Endocrine System
H   Skin/Breast
J   Subcutaneous Tissue
K   Muscles
L   Tendons
M   Bursae, Ligaments, Fasciae
N   Head and Facial Bones
P   Upper Bones
Q   Lower Bones
R   Upper Joints
S   Lower Joints
T   Urinary System
V   Female Reproductive System
W   Male Reproductive System
X   Anatomical Regions
Y   Upper Extremities
Z   Lower Extremities

The third character will represent the **objective** of the procedure. Following is a list of the available root procedures:

Fragmentation Alteration
Bypass
Change
Control
Creation
Destruction
Detachment
Dilation
Division
Drainage
Excision
Extirpation
Extraction
Fragmentation
Fusion
Insertion
Inspection
Mapping
Occlusion
Reattachment
Release
Removal
Repair
Replacement

Repositioning
Resection
Restriction
Revision
Transfer
Transplantation

Character 4 will indicate the **affected body part.**
Character 5 will code the **approach** used.
Character 6 will describe the **device** used.
A qualifier of X/Z will denote **diagnostic (X)** compared with **none (Z).**

The content of ICD-10-CM will be expanded to 21 chapters, instead of the 17 chapters that make up ICD-9-CM.

NEW FEATURES OF ICD-10-CM

The added features of ICD-10-CM are important because of their impact on medical practices and hospitals. These changes are as follows:

- More complete descriptions of disorders and treatments will be included.
- Postprocedural disorders for each specific body system will be listed at the end of each chapter.
- The book will be organized into ICD-10-CM blocks; that is, each chapter will begin with a list of subchapters or "blocks" of three-character origin.
- *Mental Disorders* will become *Mental and Behavioral Disorders;* this section will expand from 3 to 11 subchapters.
- Injury, poisoning, and other externally caused illnesses will be grouped under body region, then type of injury. These were previously classified only by type of injury.
- Victim mode of transportation will be revised in the External Causes of Morbidity/Mortality.

- Laterality codes will be changed to right/left/unspecified.
- Trimester specificity will be included for obstetrical coding.
- Expansion changes of the Alcohol/Drug codes will include:
  Fourth digit—Effects (dependence, abuse)
  Fifth digit—Aspects of Use (withdrawal)
  Sixth digit—Manifestations (delirium)
- Expansion of injury codes will include type and site of injury:
  S51.034 Puncture wound, without FB, Elbow
  S51.031 Puncture wound, without FB, Elbow, Right
  S51.032 Puncture wound, without FB, Elbow, Left
  S51.039 Puncture wound, without FB, Elbow, Unspec
- New combination codes will be included; common signs, symptoms, and complications will be added as a fifth digit.
- Manifestation codes have been eliminated through the use of combination codes that encompass the condition and the source.
- Postoperative complication codes will be expanded.
- Deactivation of some codes will take place. Consider the following:

Immunizations (there will be only one code for "encounter for immunization") will be coded differently

Nonspecific codes (unspecified diabetes, multiple superficial injuries) will be deleted from ICD-10-CM

- **Code Families** will be introduced. Each chapter will contain a three-character category:
  C Neoplasm/**(C)**ancer
  E **(E)**ndocrine Disorders
  N **(N)**ephrology Disorders
  O **(O)**bstetrical Conditions/Disorders
  P **(P)**erinatal Conditions/Disorders

TABLE 7-1	ICD-9-CM and ICD-10-CM Comparison		
Issue	ICD-9-CM	ICD-10-CM	Conversion Issue
Number of characters	3-5	3-6	Additional field
Type of characters	Numerical only (except V and E codes)	Alphanumeric	Allow for alphanumeric system; will need to distinguish between 0/1 and O/I (numbers vs letters)
Decimals	Allow third character	Allow third character	ICD-10-CM: decimals; ICD-10-PCS: no decimals
Descriptions	Tabular list shows partial descriptions, 4th/5th digits	Stand-alone descriptions	Length of field must accommodate longer descriptions
Hierarchy	4th/5th-digit codes have hierarchical relationships within 3-character category	4th/5th/6th-digit codes have hierarchical relationships within 3-character category	
Quantity	>15,000 volume 1/3	>24,000 codes; ICD-10-PCS >20,000 codes	More codes, more space
Format availability	Print/various computerized electronic formats	Print only; no electronic format at this time	May need to reformat to accept electronic file(s) in a different format

IMPLEMENTATION PLANNING FOR ICD-10-CM

Because many changes will come with the introduction of ICD-10-CM, both the coder and medical facilities must prepare for quick implementation.

COMPARISON OF ICD-9-CM AND ICD-10-CM

A comparison of ICD-9-CM with ICD-10-CM appears in Table 7-1, which also presents issues that may need to be resolved before the implementation date for ICD-10-CM.

CHAPTER IN REVIEW

CERTIFICATION REVIEW

- The format of ICD-10-CM will change significantly; however, many rules for assigning codes will remain much the same.
- ICD-10-CM codes will be assigned with six alpha-numerical digits.
- V codes and E codes will be incorporated into the regular alphabetical and tabular sections of ICD-10-CM, thereby eliminating the indexes that are used in ICD-9-CM.
- Because the codes will become more specific, the coder will be able to designate right, left, bilateral, and unspecified.
- Manifestation codes will be eliminated through the use of combination codes when necessary.
- Unspecified codes (i.e., those currently listed in ICD-9-CM as unspecified) will be eliminated.
- One code will be assigned for all immunizations, regardless of which specific immunization is administered.
- Facilities must begin preparation for ICD-10-CM implementation by identifying potential problems, eliminating staff shortages, and resolving other matters of concern before the official introduction.

STUDENT STUDY GUIDE

- Study Chapter 7.
- Review the Learning Objectives for Chapter 7.

- Complete the Certification Review for Chapter 7.
- Complete the Chapter Review exercise to reinforce concepts learned in this chapter.

CHAPTER REVIEW EXERCISE

Answer the following questions.
1. ICD-10-CM codes will be:
   a. alphabetical
   b. numerical
   c. alphanumerical
2. There will be no additional chapters in ICD-10-CM than were in ICD-9-CM.
   a. True
   b. False
3. Define code families.

   _____

   _____

4. Define service categories.

   _____

   _____

5. List three significant changes that will be made with the introduction of ICD-10-CM to the coding world.
   (1) _____
   (2) _____
   (3) _____
6. List three significant issues facilities face in implementing ICD-10-CM.
   (1) _____
   (2) _____
   (3) _____

III

PHYSICIAN PROCEDURE CODING

Section III discusses procedure and service coding for physicians and providers. Each of these services is billed according to specific coding guidelines. Physician services are billed with codes from the CPT-4 coding system. Hospital facility services are coded with the DRG (Diagnosis-Related Group) system. Outpatient hospital coding with the APG/APC (Ambulatory Payment Groups/Ambulatory Payment Classification) system began in August 2000.

This section of the textbook begins with information on physician coding. It is important for coders to understand which services are billed with CPT-4 and which with DRG. CPT-4 procedure codes are used for billing services performed by the provider; DRGs are used to bill for hospital or facility services. During the discussion of the reimbursement process later in this book, it will become apparent why this distinction is necessary.

Documentation plays a vital role in the assignment of CPT-4 codes for services. A review of this documentation involves reading and interpreting progress notes, medical histories, physical examination results, and operative reports. From these documents, the key elements needed to assign the proper CPT-4 codes to the chart must be extracted. Such elements will differ greatly on the basis of coding guidelines for each chapter of the CPT-4 coding book. An important consideration is that the CPT-4 book differs somewhat from ICD-9-CM wherein the rules remain essentially the same from one chapter to the next. For this reason, Section III is presented by CPT-4 chapter. The documents necessary for obtaining the information for coding, the specific rules for assigning codes for those services, and coding assignment exercises are introduced accordingly.

(C)urrent (P)rocedural (T)erminology, or CPT, currently in the fourth edition (thus, CPT-4), is used in much the same way as the ICD-9-CM coding book. CPT, however, provides standardization for coding billable services and procedures (i.e., **WHAT** was performed), rather than explanations of the medical necessity or diagnosis for the encounter. The information coded from CPT is also used for standardization in billing and for compilation of statistical information in much the same way as ICD-9-CM information is used.

It is important to emphasize that only by using ICD-9-CM and CPT-4 coding does the coder get the opportunity to describe **WHAT** (procedure/CPT-4) encounter took place, and to justify **WHY** (diagnosis/ICD-9-CM) the encounter took place. Claim forms do not afford the coder or the biller the opportunity to explain the circumstances surrounding an encounter. This explanation must be clearly and concisely provided with the use of CPT-4 and ICD-9-CM codes.

DETERMINING CODEABLE SERVICES

LEARNING OBJECTIVES

Following the completion of this chapter, the student will be able to:

- Understand the key elements of physician documentation that drive the assignment of CPT-4 codes.
- Follow the basic steps in the CPT-4 coding process.
- Comprehend the difference between diagnostic codes and procedural codes.
- Understand how the proper use of both diagnostic and procedural codes "tells the story" of what services were performed and gives the medical necessity (diagnosis) for those services.
- Understand the importance of properly matching the descriptions (codes) for WHAT services were performed (CPT-4) with those explaining WHY (ICD-9-CM) services were performed.

KEY TERMS

CPT (Current Procedural Terminology), 185

THE CONCEPT OF CODEABLE SERVICES

In the world of **CPT,** information on WHAT services may be coded and billed is located within appropriate subsection(s) of CPT-4, wherein individualized guidelines for specific types of service must be followed.

GENERAL DOCUMENTATION GUIDELINES

Only those services that have been documented may be charged (as is the case with ICD-9-CM diagnostic coding). In addition, signature requirements for documentation, as discussed in Section I of this text, apply to these services as well.

At a minimum, the service must be documented according to guidelines pertaining to that procedure, and it must be "authenticated" or signed. When services are ordered by a physician, the order must be authenticated. In addition, for the physician service or procedure to be billed, the provider must document his or her interpretation of these services and meet signature requirements.

Probably the most difficult part of CPT-4 procedural coding is identifying the key words in the documentation so that documentation requirements for the CPT-4 descriptor may be satisfied. Because there are a number of CPT-4 procedural codes that describe the service(s) provided, each code will need to be considered carefully; the CPT-4 descriptor will need to be compared with the information contained in the medical documentation.

The intricate nature of extracting chart components needed for coding procedures with CPT-4 are explored in later chapters.

MATCHING SERVICES AND DIAGNOSTIC CODES

The order of services provided is important for CPT-4 coding (as is the case with ICD-9-CM). The order of CPT-4 and ICD-9-CM codes together can make the difference between reimbursement and denial of payment. During earlier discussions of diagnostic coding in this text, the correct order for each procedure was demonstrated as critical.

> Patient presents to the *physician's office* because of an ongoing problem with cough, fever, and cold symptoms. *Chest x-ray* and *CBC* are ordered, which indicate the presence of an upper respiratory infection. In addition, the patient complains of urinary frequency; therefore a *urinalysis* is performed and a diagnosis of urinary tract infection is made.

Review the "story" of **WHAT** services were provided and **WHY** those services were performed.

Services (WHAT)	Diagnosis (WHY)
Physician office visit	Upper respiratory infection
	Urinary tract infection
Urinalysis	Urinary tract infection
CBC	Upper respiratory infection
Chest x-ray	Upper respiratory infection

That diagnostic and procedural codes match is imperative for obtaining proper reimbursement. Medical necessity is also delineated when the appropriate diagnostic codes are assigned for each service (CPT-4 code) provided.

Note: There will always be a **WHAT** (procedure/service) necessitated by at least one **WHY** (diagnosis/medical necessity).

BASIC STEPS IN CODING SERVICES

The basic steps for procedural coding are similar to those for diagnostic coding. The basic difference in CPT-4 coding will be to determine from which chapter of the book services will be coded.

Step 1

Determine the Appropriate Chapter from Which Services Will Be Assigned
This is discussed in detail in Chapter 9 (Using CPT-4).

Chapter 1   Evaluation and Management
Chapter 2   Anesthesia
Chapter 3   Surgery
Chapter 4   Radiology
Chapter 5   Pathology
Chapter 6   Medicine

Step 2

Identify the Key Words and Phrases Necessary to Assign Codes for Services
Important components of the documentation include information regarding location of services (e.g., hospital, office, inpatient or outpatient facility) and anatomical site for which the patient received service (e.g., humerus, radius, femur, tibia, and fibula). For the location of the codes in the CPT-4 book to be determined, knowledge of anatomy is required.

A glossary of body systems, major components, and major functions has been provided as a basic review and reference guide (Table 8-1).

Step 3

Identify Specifics about the Procedure/Service Being Performed
Specifics required in Step 3 include such information as new or established patient, the specific body area, or specific test.

TABLE 8-1	Main Body Systems		
System	Components	Major Combining Form	Major Functions
Integumentary	Skin Sweat glands Nails	cutaneo/dermo hidro onycho	Protection of body, temperature, and water regulation
Musculoskeletal	Bones Joints Cartilage Muscles Fascia Tendon	osteo arthro chondro myo fascio tendo/tendino	Support, shape, protect, store minerals, locomotion, hold body erect, movement of body fluids, generate body heat
Cardiovascular	Heart Arteries Veins Blood	cardio arterio veno/phlebo hemo/hemato	Pump blood through circulatory system
Respiratory	Nose Pharynx Trachea Larynx Lungs	naso/rhino pharyngo tracheo laryngo pneumo	Bring oxygen into body for transportation to the cells; move carbon dioxide and water waste from body
Digestive	Mouth Esophagus Stomach Small intestine Large intestine Liver Pancreas Appendix Gall bladder	oro/stomato esophago gastro entero colo/colono hepato pancreato appendico cholecysto	Digestion of food, absorption of digested food, elimination of solid wastes
Endocrine	Adrenals Pituitary Thyroid Thymus	adreno pituito thyroido thymo	Glandular and hormonal regulation and growth of the body
Urinary	Kidneys Ureters Urine Urethra Bladder	nephro/reno uretero urino urethro cysto	Filtration of blood to remove waste, maintain electrolyte balance, regulate fluid balance within body
Reproductive Male/Female	Testes Prostate Ovary Uterus Fallopian tubes	orchio/orchido prostato oophoro hystero salpingo	Production of new life
Nervous Sense Organs	Nerves Brain Spinal cord Eye Ear	neuro encephalo myelo oculo/ophthalmo acousto/oto	Coordination mechanism, reception of stimuli, transmission of messages

Step 4

Determine Additional Specific Information regarding the Services

Additional information would include documentation that addresses the level of complexity and specific approach of the surgical procedure.

Step 5

Provide Information That Supports or Clarifies

Any additional specifics should be included such as extent of the procedure, open versus closed, or with fixation or without, with respect to a fracture.

Step 6

Determine the Correct Order for Billing Services and Procedures

Correct order of services is essential for proper reimbursement. Ensuring that services are listed in the proper order protects the interests of all involved—the patient, the provider, the place of service, and the insurer.

Step 7

Assign the Correct CPT-4 Code(s) from the CPT Book

The basics of this step are similar throughout the CPT-4 code book. Some variations occur depending on which chapter the appropriate codes may be found.

CHAPTER IN REVIEW

CERTIFICATION REVIEW

- "Matching" of diagnostic and procedural codes is imperative for correct coding.
- Coding for physician services must always include a statement of services that specifies a diagnosis (WHY) and a procedure (WHAT).
- Procedural coding differs from diagnostic coding in that guidelines and rules are different for each section of the CPT-4 manual.
- Listing CPT-4 codes on the claim form in the "most significant order" is critical to maximize reimbursement.

STUDENT STUDY GUIDE

- Study Chapter 8.
- Review the Learning Objectives for Chapter 8.
- Complete the Certification Review for Chapter 8.
- Complete the Chapter Review exercise to reinforce concepts learned in this chapter.

CHAPTER REVIEW EXERCISE

Take the following services (procedures) and MATCH them to diagnoses that would be appropriate for the services.

Services	Diagnosis
1. Chest x-ray	Anemia – *CBC*
2. CBC	Pneumonia – *chest x-ray*
3. Wound repair	Bacterial infection – *Inj Antibiotic*
4. Injection antibiotic	COPD – *Bronchospasm evaluation*
5. Electrocardiogram	Schizophrenia *psychotherapy*
6. Bronchospasm evaluation	Open wound, arm – *wound repair*
7. Psychotherapy, 45 minutes	Chest pain – *Electrocardiogram*
8. Wrist x-ray	Coronary artery disease – *cardiac catherization*
9. Mammogram	Wrist sprain – *wrist x-ray*
10. Cardiac catheterization	Fibrocystic breast disease *mammogram*

9

USING CPT-4

LEARNING OBJECTIVES

Following the completion of this chapter, the student will be able to:

- Understand the levels of HCPCS codes used.
- Comprehend the basic concept and format of the CPT-4 coding book. Identify, and understand the significance of signs and symbols used in the CPT-4 coding book.
- Understand that all services in CPT-4 are broken down into six categories, with specific guidelines for each group.
- Grasp the concept of modifiers and explain their proper application to the CPT-4 coding system.
- Differentiate between global and starred procedures, and explain their impact on coding in CPT-4.

CODING REFERENCE TOOLS

Tool 24
CPT-4 Coding Guidelines

KEY TERMS

Add on Procedure, 195
AMA (American Medical Association), 189
Anesthesiology, 190
Bullet, 195
CPT (Current Procedural Terminology), 189
Evaluation and Management Codes (E & M), 189
Global Procedures, 194
HCPCS (Healthcare Common Procedure Coding System), 189
Modifiers, 192
Pathology, 191
Radiology, 191
Separate Procedure, 195
Surgery, 191
Unlisted Procedure, 194

During the early 1980s, the **American Medical Association (AMA),** with the assistance of a physician editorial panel, developed a coding methodology to standardize reporting of procedures and services, much like the standardized diagnostic coding of the ICD-9-CM. Since that time, third-party carriers have required that this procedural coding be used in billing for physician services. Effective August 2000, this methodology became required on outpatient facility (hospital) claims as well. This methodology, or coding system, is referred to as **CPT-4** or **(C)urrent (P)rocedural (T)erminology;** it is only one part of a third-party coding system known as **Healthcare Common Procedure Coding System,** or **HCPCS.** These three levels are as follows:

Level 1   Current Procedural Terminology (CPT-4)
Level 2   National Codes (referred to as HCPCS Level II)
Level 3   Local Codes

With the implementation of the Health Insurance Portability and Accountability Act (HIPAA) of 1996 and its subsequent updates, the Level 3 local codes will probably become obsolete. Under HIPAA, the law dictates that all third-party carriers in the United States will use the same code sets for billing and coding services; thus local codes would no longer be applicable.

GENERAL DOCUMENTATION REQUIREMENTS FOR CPT-4 CODING

The assignment of CPT-4 codes is perhaps the simplest part of the coding process. This chapter deals with the process of selecting the correct code(s) for services performed. Later chapters address extracting the appropriate key terms for selecting the correct code(s).

As discussed previously, medical terminology and anatomy are crucial to the process of extracting key terms from the medical documentation from which appropriate CPT-4 codes are assigned. In addition to the chapter key terms, a list of medical and anatomical terms are provided for each section of CPT-4 as it is discussed.

LAYOUT

GENERAL

The CPT-4 coding book is divided into six sections; each uses a distinctly separate set of guidelines.

Evaluation and Management (Visits)	99201-99499
Anesthesiology	00100-01999
	99100-99140
Surgery	10000-69999
Radiology	70000-79999

Pathology/Laboratory	80000-89999
Medicine	90700-99199

The layout is based on the "step" method of identifying the correct section within CPT-4, the correct components, and eventually "narrowing down" the possible selections to only the correct code. This technique was demonstrated in Chapter 8. In this chapter, the information is broken down further (see Table 9-1).

Each section within the CPT-4 book is divided into subsections by anatomical, procedural, condition, or descriptor subheadings. Procedures and services are presented in numerical order EXCEPT for the entire Evaluation and Management section, which is positioned at the front of the CPT-4 book. It is the most commonly used section and required by almost every provider at some time.

Each section is prefaced with coding guidelines specific to that section. Modifier codes are listed for that particular section, as well as any instructions unique to the section for assigning appropriate codes.

SECTION OVERVIEWS

Each section of CPT-4 is unique in regard to the requirements for assigning codes from that section, but the step-by-step process remains the same. The intricacies of each section of CPT-4 are discussed in individual chapters in this book. To get a snapshot of the components needed for each section, see Table 9-1, which shows the basic steps in assigning codes from each section of CPT-4.

Evaluation and Management (Codes 99201-99499)

This section was specifically designed to describe services provided directly by the physician or provider in the form of "visits" or evaluation services. These visits, referred to as *E & M* services, are broken down as follows:

Identify CPT-4 Chapter:	Services for Visits, Evaluations
Identify Type/Location:	Inpatient, Outpatient, Office Consultation, Office
New/Established:	New Patient, Established Patient Initial Visit, Subsequent Visit
Level of Service:	Level 1
	Level 2
	Level 3
	Level 4 (if applicable)
	Level 5 (if applicable)

This information is necessary to code E & M services, as well as all other services covered by the CPT-4 codes. As with ICD-9-CM coding, CPT-4 coding depends on the documentation by the provider. When information is not documented, the coder or biller may not assume any knowledge of the services and may need to code a lower level than is appropriate for the service.

Because all codes in the evaluation and management section begin with the number *99*, the levels are referred

TABLE 9-1   CPT-4 Coding Steps

Type Service	E & M	Anesthesia	Surgery	Radiology	Pathology	Medicine
Step 1 Identify chapter	Visits/ encounters	General Regional Spinal	Definitive Restorative Invasive	X-Rays MRI/CT Ultrasounds Nuclear med	Study of body substances	Diagnostic therapy
Range of codes	99201-99499	00100-01999 99100-99140	10021-69990	70010-79999	80048-89399	90281-99199 99500-99600
Step 2 Determine type/ location	Location Office Hospital	Anatomical location Head Upper extrem	Anatomical system Integumentary Respiratory	Type of service Diagnostic Ultrasound	Type of service Chemistry Hematology	Specialty type Allergy Pulmonary
Step 3 Specific type	Patient status New patient Established	Body area Eye Thyroid	Anatomical part Skin Finger	Anatomical part Chest Lower extremity	Specific test Hemoglobin Hematocrit	Specific test Pulmonary function test
Step 4 Specific procedure information	Level of service Level 1	Procedure Open Closed	Procedure Excision Incision	Views/contrast 2 views w/contrast	Auto/manual Automated Manual	Tests With contrast
Step 5 Extent/additional specifics	Time/other guidelines 45 min	Specifics XXXXX	Extent procedure Size/cm	Addtl guidelines	Addtl guidelines	Addtl guidelines

to simply as Level 1, Level 2, Level 3, Level 4, and Level 5. This notation is commonly used throughout this text and will likely be encountered in the physician's or provider's office.

Evaluation and Management services are subsectioned as follows:

- Outpatient/Office Visits
- Hospital Observation Services
- Hospital Inpatient Services
- Consultations
- Emergency Department Services
- Critical Care Services
- Neonatal/Pediatric Intensive Care Services
- Nursing Facility Services
- Domiciliary, Rest Home, Custodial Services
- Prolonged Services
- Physician Standby Services
- Case Management Services
- Care Plan Oversight Services
- Preventive Medicine Services
- Counseling/Risk Factor Services
- Newborn Care
- Special Evaluation and Management Services

To code services from the Evaluation and Management section of CPT-4, the coder must capture specific information from the documentation. Consider the following example:

Type/Location:	Outpatient
New/Established:	Established Patient
Level:	Level 3; based on documentation of History, Exam, Medical Decision Making (see Chapter 10)
CODE ASSIGNMENT:	99213

Anesthesiology (Codes 00100-01999/ Codes 99100-99140)

Services performed by the anesthesiologist (or under the supervision of the anesthesiologist) are listed in the **anesthesiology** section. Keep in mind that the anesthesiology provider may also perform services outside of the anesthesia section such as pain management, for example, an injection made into the spinal column and nerves. The code for this service would be found in another section of CPT-4 in such an instance.

Codes in the anesthesia section of CPT-4 are assigned based on the anatomical location of the surgery and are arranged in "anatomical order" starting at the head and progressing down the body, except for a few sections that cannot be organized in this fashion. Procedures performed on the head and neck would be found in the front portion of the anesthesia section. Keep in mind that these codes are for analgesic medications used during surgical procedures; the surgeon performing the actual surgery will use other codes.

The anesthesia codes found in this section are easily distinguishable from surgical codes for the same procedures because all codes found in the anesthesia section begin with a "0." It is clear when reviewing a claim form that a procedure code beginning with a "0" is for anesthesia services only, and not the surgery itself. The following example demonstrates how to correctly code for anesthesia by taking one step at a time:

Identify Chapter:	Induction of anesthetic substance(s)
Anatomical Location:	Where surgical procedure is being performed
	Listed as general areas such as head/neck, lower/upper abdomen
Specific Location:	Codes sometimes are specific to one body area or region (e.g., radius, ulna, femur, fibula, tibia)
Specific Procedure:	Descriptions of specifically what is performed, such as:
	Fracture Treatment/Resection/Reduction/Incision
	Resection/Reduction/Incision
Specifics:	Open/Closed Reduction

The information necessary to code or bill for anesthesia services is typically contained in the anesthesia billing card completed by the provider at the time of service. It is then returned to the provider's office for coding and billing. Keep in mind that the coder and biller are responsible for making certain that appropriately signed documentation exists for all services being billed.

Surgery (Codes 10000-69999)

Procedures that the layperson may not consider surgical may in fact have surgical codes in the CPT-4 book (e.g., laceration repairs, repair of fractures). The **surgery** section is composed of services that typically are invasive, restorative, or definitive in nature. In other words, for the services to be performed, it is usually necessary to "invade" or enter the body by some method. It is also possible that the procedure performed is definitive or corrective for the problem being treated. When codes from the surgery section of CPT-4 are assigned, all guidelines and modifiers for that section should be used when applicable. Because of the size of the surgery section, it is imperative that the coder or biller use the "breakdown" methodology built into the CPT-4 layout, particularly for locating codes in this section.

Identify Chapter:	Procedure considered invasive, definitive, or corrective in nature
Anatomical System:	Integumentary
	Musculoskeletal

	Respiratory
	Cardiovascular
	Hemic and Lymphatic
	Mediastinum and Diaphragm
	Digestive System
	Urinary System
	Male Genital System
	Intersex Surgery
	Female Genital System
	Maternity Care and Delivery
	Endocrine System
	Nervous System
	Eye and Ocular Adnexa
	Auditory system
Type of Procedure:	Incision
	Excision
	Fracture/Dislocation
	Repair, Reconstruction
	Scopy
Extent of Procedure:	EX: Fracture, Closed/Open
	With/Without Manipulation
	With/Without Fixation

Knowledge of the anatomical parts of each organ system and their function is important so that the code(s) needed for surgical services can be located. In the event a Medical Terminology or Anatomy and Physiology course has not been completed, then a review of the brief outline provided in Chapter 8 may be necessary before the surgical coding section is attempted.

Radiology (Codes 70000-79999)

The radiological section includes codes for services when imaging is performed to determine the scope or extent of a medical problem. Imaging may be performed by a number of methods, so the proper coding for **radiology** requires the following determinations in order:

Determine Chapter:	Imaging performed
Type of Service:	Diagnostic (X-Ray, CT, MRI)
	Ultrasound
	Radiation Therapy
	Nuclear Medicine
Anatomical Part:	Body Area Imaged
# Views/Contrast:	2 Views, 3 Views
	With/Without Contrast

The services found in the radiological section could include a simple chest x-ray (diagnostic section), a fetal ultrasound (ultrasound section), radiation therapy (radiation oncology), or bone scan (nuclear medicine). Information regarding the anatomical location and view/contrast information will be dependent on the radiological report because the actual films are not part of the medical record. Chapter 13 contains information about radiological reports and their necessity on reports for coding and billing purposes.

Pathology/Laboratory (Codes 80000-89399)

Services in the **Pathology** or Laboratory section typically include procedures to obtain specimens and their subsequent analysis. Such specimens may include blood, urine, cervical and vaginal fluids, semen, mucus, and other bodily fluids, as well as biopsy specimens that are sent to the laboratory for analysis and diagnosis. Because many of these tests may be performed by a number of different methods, care must be taken to select a code on the basis of the specimen and the method (e.g., automated, manual, or dipstick).

Subsections for the Pathology section are as follows:

- Organ or Disease Oriented Panels
- Drug Testing
- Therapeutic Drug Assays
- Evocative/Suppression Testing
- Consultations (Clinical Pathology)
- Urinalysis
- Chemistry
- Hematology and Coagulation
- Immunology
- Transfusion Medicine
- Microbiology
- Anatomic Pathology
- Cytopathology
- Cytogenetic Studies
- Surgical Pathology
- Reproductive Medicine Procedures

To code services from the Pathology section of CPT-4, the coder must capture the following information:

Identify Chapter:	Analysis of Body Fluids or Pathological Specimens
Procedure Performed:	Transfusion, Microbiology, Surgical Pathology
Specific Procedure:	Complete Blood Count, Blood Typing
Extent/Specifics:	Automated, Manual

Medicine (Code 90701-99199)

The Medicine section encompasses a variety of specialty services and procedures that do not meet the criteria of surgical in nature or visits/encounters. It is sometimes difficult to differentiate between medicine procedures and surgical procedures. If the coder keeps in mind that codes in the surgical section specify procedures that are invasive, definitive, or restorative in nature, and that those in the medicine section are diagnostic or therapeutic in nature, differentiation becomes straightforward. The Medicine section encompasses the following services:

- Immune Globulins
- Vaccines/Toxoids
- Injections
- Psychiatry
- Dialysis
- Gastroenterology
- Ophthalmology

- ENT (Ears, Nose, and Throat)
- Cardiovascular
- Pulmonary
- Allergy
- Neurology
- Osteopathic Procedures
- Chiropractic Services

A number of specialties are represented in the previous list. The procedures listed under each specialty are diagnostic or therapeutic in nature; that is, they do not meet the criteria for surgery or for evaluation and management. For example, such a procedure provided by a Psychiatry specialist might include psychotherapy. Note that this is a procedure and does not constitute an office visit. In the Cardiovascular section are procedures, most of which are noninvasive, such as electrocardiograms (ECGs), cardiac stress testing, and cardiac catheterizations. The reason that cardiac catheterizations are located in the medicine section rather than the surgery section is discussed later. Briefly, they are considered noninvasive because the primary purpose is for diagnosis. When cardiac catheterization involves the repair of a vessel (angioplasty), this procedure is also considered noninvasive because the advancement of a catheter is through a small incision. In comparison to a coronary artery bypass graft or a pacemaker/defibrillator insertion, such procedures seem minor and nonsurgical.

For codes from the Medicine section to be properly assigned, services should be broken down as follows:

Identify Chapter:	Diagnostic/Therapeutic Procedures (other than Radiology/Pathology)
Identify Specific Specialty:	Gastroenterology, Pulmonary, Allergy, Ophthalmology
Identify Specific Procedure:	Allergy Testing Allergy Immunotherapy Preparation of Allergan Extract
Identify Specifics:	Age/Minutes/Level

CPT-4 GUIDELINES

To select the appropriate CPT-4 codes, the coder who wishes to have a thorough understanding of CPT-4 procedure coding should know some definitions of terms and concepts that are provided in CPT-4. The coder must understand CPT-4 guidelines because they are essential for correctly coding documentation so that reimbursement is timely and uncontested.

CPT-4 guidelines are designed for each specific section. The coder must identify the procedure, ascertain which section contains the appropriate code, and follow the guidelines for that section.

MODIFIERS

Modifiers are the means by which the physician indicates that a service or procedure has been altered in some manner. Although the code itself does not change, the procedure it codes for has been modified in some respect, and an explanation of this change is required.

The coder may describe provided services using only CPT-4 codes. Therefore any changes must also be described by codes, numbers, or assignment of modifiers.

Modifier codes may be used in one of two ways. The most frequently used method is the addition of a two-digit numerical code following the CPT-4 code to represent the modifier. Modifiers have assigned codes that must be looked up, just as assigned procedure codes must be looked up.

Take note that individual modifiers may be used only for specific sections of the CPT-4. Unfortunately, the newest editions of CPT-4 do not indicate for which section(s) each modifier is appropriately used. Coders may use the "Appendix on Modifiers" located in the back of the CPT-4 book or the materials provided in Chapter 16 of this book to develop their own coding reference tools. Chapter 16 contains information about modifiers at length and provides a summary matrix of modifier codes.

Typically, modifier codes explain alterations to descriptions. Consider the following examples.

Professional versus Technical Component(s)

Modifier codes can describe situations in which only one component of a service that usually includes both professional and technical components is performed.

More Than One Physician/Location

When the same service is supplied by more than one physician or is repeated by the same physician, a modifier indicates that the service listed is not a duplicate or an error in billing. Without the use of the modifier code, the insurance carrier assumes an error in billing or a duplicate of the same service. Without such a modifier, claims with the same procedure code on the same day of service by the same provider will be disallowed or denied.

Service Performed at a Different Level Than Usual

When a service is provided at a level greater or less than usual, the change can be indicated by use of the appropriate modifier code. The use of this modifier is not intended to denote an increase or decrease in the amount charged, but rather a change in the level or type of service provided. These modifiers are usually used when the greatest or least level of service has been selected but additional description is needed. Special documenta-

tion may be required to justify the medical necessity of increased service and the requested increase in reimbursement.

Partial Service or One Portion of a Service Performed

When the service described is inclusive of several components, but not all components are performed, a modifier indicates which portion was completed. Because the total service was not performed, total reimbursement would not be appropriate. Instead, only a portion of the total reimbursement may be expected. For many years, insurance carriers did not reimburse for procedures that were started but not completed. With the introduction of a modifier code to describe this situation, however, insurance carriers now recognize that even when the procedure is not completed, the preparation and medical decision making involved should be given consideration for at least partial payment. The provider must document what portion of the service was performed.

Additional Services Performed in Conjunction with Provided Services

When coding for surgical procedures, the coder must frequently use multiple procedural codes to adequately describe the surgical case. It is necessary for the coder to specify the primary procedure, the secondary procedure, and contributing procedures. Proper use of modifiers is important because additional procedures following the first will usually be significantly discounted for reimbursement. Thus it is imperative that the most significant service be listed as the primary service. Although this service will frequently also be the most substantial charge, the coder should make certain not to select primary procedures on the basis of the charge but on their medical significance.

Bilateral Services Provided

When services are provided to both right and left extremities or to other body areas that are considered bilateral, the coder must indicate that charges are not a duplication of billing, but rather two separate and legitimate charges, by using a modifier code.

Service/Procedure Performed More Than Once

Repeat procedures must be indicated as such so that insurance carriers will not deny reimbursement for duplication of services. For instance, when a patient with myocardial infarction undergoes multiple ECGs throughout the course of treatment during a given day, the coder must indicate, by the use of a modifier, that the multiple charges are NOT a duplication error, but rather that repeat services were medically necessary.

Services Outside Those Ordinarily Provided

There are situations in which the normal postoperative period is interrupted by another procedure that may or may not have relevance to the original procedure. In other instances, additional procedures that were intended to be performed as part of the overall surgery plan may be performed during what would otherwise be considered the postoperative period. The use of modifiers explains these unusual circumstances or exceptions, which should be considered for reimbursement.

Third-Party/Insurance Carrier Significance

The use of a modifier code indicates to the insurer that the CPT-4 codes reported are not reflected in the third-party fee calculations used for averaging and statistical record keeping of charges. Modifiers also indicate that changes were made to a usual procedure so there may be differences between the usual reimbursement rate for that specific service and the reimbursement amount actually requested by a provider for services.

By placing the modifier code after a procedure code, the coder specifies that there has been a recognized exception or change in the procedure, so the request for payment differs from the usual reimbursement. Such modifiers serve as explanation for the changes and indicate to the insurance carrier that this altered service should, in fact, be considered for payment.

Think of this coding principle as follows:

CPT-4 Code + Modifier Code = CPT-4 Code (**WHAT** was provided) + (But) Modifier Code (special consideration should be made for the services/reasons identified)

DEFINITIONS/CONCEPTS

Starred Procedures

Starred procedures were eliminated from CPT-4 in the 2004 edition. As a result, all surgical procedures have a minimum follow-up of at least 10 days. The follow-up period is defined by the value or base units of the procedure as determined by the RBRVS (Resource Based Relative Value Study). This area is addressed in later chapters.

Global Procedures "Package Concept"

The **global procedures** concept is probably the most difficult concept to grasp in coding. Global procedures are defined by both insurance carriers and CPT-4 as those that follow a predetermined outline that specifically addresses services necessary to complete a surgical

procedure, including preoperative and postoperative care. Surgical procedure components include the following:

- Surgery
- Local infiltration
- Blocks (such as metacarpal or digital)
- Anesthesia performed topically
- Normal uncomplicated postoperative care
- Preoperative care

The difficulty in understanding the global procedures concept arises when it is implemented by third-party insurance carriers. Consider the concept of "global services" as it relates to purchasing an automobile. When an automobile is purchased, it comes equipped with a number of specified items that are a part of the "package price," such as a steering wheel, tires, wheels, seats, and so forth. Extras, or "upgrades," such as a CD player or special rims, are NOT included in the "package price." Therefore when they are selected, they are charged "a la carte" (Figure 9-1). Envisioning the concept of the car purchase may help the coder when the coder attempts to determine whether services are included, or "bundled," as in the package price of the car.

Global packages for procedures are much the same as the package price for an automobile. Certain items are included in the package, but "extras" must be noted as such by use of the proper modifier code. The difficulty comes from the many interpretations by third-party insurance carriers of this "package concept" or "global procedures." In the scenario of the car purchase, one dealer may include a cassette player as part of the sticker package; another may not. Air conditioning may be included in the package in some instances, but not in others. This "car" concept with its inherent variability can be applied to third-party insurance carriers and the services and procedures they may or may not reimburse.

Unlisted

When no specific procedural code has been assigned, such procedures are listed as "unspecified" or **"unlisted."** For example, because several procedures without a specific code could be indicated as "unlisted respiratory conditions," the coder should include a report for such procedures, an explanation of the procedures, and their names. With these data, the insurance carrier accumulates information about each specific procedure. At a later date, the carrier will be able to assign specific codes for high-volume procedures.

The significance of this designation for a third-party insurance carrier is that the unlisted procedure code(s) provided in each anatomical section of CPT-4 should be used ONLY when no other valid CPT-4 code is available. Should the insurance carrier decide that there is an appropriate code for the service, it may be recoded accordingly. Again, because this type of service may

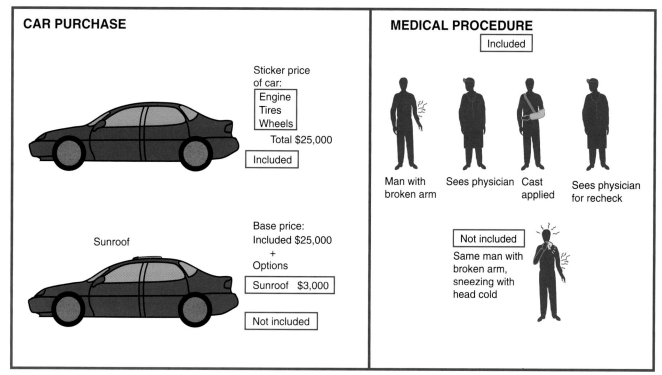

FIGURE 9-1. Compare the "package" concept of an automobile purchase to the "package" concept of global medical procedures.

encompass several procedures ranging from minor to major, a detailed report of the procedure must be attached.

Separate Procedure

There are a number of procedures, especially in the surgical section of CPT-4, that have the term **separate procedure** after the description. This designates a procedure that may be assigned a code ONLY if it is the only procedure from within that section of codes; thus, it is a "separate" procedure. Should other codes from within that subcategory be assigned, the procedures with this designation are considered included or "incidental."

FORMAT

GENERAL

In the CPT-4 manual, the coder will find stand-alone descriptions of medical procedures. When an entry in the CPT-4 book is followed by indented entries, the indented entries refer back to one or more common elements listed in the directly preceding entry. One of the tips for diagnostic coding from the ICD-9-CM was to refer back to the last entry that appears flush with the left-hand margin. This allows the coder to make certain all components have been included; the same advice holds true

for use of the CPT-4 manual. Consider the following example:

58260   Vaginal hysterectomy
58262   with removal of tube(s), and/or ovary(ies)
58263   with removal of tube(s), and/or ovary(ies) with repair of enterocele

All procedural codes listed here appear flush left; descriptors in subentries are indented past the margin of "vaginal hysterectomy." Use the index located in the back of the CPT-4 manual for cross-referencing (locating) the section in which selected codes are found.

SYMBOLS

Along with learning the format of CPT-4, the coder must become familiar with symbols used in the book. The following entries explain these symbols.

- ● **Bullet** A bullet indicates that a code is a new addition to CPT-4 with this edition.
- ▲ **Triangle** A triangle indicates that the descriptive information for a CPT-4 code has undergone revision.

In addition to learning the outline and format for the CPT-4 manual, the coder must follow some general rules for CPT-4 coding. Tool 24 identifies these important rules in the coding process.

+ **Add On**   Procedure codes are only assigned when an initial code is assigned. Procedure codes should be used only in combination with another primary code(s).

T O O L 24

CPT-4 CODING GUIDELINES

1. Identify the key words/phrases for coding purposes. Utilize medical term(s) for coding procedures and services.

2. Identify those procedural statements/services to be used for coding purposes.

3. Determine the correct order for billing services/procedures.
   Make certain the correct primary diagnosis (WHY) has been matched to the correct procedure (WHAT). Determine the most significant service provided for a given date as the primary procedure.

4. Select the correct code(s) from CPT-4/HCPCS, utilizing the following steps:
   - Locate the main term for the procedure/service in the index.
   - Locate each code listed in the CPT-4 book.
   - Follow all notes and cross-references to ensure correct selection.
   - Follow the rules for inclusion/exclusion as well as surgical packages (global).
   - Determine whether a modifier code is necessary.
   - Make certain the correct guidelines and modifiers are utilized by checking the code selected and verifying which section of CPT-4 this code originated from. Follow those guidelines and rules ONLY.

Ø	Procedure code should NOT have a modifier 51 assigned despite the fact it would be appropriate according to CPT-4 guidelines. These codes are often assigned along with other CPT-4 codes; therefore the use of modifier 51 is not necessary.
Separate Procedure	This designation is discussed in depth in Chapter 12 (Surgery). Use of this designation becomes more apparent in this chapter.
Ea/Each	This is discussed in depth in Chapter 12 (Surgery) because use of this designation becomes more apparent in this chapter.

THE FUTURE OF CPT-4/CPT-5

The CPT-5 project has been undertaken to update, revise, and add technological changes to the current CPT-4 system. Implementation of CPT-5 is currently pending. Proposed advantages of CPT-5 over CPT-4 include the following:

- Improvements in CPT long descriptors
- Codes to track new diagnostic/therapeutic technologies
- Codes to track quality of health care services
- Codes to include preventive medicine services
- Development of nonphysician evaluation and management services
- Use of Internet technology to reduce time for obtaining new codes
- Expansion of the CPT-4 Advisory Committee
- CPT-5 as a state-of-the-art database

Evaluation + mgmt
anestelogy
Surgery
Radiology
Pathology/Lab
Medicine

STOP AND PRACTICE

Locate WHERE in CPT-4 the coder would find the following procedures. This is important for assigning the correct codes and modifiers and for adhering to the guidelines for each service.

	Section Found
Ex: Physician office visit	Evaluation and Management
1. Chest x-ray	*Path/Lab*
2. CBC w/diff	*Path/Lab ok*
3. Split-thickness skin graft	*Surgery*
4. Pulmonary function testing	*med ok*
5. Placement of gastrostomy tube	*Surgery*
6. Endoscopy	*med ✓ surgery*
7. Tonsillectomy	*Surgery*
8. Cast application	*med ✓ surgery*
9. Outpatient consultation	*E + m*

10. Allergy immunotherapy	*Lab ✓ med*
11. Psychotherapy	*med*
12. Immunization(s)	*med*
13. Abdominal hysterectomy	*surgery*
14. Vaginal delivery	*med ✓ surgery*
15. Hospital visit	*E + m*
16. MRI	*Lab ✓ Radiology*
17. Emergency department visit	*E + m*
18. Allergy testing	*Lab ✓ med*
19. Laceration repair	*med*
20. Nursing home visit	*E + m*
21. Preventive medicine visit	*E + m*
22. Antibiotic injection	*med*
23. Tetanus immunization	*med*
24. Chemotherapy	*med*
25. Repair of fracture	*surgery*

After identifying the particular section from which each service should be billed, the coder must review each section's applicable guidelines or rules and modifiers. REMEMBER the importance of determining the correct section from which to select the applicable code. ONLY THOSE RULES AND GUIDELINES FOR THE SELECTED SECTION APPLY.

CHAPTER IN REVIEW

CERTIFICATION REVIEW

- The coding system used to bill for procedures is known as HCPCS (Healthcare Common Procedure Coding System).
- The HCPCS coding system consists of three levels:
  Level 1-CPT-4
  Level 2-National Codes
  Level 3-Local Codes
- CPT-4 is divided into six sections with six distinctly separate sets of guidelines:
  Evaluation and Management
  Anesthesiology
  Surgery
  Radiology
  Pathology/Laboratory
  Medicine
- Evaluation and Management services are listed first in CPT-4 because of their universal use by most physicians. These codes are used for different types and levels of physician encounters or visits.
- Anesthesiology codes are used only by the anesthesia physician or provider.
- Along with CPT-4 modifiers, anesthesia codes require a physician status modifier and additional CPT-4 codes to describe extenuating circumstances.
- The surgery section of CPT-4 encompasses a vast number of procedures, including those that the layperson might not consider as surgery. As such, the rules and guidelines for surgical procedures apply to these services as well.
- Radiology services are categorized as diagnostic radiology, diagnostic ultrasound, radiation oncology, and nuclear medicine.
- Pathology services are performed with specimens obtained from the patient to perform diagnostic services.
- The medicine section of CPT-4 includes services that are not considered surgical in nature and that do not fall under other sections of CPT-4.
- Modifier codes are the means of indicating that services described by the assignment of a CPT-4 code have been altered or modified in some fashion.

- Modifier codes are often used to justify the necessity of additional services and the need for reimbursement consideration for services not typically reimbursed.
- Global surgical procedures represent a "package" concept wherein a specified group of services, such as preoperative, operative, and postoperative services, is included in one CPT-4 procedure code, which results in reimbursement for that code.

STUDENT STUDY GUIDE

- Study Chapter 9.
- Review the Learning Objectives for Chapter 9.
- Complete the Stop and Practice exercises.
- Study the Certification Review for Chapter 9.
- Complete the Chapter Review exercise to reinforce concepts learned in this chapter.
- Chapter Review Exercise

CHAPTER REVIEW EXERCISE

Identify the sections/subsections where the services are located:

Chapter	Subsection
EX: Vaginal Hysterectomy	Surgery Female Genital
1. Chest x-ray, PA only	radiology Diag
2. CT scan, brain without contrast	radiology Diag
3. Electroencephalogram	medicine head
4. Emergency department visit	E+m emergency dept
5. Epidural anesthesia	anesteology back
6. Repair, distal radius fracture	Surgery musculoskeletal
7. Excision of lesion (skin)	Surgery integumentary
8. Office visit	E+m office/OP
9. Mastectomy	Surgery mediastinum
10. Electrocardiogram	med cardiography
11. Physical therapy	med OP
12. Manipulation, finger joint	surgery musculoskeletal
13. Bronchoscopy with biopsy	surgery respiratory
14. Tracheostomy, emergency	surgery respiratory
15. Sinus endoscopy	Surgery nose
16. Insertion of pacemaker	surgery cardiovascular
17. Colonoscopy w/removal of polyps	surgery
18. Cataract extraction	surgery eye
19. Cytoscopy	surgery
20. Hospital visit	Evm hospital/OP

EVALUATION AND MANAGEMENT SERVICES

LEARNING OBJECTIVES

Following the completion of this chapter, the student will be able to:

- Apply the concepts of evaluation and management coding to practical cases.
- Understand the different types of evaluation and management services.
- Grasp definitions of new and established patients for CPT-4 coding purposes.
- Know the differences between 1995 and 1997 evaluation and management guidelines.
- Identify and apply key concepts for determining evaluation and management levels of service.
- Identify and apply correct modifiers to evaluation and management service codes.
- Comprehend the relationship of time to levels of service for evaluation and management services.
- Understand the concept of "covering physician" as it relates to CPT-4 evaluation and management coding.
- Understand the concept of "consultation" as it relates to CPT-4 evaluation and management coding.
- Define "critical care" as it pertains to evaluation and management services.

CODING REFERENCE TOOLS

Tool 25
History Guidelines
Tool 26
Examination Guidelines
Tool 27
Risk Grid
Tool 28
Steps to Accurate Assignment of Evaluation and Management Codes
Tool 29
1995 Guidelines for New Outpatient Visits

Tool 30
1995 Guidelines for Established Outpatient
  Visits
Tool 31
1995 Guidelines for Observation Care
Tool 32
1995 Guidelines for Initial Hospital Visits
Tool 33
1995 Guidelines for Subsequent Hospital Visits
Tool 34
1995 Guidelines for Outpatient Consultation
  Codes
Tool 35
1995 Guidelines for Initial Hospital Consultations
Tool 36
Consultation Crosswalk Codes
Tool 37
New/Established Time Driven Visit Codes
Tool 38
1995 Guidelines for Emergency Department
  Visits
Tool 39
1995 Guidelines for Comprehensive Nursing Facility
  Assessments Care
Tool 40
1995 Guidelines for Subsequent Nursing Facility
  Care
Tool 41
1995 Guidelines for New Domiciliary or Rest Home
  Visits
Tool 42
1995 Guidelines for Established Domiciliary or Rest
  Home Visits
Tool 43
1995 Guidelines for New Home Visits
Tool 44
1995 Guidelines for Established Home Visits

KEY TERMS

Coordination of Care, 203
Counseling, 203
Established Patient, 201
Examination, 199
History, 199
History of Present Illness, 206
Medical Decision Making, 199
New Patient, 201
Review of Systems, 206
Risks of Morbidity/Mortality, 206

DOCUMENTATION GUIDELINES

Documentation needs for physician services have been discussed in Section I. The student will now work extensively on identifying the key components in the physician encounter: **History, Examination,** and **Medical Decision Making.** These key elements are essential in the identification of the correct Evaluation and Management procedure code for services performed.

Consistency is of the utmost importance in E & M coding. The coder must be able to substantiate the level of service coded on the basis of the documentation provided. The best way to achieve this consistency is to use some type of form to document how the coder arrives at a specific level of service. If a question arises at a later date, whether from a third-party audit or a patient inquiry, the practice or facility will be able to substantiate the level of service originally coded.

Other methods, such as developing specialty-specific coding guidelines, also assist in maintaining consistency in E & M coding. Sample grids are included with the discussion of each type of E & M service.

Look again at the E & M portion of the table in Chapter 9 at the Steps or components needed for CPT-4 coding.

CPT-4 Coding Steps E & M Example

Step 1

| Identify Chapter | Visits/Encounters |
| Range of Codes | 99201-99499 |

Step 2

Determine Type/Location	Location
	Office
	Hospital

Step 3

| Specific Type | Patient Status |
| | New Patient Established |

Step 4

| Specific Procedure Information | Level of Service |
| | Level 1 |

Step 5

| Extent/Additional Specifics | Time/Other Guidelines |
| | 45 min |

Take a sample E & M chart and evaluate that medical chart for the documentation components needed to appropriately assign the correct E & M level for the service.

CONSULTATION REPORT
GODFREY REGIONAL OUTPATIENT CLINIC

Patient:
Date of consultation: 05/14/XX
Consulting physician: **HPI (Quality)**
Referring physician:
Indication for consultation: Ventricular tachycardia

History: **PMH**

The patient is a 76-year-old female with known history of cardiac disease who underwent an outpatient knee arthroscopy yesterday. The procedure went well; however, during the postoperative period, the patient's cardiac rhythm was noted to have multiple runs of non-sustained ventricular tachycardia. The patient apparently remained asymptomatic and hemodynamically stable. Due to her significant cardiac history, it was felt she should follow up to rule out any cardiac abnormalities. Patient denies having any recent history of chest pain, PND, orthopnea, dyspnea on exertion, shortness of breath, palpitations, syncope/near syncope or lower extremity edema.   **PMH**   **PMH**   **Chief Complaint**

PMH — PAST MEDICAL HISTORY:
  1. Coronary atherosclerotic heart disease
  2. Status post myocardial infarction approximately 15 years ago
  3. S/P PTCA

PMH — ALLERGIES: Iodine

PMH — MEDICATIONS:
  1. Altace 10 mg qd
  2. Aricept 5 mg qd
  3. Amiodarone 100 mg qd
  4. Clonazepam 5 mg qhs
  5. Prevachol 40 mg qhs
  6. Spironolactone 25 q tablet qhs

FAMILY HISTORY: Non-contributory
None — SOCIAL HISTORY: Non-contributory
REVIEW OF SYSTEMS: As stated in the HPI

1E Constitutional   Exam:

PHYSICAL EXAMINATION:
The patient is a well developed, elderly white female who is alert and oriented X3 in no acute distress with pleasant demeanor. She is afebrile with stable vital signs.

2E — HEAD: Normocephalic, atraumatic
3E — NECK: Supple without evidence of JCP, mass or bruit
4E — CHEST: Clear to auscultation
5E — CARDIAC: Normal carotid upstroke with normal contour – no evidence of peristernal
Heave, lift, thrill. Auscultation reveals regular rate and rhythm without evidence of murmur, rub or gallop. Pulses are 1+ and symmetrical throughout.
6E — ABDOMEN: Soft, nontender, no evidence of pulsatile or palpable mass identified
7E — GU: Deferred
8E — EXTREM: Showed no evidence of clubbing, cyanosis, or edema
1M — NEURO: Grossly intact, nonfocal
EKG: Ectopic atrial rhythm with delayed precordial transmission and prolonged QT corrected interval. Telemetry shows no current findings suggestive of significant tachy or brady arrhythmia. No findings suggestive of any significant block or pause.
2M — LAB DATA: Hematology – WBC 4.5, hemoglobin 12.1, hematocrit 35.3, MCV 95.6, MCH 32.8, platelets 160,000. Glucose, 92, BUN 14, creatinine 1.0, calcium 8.6, alk phos 40, Potassium 3.5, Cardiac enzymes, CPK 88, CKMB 5, Troponin 0.5

Diagnosis/assessment:

MDM Risk Low

IMPRESSION:
76-year-old female with known history of coronary atherosclerotic heart disease and atrial fibrillation, now presents with run of nonsustained V tach per report. Patient has remained hemodynamically stable, no evidence of persistent cardiac arrhythmia.

We appreciate the opportunity to participate in the overall evaluation and management of this patient. We will continue the patient on her usual cardiac medications, and, should she experience any symptoms, she should follow-up immediately.

Maurice Doates, MD

Patient name: _____

Date of service: _____

GODFREY REGIONAL OUTPATIENT CLINIC
3122 Shannon Avenue • Aldon, FL 77712 • (407) 555-7654

CPT-4 Coding Steps

	E & M Example	Chart Information
Step 1		
Identify Chapter	Visits/Encounters	Evaluation and Management
Range of Codes	99201-99499	99201-99499
Step 2	**Consultation**	
Determine Type/ Location	Location Office Hospital	99241-99275 Outpatient 99241-99245
Step 3		
Specific Type	Patient Status New Patient Established	New 99241-99245
Step 4	**Will review later in chapter**	
Specific Procedure Information	Level of Service Level 1	
Step 5		
Extent/Additional Specifics	Time/Other Guidelines 45 min	

At this point, an E & M code for this service would be assigned from the range between 99241 and 99245. The exact code would be assigned based on the level of service for the Consultation. How to determine the level of service is discussed throughout this chapter. Following the discussion, this chart is reconsidered and the key components extracted that are necessary to arrive at the exact CPT-4 Evaluation and Management code for this service.

GENERAL CODING GUIDELINES

The specific definitions necessary for understanding E & M coding are as follows:

New patient—a patient who has not received any professional service from the physician or another physician of the same specialty in the same group over the past 3 years.

Established patient—a patient who has received professional services from the physician or another physician of the same specialty in the same group during the past 3 years.

In the case of "on call" physicians, or "covering physicians," the E & M service is coded and billed with the same coding that would have been used by the physician who was not available. For example, if an established patient of a family practitioner is hospitalized and is seen by a "covering physician," that E & M service would be billed as an established patient visit, despite the fact the physician attending the patient may never have seen the patient in the past.

In most instances, the physician may charge one level of service code per patient per day. Therefore when the patient is seen in the office and is referred to the hospital for admission, the provider may charge for only one service—the office visit or the hospital admission.

MODIFIERS

Take a look in Table 10-1 at the ONLY modifier codes that are applicable to the E & M section.

MODIFIER 21—PROLONGED E & M SERVICE

This modifier is defined as greater than the usual level of performance for E & M services. This modifier is typically used when the highest level of service is provided (such as Level 5) and the service provided is greater than the highest level of service codeable. Documentation must justify the use of this modifier, and a report typically is needed.

MODIFIER 24—E & M SERVICES UNRELATED TO A GLOBAL OR POSTOPERATIVE PERIOD

With modifier 24 comes the concept of global procedures. Remember, when global procedures are performed, the

TABLE 10-1   Modifiers

Modifier	Descriptor	Use
21	Prolonged E & M Service	Services greater than usually described in E & M code assigned
24	E & M Services Unrelated to Global/ Postoperative Period	Services "outside" the global package
25	Significantly Separately Identifiable E & M at the time of another service	E & M services performed distinct to another service/procedure performed at the same encounter
32	Mandated Services	Services requested by a third party
52	Reduced Services	Services less than those typically performed with code assignment
57	Decision for Surgery	E & M service performed for the sole purpose of determining whether surgery is medically indicated

normal preoperative, surgical, and postoperative services are included in the "package" price for that service. HOWEVER, when E & M services are "extras" not included in the usual package price, the coder must indicate by using a modifier that these services should be considered "outside the normal global/postoperative package." An example would be follow-up visits during the postoperative period for completely unrelated services or complications.

Without the **modifier code,** the carrier WILL NOT consider these services for payment. The **modifier code** says to the carrier: This service is not usually covered; however, the service should be considered for payment because (modifier code). A diagnosis code indicating that the chief reason for an encounter is unrelated to the initial service or that it is the result of a complication such as "infection" is also necessary to justify payment for this modified service.

The listing of an unrelated diagnosis WILL NOT serve as justification to the insurance carrier for payment. In fact, many such claims are processed by computerized systems that deny the claim owing to the fact that all services of that provider have been paid under the global/package concept for the predefined global days.

The addition of a modifier code denotes to the computerized system or manual reviewer the need for additional consideration. Consider the following example:

01/21/01 Abdominal hysterectomy for the diagnosis of ovarian cyst

01/25/01 Office visit to same physician for complaint of cough

The follow-up period allowed for the abdominal hysterectomy for purposes of the previous example is defined as 90 days. This means that any visits to that physician during those same 90 days will not be considered for payment UNLESS a modifier is attached to the E & M code to signify that the visit was not related to the surgical procedure.

MODIFIER 25—E & M SERVICE THAT IS DISTINCT AND SEPARATE ("SIGNIFICANTLY SEPARATELY IDENTIFIABLE")

When the physician performs a procedure or service that is distinct and separate from the E & M service, it can be coded separately. Following is another instance in which medical necessity (diagnosis) is crucial to coding and reimbursement.

Patient visits physician following *automobile accident. Multiple contusions of the arms and legs, a painful shoulder,* and a head laceration are examined. Laceration repair is performed for the *open wound of the head.*

Services (WHAT)	Diagnosis (WHY)
Physician visit	Shoulder pain
	Multiple contusions, legs/arms
Laceration repair	Open wound of head

The chief reason for the encounter was the laceration repair of an open wound of the head. Because the open wound medically necessitated the laceration repair, the documentation focused on significant and separately identifiable E & M services specifically for shoulder pain and multiple contusions of the arms and legs.

Note: The 25 modifier is added to the E & M service code, NOT the surgical code.

MODIFIER 32—MANDATED SERVICES

When services are requested by a third party such as a PRO (Peer Review Organization) or a third-party carrier, the services should be designated as such with the modifier 32. Often, this will be a request for an additional opinion regarding surgery. Insurance carriers may not pay for multiple physicians' opinions on the same problem; however, if insurance carriers dictate the necessity of an additional opinion, that E & M service should be coded with modifier 32.

MODIFIER 52—REDUCED SERVICES

Modifier 52 should NOT be used to reduce the charge for an E & M service. This modifier should be used to indicate that the level of a provided E & M service is partially reduced. Such an adjustment in the level of service should NOT be made for the purpose of adjusting the price for a particular service. Caution should be taken to ensure that services are billed at the level performed. If a particular service has been reduced or eliminated and a lower charge is appropriate, less may be charged with the same level of service coded and use of modifier 52. With the proper addition of modifier 52, the usual customary and reasonable (UCR) reimbursement calculation for that level of service will not be affected.

MODIFIER 57—E & M SERVICE FOR PURPOSE OF DECISION FOR SURGERY

When an E & M service is performed and the determination is made during that E & M visit that surgery is necessary, it is NOT considered part of the preoperative global package; it may be considered for reimbursement by third-party carriers with the addition of modifier 57. Care should be taken to ensure that the service in fact is not scheduled as a preoperative visit, and that the decision to proceed with surgery has not already made before the time of the visit. These E & M services are considered part of the global surgical package and would be considered as included or BUNDLED. If the surgical procedure is global and no modifier is appended to services, a visit on the same day or on the day(s) preceding surgery typically will be denied as part of the global surgical package.

Not all insurance carriers agree with the use of this modifier, and some may still include this visit as part of the global package. Check the individual contract(s) with each carrier to determine whether this service is reimbursable.

Remember that the coder should code and bill services according to CPT-4 and not third-party guidelines. Despite the possibility that the carrier may include this service in the global package, if appropriate, the coder should code and bill the service. Third-party carrier inclusion or exclusion of payment should not determine how services are coded.

E & M SERVICE DETERMINATION

GENERAL GUIDELINES

CPT-4 guidelines are given for each type and level of service. The evaluation and management section (E & M) offers perhaps the greatest coding diversity of any section in the CPT-4 book. If the selection of codes from this section is made in a methodical step-by-step manner, then these services will be coded accurately.

The E & M section may also be the most controversial section of CPT-4. Many of the guidelines in this section are subject to interpretation; however, the coder must be consistent and capable of documenting and defending his or her choice of codes. Despite accurate E & M coding, some insurance carriers will not pay for some services that have been coded and billed appropriately. Inclusion of codes in CPT-4 does not imply that health insurance coverage will be provided for these services. These codes simply identify provided services; the medical necessity for those services is explained by the use of ICD-9-CM codes.

Services within the E & M section are assigned "levels." E & M services encompass those provided directly to the patient during a visit or encounter that does not involve diagnostic testing or services. This means that within the outpatient office visit section, the patient may be given a numerical level, typically from 1 to 5, depending on what services are performed. Each E & M service is coded according to the following criteria:

- New patient versus established patient
- Level of service
- Location of service (e.g., outpatient setting, hospital, nursing home)

Key E & M Components

The definition of "new versus established patient" has been discussed previously. Location of service, as it per-

tains to this definition, is discussed later in the chapter. The key components that determine levels for all E & M services, despite "new versus established" status and location of service are as follows:

- (H)istory
- Physical (E)xamination
- (M)edical decision making

In certain instances, other factors are taken into consideration as well. These include the following:

- **Counseling**
- **Coordination of care**
- Nature of presenting problem
- Time

The first three components are considered KEY COMPONENTS. They are always considered in making the initial determination of level of service. The last four factors apply in certain circumstances that are discussed later.

Level of Service According to 1995 and 1997 Guidelines

There are two separate sets of guidelines that may be followed for determining the level of service. In 1995, guidelines were established that define history, physical examination, and medical decision making components necessary for each level. New guidelines were introduced in 1997; however, their implementation has been delayed and they have not been officially adopted at this time. According to the 1997 guidelines, history, physical examination, and medical decision making criteria must still be met as outlined in the 1995 guidelines. Additionally, specific elements or "bullets" must be present in the documentation for the minimum requirement for each level to be met. Under the 1997 guidelines, the provider has the choice of using the key elements or bullets from either the multisystem or body organ system review that are pertinent to the patient's complaint.

Figure 10-1 provides a comparison of the 1995 and 1997 guidelines for outpatient office visits. The requirements of the 1995 and the 1997 guidelines are similar, except that the 1997 guidelines are more specific about the documentation that must be included. Because the 1995 guidelines are less specific, third-party carriers often disagree with the level the coder has assigned. Currently, the coder may use whichever guidelines he or she wishes to use for each case; however, it is advisable to stick with one set of guidelines to avoid confusion. Make certain that the physicians, the third-party carriers, and any entity performing chart audits are aware of which guidelines the facility has chosen to follow.

Facilities with many physicians may choose to use both sets of guidelines. A specific specialty or a physician may choose to use the 1997 guidelines. Other providers in the same group may wish to follow the 1995 guidelines.

Page 1

1995/1997 E & M CODING GUIDELINES COMPARISON
OFFICE/OTHER OUTPATIENT SERVICES, NEW PATIENT

	1995 Guidelines	1997 Guidelines
99201 **History:**	CC/brief HPI	Same
Exam:	Limited exam of affected body area/organ system	1-5 bullet elements in >1 body area/organ system
MDM:	Dx/Mgt minimal; Quantity/complex data minimal/none Risk minimal	Same
99202 **History:**	CC/brief HPI/problem pertinent ROS	Same
Exam:	Limited exam of affected body area/organ system Other related/symptomatic system(s)	6 bullet elements in >1 body area/organ system
MDM:	Dx/Mgt minimal; Quantity/complex data minimal/none Risk minimal	Same
99203 **History:**	CC/extended HPI/problem pertinent ROS including review of limited number of additional systems	Same 2-9 systems ROS/PFSH 1 item any history area
Exam:	Pertinent PFSH directly related to problem(s) Extend exam of affected body area/organ system Other related/symptomatic system(s)	2 bullet elements in at least 6 body areas/organ systems OR 12 bullet elements in >2 body areas/organ systems Single system (eye/psych): 9 bullet items required
MDM:	Dx/Mgt limited; Quantity/complex data limited Risk low	Same
99204 **History:**	CC/extended HPI/problem pertinent ROS + review of all additional systems/complete PFSH	Same 4 elements of HPI or 3 chronic/inactive conditions ROS at least 10 body areas/organ systems
Exam:	General multisystem exam OR complete exam of one organ system	All bullet elements in at least 9 body areas/organ systems No fewer than 2 bullet elements in each area/system Single system: All bullet items in shaded boxes and at least one bullet in each unshaded box
MDM:	Dx/Mgt multiple; Quantity/complex data moderate Risk moderate	Same
99205 **History:**	CC/extended HPI/problem pertinent ROS + review of all additional systems/complete PFSH	Same 4 elements of HPI or 3 chronic/inactive conditions ROS at least 10 body areas/organ systems
Exam:	General multisystem exam OR complete exam of one organ system	All bullet elements in at least 9 body areas/organ systems No less than 2 bullet elements in each area/system Single system: All bullet items in shaded boxes and at least one bullet in each unshaded box
MDM:	Dx/Mgt extensive; Quantity/complex data extensive Risk high	Same

FIGURE 10-1. 1995/1997 E&M Coding Guidelines Comparison.

Page 2

1995/1997 E & M CODING GUIDELINES COMPARISON		
OFFICE/OTHER OUTPATIENT SERVICES, ESTABLISHED PATIENT		
	1995 Guidelines	**1997 Guidelines**
99211 **History:**	No key elements required	Same
Exam:	Problem severity does not require physician presence; however, service provided under physician's care	
MDM:	None specified	
99212 **History:**	CC/brief HPI	Same
Exam:	Limited exam of affected body area/organ system	1-5 bullet elements in >1 body area/organ system
MDM:	Dx/Mgt minimal; Quantity/complex data minimal/none Risk minimal	Same
99213 **History:**	CC/extended HPI/problem pertinent ROS	Same
Exam:	Limited exam of affected body area/organ system Other related/symptomatic system(s)	6 bullet elements in >1 body area/organ system
MDM:	Dx/Mgt limited; Quantity/complex data limited Risk low	Same
99214 **History:**	CC/extended HPI/problem pertinent ROS Review of limited additional systems Pertinent PFSH related to problem(s)	Same Document 2-9 systems for ROS PFSH document 1 item any history area
Exam:	Extend exam of affected body area/organ system Other related/symptomatic system(s)	2 bullet elements in at least 6 body areas/organ systems OR 12 bullet elements in >2 body areas/organ systems Single system (eye/psych): 9 bullet elements required and at least 1 bullet in each unshaded box
MDM:	Dx/Mgt multiple; Quantity/complex data moderate Risk moderate	Same
99215 **History:**	CC/extended HPI/problem pertinent ROS + review of all additional systems/complete PFSH	Same 4 elements of HPI or 3 chronic/inactive conditions ROS at least 10 body areas/organ systems
Exam:	General multisystem exam OR complete exam of one organ system	All bullet elements in at least 9 body areas/organ systems No fewer than 2 bullet elements in each area/system Single system: All bullet items in shaded boxes and at least one bullet in each unshaded box
MDM:	Dx/Mgt extensive; Quantity/complex data extensive Risk high	Same

FIGURE 10-1, cont'd

Much controversy ensued when Medicare originally attempted to implement the 1997 guidelines in that same year. Additional attempts to implement these guidelines have been made since that time, but they have been thwarted by physicians nationwide. Time will tell whether the 1997 guidelines, with some adaptations, will eventually be adopted.

No matter which guidelines the facility or provider chooses to use for determining levels of service, the primary factors of HISTORY, PHYSICAL EXAMINATION, and MEDICAL DECISION MAKING still guide the assignment of those levels. Following is a discussion of the components needed in documentation so that E & M services can be coded appropriately.

HISTORY

History components provide information about the chief complaint and the history of the present illness such as:

- Chief complaint
- **History of present illness**
- Medical history
- Family and social history
- Review of systems

For specific examples of the documentation used to record these elements, refer to Tool 25.

By now, it should be apparent to the reader why proper physician documentation is so crucial. If these elements of documentation are omitted or are not recorded adequately, the code assigned may reflect a reduced level of service, and reimbursement may be adversely affected. Remember that the physician may bill only for what can be substantiated by the medical documentation. Tool 25 presents a listing of elements that make up all the history components of medical documentation.

PHYSICAL EXAMINATION

The physical examination, which reflects both the clinical judgment of the physician and the nature of the patient complaints at the time of the examination, is based on a number of elements that are reviewed AND documented during the course of the examination. These elements are defined by the number of organ systems or body areas that are examined on the basis of the complaint(s) and medical history.

Tool 26 demonstrates the elements included in the examination components.

The following BODY AREAS are recognized by CPT-4:

- Head
- Neck
- Chest (body area includes breasts, axillae)
- Abdomen
- Genitalia, groin, buttocks
- Back
- *Each* extremity

The following ORGAN SYSTEMS are recognized as physical examination elements:

- Eyes
- Ears, nose, mouth, throat

- Cardiovascular
- Respiratory
- Gastrointestinal
- Genitourinary
- Musculoskeletal
- Skin
- Neurological
- Psychiatric
- Hematological/lymphatic/immunological

Keep in mind that the components for the examination portion of the evaluation and management service are those gathered as the result of the hands-on examination by the provider. The review of systems portion of the History is facts gathered from information or taken from the patient. Care should be taken not to confuse these two E & M components.

MEDICAL DECISION MAKING

The third and final primary component of levels of service determination is medical decision making. Within the medical decision making component, there are three subcomponents, two of which must be met at the level assigned for medical decision making. These three subcomponents are (1) the number of diagnoses or management options, (2) the quantity and complexity of data, and (3) the risks of morbidity and mortality.

Number of Diagnoses or Management Options

The number of diagnoses or presenting problems treated is considered in the overall evaluation of medical decision making. Documented differential diagnoses are essential in achieving the highest level of diagnosis or management options possible.

Quantity and Complexity of Data

The quantity and complexity of data attained are based on the tests ordered and interpreted, as well as on medical records from or discussion of results with other health professionals.

Risks of Morbidity and Mortality

The **risks of morbidity and mortality** are determined by the complexity of the diagnosis and treatment plans. For instance, treatment with over-the-counter or prescription medications would be considered of low complexity, whereas the infusion of medications would increase patient risk.

Tool 27 illustrates the key components in determining the level of risk or mortality associated with the encounter. As opposed to the other components in the history, examination, and medical decision making process, only

T O O L 25

HISTORY GUIDELINES

HISTORY OF PRESENT ILLNESS			
Location	(where, radiation from-to)	**Timing**	(start, steady, intermitt, constant)
Quality	(sharp, burning, dull, productive, color)	**Context**	(activity at onset, causation)
Severity	(scale 1-10, severe, mild, progressive)	**Duration**	(length of time, time of present)
Assoc S & S	(swelling, nausea, vomiting)	**Modifying Factors**	(what helps, worsens, relieves)

MEDICAL HISTORY		
Adult medical illnesses	Trauma	Date of most recent medical exam/results
Childhood illnesses	Surgical hx	Age-appropriate feeding/dietary

FAMILY HISTORY	
Marital status	Health status/cause of death of parents, siblings, children
Genetic diseases	Specific diseases related to chief complaint
Parents/children/siblings	Family hx of chronic diseases such as: HTN, diabetes, cancer, heart dz, cardiovascular
	dz, psych

SOCIAL HISTORY	
Smoking	Heterosexual/homosexual/bisexual
Alcohol	Place of birth/residence/occupation/education
Caffeine	Marital status/living arrangements
Drug usage	Level of education
Occupational hx	Other relevant social factors

ALLERGIES		
Medications	Insects	Occupational allergies
Foods	Animals	

MEDICATIONS	
Prescription	Doses, frequencies
OTC medications	Immunizations

REVIEW OF SYSTEMS	
Constitutional	General appearance, vital signs, current state of health
Integumentary	Rash, color, sores, dryness
Eyes	Vision, cataracts, pain, redness, tearing, double/blurred vision
ENT/Mouth	Ears: hearing, vertigo, earaches, infections, discharge
	Nose: colds, stuffiness, discharge, itching, nosebleeds
	Mouth/throat: teeth, gums, dentures, dry mouth, sore throat, hoarseness, bleeding
Cardiovascular	Shortness of breath, dizziness, HTN, heart murmurs, chest pains, palpitations,
	dyspnea, orthopnea, rheumatic fever
Respiratory	Cough, sputum, wheezing, asthma, bronchitis, TB, emphysema, pneumonia
Gastrointestinal	Heartburn, appetite, vomiting, indigestion, frequency/change in bowel habits, gas,
	food intolerance, excessive bleeding, jaundice, hepatitis, gallbladder prob, weight diff
Genitourinary	Frequent urination, nocturia, hematuria, urgency
	Male specific: hernia, discharge, hx STD
	Female specific: age at menarche, menstrual hx, pregnancies, hx STD
Musculoskeletal	Muscle/joint pain, arthritis, gout, backache
Neurologic	Fainting, seizures, weakness, paralysis, numbness, loss of sensation, tremors,
	blackouts
Hema/Lymphatic	Anemia, bruising, bleeding, transfusion
Endocrine	Thyroid problems, heat/cold intolerance, diabetes
Psychiatric	Nervousness, tension, mood swings, panic, anxiety
Allerg/Immunologic	Immunizations, allergies to meds, immune suppression, blood transfusion

T O O L   26

EXAMINATION GUIDELINES

Constitutional	Measurement of certain number of vital signs with notation of abnormal findings General appearance of patient at time of exam
Eyes	Conjunctivae, lids, extraocular movement Reaction to light/accommodation Ophthalmic examination of retinal discs
ENT/Teeth	External inspection of ears and nose Otoscopic exam of external auditory canals/tympanic membranes Assessment of hearing Inspection of nasal mucosa, septum, turbinates Inspection of lips, teeth, gums Examination of oropharynx (salivary glands, palates, tongue, tonsils, post pharynx)
Neck	General exam of neck (masses, overall appearance) Exam of thyroid (enlargement, tenderness, mass)
Respiratory	Assessment of respiratory effort Percussion of chest (dullness, flatness) Palpation of chest Auscultation of lungs (breath sounds, rubs, clicks)
Cardiovascular	Palpation of heart Auscultation of heart Carotid arteries (pulse, amplitude, bruits) Abdominal aorta (size, bruits) Femoral arteries (pulse, amplitude, bruits) Pedal pulses (pulse, amplitude) Exam of extremities for edema and varicosities
Chest	Inspection of breasts Palpation of breasts/axillae (lumps, masses, tenderness)
Gastrointestinal	Examination of abdomen (masses, tenderness) Examination of liver/spleen Examination for presence/absence of hernia BOWEL SOUNDS ARE NOT PHYSICAL EXAM ELEMENT
Genitourinary	**MALE:** Examination of scrotal contents Examination of penis Digital rectal exam of prostate **FEMALE:** Pelvic examination Exam of external genitalia Exam of urethra (masses, tenderness) Exam of bladder (fullness, masses, tenderness) Cervical exam (general appearance, discharge) Exam of uterus (contour, mobility, tenderness) Adnexa/parametria (masses, tenderness, nodularity)
Lymphatic	Palpation of lymph nodes of two or more areas: Neck Axillae Groin Other
Musculoskeletal	Examination of gait/station Inspection of nails/digits (ischemia, infections, cyanosis) Assessment of stability of any dislocation Assessment of muscle strength and tone
Integumentary	Inspection of skin/subcutaneous tissue Palpation of skin/subcutaneous tissue
Neurologic	Test cranial nerves (note deficits) Examination of deep tendon reflexes Examination of sensation Examination of motor strength
Psychiatric	Evaluation of patient's judgment and insight Brief assessment of mental status to include: Orientation to time, place, person Recent/remote memory Mood and affect Review of former mental status

T O O L   27

TABLE OF RISK (MEDICAL DECISION MAKING)

Level of Risk	Presenting Problem	Diagnostic Data	Management/Diagnostic Options
Minimal	1 self-limited or minor problem	Lab test Chest x-rays ECG/EEG Ultrasound	Rest/gargle Elastic bandages Superficial dressings
Low	2> self-limited or minor problem 1 stable chronic illness Acute, uncomplicated illness/injury Physiological tests not under stress	Noncardiovascular imaging study with contract Superficial needle biopsies Lab tests req arterial puncture Skin biopsies	Over-the-counter drugs Physical therapy Occupational therapy IV fluids w/o additives Minor surgery with no risk
Moderate	1> chronic illnesses w/mild exacerbation 2> stable chronic illnesses Undiagnosed new problem w/uncertain prognosis Acute illness with systemic symptoms Acute complicated injury	Physiological tests under stress Diagnostic endoscopies with no risk Deep needle or incisional biopsy Cardiovascular imaging w/contrast, no identified risk Obtain fluid from body cavity	Minor surgery w/risk Elective major surgery Prescription drug management Therapeutic nuclear medicine Closed treatment fracture/dislocation without manipulation

High	1> chronic illness with severe exacerbation
	
	Acute/chronic illness/injury posing threat to life/bodily function
	Abrupt change in neurological status
		Cardiovascular imaging studies with contract with identified risk
		Cardiac electrophysiological test
		
		Diagnostic endoscopies with identified risk
		Discography
			Elective major surgery
			
			Emergency major surgery
			
			Parenteral controlled substances
			
			Drug therapy requiring
			  Intensive monitoring
			  Decision not to resuscitate or
			  De-escalate care due to
			  poor prognosis

one component of risk must be met (choose the highest level of risk associated with the visit).

Other Elements

Other elements that can be used for determining additional level(s) of service in special circumstances include the following:

- Counseling
- Coordination of care
- Nature of presenting problem
- Time

In those instances in which counseling or coordination of care represents 50% or more of the time spent in completion of the visit or encounter, the provider may use the time element toward determining level of service. Again, the correct code will vary by location of service and new/established patient status. ONLY IN THESE INSTANCES DOES TIME BECOME THE CONTROLLING FACTOR IN DETERMINING LEVEL OF SERVICE.

As with all elements discussed so far, documentation is crucial to authenticating that the time element is the key factor in determining level of service. At a minimum, the amount of time spent in counseling or coordination of care must be documented, along with an explanation of the extent of that part of the service. Counseling may include such services as educating, instructing, or advising about care of the patient's condition or resolution of problem(s) presented. Coordination of care may include such services as setting up and monitoring home health care or making arrangements for other care to be provided outside the realm of the physician office visit.

Each of these identified components is then evaluated to determine what level of history, physical examination, and medical decision making may be coded, or whether time is to be considered a factor in this determination.

In the example that follows, identify the key components and others:

1. History components
2. Physical examination elements
3. Medical decision making process
4. Modifying circumstances (e.g., counseling, coordination of care)

PROGRESS NOTE

Chief complaint: _____

Date: _____

Vital signs: BP_____ P_____ R_____

History:

This 4-year-old child presents with a 2-day history of cough, fever, and earache. The mother reports a temperature as high as 104° in the evening, relieved only somewhat by Tylenol. Medical history includes recurrent ear infections since birth. No smoking occurs in the household.

Exam:

Tympanic membranes are dull and surrounded by serous fluid. Remainder of HEENT is normal. Child appears to be in no acute distress, behaving normally and interacting with the mother. Labs are normal and there appears to be no medical justification for performing a chest x-ray at this time.

Diagnosis/assessment:

Patient will be given amoxicillin for otitis media and mother is informed to return with the child in approximately 10 days for recheck.

Patient name: _____

Date of service: _____

GODFREY MEDICAL ASSOCIATES
1532 Third Avenue, Suite 120 • Aldon, FL 77713 • (407) 555-4000

Note: The E & M coding grid (Figure 10-2) and the workbook may be of assistance in identifying and documenting the appropriate information for the service. Use of this grid or a similar document is advisable until one is comfortable with locating and categorizing all documentation elements. Use of a similar format even after that time is advantageous because compliance programs required by some third-party carriers consider consistency to be one of the most important factors of a chart audit.

Step 1 in the CPT-4 coding process **(Identify the key words and phrases for coding purposes.)** has already been discussed. On the basis of the documentation, **pinpoint or eliminate those elements necessary for**

EVALUATION AND MANAGEMENT LEVEL WORKSHEET

History	1	2	3	4	5
HPI:					
PMH:					
SH/FH:					
ROS:					
Level history assigned:					

Examination	1	2	3	4	5
Body organ(s):					
Organ system(s):					
Level exam assigned:					

Medical Decision-making	1	2	3	4	5
Diagnosis/management options:					
Amount/complexity data:					
Risk/morbidity/mortality:					
Level medical decision-making assigned:					

OTHER FACTORS DOCUMENTED (TIME, COUNSELING):

Location of service (circle one)

Office/outpatient	Emergency department	Domiciliary, rest home	Care plan oversight
Hospital observation	Critical care	Home services	Preventative medicine
Hospital inpatient	Neonatal ICU	Prolonged services	Newborn care
Consultations	Nursing facility	Case management	Special E & M service

Type of service (circle one)

New patient   Established patient

Patient name: _____   Level assigned: _____

Date: _____   Coder: _____

GODFREY MEDICAL ASSOCIATES
1532 Third Avenue, Suite 120 • Aldon, FL 77713 • (407) 555-4000

FIGURE 10-2. Evaluation and Management Level Worksheet Tables.

determining what services should be coded (Step 2). Step 3 is to **assign the order of services for coding.**

Because only one E & M service is usually provided on a daily basis, only one service from this section is reported. In the event that more than one E & M service is provided, the coder should review the guidelines to ensure that these services are not provided as part of another E & M service. If more than one E & M service is reportable, the service that is most significant and reflects the greatest level and complexity should be reported.

After the key components within the medical documentation are identified, **Step 4** of the step-by-step process of CPT-4 coding, **selecting the correct code(s),** should be completed. In the case of E & M services, this will provide the appropriate factors for determining level of service. Take a look at the different levels for each of these components.

LEVELS OF E & M COMPONENTS

LEVELS OF HISTORY

Problem focused	Chief complaint
	Brief history of present illness/ problem(s)
Expanded problem focused	Chief complaint
	Brief history of present illness/ problem(s)
	Problem-pertinent system review
Detailed	Chief complaint
	Extended history of present illness
	Problem-pertinent system review extended to include review of a limited number of additional systems
	Pertinent medical, family, and/or social history directly related to patient problem(s)
Comprehensive	Chief complaint
	Extended history of present illness
	Review of systems directly related to problem(s) identified in history of present illness
	Review of all additional body systems
	Complete medical, family, social history

LEVELS OF PHYSICAL EXAMINATION

Problem focused	Limited to part of body area or organ system affected, usually one area is identified
Expanded problem focused	Limited examination of affected body area/organ systems and of other body area/organ systems that may contribute to the presenting complaint(s); two to four elements are required
Detailed	Extensive examination of affected body areas/organ systems and of other body

areas/organ systems that may contribute to the presenting complaint(s); five to seven elements are required

Comprehensive	Either a multisystem physical examination or complete examination of a single organ/body system; eight or more elements are required

The elements of physical examination are as follows:

Body Areas	**Organ Systems**
Head (including face)	Eyes
Neck	Ears, nose, mouth, throat
Chest (including breasts/ axillae)	Cardiovascular
	Respiratory
Abdomen	Gastrointestinal
Genitalia, groin, buttocks	Genitourinary
Back	Musculoskeletal
Each extremity	Skin
	Neurological
	Psychiatric
	Hematological/immunological/ lymphatic

LEVELS OF MEDICAL DECISION MAKING

Straightforward	A minimum number of diagnosis or management options for the problem
	Minimal medical data to be reviewed and considered
	Minimal or no risk of morbidity or mortality
Low	Limited diagnosis and options for management of the medical problem
	Limited data to be reviewed
	Low risk of morbidity or mortality
Moderate	Diagnosis and medical management options are multiple
	Data to be reviewed are moderate in complexity and volume
	Morbidity/mortality risks are moderate
High	Medical Decision Making Options for management of the medical problem are extensive
	Review of data is extensive in terms of volume and complexity
	Problem presents a high risk of morbidity/mortality

STEPS IN ASSIGNMENT OF E & M CODES

Take a look at the specific steps involved in the coding of E & M services, as shown in Tool 28 (Step 4 of the overall coding process). These steps are discussed and applied to completion of the E & M grid for the sample chart.

Step 1. Identify relevant components within the medical documentation and highlight or mark these items. Once the information that includes these components has been determined, plot them in the coding grid under the appropriate area.

Step 2. Determine the location of service. Circle the location on the grid.

Step 3. Determine whether the patient was new or established as defined by the E & M guidelines. **If it is not stated, the coder must assume that the patient is an established patient because that is the least significant.**

- Two of three components are required for established patient services.
- Three of three components are required for new patient services.

    Document this information on the coding grid as well.

Step 4. Take the information gathered on the grid and determine the correct level of service, according to the status and location of the new and established patient. Because there are a multitude of components for location and status, the use of grids for each of these is a concise method of describing the elements necessary for each. Grids that include documentation requirements follow.

After plotting the elements using the grid, determine whether the level of one or more elements seems ambiguous (could be higher or lower). If so, place a mark on the line. It may not be that important to determine the exact level for that specific component, because the other two components may reach levels that will determine assignment of level of service.

Finally, after plotting the level of service, determine whether time, counseling, or coordination of care drives the assignment of the level of service. Use the time elements listed in the grid for the appropriate level of service. Make certain that documentation supports this decision.

The following is a completed grid of the components identified in a sample chart.

TOOL 28

STEPS TO ACCURATE ASSIGNMENT OF EVALUATION AND MANAGEMENT CODES

1. **Identify history, physical examination, medical decision making, or modifying factors (time, counseling, coordination of care).** This involves the steps of the overall coding process up to assignment of the CPT code.

2. **Determine the type/location of service.**

3. **Determine the status of the patient — new or established.** Also note that new patient criteria require that all 3 components of history, exam, and medical decision making must meet the criteria for the level selected; established patient criteria require only 2 of 3 components for the level selected.

4. **Determine the correct level of service.**

5. **Determine whether modifying factors (time, counseling, coordination of care) or key elements will determine level of service.**

1995 Guidelines
OUTPATIENT CONSULTATION CODES (New/Established)
LEVELS OF SERVICE DOCUMENTATION REQUIREMENTS
(3 of 3 elements must be met)

		Level 1	Level 2	Level 3	Level 4	Level 5
HISTORY		*Problem Focused*	*Exp Problem Foc*	*Detailed*	*Comprehensive*	*Comprehensive*
Hx= 1	Hx Present Illness	Brief 1–3 elements	Brief 1–3 elements	Extended 4> elements	Extended 4> elements	Extended 4> elements
	Fam Hx/Social Hx	Not required	Not required	Pertinent Stmt Re Minimum 1 component	Complete Stmt Re: Minimum 2/3 components	Complete Stmt Re: Min 2/3 components
	Review of Systems	Not required	Prob pertinent 1 affected system Related to chief complaint	Extended 2–9 systems	Complete 10> systems OR pert positive & "all sys review & neg"	Complete 10> systems OR pert positive & "all sys review & neg"
Exam= 4	**EXAM**	*Problem Focused*	*Exp Problem Foc*	*Detailed*	*Comprehensive*	*Comprehensive*
		1 element Body area/organ system	2–4 elements Body area/organ system	5–7 elements Body area/organ system	8 or more Body area/organ system	8 or more Body area/organ system
MDM= 3	**MDM (2 of 3)**	*Straightforward*	*Straightforward*	*Low*	*Moderate*	*High*
	Amt Data	Minimal/None	Minimal/None	Limited	Moderate	Extensive
	Trt/Dx Options	Minimal	Minimal	Limited	Multiple	Extensive
	Risk	Minimal	Minimal	Low	Moderate	High
	Time *	15 minutes	30 minutes	40 minutes	60 minutes	80 minutes

ELEMENTS COMPRISING HISTORY, EXAM, MEDICAL DECISION MAKING
(Circle those elements present in documentation)

Elements HX PRES ILLNESS	Elements REVIEW OF SYSTEMS	Exam Elements BODY AREAS	Elements — Medical Decision Making (2 of 3)		
			AMT/ COMPLEX DATA	DX/TREAT OPTIONS	RISKS
Location Duration (Quality) Ventricular Severity Timing Modifying Context factors Assoc S/S: **ELEMENT COUNT: 1**	Eyes Neuro Card Psych Resp Endo GI GU MS Integum Constitutional Ear, Nose, Mouth, Throat Hema/Lymph Aller/Immuno **ELEMENT COUNT: 0**	Head (inc face) 2E Neck 3E Chest (inc breast) Abdomen Genitalia, groin, buttocks Back, inc spine Each extremity 7E(1) **Exam Elements ORGAN SYSTEMS** Eyes GU Skin Neuro 8E Card 5E Psych Resp 4E GI 6E MS Ear, Nose, Mouth Constitutional 1E Hema/Lymph/Immuno **ELEMENT COUNT: 8**	Path/Lab 1 2M Radiology 1 Other Dx 1 1M Comp Test Ea 2 Old Records: Need for 1 Review of 2 Scoring: Minimal = 0-1 Limited = 2 Moderate = 3 Extensive = 4 **ELEMENT COUNT: 2**	Self Lmtd/Minor 1 Est Prob Stable 1 Est Prob Worse 2 New Problem No Addtl W/Up 3 New Problem Addtl W/Up 4 Scoring: Minimal = 1 Limited = 2 Multiple = 3 Extensive = 4 **ELEMENT COUNT: 3**	Minimal (Low) Moderate High Based On: Presenting Prob Dx Proc Ordered Mgt Option Selected **ELEMENT LEVEL: Low**

* Time is determinant factor ONLY when documented counseling/coordination of care >50% of total face-to-face time.

TYPES OF E & M SERVICE CATEGORIES

The following discussion and corresponding Coding Reference Tools detail information regarding each type of E & M services listed in CPT-4. A grid outlining the components is included with each section. The level of service (e.g., Level 1, Level 2) has been designated on the grids provided. The designated CPT-4 code number may be added onto the grids for reference purposes. The grids provided in this section are specific to the type and location of services in contrast to the general Evaluation and Management grid used in Figure 10-2.

OUTPATIENT/OFFICE VISITS

Outpatient or office visits (Tools 29 and 30) should take place in the physician's office or outpatient setting.

Remember that in the hospital setting, the patient is still considered an outpatient until such time as he or she is officially admitted. If the patient is admitted to the facility or hospital by the same physician during that day's encounter in the office or outpatient setting, hospital inpatient care codes or comprehensive nursing facility assessments should be used, because these represent the more significant service performed by the physician.

In the event both the office/outpatient visit and the initial hospital care visit are significant, the provider may incorporate the documentation from both visits to determine the level of service. Make certain, however, that the provider is aware of the necessity of documenting this information.

HOSPITAL OBSERVATION SERVICES

Patients must be designated as on "observation status" while they are in the hospital. Coding staff members may not choose to code observation status instead of inpatient

TOOL 29

1995 Guidelines
NEW OUTPATIENT VISITS
LEVELS OF SERVICE DOCUMENTATION REQUIREMENTS
(3 of 3 elements must be met)

	99201/Level 1	99202/Level 2	99203/Level 3	99204/Level 4	99205/Level 5
HISTORY	*Problem Focused*	*Exp Problem Foc*	*Detailed*	*Comprehensive*	*Comprehensive*
Hx Present Illness	Brief 1-3 elements	Brief 1-3 elements	Extended ≥4 elements	Extended ≥4 elements	Extended ≥4 elements
Past Med Hx/ Fam Hx/Social Hx (PMH/FH/SH)	Not required	Not required	Pertinent Stmt Re: Minimum 1 component	Complete Stmt Re: Minimum 2/3 components	Complete Stmt Re: Minimum 2/3 components
Review of Systems (ROS)	Not required	Prob pertinent 1 affected system Related to Chief Complaint	Extended 2-9 systems	Complete ≥10 systems OR pert positive & "all sys review & neg"	Complete ≥10 systems OR pert positive & "all sys review & neg"
	Problem Focused	*Exp Problem Foc*	*Detailed*	*Comprehensive*	*Comprehensive*
EXAM	1 element Body area/organ system	2-4 elements Body area/organ system	5-7 elements Body area/organ system	8 or more elements Body area/organ system	8 or more elements Body area/organ system
MDM (2 of 3)	*Straightforward*	*Straightforward*	*Low*	*Moderate*	*High*
Quantity Data	Minimal/None	Minimal/None	Limited	Moderate	Extensive
Trt/Dx Options	Minimal	Minimal	Limited	Multiple	Extensive
Risk	Minimal	Minimal	Low	Moderate	High
Time *	10 minutes	20 minutes	30 minutes	45 minutes	60 minutes

ELEMENTS OF HISTORY, EXAM, MEDICAL DECISION MAKING
(Circle those elements present in documentation)

Elements HX PRES ILLNESS	Elements REVIEW OF SYSTEMS	Exam Elements BODY AREAS	Elements — Medical Decision Making (2 of 3)		
			QUANTITY/ COMPLEX DATA	DX/TREAT OPTIONS	RISKS
Location Duration Quality Timing Severity Context Modifying Factors Assoc S/S **ELEMENT COUNT:**	Eyes Neuro Card Psych Resp Endo GI GU MS Integum Constitutional Ear, Nose, Mouth, Throat Hema/Lymph Aller/Immuno **ELEMENT COUNT:**	Head (incl face) Neck Chest (incl breast) Abdomen Genitalia, groin, buttocks Back, incl spine Each extremity **Exam Elements ORGAN SYSTEMS** Eyes GU Skin Neuro Card Psych Resp GI MS Ear, Nose, Mouth Constitutional Hema/Lymph/Immuno **ELEMENT COUNT:**	Path/Lab 1 Radiology 1 Other Dx 1 Comp Test ea 2 Old Records: Need for 1 Review of 2 Discussion of Results 1 Scoring: Minimal = 0-1 Limited = 2 Moderate = 3 Extensive = 4 **ELEMENT COUNT:**	Self-Lmtd/Minor 1 Est Prob Stable 1 Est Prob Worse 2 New Problem No Addtl W/Up 3 New Problem Addtl W/Up 4 Scoring: Minimal = 1 Limited = 2 Multiple = 3 Extensive = 4 **ELEMENT COUNT:**	Minimal Low Moderate High Based On: Presenting Prob Dx Proc Ordered Mgt Option Selected **ELEMENT LEVEL:**

* Time is determinant factor ONLY when documented counseling/coordination of care >50% of total face-to-face time.

T O O L   30

1995 Guidelines
ESTABLISHED OUTPATIENT VISITS
LEVELS OF SERVICE DOCUMENTATION REQUIREMENTS
(2 of 3 elements must be met)

	99211/Level 1	99212/Level 2	99213/Level 3	99214/Level 4	99215/Level 5
HISTORY	*Straightforward*	*Problem Focused*	*Exp Problem Foc*	*Detailed*	*Comprehensive*
Hx Present Illness	May not req presence of physician	Brief 1-3 elements	Brief 1-3 elements	Extended ≥4 elements	Extended ≥4 elements
Past Med Hx/ Fam Hx/Social Hx (PMH/FH/SH)	Not required	Not required	Not required	Pertinent Stmt Re: Minimum 1 component	Complete Stmt Re: Minimum 2/3 components
Review of Systems (ROS)	Not required	Not required	Prob pertinent 1 affected system Related to Chief Complaint	Extended 2-9 systems	Complete ≥10 systems OR pert positive & "all sys review & neg"
	Straightforward	*Problem Focused*	*Exp Problem Foc*	*Detailed*	*Comprehensive*
EXAM	May not req presence of physician	1 element Body area/organ system	2-4 elements Body area/organ system	5-7 elements Body area/organ system	8 or more elements Body area/organ system
MDM (2 of 3)	*Straightforward*	*Straightforward*	*Low*	*Moderate*	*High*
Quantity Data	Minimal/None	Minimal/None	Limited	Moderate	Extensive
Trt/Dx Options	Minimal	Minimal	Limited	Multiple	Extensive
Risk	Minimal	Minimal	Low	Moderate	High
Time *	None specified	10 minutes	15 minutes	25 minutes	40 minutes

ELEMENTS OF HISTORY, EXAM, MEDICAL DECISION MAKING
(Circle those elements present in documentation)

Elements HX PRES ILLNESS	Elements REVIEW OF SYSTEMS	Exam Elements BODY AREAS	Elements — Medical Decision Making (2 of 3)		
			QUANTITY/ COMPLEX DATA	DX/TREAT OPTIONS	RISKS
Location Duration Quality Timing Severity Context Modifying Factors Assoc S/S **ELEMENT COUNT:**	Eyes Neuro Card Psych Resp Endo GI GU MS Integum Constitutional Ear, Nose, Mouth, Throat Hema/Lymph Aller/Immuno **ELEMENT COUNT:**	Head (incl face) Neck Chest (incl breast) Abdomen Genitalia, groin, buttocks Back, incl spine Each extremity	Path/Lab 1 Radiology 1 Other Dx 1 Comp Test ea 2 Old Records: Need for 1 Review of 2 Discussion of Results 1	Self-Lmtd/Minor 1 Est Prob Stable 1 Est Prob Worse 2 New Problem No Addtl W/Up 3 New Problem Addtl W/Up 4	Minimal Low Moderate High Based On: Presenting Prob Dx Proc Ordered Mgt Option Selected
		Exam Elements ORGAN SYSTEMS	Scoring: Minimal = 0-1 Limited = 2 Moderate = 3 Extensive = 4 **ELEMENT COUNT:**	Scoring: Minimal = 1 Limited = 2 Multiple = 3 Extensive = 4 **ELEMENT COUNT:**	**ELEMENT LEVEL:**
* Time is determinant factor ONLY when documented counseling/coordination of care >50% of total face-to-face time.		Eyes GU Skin Neuro Card Psych Resp GI MS Ear, Nose, Mouth Constitutional Hema/Lymph/Immuno **ELEMENT COUNT:**			

visit simply because of reimbursement issues. This practice has been targeted by third-party audits for fraud and abuse. Only the admitting physician for the "observation" may change the patient's status.

It is not necessary for the patient to be admitted to an "observation area" if none is available within the facility. It is only required that the patient's status be designated as "observation" in an area so determined by the hospital.

Other than the admitting physician for observation status, physicians billing for E & M services should use outpatient codes. In many instances, other E & M services may have been performed on the same day. Below is the designation of which service should be billed:

Admit and observation code	Bill *Hospital Admit*
ED visit and observation code	Bill *Observation Care*
Office visit and observation code	Bill *Observation Care*
E & M services at site related to initiating observation status	Bill *Observation Care*

There are three levels of initial observation care delineated in the Initial Observation Care grid (Tool 31). These are used when the patient is admitted to observation care and discharged on a subsequent date of service.

When subsequent days are provided in the observation unit, other than the initial observation day and the discharge day, these would be coded as office/outpatient visits because they are performed in the outpatient setting. Observation units in the hospital facility are considered to be outpatient in nature rather than inpatient.

HOSPITAL INPATIENT SERVICES

Initial Inpatient Services

Initial inpatient service codes may be assigned by the admitting physician for the first hospital visit whether the patient is established or new to that physician. When physicians other than the admitting physician initially see the patient, these encounters should be coded with consultation codes. If the consultation definitions are not met, then subsequent visit codes should be used.

All services provided by the admitting physician on the same date, including those performed in another facility or setting, are included in the coding for initial inpatient hospital care. Also, there are three levels of initial hospital care included in the Inpatient Hospital Visits grid (Tool 32).

Subsequent Inpatient Hospital Care

Subsequent inpatient hospital care codes are assigned by the admitting provider for additional inpatient visits occurring during the same admission or for services of

other consulting physicians when consultation guidelines have not been met.

Make certain that documentation is included in the hospital medical record for EACH DAY billed. Another focus of fraud and abuse investigation is the provider who bills multiple consecutive days of subsequent care, when the provider may have not seen the patient on each of those days. There are three levels of subsequent inpatient hospital care included in the Subsequent Hospital Visits grid (Tool 33).

Observation/Inpatient Care (Including Admission/Discharge Same Day)

When patients are admitted and discharged the same day from the inpatient on observation status, these codes should be used. Do not bill by assigning individual discharge services or initial hospital care codes.

CONSULTATIONS

For an evaluation and management service to be billed as a consultation, it must meet the following three criteria (referred to as the *3 R's*)

1. A documented REQUEST for the consultation must be included in the patient record.
2. This should be submitted by a REFERRING provider/physician or a provider agency (e.g., Division of Blind Services, Vocational Rehabilitation) in which the requesting agency has a physician overseeing the requests.
3. A REPORT back to the requesting physician must also be a part of the medical documentation.

Although diagnostic and therapeutic services may be initiated by the consulting physician, the patient's care may not be assumed by the consulting physician. If subsequent to the E & M service the physician assumes management of the patient's care, however, consultation codes cannot be used.

"Patient-requested" consultations may not be billed with the outpatient/inpatient consultation codes but instead should be billed with the visit codes appropriate to the location of service. Types of consultations include the following.

Office/Outpatient Consultations

When consultations are performed in the office or outpatient location, codes from this subsection should be used. If after the initial consultation, additional advice or specialty opinions are requested, these may be coded as office consultations as well.

There are five levels of office/outpatient consultation outlined in the Outpatient Consultation Codes grid (Tool 34).

Think back to the original chart that was reviewed at the beginning of the chapter. It was

TOOL 31

1995 Guidelines
INITIAL OBSERVATION CARE
LEVELS OF SERVICE DOCUMENTATION REQUIREMENTS
(3 of 3 elements must be met)

			99218	99219	99220
HISTORY			*Detailed*	*Comprehensive*	*Comprehensive*
Hx Present Illness			Extended ≥4 elements	Extended ≥4 elements	Extended ≥4 elements
Past Med Hx/ Fam Hx/Social Hx (PMH/FH/SH)			Pertinent Stmt Re: Minimum 1 component	Complete Stmt Re: Minimum 2/3 components	Complete Stmt Re: Minimum 2/3 components
Review of Systems (ROS)			Extended 2-9 systems	Complete ≥10 systems OR pert positive & "all sys review & neg"	Complete ≥10 systems OR pert positive & "all sys review & neg"
EXAM			*Detailed*	*Comprehensive*	*Comprehensive*
			5-7 elements Body area/organ system	8 or more elements Body area/organ system	8 or more elements Body area/organ system
MDM (2 of 3)			*Straightforward/Low*	*Moderate*	*High*
Quantity Data			Minimal/Limited	Moderate	Extensive
Trt/Dx Options			Minimal/Limited	Multiple	Extensive
Risk			Minimal/Low	Moderate	High

ELEMENTS OF HISTORY, EXAM, MEDICAL DECISION MAKING
(Circle those elements present in documentation)

Elements HX PRES ILLNESS	Elements REVIEW OF SYSTEMS	Exam Elements BODY AREAS	Elements — Medical Decision Making (2 of 3)		
			QUANTITY/ COMPLEX DATA	DX/TREAT OPTIONS	RISKS
Location Duration Quality Timing Severity Context Modifying Factors Assoc S/S **ELEMENT COUNT:**	Eyes Neuro Card Psych Resp Endo GI GU MS Integum Constitutional Ear, Nose, Mouth, Throat Hema/Lymph Aller/Immuno **ELEMENT COUNT:**	Head (incl face) Neck Chest (incl breast) Abdomen Genitalia, groin, buttocks Back, incl spine Each extremity **Exam Elements ORGAN SYSTEMS** Eyes GU Skin Neuro Card Psych Resp GI MS Ear, Nose, Mouth Constitutional Hema/Lymph/Immuno **ELEMENT COUNT:**	Path/Lab 1 Radiology 1 Other Dx 1 Comp Test ea 2 Old Records: Need for 1 Review of 2 Discussion of Results 1 Scoring: Minimal = 0-1 Limited = 2 Moderate = 3 Extensive = 4 **ELEMENT COUNT:**	Self-Lmtd/Minor 1 Est Prob Stable 1 Est Prob Worse 2 New Problem No Addtl W/Up 3 New Problem Addtl W/Up 4 Scoring: Minimal = 1 Limited = 2 Multiple = 3 Extensive = 4 **ELEMENT COUNT:**	Minimal Low Moderate High Based On: Presenting Prob Dx Proc Ordered Mgt Option Selected **ELEMENT LEVEL:**

determined to be a consultation, based on the request by a referring physician for an expert opinion; it would therefore be assigned a code from this section. Because the consultation was performed on an outpatient basis, the code range 99241 to 99245 would be appropriate.

Take another look at the same chart and attempt to extract the history, examination, and medical decision making components necessary to determine the exact E & M code for this service. Use Tool 34 to record this information and determine the appropriate level. Compare the answer to that provided previously on page 214.

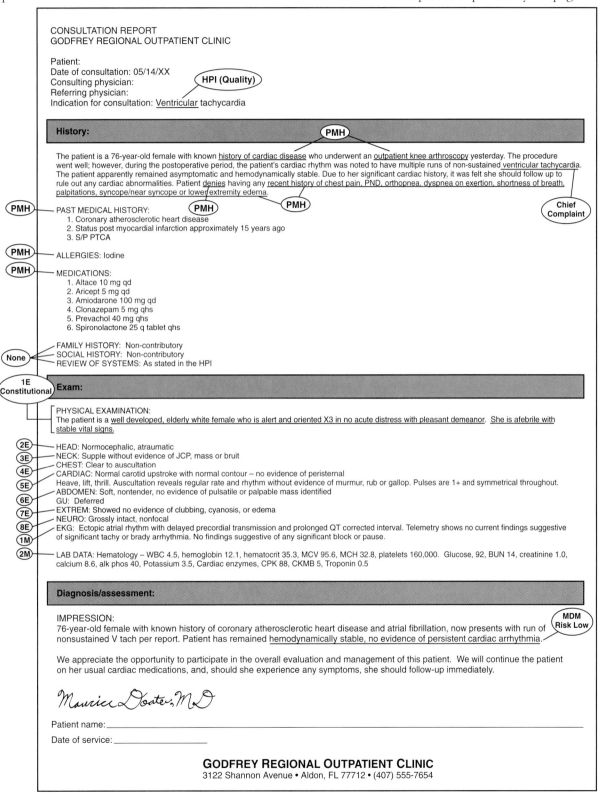

CONSULTATION REPORT
GODFREY REGIONAL OUTPATIENT CLINIC

Patient:
Date of consultation: 05/14/XX
Consulting physician: — HPI (Quality)
Referring physician:
Indication for consultation: <u>Ventricular</u> tachycardia

History: — PMH

The patient is a 76-year-old female with known <u>history of cardiac disease</u> who underwent an <u>outpatient knee arthroscopy</u> yesterday. The procedure went well; however, during the postoperative period, the patient's cardiac rhythm was noted to have multiple runs of non-sustained <u>ventricular tachycardia</u>. The patient apparently remained asymptomatic and hemodynamically stable. Due to her significant cardiac history, it was felt she should follow up to rule out any cardiac abnormalities. Patient <u>denies</u> having any <u>recent history of chest pain, PND, orthopnea, dyspnea on exertion, shortness of breath, palpitations, syncope/near syncope or lower extremity edema.</u>

— PMH — PMH — Chief Complaint

PMH — PAST MEDICAL HISTORY:
    1. Coronary atherosclerotic heart disease
    2. Status post myocardial infarction approximately 15 years ago
    3. S/P PTCA

PMH — ALLERGIES: Iodine

PMH — MEDICATIONS:
    1. Altace 10 mg qd
    2. Aricept 5 mg qd
    3. Amiodarone 100 mg qd
    4. Clonazepam 5 mg qhs
    5. Prevachol 40 mg qhs
    6. Spironolactone 25 q tablet qhs

FAMILY HISTORY: Non-contributory
None — SOCIAL HISTORY: Non-contributory
REVIEW OF SYSTEMS: As stated in the HPI

1E Constitutional — **Exam:**

PHYSICAL EXAMINATION:
The patient is a <u>well developed, elderly white female who is alert and oriented X3 in no acute distress with pleasant demeanor.</u> <u>She is afebrile with stable vital signs.</u>

2E — HEAD: Normocephalic, atraumatic
3E — NECK: Supple without evidence of JCP, mass or bruit
4E — CHEST: Clear to auscultation
5E — CARDIAC: Normal carotid upstroke with normal contour – no evidence of peristernal
    Heave, lift, thrill. Auscultation reveals regular rate and rhythm without evidence of murmur, rub or gallop. Pulses are 1+ and symmetrical throughout.
6E — ABDOMEN: Soft, nontender, no evidence of pulsatile or palpable mass identified
    GU: Deferred
7E — EXTREM: Showed no evidence of clubbing, cyanosis, or edema
    NEURO: Grossly intact, nonfocal
8E — EKG: Ectopic atrial rhythm with delayed precordial transmission and prolonged QT corrected interval. Telemetry shows no current findings suggestive
1M — of significant tachy or brady arrhythmia. No findings suggestive of any significant block or pause.
2M — LAB DATA: Hematology – WBC 4.5, hemoglobin 12.1, hematocrit 35.3, MCV 95.6, MCH 32.8, platelets 160,000. Glucose, 92, BUN 14, creatinine 1.0, calcium 8.6, alk phos 40, Potassium 3.5, Cardiac enzymes, CPK 88, CKMB 5, Troponin 0.5

Diagnosis/assessment:

IMPRESSION: — MDM Risk Low
76-year-old female with known history of coronary atherosclerotic heart disease and atrial fibrillation, now presents with run of nonsustained V tach per report. Patient has remained <u>hemodynamically stable, no evidence of persistent cardiac arrhythmia.</u>

We appreciate the opportunity to participate in the overall evaluation and management of this patient. We will continue the patient on her usual cardiac medications, and, should she experience any symptoms, she should follow-up immediately.

Maurice Doater, MD

Patient name: _____

Date of service: _____

GODFREY REGIONAL OUTPATIENT CLINIC
3122 Shannon Avenue • Aldon, FL 77712 • (407) 555-7654

T O O L   32

1995 Guidelines
INITIAL HOSPITAL VISITS
LEVELS OF SERVICE DOCUMENTATION REQUIREMENTS
(3 of 3 elements must be met)

	99221/Level 1	99222/Level 2	99223/Level 3	No Level 4	No Level 5
HISTORY	*Detailed/Comprehensive*	*Comprehensive*	*Comprehensive*		
Hx Present Illness	Extended ≥4 elements	Extended ≥4 elements	Extended ≥4 elements		
Past Med Hx/ Fam Hx/Social Hx (PMH/FH/SH)	Pertinent Stmt Re: Minimum 1 component	Complete Stmt Re: Minimum 2/3 components	Complete Stmt Re: Minimum 2/3 components		
Review of Systems (ROS)	Extended 2-9 systems	Complete ≥10 systems OR pert positive & "all sys review & neg"	Complete ≥10 systems OR pert positive & "all sys review & neg"		
EXAM	*Detailed*	*Comprehensive*	*Comprehensive*		
	5-7 elements Body area/organ system	8 or more elements Body area/organ system	8 or more elements Body area/organ system		
MDM (2 of 3)	*Straightforward/Low*	*Moderate*	*High*		
Quantity Data	Minimal/Limited	Moderate	Extensive		
Trt/Dx Options	Minimal/Limited	Multiple	Extensive		
Risk	Minimal/Low	Moderate	High		
Time *	30 minutes	50 minutes	70 minutes		

ELEMENTS OF HISTORY, EXAM, MEDICAL DECISION MAKING
(Circle those elements present in documentation)

Elements HX PRES ILLNESS	Elements REVIEW OF SYSTEMS	Exam Elements BODY AREAS	QUANTITY/ COMPLEX DATA	DX/TREAT OPTIONS	RISKS
Location Duration Quality Timing Severity Context Modifying Factors Assoc S/S **ELEMENT COUNT:**	Eyes Neuro Card Psych Resp Endo GI GU MS Integum Constitutional Ear, Nose, Mouth, Throat Hema/Lymph Aller/Immuno **ELEMENT COUNT:**	Head (incl face) Neck Chest (incl breast) Abdomen Genitalia, groin, buttocks Back, incl spine Each extremity **Exam Elements ORGAN SYSTEMS** Eyes GU Skin Neuro Card Psych Resp GI MS Ear, Nose, Mouth Constitutional Hema/Lymph/Immuno **ELEMENT COUNT:**	Path/Lab 1 Radiology 1 Other Dx 1 Comp Test ea 2 Old Records: Need for 1 Review of 2 Discussion of Results 1 Scoring: Minimal = 0-1 Limited = 2 Moderate = 3 Extensive = 4 **ELEMENT COUNT:**	Self-Lmtd/Minor 1 Est Prob Stable 1 Est Prob Worse 2 New Problem No Addtl W/Up 3 New Problem Addtl W/Up 4 Scoring: Minimal = 1 Limited = 2 Multiple = 3 Extensive = 4 **ELEMENT COUNT:**	Minimal Low Moderate High Based On: Presenting Prob Dx Proc Ordered Mgt Option Selected **ELEMENT LEVEL:**

* Time is determinant factor ONLY when documented counseling/coordination of care >50% of total unit/floor time.

T O O L   33

1995 Guidelines
SUBSEQUENT HOSPITAL VISITS
LEVELS OF SERVICE DOCUMENTATION REQUIREMENTS
(2 of 3 elements must be met)

	99231/Level 1	99232/Level 2	99233/Level 3	No Level 4	No Level 5
HISTORY (Interval)	*Prob Focused*	*Exp Problem Foc*	*Detailed*		
Hx Present Illness	Brief 1-3 elements	Brief 1-3 elements	Extended ≥4 elements		
Past Med Hx/ Fam Hx/Social Hx (PMH/FH/SH)	Not required	Not required	Pertinent Stmt Re: Minimum 1 component		
Review of Systems (ROS)	Not required	Prob pertinent 1 affected system Related to Chief Complaint	Extended 2–9 systems		
EXAM	*Prob Focused*	*Exp Problem Foc*	*Detailed*		

	1 element
	Body area/organ
	  system
		2-4 elements
		Body area/organ
		  system
			5-7 elements
			Body area/organ
			  system		

MDM (2 of 3)	*Straightforward/Low*	*Moderate*	*High*		
Quantity Data	Minimal/Limited	Moderate	Extensive		
Trt/Dx Options	Minimal/Limited	Multiple	Extensive		
Risk	Minimal/Low	Moderate	High		
Time *	15 minutes	25 minutes	35 minutes		

ELEMENTS OF COMPRISING HISTORY, EXAM, MEDICAL DECISION MAKING
(Circle those elements present in documentation)

Elements HX PRES ILLNESS	Elements REVIEW OF SYSTEMS	Exam Elements BODY AREAS	Elements — Medical Decision Making (2 of 3)		
			QUANTITY/ COMPLEX DATA	DX/TREAT OPTIONS	RISKS

Location   Duration
Quality   Timing
Severity   Context
Modifying Factors
Assoc S/S
**ELEMENT
COUNT:**
	Eyes Neuro
	Card Psych
	Resp Endo
	GI GU
	MS Integum
	Constitutional
	Ear, Nose, Mouth,
	  Throat
	Hema/Lymph
	Aller/Immuno
	**ELEMENT
	COUNT:**
		Head (incl face)
		Neck
		Chest (incl breast)
		Abdomen
		Genitalia, groin, buttocks
		Back, incl spine
		Each extremity
			Path/Lab 1
			Radiology 1
			Other Dx 1
			Comp Test ea 2
			Old Records:
			  Need for 1
			  Review of 2
			  Discussion of
			  Results 1
				Self-Lmtd/Minor 1
				Est Prob Stable 1
				Est Prob Worse 2
				New Problem
				  No Addtl W/Up 3
				New Problem
				  Addtl W/Up 4
					Minimal
					Low
					Moderate
					High
					Based On:
					Presenting Prob
					Dx Proc Ordered
					Mgt Option
					  Selected

		**Exam Elements
		ORGAN SYSTEMS**
			Scoring:
			  Minimal = 0-1
			  Limited = 2
			  Moderate = 3
			  Extensive = 4
				Scoring:
				  Minimal = 1
				  Limited = 2
				  Multiple = 3
				  Extensive = 4
					**ELEMENT
					LEVEL:**

		Eyes GU Skin Neuro Card Psych Resp GI MS Ear, Nose, Mouth Constitutional Hema/Lymph/Immuno **ELEMENT COUNT:**	**ELEMENT COUNT:**	**ELEMENT COUNT:**	

* Time is determinant factor ONLY when
  documented counseling/coordination
  of care >50% of total unit/floor time.

T O O L   34

1995 Guidelines
OUTPATIENT CONSULTATION CODES (New/Established)
LEVELS OF SERVICE DOCUMENTATION REQUIREMENTS
(3 of 3 elements must be met)

	99241/Level 1	99242/Level 2	99243/Level 3	99244/Level 4	99245/Level 5
HISTORY	*Problem Focused*	*Exp Problem Foc*	*Detailed*	*Comprehensive*	*Comprehensive*
Hx Present Illness	Brief 1-3 elements	Brief 1-3 elements	Extended ≥4 elements	Extended ≥4 elements	Extended >4 elements
Past Med Hx/ Fam Hx/Social Hx (PMH/FH/SH)	Not required	Not required	Pertinent Stmt Re: Minimum 1 component	Complete Stmt Re: Minimum 2/3 components	Complete Stmt Re: Minimum 2/3 components
Review of Systems (ROS)	Not required	Prob pertinent 1 affected system Related to Chief Complaint	Extended 2-9 systems	Complete ≥10 systems OR pert positive & "all sys review & neg"	Complete ≥10 systems OR pert positive & "all sys review & neg"
EXAM	*Problem Focused*	*Exp Problem Foc*	*Detailed*	*Comprehensive*	*Comprehensive*
	1 element Body area/organ system	2-4 elements Body area/organ system	5-7 elements Body area/organ system	8 or more elements Body area/organ system	8 or more elements Body area/organ system
MDM (2 of 3)	*Straightforward*	*Straightforward*	*Low*	*Moderate*	*High*
Quantity Data	Minimal/None	Minimal/None	Limited	Moderate	Extensive
Trt/Dx Options	Minimal	Minimal	Limited	Multiple	Extensive
Risk	Minimal	Minimal	Low	Moderate	High
Time *	15 minutes	30 minutes	40 minutes	60 minutes	80 minutes

ELEMENTS OF HISTORY, EXAM, MEDICAL DECISION MAKING
(Circle those elements present in documentation)

Elements HX PRES ILLNESS	Elements REVIEW OF SYSTEMS	Exam Elements BODY AREAS	QUANTITY/ COMPLEX DATA	DX/TREAT OPTIONS	RISKS

Location   Duration
Quality   Timing
Severity   Context
Modifying Factors
Assoc S/S
ELEMENT COUNT:
	Eyes Neuro
	Card Psych
	Resp Endo
	GI GU
	MS Integum
	Constitutional
	Ear, Nose, Mouth, Throat
	Hema/Lymph
	Aller/Immuno
	ELEMENT COUNT:
		Head (incl face)
		Neck
		Chest (incl breast)
		Abdomen
		Genitalia, groin, buttocks
		Back, incl spine
		Each extremity
		Exam Elements ORGAN SYSTEMS
		Eyes GU
		Skin Neuro
		Card Psych
		Resp GI
		MS
		Ear, Nose, Mouth
		Constitutional
		Hema/Lymph/Immuno
		ELEMENT COUNT:
			Path/Lab 1
			Radiology 1
			Other Dx 1
			Comp Test ea 2
			Old Records:
			  Need for 1
			  Review of 2
			Discussion of
			Results 1
			Scoring:
			  Minimal = 0-1
			  Limited = 2
			  Moderate = 3
			  Extensive = 4
			ELEMENT COUNT:
				Self-Lmtd/Minor 1
				Est Prob Stable 1
				Est Prob Worse 2
				New Problem
				  No Addtl W/Up 3
				New Problem
				  Addtl W/Up 4
				Scoring:
				  Minimal = 1
				  Limited = 2
				  Multiple = 3
				  Extensive = 4
				ELEMENT COUNT:
					Minimal
					Low
					Moderate
					High
					Based On:
					Presenting Prob
					Dx Proc Ordered
					Mgt Option
					Selected
					ELEMENT LEVEL:

Elements — Medical Decision Making (2 of 3) spans the QUANTITY/COMPLEX DATA, DX/TREAT OPTIONS, and RISKS columns.

* Time is determinant factor ONLY when documented counseling/coordination of care >50% of total face-to-face time.

CPT-4 Coding Steps

	E & M Example	Chart Information
Step 1		
Identify Chapter	Visits/Encounters	Evaluation and Management
Range of Codes	99201-99499	99201-99499
Step 2	**Consultation**	
Determine Type/ Location	Location Office Hospital	99241-99275 Outpatient 99241-99245
Step 3		
Specific Type	Patient Status New Patient Established	New 99241-99245
Step 4		
Specific Procedure Information	Level of Service Level 1	
Step 5		
Extent/Additional Specifics	Time/Other Guidelines 45 min	

Initial Inpatient Consultations

Because these codes specify "initial," only one initial consultation may be charged by each consultant per hospital admission. This code includes both the initial consultation, which is perhaps requested at the time of admission, and a later session during the hospitalization, in which the same physician is consulted again.

There are five levels of initial inpatient consultation codes included in the Initial Hospital Consultations grid (Tool 35).

Follow-up Inpatient Consultations

When additional consultative services are requested during the same hospitalization, codes from the subsequent hospital care range would be assigned.

Follow-up consultation codes and confirmatory consultations were deleted in the 2006 CPT code book. As a result, established coders will have to adapt to these changes. Tool 36 provides a crosswalk of old consultation codes to codes for use beginning January 1, 2006.

It is often difficult to differentiate those visits considered new/initial, which require all three key components to be met, and established/subsequent visits, which require only two of the three key components. Tool 37 contains those code ranges contained in each category for convenient reference.

EMERGENCY DEPARTMENT VISITS

Each visit to the emergency department is considered new, because the physician staff changes or presenting problems differ from visit to visit. Therefore all three key components must be met before a specific level of emergency department service can be billed.

To qualify as an emergency facility, the facility must be available 24 hours a day and must provide unscheduled episodic services to patients who present for immediate medical care. There are five levels of emergency department services outlined in the Emergency Department Visits grid (Tool 38).

In addition to the usual levels of service documentation necessary with all E & M services, emergency department services for levels 4 and 5 require the following:

Level 4   Documentation of the necessity for urgent evaluation
Level 5   Documentation of the necessity for urgent treatment

This documentation may be implied. Keep in mind that the third party auditing records must be able to identify clearly the presence of this documentation. The easiest way to meet this requirement is to make certain that the provider documents the information, either in dictation or somewhere on the emergency record.

Level 5 emergency room visits may also be assigned when the history and examination components cannot be met because of the patient's medical or psychiatric condition. Documentation should support that the patient was unable to provide the history or that a comprehensive examination was not possible because of the patient's condition, but the medical decision making still met high complexity requirements.

In addition to the five levels of emergency department service, there is another code used by the hospital emergency department. **Code 99288,** Direction of Emergency Medical Systems (EMS), is used when the physician directs personnel outside the facility, such as ambulance or paramedic personnel, by providing medical directives and instructions. Note that this code often is not reimbursed by third-party insurance carriers. Codeable services must be coded, however, whether or not there is a possibility of reimbursement.

PEDIATRIC CRITICAL CARE PATIENT TRANSPORT

Codes 99289 and 99290 are used for critical care services provided during transport from one facility to another for a critically ill or injured pediatric patient (24 months

T O O L   35

1995 Guidelines
INITIAL HOSPITAL CONSULTATIONS
LEVELS OF SERVICE DOCUMENTATION REQUIREMENTS
(3 of 3 elements must be met)

	99251/Level 1	99252/Level 2	99253/Level 3	99254/Level 4	99255/Level 5
HISTORY	*Prob Focused*	*Exp Problem Foc*	*Detailed*	*Comprehensive*	*Comprehensive*
Hx Present Illness	Brief 1-3 elements	Brief 1-3 elements	Extended ≥4 elements	Extended ≥4 elements	Extended ≥4 elements
Past Med Hx/ Fam Hx/Social Hx (PMH/FH/SH)	Not required	Not required	Pertinent Stmt Re: Minimum 1 component	Complete Stmt Re: Minimum 2/3 components	Complete Stmt Re: Minimum 2/3 components
Review of Systems (ROS)	Not required	Prob pertinent 1 affected system Related to Chief Complaint	Extended 2-9 systems	Complete ≥10 systems OR pert positive & "all sys review & neg"	Complete ≥10 systems OR pert positive & "all sys review & neg"
EXAM	*Prob Focused*	*Exp Problem Foc*	*Detailed*	*Comprehensive*	*Comprehensive*
	1 element Body area/organ system	2-4 elements Body area/organ system	5-7 elements Body area/organ system	8 or more elements Body area/organ system	8 or more elements Body area/organ system
MDM (2 of 3)	*Straightforward*	*Straightforward*	*Low*	*Moderate*	*High*
Quantity Data	Minimal/None	Minimal/None	Limited	Moderate	Extensive
Trt/Dx Options	Minimal	Minimal	Limited	Multiple	Extensive
Risk	Minimal	Minimal	Low	Moderate	High
Time *	20 minutes	40 minutes	55 minutes	80 minutes	110 minutes

ELEMENTS OF HISTORY, EXAM, MEDICAL DECISION MAKING
(Circle those elements present in documentation)

Elements HX PRES ILLNESS	Elements REVIEW OF SYSTEMS	Exam Elements BODY AREAS	Elements — Medical Decision Making (2 of 3)		
			QUANTITY/ COMPLEX DATA	DX/TREAT OPTIONS	RISKS
Location Duration Quality Timing Severity Context Modifying Factors Assoc S/S **ELEMENT COUNT:**	Eyes Neuro Card Psych Resp Endo GI GU MS Integum Constitutional Ear, Nose, Mouth, Throat Hema/Lymph Aller/Immuno **ELEMENT COUNT:**	Head (incl face) Neck Chest (incl breast) Abdomen Genitalia, groin, buttocks Back, incl spine Each extremity	Path/Lab 1 Radiology 1 Other Dx 1 Comp Test ea 2 Old Records: Need for 1 Review of 2 Discussion of Results 1	Self-Lmtd/Minor 1 Est Prob Stable 1 Est Prob Worse 2 New Problem No Addtl W/Up 3 New Problem Addtl W/Up 4	Minimal Low Moderate High Based On: Presenting Prob Dx Proc Ordered Mgt Option Selected
		Exam Elements ORGAN SYSTEMS	Scoring: Minimal = 0-1 Limited = 2 Moderate = 3 Extensive = 4 **ELEMENT COUNT:**	Scoring: Minimal = 1 Limited = 2 Multiple = 3 Extensive = 4 **ELEMENT COUNT:**	**ELEMENT LEVEL:**
		Eyes GU Skin Neuro Card Psych Resp GI MS Ear, Nose, Mouth Constitutional Hema/Lymph/Immuno **ELEMENT COUNT:**			

* Time is determinant factor ONLY when documented counseling/coordination of care >50% of total unit/floor time.

T O O L   36

CONSULTATION CROSSWALK CODES

Location/Type	Pre 2006	2006 Code Range
Office	99241-99245	same
Outpatient	99241-99245	same
Initial Inpatient	99251-99255	same
Subsequent Inpatient	99261-99263	99231-99233
Confirmatory/Office	99271-99275	99201-99205
Confirmatory/Inpatient	99271-99275	99231-99233

old or younger). These codes are assigned based on time as follows:

99289	First 30 to 74 minutes
99290	Each additional 30 minutes

CRITICAL CARE SERVICES

The critical care services category has been misused and abused by physicians throughout the country for some time. In Pennsylvania, for example, one carrier banned the use of these codes because of the high volume of inappropriate usage by physicians. Therefore the coder can add these codes to the growing list of those watched closely for potential fraud and abuse.

Critical care services must meet ALL of the following guidelines:

- An unstable and/or critically ill patient
- Constant attention required from the provider for the time(s) coded and billed

Note that NOT ALL patients who are treated in the intensive care unit (ICU) of the hospital will qualify for critical care services. Care should be taken to make certain all requirements are met before these codes are used.

Critical care service comprises several comprehensive services that make up the critical care charge. They include the following:

- Cardiac output measurement interpretation
- Chest x-rays
- Blood gases
- Use of computer-stored information
- Gastric intubation
- Temporary transcutaneous pacing
- Ventilation management
- Vascular access procedures

If additional services beyond those listed are provided, they may be billed along with the critical care code(s).

Because each code is based on the amount of time spent rendering critical care, this series of E & M codes may have more than one code billed per day. The documented time spent by the physician providing constant attention to unstable, critically ill, or injured patients is billed with these codes. The critical care time is calculated according to the total time spent with a patient on a specific date. It may include critical care time that is not continuous for the same calendar date.

For the criteria for each component of critical care to be met, a minimum of one half of the specified time element must be met. For instance, code 99291 is specified as the first hour of critical care provided on a given calendar date. If the time spent is less than 30 minutes (or less than one half of the total critical care time), it may not be billed as critical care code 99291. In this case, the appropriate level based on location of service would be billed, such as a hospital visit or an office visit.

The coder should also remember that critical care may be provided in ANY location as long as the requirements of constant attention for an unstable, critically ill/injured patient are met. The following example illustrates this concept.

A patient arrives at the pediatric office in acute respiratory distress as the result of an acute asthmatic exacerbation. The patient is documented as unstable and critically ill, and requires the constant attention of the physician for care. An ambulance is summoned, and the provider continues to provide constant care to

T O O L   37

NEW/INITIAL VISIT CODES (3/3 COMPONENTS REQUIRED)
ESTABLISHED/SUBSEQUENT VISIT CODES (2/3 COMPONENTS REQUIRED:
TIME DRIVE VISIT CODES

New/Initial Visits (3/3 components required)	Code Ranges
Office/Outpatient	99201-99205
Hospital Observation	99218-99220
Initial Hospital Care	99221-99223
Observation/Inpatient Admit/Discharge Same Day	99234-99236
Office/Outpatient Consultations	99241-99245
Initial Inpatient Consultations	99251-99255
Emergency Department Services	99281-99285
Initial Nursing Facility Care	99304-99306
Domiciliary, Rest Home, Custodial Care	99324-99328
Home Services	99341-99345

Established/Subsequent Visits (2/3 components required)	Code Ranges
Office/Outpatient	99211-99215
Subsequent Hospital Care	99231-99233
Subsequent Nursing Facility Care	99307-99310
Domiciliary, Rest Home, Custodial Care	99334-99337
Home Services	99347-99350

Time Drive Codes	Code Ranges
Observation Discharge Services	99217
Hospital Discharge Services	99238-99239
Pediatric Critical Care Transport	99289-99290
Critical Care	99291-99292
Inpatient Neonatal/Pediatric Critical Care	99293-99296 (Per Day Codes)
Continuing Intensive Care	99298-99300 (Per Day Codes)
Nursing Facility Discharge Services	99315-99316
Prolonged Services	99354-99359
Physician Standby Services	99360
Case Management Services	99361-99362
Care Plan Oversight Services	99374-99380
Counseling/Risk Factor Intervention	99401-99412

TOOL 38

1995 Guidelines
EMERGENCY DEPARTMENT VISITS
LEVELS OF SERVICE DOCUMENTATION REQUIREMENTS
(3 of 3 elements must be met)

	99281/Level 1	99282/Level 2	99283/Level 3	99284/Level 4	99285/Level 5
HISTORY	*Problem Focused*	*Exp Problem Foc*	*Exp Problem Foc*	*Detailed*	*Comprehensive*
Hx Present Illness	Brief 1-3 elements	Brief 1-3 elements	Brief 1-3 elements	Extended ≥4 elements	Extended ≥4 elements
Past Med Hx/ Fam Hx/Social Hx (PMH/FH/SH)	Not required	Not required	Not required	Pertinent Stmt Re: Minimum 1 component	Complete Stmt Re: Minimum 2/3 components
Review of Systems (ROS)	Not required	Prob pertinent 1 affected system Related to Chief Complaint	Prob pertinent 1 affected system Related to Chief Complaint	Extended 2-9 systems	Complete ≥10 systems OR pert positive & "all sys review & neg"
EXAM	*Problem Focused*	*Exp Problem Foc*	*Exp Problem Foc*	*Detailed*	*Comprehensive*
	1 element Body area/organ system	2-4 elements Body area/organ system	2-4 elements Body area/organ system	5-7 elements Body area/organ system	8 or more elements Body area/organ system
MDM (2 of 3)	*Straightforward*	*Low*	*Moderate*	*Moderate*	*High*
Quantity Data	Minimal/None	Limited	Moderate	Moderate	Extensive
Trt/Dx Options	Minimal	Limited	Multiple	Multiple	Extensive
Risk	Minimal	Low	Moderate	Moderate	High

ELEMENTS OF HISTORY, EXAM, MEDICAL DECISION MAKING
(Circle those elements present in documentation)

Elements HX PRES ILLNESS	Elements REVIEW OF SYSTEMS	Exam Elements BODY AREAS	Elements — Medical Decision Making (2 of 3)		
			QUANTITY/ COMPLEX DATA	DX/TREAT OPTIONS	RISKS

Location   Duration
Quality   Timing
Severity   Context
Modifying Factors
Assoc S/S
**ELEMENT
COUNT:**
	Eyes Neuro
	Card Psych
	Resp Endo
	GI GU
	MS Integum
	Constitutional
	Ear, Nose, Mouth,
	  Throat
	Hema/Lymph
	Aller/Immuno
	**ELEMENT
	COUNT:**
		Head, incl face
		Neck
		Chest (incl breast)
		Abdomen
		Genitalia, groin, buttocks
		Back, incl spine
		Each extremity
			Path/Lab 1
			Radiology 1
			Other Dx 1
			Comp Test ea 2
			Old Records:
			  Need for 1
			  Review of 2
			Discussion of
			  Results 1
				Self-Lmtd/Minor 1
				Est Prob Stable 1
				Est Prob Worse 2
				New Problem
				  No Addtl W/Up 3
				New Problem
				  Addtl W/Up 4
					Minimal
					Low
					Moderate
					High
					Based On:
					Presenting Prob
					Dx Proc Ordered
					Mgt Option
					  Selected

		**Exam Elements
		ORGAN SYSTEMS**
			Scoring:
			  Minimal = 0-1
			  Limited = 2
			  Moderate = 3
			  Extensive = 4
				Scoring:
				  Minimal = 1
				  Limited = 2
				  Multiple = 3
				  Extensive = 4
					**ELEMENT
					LEVEL:**

		Eyes GU Skin Neuro Card Psych Resp GI MS Ear, Nose, Mouth Constitutional Hema/Lymph/Immuno **ELEMENT COUNT:**	**ELEMENT COUNT:**	**ELEMENT COUNT:**	

the unstable, critically ill patient while en route to the hospital and in the emergency department.

Total time: 2 hours, 15 minutes
Office time: 30 minutes
Ambulance: 1 hour
Emergency department: 45 minutes

The following codes are used for billing critical care services:

99291   Critical care, first hour (at least 30 minutes up to 60 minutes)
99292   Critical care, each additional 30 minutes (at least 15 minutes up to 30 minutes)

These are all critical care services performed on the same calendar date. It is advisable that the provider document the time(s) spent with the patient, preferably by indicating "start" and "stop" times, or actual blocks of time (e.g., 3:10 PM to 3:55 PM). Should additional clarification of time units for critical care visits be needed, the CPT-4 manual has an excellent chart for reference purposes.

Make certain the physician understands the importance of documenting the unstable, critically ill/injured nature of the patient. Words such as "doing well," "stable," "without complaints," or "no acute distress" are not acceptable terminology for documenting the critical care visit.

INPATIENT PEDIATRIC CRITICAL CARE AND NEONATAL INTENSIVE CARE

Code 99293 and 99294 are used for pediatric critical care when provided on an inpatient basis. These codes are assigned on a "per day" basis, with 99293 for the initial day, and code 99294 for each additional day. When codes are stated as "each, each additional," the services should be assigned codes that are based on units of service rather than each day as a separate line item. Consider the following example:

Pediatric patient admitted to Pediatric ICU on 01/01/xx and remained in Pediatric ICU 01/02/xx, 01/03/xx, 01/04/xx, and 01/05/xx. These services would be assigned codes as follows:

01/01/xx   Code 99294 X   1 unit
01/02–01/05/xx   Code 992925 X   4 units

Codes 99295 through 99299 are the "critical care" codes for neonates. They may be used only for the critically ill or very low-birth-weight neonate. As with regular critical care codes, when the criteria for neonatal intensive care services can no longer be met, the appropriate location and level of service should be coded, such as a hospital visit.

Unlike the regular critical care codes, these neonatal codes should be reported only ONCE per calendar day, regardless of the amount of time or number of visits made per calendar day.

Neonatal intensive care services comprise a number of comprehensive medical services. They include the following:

- Monitoring and treatment of the patient
- Enteral/parenteral nutritional maintenance
- Metabolic/hematological maintenance
- Pharmacological control of the circulatory system
- Counseling of parents
- Case management services
- Personal direct supervision of health care team
  All the following listed services are included in the charge for neonatal intensive care:
  - Umbilical, central, or peripheral vessel catheterization
  - Oral or nasogastric tube placement
  - Endotracheal intubation
  - Lumbar puncture
  - Suprapubic bladder aspiration
  - Bladder catheterization
  - Initiation/management of mechanical ventilation of continuous positive airway pressure (CPAP)
  - Surfactant administration
  - Intravascular fluid administration
  - Transfusion of blood components
  - Vascular puncture
  - Invasive or noninvasive electronic monitoring, including vital signs, bedside pulmonary function testing, and monitoring or interpretation of gases or oxygen saturation

Critically ill neonates are defined as those requiring life support, such as respiratory or cardiac assistance, frequent to continuous vital sign monitoring, laboratory and blood gas interpretations, and frequent reevaluations by the provider (including constant observation by members of the health care team under the provider's supervision). Two categories of codes are used for coding neonatal intensive care services.

Initial Neonatal Intensive Care

This code is used only for the initial date of admission of the critically ill neonate.

Subsequent Neonatal Intensive Care

The neonate must remain critically ill and unstable for this code to be used. This code is assigned for EACH subsequent calendar day. In addition, codes exist for critically ill but stable neonatal visits and for low-birth-weight infant care. These may be used as long as the neonatal intensive care requirements are met.

When the neonate no longer meets the guidelines for neonatal intensive care services, but still remains hospitalized, regular inpatient hospital codes are appropriate.

NURSING FACILITY SERVICES

When services are provided in nursing facilities, skilled nursing facilities (SNFs), intermediate-care facilities (ICFs), and long-term care facilities, and when E & M services are provided in the psychiatric residential treatment facility, the following codes are billed.

Initial Nursing Facility Assessments (New/Established)

When comprehensive nursing facility assessment codes are billed, all other E & M services provided for the same day are included. In the case of nursing facility services, codes are assigned on the basis of the performance of a comprehensive nursing assessment or with subsequent nursing facility codes.

Comprehensive nursing facility assessment codes require the formulation or reformulation of a medical plan of care. One of the three levels of comprehensive nursing assessment codes may be used as outlined in the Comprehensive Nursing Facility Assessment grid (Tool 39).

Subsequent Nursing Facility Assessments

These codes are used to report services provided to patients in this type of facility when no further comprehensive assessment is required. This is an established visit code; only two of the three key components must be met for the particular level of service assigned. Three subsequent nursing facility codes are used as outlined on the Subsequent Nursing Facility Care grid (Tool 40).

Nursing Facility Discharge

These codes are used for services performed in conjunction with the final examination of the patient before discharge from the nursing facility. These services may include such items as final examination of the patient; discussion of the nursing facility stay with the patient or patient's family; continuing care instructions provided to caregivers; discharge preparation; and final preparation of discharge records, prescriptions, and referral forms. This set of codes is time driven, as are other discharge services; therefore the rounding rule applies to these codes. One half or more of the time must be documented to justify the use of these codes. The documented time may not necessarily be continuous, but it must fall on the same calendar day. The following codes are used for billing nursing facility discharge services:

99315 Nursing facility discharge 30 minutes or less
99316 Nursing facility discharge more than 30 minutes

DOMICILIARY, REST HOME, AND CUSTODIAL SERVICES

When services occur in a facility in which room, board, and other personal assistance services are provided, the codes from the domiciliary, rest home, or custodial care services should be assigned. These facilities typically offer long-term care of the patient or boarder. New and established patient visit codes exist. As with other E & M codes, all three key elements must be met for new patients; only two of the three key elements must be met for established patients.

Remember that the facility charges for the care and upkeep of the patient or boarder. This reimbursement billed by the facility does not include any medical services provided by the physician.

Domiciliary, rest home, and custodial care new and established services are outlined in the New and Established Domiciliary or Rest Home Visits grids (Tools 41 and 42).

HOME SERVICES

Home service codes are reserved for E & M services provided in the residential setting. These services do not have to be provided specifically in the patient's home, but merely in a residential setting. For instance, this could include a hotel or motel in which a patient is temporarily residing. Home services are outlined in the New and Established Home Visits grids (Tools 43 and 44).

PROLONGED SERVICES

When provider services are given over and above the usual E & M services outlined in the E & M section, they may be billed as follows:

With face-to-face prolonged services
Without face-to-face prolonged services

The differentiation between face-to-face and non–face-to-face services is the patient contact made during the face-to-face encounter. Non–face-to-face codes typically are used for services provided on behalf of the patient, without the presence of the patient (i.e., contact with health providers, arranging for health care outside of the office or hospital setting, or meeting with family members regarding the care of the patient).

Because these codes are based on time, the rounding rules apply. To meet the stated criteria and bill for these services, the coder must document a minimum of one half of the stated time.

Text continued on p. 236

TOOL 39

1995 Guidelines
INITIAL NURSING FACILITY ASSESSMENTS
LEVELS OF SERVICE DOCUMENTATION REQUIREMENTS
(3 of 3 elements must be met)

	99304	99305	99306		
HISTORY	*Detailed*	*Comprehensive*	*Comprehensive*		
Hx Present Illness	Extended ≥4 elements	Extended ≥4 elements	Extended ≥4 elements		
Past Med Hx/ Fam Hx/Social Hx (PMH/FH/SH)	Pertinent Stmt Re: Minimum one component	Complete Stmt Re: Minimum 2/3 components	Complete Stmt Re: Minimum 2/3 components		
Review of Systems (ROS)	Extended 2-9 systems	Complete ≥10 systems OR pert positive & "all sys review & neg"	Complete ≥10 systems OR pert positive & "all sys review & neg"		
EXAM	*Comprehensive*	*Comprehensive*	*Comprehensive*		
	Complete ≥10 systems OR pert positive & "all sys review & neg"	Complete ≥10 systems OR pert positive & "all sys review & neg"	Complete ≥10 systems OR pert positive & "all sys review & neg"		
MDM (2 of 3)	*Straightforward/Low*	*Moderate/High*	*Moderate/High*		
Quantity Data	Minimal/Limited	Moderate	Extensive		
Trt/Dx Options	Minimal/Limited	Multiple	Extensive		
Risk	Minimal/Low	Moderate	High		

ELEMENTS OF HISTORY, EXAM, MEDICAL DECISION MAKING
(Circle those elements present in documentation)

Elements HX PRES ILLNESS	Elements REVIEW OF SYSTEMS	Exam Elements BODY AREAS	Elements — Medical Decision Making (2 of 3)		
			QUANTITY/ COMPLEX DATA	DX/TREAT OPTIONS	RISKS
Location Duration Quality Timing Severity Context Modifying Factors Assoc S/S **ELEMENT COUNT:**	Eyes Neuro Card Psych Resp Endo GI GU MS Integum Constitutional Ear, Nose, Mouth, Throat Hema/Lymph Aller/Immuno **ELEMENT COUNT:**	Head (incl face) Neck Chest (incl breast) Abdomen Genitalia, groin, buttocks Back, incl spine Each extremity **Exam Elements ORGAN SYSTEMS** Eyes GU Skin Neuro Card Psych Resp GI MS Ear, Nose, Mouth Constitutional Hema/Lymph/Immuno **ELEMENT COUNT:**	Path/Lab 1 Radiology 1 Other Dx 1 Comp Test ea 2 Old Records: Need for 1 Review of 2 Discussion of Results 1 Scoring: Minimal = 0-1 Limited = 2 Moderate = 3 Extensive = 4 **ELEMENT COUNT:**	Self-Lmtd/Minor 1 Est Prob Stable 1 Est Prob Worse 2 New Problem No Addtl W/Up 3 New Problem Addtl W/Up 4 Scoring: Minimal = 1 Limited = 2 Multiple = 3 Extensive = 4 **ELEMENT COUNT:**	Minimal Low Moderate High Based On: Presenting Prob Dx Proc Ordered Mgt Option Selected **ELEMENT LEVEL:**

1995 Guidelines
SUBSEQUENT NURSING FACILITY CARE
LEVELS OF SERVICE DOCUMENTATION REQUIREMENTS
(2 of 3 elements must be met)

	99307	99308	99309	99310	
HISTORY (Interval)	*Problem Focused*	*Exp Problem Focused*	*Detailed*	*Comprehensive*	
Hx Present Illness	Brief 1-3 elements	Brief 1-3 elements	Extended ≥4 elements	Extended ≥4 elements	
Past Med Hx/ Fam Hx/Social Hx (PMH/FH/SH)	Not required	Not required	Pertinent Stmt Re: Minimum 1 component	Complete Stmt Re: Minimum 2/3 components	
Review of Systems (ROS)	Not required	Prob pertinent 1 affected system Related to Chief Complaint	Extended 2-9 systems	Complete ≥10 systems OR pert positive & "all sys review & neg"	
EXAM	*Problem Focused*	*Exp Problem Foc*	*Detailed*	*Comprehensive*	
	1 element Body area/organ system	2-4 elements Body area/organ system	5-7 elements Body area/organ system	Complete ≥10 systems OR pert positive & "all sys review & neg"	
MDM (2 of 3)	*Straightforward/Low*	*Low*	*Moderate*	*High*	
Quantity Data	Minimal/Limited	Limited	Moderate	Extensive	
Trt/Dx Options	Minimal/Limited	Limited	Multiple	Extensive	
Risk	Minimal/Low	Low	Moderate	High	

ELEMENTS OF HISTORY, EXAM, MEDICAL DECISION MAKING
(Circle those elements present in documentation)

Elements HX PRES ILLNESS	Elements REVIEW OF SYSTEMS	Exam Elements BODY AREAS	Elements — Medical Decision Making (2 of 3)		
			QUANTITY/ COMPLEX DATA	DX/TREAT OPTIONS	RISKS
Location Duration Quality Timing Severity Context Modifying Factors Assoc S/S **ELEMENT COUNT:**	Eyes Neuro Card Psych Resp Endo GI GU MS Integum Constitutional Ear, Nose, Mouth, Throat Hema/Lymph Aller/Immuno **ELEMENT COUNT:**	Head (incl face) Neck Chest (incl breast) Abdomen Genitalia, groin, buttocks Back, incl spine Each extremity	Path/Lab 1 Radiology 1 Other Dx 1 Comp Test ea 2 Old Records: Need for 1 Review of 2 Discussion of	Self-Lmtd/Minor 1 Est Prob Stable 1 Est Prob Worse 2 New Problem No Addtl W/Up 3 New Problem Addtl W/Up 4	Minimal Low Moderate High Based On: Presenting Prob Dx Proc Ordered Mgt Option
		Exam Elements ORGAN SYSTEMS	Results 1 Scoring:	Scoring: Minimal = 1	Selected
		Eyes GU Skin Neuro Card Psych Resp GI MS Ear, Nose, Mouth Constitutional Hema/Lymph/Immuno **ELEMENT COUNT:**	Minimal = 0-1 Limited = 2 Moderate = 3 Extensive = 4 **ELEMENT COUNT:**	Limited = 2 Multiple = 3 Extensive = 4 **ELEMENT COUNT:**	**ELEMENT LEVEL:**

TOOL 41

1995 Guidelines
NEW DOMICILIARY OR REST HOME VISITS
LEVELS OF SERVICE DOCUMENTATION REQUIREMENTS
(3 of 3 elements must be met)

	99324	99325	99326	99327	99328
HISTORY	*Problem Focused*	*Exp Problem Foc*	*Detailed*	*Comprehensive*	*Comprehensive*
Hx Present Illness	Brief 1-3 elements	Brief 1-3 elements	Extended ≥4 elements	Extended ≥4 elements	Extended ≥4 elements
Past Med Hx/ Fam Hx/Social Hx (PMH/FH/SH)	Not required	Not required	Pertinent Stmt Re: Minimum 1 component	Complete Stmt Re: Minimum 2/3 components	Complete Stmt Re: Minimum 2/3 components
Review of Systems (ROS)	Not required	Prob pertinent 1 affected system Related to Chief Complaint	Extended 2-9 systems	Complete ≥10 systems OR pert positive & "all sys review & neg"	Complete ≥10 systems OR pert positive & "all sys review & neg"
EXAM	*Problem Focused*	*Exp Problem Foc*	*Detailed*	*Comprehensive*	*Comprehensive*
	1 element Body area/organ system	2-4 elements Body area/organ system	5-7 elements Body area/organ system	8 or more elements Body area/organ system	8 or more elements Body area/organ system
MDM (2 of 3)	*Straightforward/Low*	*Low*	*Moderate*	*Moderate*	*High*
Quantity Data	Minimal/Limited	Limited	Moderate	Moderate	Extensive
Trt/Dx Options	Minimal/Limited	Limited	Multiple	Multiple	Extensive
Risk	Minimal/Low	Low	Moderate	Moderate	High

ELEMENTS OF HISTORY, EXAM, MEDICAL DECISION MAKING
(Circle those elements present in documentation)

Elements HX PRES ILLNESS	Elements REVIEW OF SYSTEMS	Exam Elements BODY AREAS	Elements — Medical Decision Making (2 of 3)		
			QUANTITY/ COMPLEX DATA	DX/TREAT OPTIONS	RISKS

Location   Duration
Quality   Timing
Severity   Context
Modifying Factors
Assoc S/S
**ELEMENT
COUNT:**
	Eyes Neuro
	Card Psych
	Resp Endo
	GI GU
	MS Integum
	Constitutional
	Ear, Nose, Mouth,
	  Throat
	Hema/Lymph
	Aller/Immuno
	**ELEMENT
	COUNT:**
		Head (incl face)
		Neck
		Chest (incl breast)
		Abdomen
		Genitalia, groin, buttocks
		Back, incl spine
		Each extremity
		**Exam Elements
		ORGAN SYSTEMS**
		Eyes GU
		Skin Neuro
		Card Psych
		Resp GI
		MS
		Ear, Nose, Mouth
		Constitutional
		Hema/Lymph/Immuno
		**ELEMENT
		COUNT:**
			Path/Lab 1
			Radiology 1
			Other Dx 1
			Comp Test ea 2
			Old Records:
			  Need for 1
			  Review of 2
			Discussion of
			Results 1
			Scoring:
			  Minimal = 0-1
			  Limited = 2
			  Moderate = 3
			  Extensive = 4
			**ELEMENT
			COUNT:**
				Self-Lmtd/Minor 1
				Est Prob Stable 1
				Est Prob Worse 2
				New Problem
				  No Addtl W/Up 3
				New Problem
				  Addtl W/Up 4
				Scoring:
				  Minimal = 1
				  Limited = 2
				  Multiple = 3
				  Extensive = 4
				**ELEMENT
				COUNT:**
					Minimal
					Low
					Moderate
					High
					Based On:
					Presenting Prob
					Dx Proc Ordered
					Mgt Option
					  Selected
					**ELEMENT
					LEVEL:**

TOOL 42

1995 Guidelines
ESTABLISHED DOMICILIARY OR REST HOME VISITS
LEVELS OF SERVICE DOCUMENTATION REQUIREMENTS
(2 of 3 elements must be met)

	99334	99335	99336	99337	
HISTORY	*Problem Foc Interval*	*Exp Prob Foc Inter*	*Detailed interval*	*Comprehensive Interval*	
Hx Present Illness	Brief 1-3 elements	Brief 1-3 elements	Extended ≥4 elements	Extended ≥4 elements	
Past Med Hx/ Fam Hx/Social Hx (PMH/FH/SH)	Not required	Not required	Pertinent Stmt Re: Minimum 1 component	Complete Stmt Re: Minimum 2/3 components	
Review of Systems (ROS)	Not required	Prob pertinent 1 affected system Related to Chief Complaint	Extended 2-9 systems	Complete ≥10 systems OR pert positive & "all sys review & neg"	
EXAM	*Problem Focused*	*Exp Problem Foc*	*Detailed*	*Comprehensive*	
	1 element Body area/organ system	2-4 elements Body area/organ system	5-7 elements Body area/organ system	8 or more elements Body area/organ system	
MDM (2 of 3)	*Straightforward/Low*	*Moderate/Low*	*Moderate*	*Moderate/High*	
Quantity Data	Minimal/Limited	Moderate/Limited	Moderate	Moderate/Extensive	
Trt/Dx Options	Minimal/Limited	Multiple/Limited	Multiple	Multiple/Extensive	
Risk	Minimal/Low	Moderate/Low	Moderate	Moderate/High	
Time *	15 minutes	25 minutes	40 minutes	60 minutes	

ELEMENTS OF HISTORY, EXAM, MEDICAL DECISION MAKING
(Circle those elements present in documentation)

Elements HX PRES ILLNESS	Elements REVIEW OF SYSTEMS	Exam Elements BODY AREAS	Elements — Medical Decision Making (2 of 3)		
			QUANTITY/ COMPLEX DATA	DX/TREAT OPTIONS	RISKS

Location   Duration
Quality   Timing
Severity   Context
Modifying Factors
Assoc S/S
**ELEMENT
COUNT:**
	Eyes Neuro
	Card Psych
	Resp Endo
	GI GU
	MS Integum
	Constitutional
	Ear, Nose, Mouth,
	   Throat
	Hema/Lymph
	Aller/Immuno
	**ELEMENT
	COUNT:**
		Head (incl face)
		Neck
		Chest (incl breast)
		Abdomen
		Genitalia, groin, buttocks
		Back, incl spine
		Each extremity
		**Exam Elements
		ORGAN SYSTEMS**
		Eyes GU
		Skin Neuro
		Card Psych
		Resp GI
		MS
		Ear, Nose, Mouth
		Constitutional
		Hema/Lymph/Immuno
		**ELEMENT
		COUNT:**
			Path/Lab 1
			Radiology 1
			Other Dx 1
			Comp Test ea 2
			Old Records:
			   Need for 1
			   Review of 2
			Discussion of
			   Results 1
			Scoring:
			   Minimal = 0-1
			   Limited = 2
			   Moderate = 3
			   Extensive = 4
			**ELEMENT
			COUNT:**
				Self-Lmtd/Minor 1
				Est Prob Stable 1
				Est Prob Worse 2
				New Problem
				   No Addtl W/Up 3
				New Problem
				   Addtl W/Up 4
				Scoring:
				   Minimal = 1
				   Limited = 2
				   Multiple = 3
				   Extensive = 4
				**ELEMENT
				COUNT:**
					Minimal
					Low
					Moderate
					High
					Based On:
					   Presenting Prob
					   Dx Proc Ordered
					   Mgt Option
					   Selected
					**ELEMENT
					LEVEL:**

* Time is determinant factor ONLY when
documented counseling/coordination
of care >50% of total face-to-face time.

T O O L   43

1995 Guidelines
NEW HOME VISITS
LEVELS OF SERVICE DOCUMENTATION REQUIREMENTS
(3 of 3 elements must be met)

	99341	99342	99343	99344	99345
HISTORY	*Problem Focused*	*Exp Problem Foc*	*Detailed*	*Comprehensive*	*Comprehensive*
Hx Present Illness	Brief 1-3 elements	Brief 1-3 elements	Extended ≥4 elements	Extended ≥4 elements	Extended ≥4 elements
Past Med Hx/ Fam Hx/Social Hx (PMH/FH/SH)	Not required	Not required	Pertinent Stmt Re: Minimum 1 component	Complete Stmt Re: Minimum 2/3 components	Complete Stmt Re: Minimum 2/3 components
Review of Systems (ROS)	Not required	Prob pertinent 1 affected system Related to Chief Complaint	Extended 2-9 systems	Complete ≥10 systems OR pert positive & "all sys review & neg"	Complete ≥10 systems OR pert positive & "all sys review & neg"
EXAM	*Problem Focused*	*Exp Problem Foc*	*Detailed*	*Comprehensive*	*Comprehensive*
	1 element Body area/organ system	2-4 elements Body area/organ system	5-7 elements Body area/organ system	8 or more elements Body area/organ system	8 or more elements Body area/organ system
MDM (2 of 3)	*Straightforward*	*Low*	*Moderate*	*Moderate*	*High*
Quantity Data	Minimal	Limited	Moderate	Moderate	Extensive
Trt/Dx Options	Minimal/None	Limited	Multiple	Multiple	Extensive
Risk	Minimal	Low	Moderate	Moderate	High
Time *	20 minutes	30 minutes	45 minutes	60 minutes	75 minutes

ELEMENTS OF HISTORY, EXAM, MEDICAL DECISION MAKING
(Circle those elements present in documentation)

Elements HX PRES ILLNESS	Elements REVIEW OF SYSTEMS	Exam Elements BODY AREAS	Elements — Medical Decision Making (2 of 3)		
			QUANTITY/ COMPLEX DATA	DX/TREAT OPTIONS	RISKS
Location Duration Quality Timing Severity Context Modifying Factors Assoc S/S **ELEMENT COUNT:**	Eyes Neuro Card Psych Resp Endo GI GU MS Integum Constitutional Ear, Nose, Mouth, Throat Hema/Lymph Aller/Immuno **ELEMENT COUNT:**	Head (incl face) Neck Chest (incl breast) Abdomen Genitalia, groin, buttocks Back, incl spine Each extremity	Path/Lab 1 Radiology 1 Other Dx 1 Comp Test ea 2 Old Records: Need for 1 Review of 2 Discussion of Results 1	Self-Lmtd/Minor 1 Est Prob Stable 1 Est Prob Worse 2 New Problem No Addtl W/Up 3 New Problem Addtl W/Up 4	Minimal Low Moderate High Based On: Presenting Prob Dx Proc Ordered Mgt Option Selected
		Exam Elements ORGAN SYSTEMS Eyes GU Skin Neuro Card Psych Resp GI MS Ear, Nose, Mouth Constitutional Hema/Lymph/Immuno **ELEMENT COUNT:**	Scoring: Minimal = 0-1 Limited = 2 Moderate = 3 Extensive = 4 **ELEMENT COUNT:**	Scoring: Minimal = 1 Limited = 2 Multiple = 3 Extensive = 4 **ELEMENT COUNT:**	**ELEMENT LEVEL:**

* Time is determinant factor ONLY when documented counseling/coordination of care >50% of total face-to-face time.

T O O L   44

1995 Guidelines
ESTABLISHED HOME VISITS
LEVELS OF SERVICE DOCUMENTATION REQUIREMENTS
(2 of 3 elements must be met)

	99347	99348	99349	99350	No Addtl Level
HISTORY	*Prob Foc Interval*	*Exp Prob Foc Interv*	*Detailed Interval*	*Comprehensive*	
Hx Present Illness	Brief 1-3 elements	Brief 1-3 elements	Extended ≥4 elements	Extended ≥4 elements	
Past Med Hx/ Fam Hx/Social Hx (PMH/FH/SH)	Not required	Not required	Pertinent Stmt Re: Minimum 1 component	Complete Stmt Re: Minimum 2/3 components	
Review of Systems (ROS)	Not required	Prob pertinent 1 affected system Related to Chief Complaint	Extended 2-9 systems	Complete ≥10 systems OR pert positive & "all sys review & neg"	
EXAM	*Problem Focused*	*Exp Prob Foc*	*Detailed*	*Comprehensive*	
	1 element Body area/organ system	2-4 elements Body area/organ system	5-7 elements Body area/organ system	8 or more elements Body area/organ system	
MDM (2 of 3)	*Straightforward*	*Low*	*Moderate*	*Moderate/High*	
Quantity Data	Minimal/None	Limited	Moderate	Moderate/Extensive	
Trt/Dx Options	Minimal	Limited	Multiple	Multiple/Extensive	
Risk	Minimal	Low	Moderate	Moderate/High	
Time *	15 minutes	25 minutes	40 minutes	60 minutes	

ELEMENTS OF HISTORY, EXAM, MEDICAL DECISION MAKING
(Circle those elements present in documentation)

Elements HX PRES ILLNESS	Elements REVIEW OF SYSTEMS	Exam Elements BODY AREAS	Elements — Medical Decision Making (2 of 3)		
			QUANTITY/ COMPLEX DATA	DX/TREAT OPTIONS	RISKS
Location Duration Quality Timing Severity Context Modifying Factors Assoc S/S **ELEMENT COUNT:**	Eyes Neuro Card Psych Resp Endo GI GU MS Integum Constitutional Ear, Nose, Mouth, Throat Hema/Lymph Aller/Immuno **ELEMENT COUNT:**	Head (incl face) Neck Chest (incl breast) Abdomen Genitalia, groin, buttocks Back, incl spine Each extremity **Exam Elements ORGAN SYSTEMS** Eyes GU Skin Neuro Card Psych Resp GI MS Ear, Nose, Mouth Constitutional Hema/Lymph/Immuno **ELEMENT COUNT:**	Path/Lab 1 Radiology 1 Other Dx 1 Comp Test ea 2 Old Records: Need for 1 Review of 2 Discussion of Results 1 Scoring: Minimal = 0-1 Limited = 2 Moderate = 3 Extensive = 4 **ELEMENT COUNT:**	Self-Lmtd/Minor 1 Est Prob Stable 1 Est Prob Worse 2 New Problem No Addtl W/Up 3 New Problem Addtl W/Up 4 Scoring: Minimal = 1 Limited = 2 Multiple = 3 Extensive = 4 **ELEMENT COUNT:**	Minimal Low Moderate High Based On: Presenting Prob Dx Proc Ordered Mgt Option Selected **ELEMENT LEVEL:**

* Time is determinant factor ONLY when documented counseling/coordination of care >50% of total face-to-face time.

These codes are assigned according to cumulative time spent and documented on each calendar date; therefore the initial code is coded only once per day. Time does not need to be continuous but is correctly coded by the time spent per calendar date.

These codes are intended to be used in addition to the regular E & M services provided. Make certain to list the regular E & M services first because these indicate the most significant service and the chief reason for the encounter. In the event the prolonged service is not reimbursed, the primary E & M service is still considered for reimbursement.

Note: Many third-party carriers do not recognize these codes or do not reimburse for these services.

PHYSICIAN STANDBY SERVICES

In many instances, a provider may be requested to be available in the event services are needed. For example, in the case of a high-risk obstetrical delivery, the neonatologist may be requested by the obstetrician to be available. This physician standby service code is intended for use ONLY when the physician ultimately does not provide any other service. As in the earlier case, if the neonatologist provides NICU services, the code for physician standby services is not applicable. In addition, the standby service physician may NOT provide services to other patients at the time the physician standby service is being billed. It is imperative that the provider coding and billing for this service makes certain that documentation by the requesting physician for this service is available, and that the time of service is documented.

In the case of physician standby services, ALL of the full 30 minutes MUST BE PROVIDED before this service can be billed. Any standby services totaling less than a full 30 minutes may not be coded and billed. For **Code 99360,** Physician Standby Service, each 30 minutes, is the ONLY code used for billing physician standby services.

Examples of physician standby services include operative standby, high-risk obstetrical delivery, and standby for cesarean section. Remember that the physician standby service must be requested and documented.

Physician standby services may not be reimbursable by many third-party carriers, but they still should be coded and billed when appropriate.

CASE MANAGEMENT SERVICES

When the provider is designated as responsible for coordinating, supervising, and initiating health care for the patient, the case management codes are used. Again, note that inclusion of these codes does not indicate

guaranteed reimbursement for these services, even when they have been documented, coded, and billed correctly.

Case management services are divided into the two following categories:

Team conferences
Telephone calls

Team Conferences

Team conferences involve the participation of multiple health care providers in discussing, planning, and instituting the coordination, supervision, and initiation of health care services for a specified patient. The rounding factor may also apply here, according to the time, with one half of the time documented before the specific code can be used. The following categories fall under team conference billing:

Medical conference with interdisciplinary team, approximately 30 minutes
Medical conference with interdisciplinary team, approximately 60 minutes

Telephone Calls

Telephone call services, as with all other services, must be documented. Documentation should include the date and time of the phone call, the content and complexity of the call, and the name of the person who spoke with the provider. These provider notes should be signed in the usual fashion. Telephone calls are categorized as follows:

Telephone call, simple or brief for the purpose of:	Reporting on tests/laboratory results Clarifying/altering previous instructions Combining new information into the patient's treatment
Telephone call, intermediate for the purpose of:	Advising patient on new problem Discussing test results in detail Coordinating a new problem Discussing evaluating the combination of new information into the patient's treatment
Telephone call, complex or lengthy for the purpose of:	Counseling (for instance, in the case of the extremely anxious/distraught patient) Discussing the care of a seriously ill patient with family members Coordinating complex services with a number of professionals

CARE PLAN OVERSIGHT SERVICES

When a provider oversees the care of a patient requiring multiple services over a prolonged period, the care plan oversight codes should be considered. Typically, the provider is involved in the revision of care plans and the review of a number of reports, including laboratory and other studies. These services must be documented as extending over and above the usual services provided in the billed E & M services.

Caution should be used in coding these services: only ONE physician may oversee the care of the patient using these codes ONLY when documentation that substantiates care beyond the usual services is provided. Infrequent service or lower levels of service are considered a part of the usual evaluation and management services coded.

As with the other "times" recorded for evaluation and management services, the coder must make certain the time is documented and the rounding rule is followed (one half of the amount of time specified must be documented before the code can be used).

The care plan oversight codes are subcategorized into locations of service: home health agency, hospice, and nursing facility. Coding and reimbursement for these services are based on the total cumulative time spent in supervision of the patient's care during a calendar month.

FRAUD ALERT: Specific Medicare regulations prohibit any physician who is the Medical Director of these facilities, or who is paid by the entity who owns them, from receiving compensation for "care plan oversight services." Because these individuals have already been paid for direction of services, reimbursement of the care plan oversight services would represent duplication of payment.

Care plan oversight services are outlined as follows:

Home health agency patient	15 to 29 minutes per calendar month
	30 minutes or more per calendar month
Hospice patient	15 to 29 minutes per calendar month
	30 minutes or more per calendar month
Nursing facility patient	15 to 29 minutes per calendar month
	30 minutes or more per calendar month

PREVENTIVE MEDICINE SERVICES

When medical care is provided for the purpose of progress evaluation or preventive care of the patient, the preventive medicine service codes are appropriate. These codes are divided between new and established patient encounters, and are further subdivided by age groups. Reimbursement varies according to the categories and subcategories, because certain age group evaluations are considered more involved than others.

Many third-party carriers abide by varying interpretations of the preventive medicine CPT-4 codes. Some do not reimburse for any preventive care; others do not recognize the preventive medicine codes in

CPT-4. Always check with specific carrier contracts to make certain of acceptable practice for coding these appropriately.

When a problem, complaint, or abnormality is noted during the course of the preventive medicine examination, it may be considered significant enough to warrant the coding of an additional E & M service code. These services are billed with modifier 25 to denote that significantly separate and distinct services have been performed. The diagnosis for the complaint, problem, or abnormality should be included in the other E & M service to further justify the request for reimbursement. Other insignificant services or E & M services for insignificant problems or complaints are not codeable or reimbursable in combination with the preventive medicine services already coded.

If immunizations, other separate services, or ancillary services are performed at the time of the preventive medicine service, these services are coded and billed as usual. In most instances, third-party consideration for reimbursement is made for these services, even when the third-party carrier may not reimburse for the actual preventive medicine service.

Preventive medicine services are outlined as follows:

New patients	Preventive Medicine Visit, Under 1 Year (Infant)
	Preventive Medicine Visit, Early Childhood (Ages 1-4)
	Preventive Medicine Visit, Late Childhood (Ages 5-11)
	Preventive Medicine Visit, Adolescent (Ages 12-17)
	Preventive Medicine Visit, Ages 18-39
	Preventive Medicine Visit, Ages 40-64
	Preventive Medicine Visit, Ages 65 and older
Established patients	Preventive Medicine, Under 1 Year (Infant)
	Preventive Medicine, Early Childhood (Ages 1-4)
	Preventive Medicine, Late Childhood (Ages 5-11)
	Preventive Medicine, Adolescent (Ages 12-17)
	Preventive Medicine, Ages 18-39
	Preventive Medicine, Ages 40-64
	Preventive Medicine, Ages 65 and older

COUNSELING/RISK FACTOR INTERVENTION

These E & M codes are used ONLY for intervention purposes, not when patients have specific symptoms, problems, or complaints related to the risk factor. Counseling or risk factor intervention services are outlined as follows:

Individual counseling	15 minutes
	30 minutes
	45 minutes
	60 minutes
Group counseling	30 minutes
	60 minutes

NEWBORN CARE

For care of the neonate, services are categorized by setting and type of service provided. Newborn care services are outlined as follows:

History and examination	Normal newborn infant, hospital and birthing room
	Normal newborn infant, other than hospital or birthing room
Subsequent newborn care	Normal newborn care, per subsequent day
History, examination, discharge and newborn care on same day	Normal newborn history, examination, discharge from hospital or birthing room, all on the same date
Attendance at delivery	Initial attendance at delivery and stabilization of neonate (when documented and requested by delivering physician); may be reported also as 99431, Normal newborn care
Newborn resuscitation	Neonate requires chest compressions, positive-pressure ventilation, or other newborn resuscitation; when this service is billed, it is inappropriate to bill Attendance at delivery (99436)

SPECIAL EVALUATION AND MANAGEMENT SERVICES

In response to the increasing demand for evaluative services other than for specific complaints or problems, evaluation codes were established a few years ago for the purpose of administrative evaluations. These evaluative services are used for establishing baseline information before the initiation of insurance policies or for approval of disability or Workers' Compensation benefits.

During the administration of these services, no medical management is instituted, nor is any modification made to the current treatment plan by the provider. These examinations are not intended to address the disability, but simply to evaluate the progress or lack thereof and to make recommendations for further evaluation and treatment.

These services typically are billed to the requesting entity (e.g., disability insurance agency, life insurance company) rather than to the patient's current health insurance carrier. These services usually are requested by the entity and are authorized in advance.

Special evaluation and management services are categorized as follows and include life/disability evaluation and work related/medical disability.

Life/disability evaluation	Height, weight, blood pressure
	Medical history
	Blood sample/urinalysis following "chain of command"
	Completion of necessary forms/reports
Work related/ medical disability (treating physician)	Completion of the medical history
	Examination commensurate with patient's condition
	Formulation of diagnosis, assessment of capabilities, calculation of impairment
	Development of future medical options
	Completion of necessary forms
Work related/ medical disability (other than treating physician)	Completion of the medical history
	Examination commensurate with patient's condition
	Formulation of diagnosis, assessment of capability, calculation of impairment
	Development of future medical options
	Completion of necessary forms

This code is used ONLY by the consultant, not the treating physician. Code 99455 should be used by the treating physician.

OTHER EVALUATION AND MANAGEMENT SERVICES

Unlisted evaluation and management services are billed with code 99499 (Unlisted Evaluation and Management Services). As with any unlisted procedure in CPT-4, this code must include a description of the service performed and a written report to accompany the claim to the insurance carrier.

STOP AND PRACTICE

Now that all the types of Evaluation and Management service have been discussed, identify the history, examination, and medical decision making components and determine what level of service should be coded in the following encounter scenarios. Use the appropriate grid for the location of service and the type of patient (new/established) and determine the correct level of service.

1. Office visit for an established patient who presents with new onset of left upper quadrant pain following fall. Past medical history of gallbladder disease. Exam of the abdomen and pelvic exam were performed. Abdomen series negative. Diagnosis: Abdominal pain.

   Location: _____

   New/estab: _____

Range of codes: _____
Grid selected: _____
Level of service: _____

2. Office visit for follow-up for stable diabetes mellitus. Patient has multiple medical problems; however, all appear stable at this time. No complaints of diplopia; excessive thirst of possible diabetic symptoms at this time. She notes that she has been symptom free, except for some lower back pain in the last couple of weeks. Exam completed of the back, heart, and lungs. Glucose level taken, which was normal. Assessment: Diabetes Type II.
Location: _____
New/estab: _____
Range of codes: _____
Grid selected: _____
Level of service: _____

3. Patient known to the physician is admitted to the inpatient hospital facility for possible stroke. History of right-sided numbness and weakness, 2 weeks' duration. No cough, no chest pain. Exam of respiratory, cardiovascular, neurological performed. CT of brain with contrast performed as well as labs, x-rays. Patient admitted for cardiovascular accident with neurological symptoms.
Location: _____
New/estab: _____
Range of codes: _____
Grid selected: _____
Level of service: _____

4. Office visit for complaint of pain and swelling in knee. Patient presents with 2-week duration of red and painful swollen knee. No swelling or pain in other joints, no fever, no fatigue. Exam of both knees are performed as well as neurological exam. X-rays reveal osteoarthritis of both knee joints.
Location: _____
New/estab: _____
Range of codes: _____
Grid selected: _____
Level of service: _____

5. Office visit for patient with known diagnosis of hypertension who now presents with symptoms of fatigue and 2-week history of headaches. Past history of diabetes and CAD. Cardiovascular, respiratory, and neurological exam are negative. Patient given new beta blocker for hypertension and hypertension-associated headaches.
Location: _____
New/estab: _____
Range of codes: _____
Grid selected: _____
Level of service: _____

6. 56-year-old patient with ear pain for the past 2 days following swimming over the weekend. Ear pain

accompanied by fever, up to 102. No respiratory symptoms; however, patient has past history of extensive otitis media. Exams of ears, nose, and throat as well as chest are performed with a diagnosis of otitis media.
Location: _____
New/estab: _____
Range of codes: _____
Grid selected: _____
Level of service: _____

7. 3-year-old patient with complaints of stomachache following dinner at home. Patient had spaghetti approximately 3-4 hours ago and began experiencing nausea and vomiting. No respiratory symptoms. No past history of abdominal problems; however, patient has bilateral ear tube placement. Exams of ENT, abdomen, and chest are performed. Abdomen series negative, labs negative. Patient prescribed Compazine for N/V, with diagnosis of food poisoning.
Location: _____
New/estab: _____
Range of codes: _____
Grid selected: _____
Level of service: _____

8. 21-year-old patient seen in follow-up for otitis media following 10 days of antibiotic treatment. No complaints. ENT are clear. Resolved otitis media.
Location: _____
New/estab: _____
Range of codes: _____
Grid selected: _____
Level of service: _____

9. Office visit for a known asthmatic for regular follow-up. No complaints other than shortness of breath with exercise, resolving with nebulizer treatment ×2. No fatigue, chest pain. Exam includes respiratory, cardiovascular, ENT. Asthma controlled.
Location: _____
New/estab: _____
Range of codes: _____
Grid selected: _____
Level of service: _____

10. 43-year-old patient with complaints of rash appeared approximately 2-3 days ago following trip to the country with her children. No other problems such as fatigue, joint pain. Exam reveals diffuse rash over the legs, arms, and back. Assessment: Rash of unknown etiology.
Location: _____
New/estab: _____
Range of codes: _____
Grid selected: _____
Level of service: _____

REVIEW OF THE E & M CODING PROCESS

Briefly review the steps used in selecting correct codes from the E & M section:

Step 1

Identify History, Physical Examination, and Medical Decision Making Components, and Explain Modifying Circumstances
Highlight or mark these components within the documentation and plot them on the E & M coding grid.

Step 2

Determine Location of Service
Determine the location where service was performed and mark this on the E & M coding grid.

Step 3

Determine Patient Status (New/Established)
If it is not stated, the coder assumes the patient is established. Select the correct coding grid for determining level of service, which is based on location and patient status.

Step 4

Determine the Correct Level of Service
According to the components plotted on the E & M grid, determine the correct level of service.

Step 5

Determine Whether Modifying Factors Are Key Elements
Determine whether history, physical examination, and medical decision making components are the determining factors or whether modifying circumstances control the level of service.

If the five basic steps for coding E & M services are followed, regardless of the complexity of the services performed, E & M service coding is as simple as diagnostic coding. The idea is to keep basic guidelines in mind no matter how complicated the documentation or procedures appear to be. Using the step-by-step accumulation of only the needed components makes even the most complex and detailed case a simple one.

COMMON PROBLEMS IN ASSIGNING E & M CODES

In the event the student finds that he or she consistently assigns a level of service that is too high or too low, some suggestions may help.

Code too **HIGH:** After coding the service, attempt to code to the next lower level and see if the criteria there more accurately reflect the case.

Code too **LOW:** After coding the service, attempt to code to the next higher level. If the criteria for the higher level more accurately reflect the case presented, code higher. If the criteria do not reflect a higher level, the student can feel comfortable that the level selected is the most appropriate.

OTHER COMMON E & M CODING ERRORS

Examination criteria are NOT the same as a review of systems. Make sure to choose as physical examination criteria those elements for which the physician actually performed an examination. Elements reviewed verbally or covered in a questionnaire format with the patient (typically before the examination) are a review of symptom components.

- Remember, new visits require three of three key elements for criteria to be met. Established visits require two of three key elements. Visits not specified as new are assumed to be established visits.
- Remember not to use chart notes indicating "probable," "possible," or other notations that are not definitive diagnoses.
- Only documented material may be used in the consideration of key factors.
- Codes involving time elements must be documented as to the specific amount of time and the nature of the counseling or coordination of care.

CHAPTER IN REVIEW

CERTIFICATION REVIEW

- New patients are those who have not visited the physician or physician group or specialty within the last 3 years. This includes all services provided to the patient regardless of location of service.
- "On call" or "covering physicians" assign E & M levels in the same manner as the physicians for whom they cover.
- Guidelines for each location of service and for levels of service are defined by the number of documented components required in the physician documentation.
- The HISTORY component comprises history of present illness; chief complaint; review of systems; and past medical, social, and family history.
- The EXAMINATION component comprises body areas and organ systems as follows:
  Body areas: Head, neck, chest, abdomen, genitalia, back, each extremity
  Organ systems: Eyes; ENT/mouth; cardiovascular, respiratory, gastrointestinal, genitourinary, musculoskeletal, neurological, psychiatric, and hematological/lymphatic/immunological systems; skin
- The component MEDICAL DECISION MAKING includes three elements, two of which must be met: diagnosis/management options, amount/complexity of data, risk of morbidity/mortality.
- Time is a factor in the determination of E & M levels of service ONLY when more than 50% of time is spent in counseling and coordination of care.
- Types of E & M services include the following:
  Outpatient/office visits
  Hospital observation services
  Hospital inpatient services
  Consultations (inpatient/outpatient/confirmatory)
  Emergency department services
  Critical care services
  Neonatal intensive care services
  Nursing facility services
  Domiciliary, rest home, custodial services
  Home services
  Prolonged services
  Physician standby services
  Case management services
  Care plan oversight services
  Preventive medicine services
  Counseling/risk factor intervention
  Newborn care services
  Special evaluation and management services
- Basic steps for E & M coding are the following:

Identify history, physical examination, and medical decision making components
Determine location of service
Determine patient status
Determine level of service
Determine whether modifying factors (such as time or modifier codes needed) are key elements

STUDENT STUDY GUIDE

- Study Chapter 10.
- Review the Learning Objectives for Chapter 10.
- Complete the Stop and Practice exercises, which include Workbook exercises 1 through 20 on procedure coding.
- Review the Certification Review for Chapter 10.
- Complete the Chapter Review exercise to reinforce concepts learned in the chapter. Try the Practical Application exercises to apply all the concepts to actual medical documentation.

CHAPTER REVIEW EXERCISE

For each of the following services, determine the location of service, determine new and established patient, and list the range of codes that would be used for coding these services.

Range of codes:

1. Initial nursing home visit
   Location: _nursing home_
   New/established: _established_
   Range of codes: _99304 - 99306_
2. Visit to the outpatient clinic
   Location: _Outpatient clinic_
   New/established: _established_
   Range of codes: _99211 - 99215_
3. Hospital consultation
   Location: _Hospital_
   New/established: _established_
   Range of codes: _99251 - 99255_
4. Patient requested consult
   Location: _Office/outpatient_
   New/established: _established_
   Range of codes: _99211 - 99215_
5. Emergency department visit
   Location: _Emergency Dept._
   New/established: _new_
   Range of codes: _99281 - 99285_

In each of the following, assign the same information and the appropriate E & M code.

6. Office visit, established patient
   Problem-focused history
   Problem-focused examination
   Straightforward MDM

Location: _____office_____
New/established: _____established_____
Range of codes: _____99211 - 99215_____
Code selected: _____99212_____

7. Emergency department visit
   Detailed history
   Expanded problem-focused examination
   Moderate medical decision making
   Location: _____Emergency Dept_____
   New/established: _____new_____
   Range of codes: _____99281 - 99285_____
   Code selected: _____99283_____

8. Outpatient consultation, established patient
   Comprehensive history
   Comprehensive examination
   Moderate medical decision making
   Location: _____
   New/established: _____
   Range of codes: _____
   Code selected: _____

9. Hospital admit
   Comprehensive history
   Comprehensive examination
   High medical decision making

Location: _____
New/established: _____
Range of codes: _____
Code selected: _____

10. Hospital observation care
    Comprehensive history
    Detailed examination
    Moderate medical decision making
    Location: _____
    New/established: _____
    Range of codes: _____
    Code selected: _____

PRACTICAL APPLICATION

Review the following medical records and determine the appropriate type, location, and level of service, finally assigning the appropriate E & M code(s). After making the determination of the type/location of service, select the appropriate E & M grid to capture the history, examination, and medical decision making components to determine the level of service.

1.

EMERGENCY ROOM RECORD

Name:		Age:	ER physician:
		DOB:	06/16/XXXX

Allergies/type of reaction:	Usual medications/dosages:

Triage/presenting complaint:	The patient is a 56-year-old female with a rather complex medical history including anemia, thrombocytopenia, recurrent fevers, and a chronic cough that has been bothering her for about the past 2 months. Tonight, the patient presents because the cough has worsened, and constantly bothers her. Felt that it is a little more productive. Sputum is sometimes gray, but saw no blood streaks or frank hemoptysis. Denies pleuritic chest pain, shortness of breath or other
Initial assessment:	respiratory symptoms. Has felt weaker and generalized malaise, but has not noticed any chills. Denies decreased appetite or weight loss recently. She has been unable to sleep due to the increased cough and states that she is extremely tired. Also states has been diagnosed with a recent history of microhematuria. Today noticed urine was blood tinged when she urinated. No difficulty starting urine flow, no dysuria, no frequency, no flank pain or fever. Stated she does bruise easily, particularly since she has been on Deltasone for the past 2 years.

Time	T	P	R	BP	Other:					
Medication orders:										

Lab work:	

X-Ray:	

Physician's report:

Pleasant, in no acute distress. Full oriented and cooperative. Blood pressure is slightly elevated with 170/85. Saturations at 92 to 94% in room air. Slight tachycardic and her temperature was around 100.
Head: NO pallor, no jaundice, hydration well-maintained, no facial asymmetries, PERRLA, EOMI
Neck: Supple without lymphadenopathies
Chest: Lungs, good equal air entry bilaterally with some scattered expiratory rhonchi. These changed with cough. No decreased breath sounds. No fixed crackles. No wheezes or rales.
Heart: Regular, rate and rhythm. Heart sounds somewhat distant. No murmurs, no gallops, slightly tachycardic with a few premature beats.
Abdomen: Obese, but otherwise benign. Lower extremities, no pedal edema
Skin: No suspicious lesions
Neurologic: Nonfocal, has a severely deformed right foot and walks with a limp, which is not new.
Urinalysis showed a 3+ bilirubin, 3+ protein, nitrite positive, leukocyte esterase was negative. 3+ hemoglobin, 30-40 RBCs and 3-5 WBCs.
IMPRESSION:
1. Upper Respiratory Infection possibly bronchitis per clinical history.
2. Microhematuria of unclear etiology
UTI vs cystitis
3. Complex past medical history

Diagnosis:	Physician sign/date
Patient was given Rocephin 1 gram IM in the ER and will start a Z-pack tomorrow morning for her upper respiratory infection. Robitussin AC recommended for night time, 2 t qhs. With regards to urine, will await culture results.	*Robert Rai MD*

Discharge	Transfer	Admit	Good	Satisfactory	Other:

GODFREY REGIONAL HOSPITAL
123 Main Street • Aldon, FL 77714 • (407) 555-1234

Location: _____

New/estab: _____

Range of codes: _____

Grid selected: _____

Level of service: _____

2.

HISTORY AND PHYSICAL EXAMINATION

Patient name:
Date of admission: 10/10/XXXX
Admitting physician:

Patrick Chung, MD

CHIEF COMPLAINT:
Pain, left knee

HISTORY:
Patient is a 23-year-old male with a large osteochrondritic defect of the weight bearing portion of the medial femoral condyle of the left knee. He underwent an arthroscopic evaluation of the knee, which revealed an osteochrondritic defect consisting of a non-attached pure cartilaginous fragment of the medial femoral condyle which was removed. Decision was made to hold off any future surgical procedures, however, the patient presented in the Emergency Room in extreme pain, unable to walk. He is being seen to evaluate further intervention for his osteochrondritic defect at this time.

Past medical history:

ALLERGIES: None
MEDICATION: None
PAST SURGICAL HISTORY: Left knee arthroscopy as mentioned above

Family and social history

Nonsmoker and nondrinker

Review of systems:

Physical exam

HEENT:	Atraumatic, normocephalic
LUNGS:	Clear
HEART:	Regular rate and rhythm
ABDOMEN:	Soft nontender
LEFT KNEE:	2+ effusion with full range of motion, however, painful when put through range of motion and gait unsteady when full weight bearing.

Laboratory/radiology:

X-ray:

X-rays of the knee show a large osteochrondritic defect of the lateral aspect of the medial femoral condyle. Discussed the possibility of an osteochondral allograft procedure.

Assessment:

Plan:

The patient wishes to proceed with the surgery so we will plan for tomorrow.
He understands that he may also have an element of chronic pain, stiffness, numbness and/or weakness which may limit his activities and lifestyle with or without the surgery. He appears to understand and we will proceed with arrangements for surgery tomorrow.

Patrick Chung, MD

GODFREY REGIONAL HOSPITAL
123 Main Street • Aldon, FL 77714 • (407) 555-1234

Location: _____

New/estab: _____

Range of codes: _____

Grid selected: _____

Level of service: _____

3.

PROGRESS NOTE

Date: 05/11/XXXX	Vital signs:	T		R	
Chief complaint:		P		BP	

05/11/XXXX	SUBJECTIVE: This 64-year-old white male presents with severe epigastric cramping for the past 1–2 days. He states he feels as if nothing is moving in his abdomen. The pain started 2 days ago after eating a large dinner of seafood. He has had cramping and severe abdominal discomfort which has been unrelenting for the past 24–48 hours. Has had 1 episode of emesis but has not had any fever and does not feel nauseated at the present time. He states he has been able to pass gas.
	Physical examination:
	OBJECTIVE: Temperature 97, Pulse 70, Respirations 16, BP 182/98. Patient unable to lie on the cot, walking back and forth holding his abdomen in distress. Lungs are clear, heart regular, abdomen is minimally distended but soft. More tenderness in the epigastrium than the lower abdomen. Lab shows white count of 4.5, hemoglobin of 12, platelet count 85, sodium 141, BUN 21, creatinine 1.2, glucose 115.
	Assessment:
	IMPRESSION: Abdominal pain unclear etiology Anxiety
	Plan:
	Follow-up in 3–4 days or sooner if worsened symptoms Prescribed Reglan 10 mg *Patk Adam MD*
	Patient name: DOB: MR/Chart #:

GODFREY REGIONAL OUTPATIENT CLINIC
3122 Shannon Avenue • Aldon, FL 77712 • (407) 555-7654

Location: _____ Grid selected: _____
New/estab: _____ Level of service: _____
Range of codes: _____

4.

PROGRESS NOTE

Chief complaint: Left Hip Pain, radiating to left lower abdomen

Date: 01/XX/XXXX

Vital signs: BP_____ P_____ R_____

History:

HISTORY OF PRESENT ILLNESS:
This 29-year-old female presents for the first time with complaints of left hip pain, which has lasted for approximately 2 weeks, Starting yesterday, the pain seems to radiate down her lower abdomen along the left side. Reports the last time she experienced such pain, she was diagnosed to have a kidney infection. She denies any fever, urinary frequency, or dysuria. Her left hip hurts more with coughing and taking deep breaths.
MEDICAL HISTORY: Unremarkable
CURRENT MEDICATIONS: None
ALLERGIES: None
SOCIAL: She is sexually active, and has 2 children
FAMILY: Positive for diabetes
REVIEW OF SYSTEMS: Has regular periods, but is on Depo-Provera, every 3 months

Exam:

PHYSICAL EXAMINATION:
Vital signs: Temperature 98.5, Pulse 88, Respiratory Rate 15, BP 127/82
She rates pain 6 on a scale of 1–20
Head: Atraumatic
Neck: Supple
Eyes: No pallor
HEENT: Unremarkable
Chest: Clear to auscultation
Cardio: Normal
Abdomen: Mild tenderness, left lower abdomen, no rebound, guarding, tender along her left flank.
Extrem: Unremarkable
Skin: Free of rash

Labs/X-Ray: UA shows 2+ hemoglobin but normal RBC counts. White cells normal. 1+bacteria. Pregnancy test is negative.

Diagnosis/assessment:

IMPRESSION:
Microscopic hematuria and possibly hemoglobinuria with left flank pain

PLAN:
Will order KUB and be scheduled for an IVP. If develops fever or chills needs to seek evaluation and treatment.

Patient name: _____
Date of service: _____

GODFREY MEDICAL ASSOCIATES
1532 Third Avenue, Suite 120 • Aldon, FL 77713 • (407) 555-4000

Location: _____   Grid selected: _____
New/estab: _____   Level of service: _____
Range of codes: _____

5.

PROGRESS NOTE

Date: 08/17/XXXX	Vital signs:	T	R
Chief complaint:		P	BP

This patient returns with complaints of fatigue, nausea and concern for Hepatitis C infection. His girlfriend has tested positive, and he is concerned that his recent tiredness and fatigue plus nausea may be related to infection himself. He has never been tested for Hepatitis C.
PAST MEDICAL HISTORY: Sleep apnea, diabetes, hypertension, atrial fibrillation
CURRENT MEDICATIONS: Zestril and Trazodone. Does not take any meds for diabetes
SOCIAL HISTORY: Not married, smokes 2 packs per day. Currently not employed. Quit drinking several years ago but does drink once in a while
FAMILY HISTORY: Noncontributory

Examination:

Vital Signs: Temperature 98.3, pulse 75, respirations 24, BP 136/99
He smells of heavy smoke
Head: Atraumatic, unshaved, poor hygiene
Neck: Supple
Eyes: No pallor
HEENT: Unremarkable
Chest: Clear to auscultation, no rhonchi, wheezing
C/V: Normal heart sounds, no murmurs, pulses regular
Abdomen: Soft, nontender. No hepatosplenomegaly, no masses palpable. Bowel sounds active.
Extremities: Unremarkable, free of ankle edema
Skin: No skin rash
CNS: Alert, oriented with normal speech, normal gait. No focal neurological deficits and appears alert and oriented
Labs/X-Ray: CBC shows white count of 9.3, hemoglobin is 18.8 with hematocrit 54.6. CMP is normal, except for random glucose of 211, consistent with his diabetes.

Impression:

Fatigue likely due to chronic polycythemia in a patient with smoking and sleep apnea

Plan:

Advised on smoking cessation, take his medications, including diabetes medication regularly. Will check for Hepatitis C since he has been exposed via his girlfriend. However, there is no liver inflammation at this point.

Patrick Adam MD

	Patient name:
	DOB:
	MR/Chart #:

GODFREY REGIONAL OUTPATIENT CLINIC
3122 Shannon Avenue • Aldon, FL 77712 • (407) 555-7654

Location: _____
New/estab: _____
Range of codes: _____

Grid selected: _____
Level of service: _____

11

ANESTHESIA SERVICES

LEARNING OBJECTIVES

Following the completion of this chapter, the student will be able to:

- Comprehend the documentation used for anesthesia coding.
- Understand the types of anesthesia providers.
- Know the types of care provided by anesthesia providers.
- Understand and apply the principal elements of anesthesia coding.
- Comprehend the proper use of modifier codes for anesthesia services.
- Know the basic differences that make anesthesia coding unique.

CODING REFERENCE TOOLS

Tool 45
Anesthesia Coding Elements

KEY TERMS

Anesthesia Assistant (AA), 253
Anesthesia Time Units, 256
Anesthesiologist, 253
ASA (American Society of Anesthesiologists), 249
Base Units, 256
Certified Registered Nurse Anesthetist (CRNA), 253
General Anesthesia, 254
Monitored Anesthesia Care (MAC), 253
Moribund, 255
Physical Status Modifier, 255
Qualifying Circumstance, 255
Regional Anesthesia, 254
Systemic Disease, 255

ANESTHESIA DOCUMENTATION AND CODING GUIDELINES

The anesthesia record serves as the main document for information pertaining to services performed before, during, and after the administration of anesthesia. The procedure and documentation are usually provided by the health care professional and consist of the following information:

- Preanesthesia Evaluation

  A patient interview that includes medical, anesthesia, and medication history, and an appropriate physical examination, is usually performed before the administration of anesthesia. In addition, the provider will typically review any diagnostic data, such as x-rays, laboratory test results, and ECGs. The plan for anesthesia care will be formulated and discussed with the patient or responsible party. At the conclusion of the evaluation, the provider will also assign a code to the physical status of the patient based on the information gathered and pursuant to **ASA (American Society of Anesthesiologists).**

- Perianesthesia Record

  A record will be kept during the actual anesthesia administration and patient monitoring throughout the surgical procedure. The review immediately before anesthetic administration, patient monitoring by qualified anesthesia personnel, the patient's vital signs, amount of drugs and agents used, times given, technique, and patient status at the conclusion of the anesthetic event are all documented on the Anesthesia Record. Although anesthesia billing is usually by means of a billing card, codes that are assigned and billed must be substantiated by the anesthesia provider's documentation before, during, and after surgery.

- Postanesthesia Record

  After the completion of the surgical procedure, the anesthesia provider will continue to monitor the patient for vital signs, level of consciousness, additional drugs administered, all postanesthesia visits, and any prescribed follow-up.

All of the aforementioned services are included in the code(s) assigned for anesthesia care.

Figure 11-1 represents an example of a Preanesthesia Evaluation record. Note that the anesthesia provider also obtains information such as review of systems and medical history (discussed in Chapter 10, Evaluation and Management). Figure 11-2 represents an example of an Anesthesia Record, wherein the provider documents the monitors, equipment, technique for anesthesia administration, start/stop time, vital signs, and other output measurements. Take a look at the portion of the table that was reviewed in Chapter 9 of the steps or components needed for CPT-4 coding, especially the anesthesia portion of that table.

CPT-4 Coding Steps

	Anesthesia
Step 1	
Identify	General
	Regional
	Spinal
Range of Codes	00100-01999
	99100-99140
Step 2	
Determine Type/Location	Anatomical
	Location
	Head
	Upper Extrem
Step 3	
Specific Type	Body Area
	Eye
	Thyroid
Step 4	
Specific Procedure Information	Procedure
	Open
	Closed
Step 5	
Extent/Specifics	Specifics

Using a sample anesthesia record such as that on page 252, in the Chapter Review exercise, or in the workbook, evaluate it for documentation necessary to assign the correct anesthesia code(s) for the service(s) provided. In addition to capturing the actual procedure performed, capture the patient's medical status and any extenuating circumstances during this review.

| History from: ☐ Patient ☐ Chart
☐ Parent/guardian ☐ Poor historian
☐ Significant other ☐ Language barrier | PRE-ANESTHESIA EVALUATION | ☐ | See previous anesthesia record dated
_____ for information |

Proposed procedure	Age	Sex	Height	Weight
P/E Tubes	5	☐ M ☒ F	in/cm	42 lb lb/kg

Pre-procedure vital signs
B/P: 120/80   P: 80   R: 18   T: 98^8 O_2 SAT %: 98

Current medications	☐ None

Previous anesthesia/operations ☐ None

n/a

None

Airway	☐ MP1 ☐ Unrestricted neck ROM	☐ ↓ mouth opening/TMJ	☐ Edentulous
	☐ MP2 ☐ T-M distance = _____	☐ Hx difficult airway	☐ Facial hair
	☐ MP3 ☐ Obesity	☐ Teeth poor repair	☐ Short muscular neck
	☐ MP4 ☐ ↓ neck ROM:	☐ Teeth chipped/loose:	

Family HX anes. problems

Allergies ☐ None

System	Comments	Diagnostic studies

☒ WNL   **Respiratory**
Asthma/RAD   Chronic tonsillitis
Bronchiolitis   Chronic OM
COPD   Recent URI
  Emphysema   TB/+PPD
  Bronchitis   Pneumonia
Respiratory failure Productive cough
Pleural effusion   SOB/dyspnea
Pulmonary embolism OSA
Sinusitis/rhinitis   Orthopnea
Environ. allergies   Wheezing
	Tobacco use: ☐ Yes ☐ No ☐ Quit _____ Packs/Day for_____Years
	
	Pre-procedure pulmonary assessment:
		ECG
		
		Chest X-ray

☒ WNL   **Cardiovascular**
Hypertension   Abnormal ECG
Hyperlipoproteinemia Dysrhythmia
CAD/cardiomyopathy Hypovolemia
Angina   Chronic fatigue
  Stable/unstable   Pacemaker/AICD
Myocardial infarction Murmur
CHF DOE PND   Valvular Dz/MVP
Peripheral vascular Dz Rheumatic fever
Exercise tolerance   Endocarditis
  Excellent/fair/poor Aneurysm
	
	Pulmonary studies
	
	Pre-procedure cardiac assessment:
		Pulmonary studies

☒ WNL **Hepato/gastrointestinal** Obesity N & V Cirrhosis Diarrhea Hepatitis/jaundice IBS Bowel obstruction Pancreatitis Ulcers Gallbladder Dz Hiatal hernia Diverticulum GERD Colon polyps	Ethanol use: ☐ Yes ☐ No ☐ Quit Frequency_____ ☐ Hx ETOH abuse	**Laboratory studies**
☒ WNL **Neuro/musculoskeletal** Arthritis/DJD Muscle weakness Back problems (LBP) Neuromuscular Dz CVA/TIA Paralysis Psychiatric disorder Paresthesia(s) Headaches Syncope ↑ ICP/head injury Seizures Loss of consciousness Epilepsy		PT/PTT/INR: T&S/T&C: HCG: U/A: LMP:
☒ WNL **Renal/endocrine** Thyroid disease Prostate Cushing's syndrome BPH/CA Renal failure/dialysis Diabetes mellitus Renal insufficiency Type I/II/Gest. Renal stones UTI Adrenocortical insuff. Pituitary disorder		**Other diagnostic tests**
☒ WNL **Other** Anemia Immunosuppressed Bleeding disorder Sickle cell Dz/trait Cancer Recent steroids Chemotherapy Transfusion Hx Radiation Tx Weight loss/gain Dehydration Herbal/OTC drug use HIV/AIDS Illicit drug use		
☒ WNL **Pregnancy** TIUP SGA Multiple gestation Pre-eclampsia LGA VBAC HELLP PROM IUGR	☐ AROM ☐ Mg drip ☐ SROM _____gm/hr Weeks gest: ☐ Pitocin drip ☐ Induction G: P: EDC:	

Surgical diagnosis/problem list		Post-anesthesia care notes				
SOM		Location	Time	**Controlled medications**		
				Medication	Used	Destroyed	Returned
		B/P	O_2 Sat %				

Planned anesthesia/special monitors		Physical status 1 2 3 4 5 E	Pulse	Resp	Temp	Provider Witness

☐ Awake ☐ Stable ☐ Mask O_2
☐ Somnolent ☐ Unstable ☐ NC O_2
☐ Unarousable ☐ Oral/nasal airway
Intubated - ☐ T-piece ☐ Ventilator
Regional - dermatome level:
☐ Continuous epidural analgesia
☐ Direct admit to hospital ward
  (PACU recovery not required)
☐ Recovery recorded on anes. form

☐ No anesthesia related complications noted
☐ Satisfactory post anesthesia/analgesia recovery
☐ See progress notes for anesthesia related concerns

Pre-anesthesia medications ordered
Fenatol

Evaluator signature   Date

Provider   Date
            Time

GODFREY REGIONAL HOSPITAL
123 Main Street • Aldon, FL 77714 • (407) 555-1234

FIGURE 11-1. Preanesthesia Evaluation Form.

Authorized for local reproduction

MEDICAL RECORD–ANESTHESIA				Procedure P/E Tubes			Item	Start	Stop
							Anesthesia	0700	0730
Date	OR no.	Page of	Surgeon(s)				Procedure	0710	0725

Pre-procedure	Monitors and equipment	Anesthetic techniques	Airway management	Recovery room
☒ Identified ☐ ID band ☐ Questioned	☒ Steth ☐ Esoph ☐ Precord ☐ Other	Method: ☒ General ☐ Spinal	☐ Intubation ☐ Oral ☐ Nasal	Time 755 ᴮ/ᴾ 120/80 O₂ Sat. 97
☒ Chart review ☐ Permit signed	☐ Non-invasive B/P ☐ Nerve stimulator	☐ Epidural ☐ Caudal ☐ Brachial	☐ Direct vision ☐ Magill's ☐ Blind	☒ PACU ᴾ 80 ᴿ 18 ᵀ 98.8
☒ NPO since ___PM___	☐ Continuous EKG ☒ V lead EKG	☐ Bier block ☐ Ankle blk ☐ M.A.C.	☐ Diff. see rmks ☐ Fiber op ☐ Stylet	☐ ICU ☐ L&D
Pre-anesthetic state: ☐ Calm	☐ Pulse oximeter ☐ Oxygen analyzer	General: ☐ Pre-O₂ ☐ L.T.A.	☐ Attemps x ___ ☐ Blade ___	☐ Awake ☐ Spont resp ☐ Oral airway
☐ Awake ☐ Asleep	☐ End tidal CO₂ ☐ Resp gas anlyzr	☐ Rapid sequence ☐ Cricoid pressure	☐ Tube size___ ☐ Endobronchial	☒ Asleep ☐ Ventilator ☐ Nasal airway
☒ Apprehensive ☐ Confused	☐ Temp ___ ☐ EEG	☐ Intravenous ☐ Inhalation	☐ Regular☐ RAE ☐ Armored ☐ Laser	☐ Stable ☐ Extubated ☐ Face shield O₂
☐ Uncooperative ☐ Unresponsive	☐ Warming blanket ☐ Fluid warmer	☐ Intramuscular ☐ Rectal	☐ Cuffed ☐ Min. occ. pres. ☐ Air ☐NS	☐ Unstable☐ Intubated ☐ T-piece O₂
Patient safety	☐ Airway humidifier ☐ ___	Regional: ☐ Position ___	☐ Uncuffed, leaks at ___ cm H₂O	**Controlled drugs**
☐ Anes. machine #___ checked	☐ NG/OG tube ☐ Foley catheter	☐ Prep ___ ☐ Local ___	☐ Secured at___ ☐ ET CO₂ present	Drug / Used / Destroyed / Returned
☒ Safety belt on ☐ Axillary roll	☐ Art line ___	☐ Needle ___	☐ Breath sounds ___	
☒ Arm restraints ☐ Arms tucked	☐ CVP ___	☐ Drug(s) ___	☐ Circuit: ☐ Circle ☐ Non-rebreathing	
☐ Pressure points checked and padded	☐ PA line ___	☐ Dose ___ ☐ Attempts x ___	☐ Airway:☐ Oral ☐ Nasal ☐ Natural	
☐ Eye care: ☐ Ointment ☐ Saline	☐ IV(s) ___	☐ Site ___ ☐ Level ___	☐ Mask case ☐ Via tracheostomy	Provider / Witness
☐ Taped ☐ Pads ☐ Goggles	☐ ___	☐ Catheter ___ ☐ See remarks	☐ Nasal cannula ☐ Simple O₂ mask	

Time:

Agents														Totals
☐ Hal ☐ Enf☐ Iso (%)														
☐ N₂O ☐ Air (L/min)														
Oxygen (L/min)														
( )														
( )														
( )														
( )														

Fluids														

Monitors												
Urine (ml)												
EBL (ml)												
EKG												
% O₂ inspired (FIO₂)												
O₂ saturation (SaO₂)												
End Tidal CO₂												
Temp: ☐ C ☐ F												

Vital signs

	Baseline values	200															Symbols
		180															x Anesthesia
		160															⊙ Operation
		140															v ∧ B/P cuff pressure
	B/P	120															⊥ ⊤ Arterial line pressure
		100															Δ Mean arterial pressure
	P	80															● Pulse
		60															○ Spontaneous resp
		40															Ø Assisted resp
	R	20															⊗ Controlled resp
																	τ Tourniquet

Vent

Tidal vol. (ml)												
Resp. rate												
Peak pres. (cm H₂O)												
PEEP (cm H₂O)												

Symbols for remarks

Position

Anesthesia provider(s) | **Remarks:**

Patient's identification (For typed or written entries give: Name–last, first, middle; ID no. (SSN or other); hospital or medical facility.)

Helen Smith

Anesthesia
Medical record
Optional form 517 (7–95)
Prescribed by GSA/ICMR,
FPMR (41 CFR) 101–11.203(b)(10)

GODFREY REGIONAL HOSPITAL
123 Main Street • Aldon, FL 77714 • (407) 555-1234

FIGURE 11-2. Anesthesia Record.

Authorized for local reproduction

MEDICAL RECORD–ANESTHESIA	Procedure	Item	Start	Stop
	P/E Tubes	Anesthesia	0700	0730

Date	OR no.	Page	of	Surgeon(s)		Procedure	0710	0725

Pre-procedure
- ☒ Identified ☐ ID band ☐ Questioned
- ☒ Chart review ☐ Permit signed
- ☒ NPO since _____ PM
- Pre-anesthetic state: ☐ Calm
- ☐ Awake ☐ Asleep
- ☒ Apprehensive ☐ Confused
- ☐ Uncooperative ☐ Unresponsive

Patient safety
- ☐ Anes. machine # _____ checked
- ☒ Safety belt on ☐ Axillary roll
- ☒ Arm restraints ☐ Arms tucked
- ☐ Pressure points checked and padded
- ☐ Eye care: ☐ Ointment ☐ Saline
- ☐ Taped ☐ Pads ☐ Goggles

Time:

Monitors and equipment
- ☒ Steth ☐ Esoph ☐ Precord ☐ Other
- ☐ Non-invasive B/P ☐ Nerve stimulator
- ☐ Continuous EKG ☒ V lead EKG
- ☐ Pulse oximeter ☐ Oxygen analyzer
- ☐ End tidal CO$_2$ ☐ Resp gas anlyzr
- ☐ Temp _____ ☐ EEG
- ☐ Warming blanket ☐ Fluid warmer
- ☐ Airway humidifier ☐ _____
- ☐ NG/OG tube ☐ Foley catheter
- ☐ Art line _____
- ☐ CVP _____
- ☐ PA line _____
- ☐ IV(s) _____
- ☐ _____

Anesthetic techniques
- Method: ☒ General ☐ Spinal
- ☐ Epidural ☐ Caudal ☐ Brachial
- ☐ Bier block ☐ Ankle blk ☐ M.A.C.
- General: ☐ Pre-O$_2$ ☐ L.T.A.
- ☐ Rapid sequence ☐ Cricoid pressure
- ☐ Intravenous ☐ Inhalation
- ☐ Intramuscular ☐ Rectal
- Regional: ☐ Position _____
- ☐ Prep _____ ☐ Local _____
- ☐ Needle _____
- ☐ Drug(s) _____
- ☐ Dose _____ ☐ Attempts x _____
- ☐ Site _____ ☐ Level _____
- ☐ Catheter _____ ☐ See remarks

Airway management
- ☐ Intubation ☐ Oral ☐ Nasal
- ☐ Direct vision ☐ Magill's ☐ Blind
- ☐ Diff. see rmks ☐ Fiber op ☐ Stylet
- ☐ Attemps x _____ ☐ Blade _____
- ☐ Tube size ___ ☐ Endobronchial
- ☐ Regular☐ RAE ☐ Armored ☐ Laser
- ☐ Cuffed ☐ Min. occ. pres. ☐ Air☐NS
- ☐ Uncuffed, leaks at _____ cm H$_2$O
- ☐ Secured at _____ ☐ ET CO$_2$ present
- ☐ Breath sounds _____
- ☐ Circuit: ☐ Circle ☐ Non-rebreathing
- ☐ Airway: ☐ Oral ☐ Nasal ☐ Natural
- ☐ Mask case ☐ Via tracheostomy
- ☐ Nasal cannula ☐ Simple O$_2$ mask

Recovery room
Time 755	B/P 120/80	O$_2$ Sat. 97
☒ PACU	P 80 R 18	T 98.8
☐ ICU ☐ L&D		

- ☐ Awake ☐ Spont resp ☐ Oral airway
- ☒ Asleep ☐ Ventilator ☐ Nasal airway
- ☐ Stable ☐ Extubated ☐ Face shield O$_2$
- ☐ Unstable ☐ Intubated ☐ T-piece O$_2$

Controlled drugs
Drug	Used	Destroyed	Returned
Provider		Witness	

Agents
- ☐ Hal ☐ Enf☐ Iso (%)
- ☐ N$_2$O ☐ Air (L/min)
- Oxygen (L/min)

Totals

Fluids

- Urine (ml)
- EBL (ml)

Monitors
- EKG
- % O$_2$ inspired (FIO$_2$)
- O$_2$ saturation (SaO$_2$)
- End Tidal CO$_2$
- Temp: ☐ °C ☐ °F

Vital signs

Baseline values	200
	180
	160
	140
B/P	120
	100
P	80
	60
	40
R	20

Symbols
- **x** Anesthesia
- **⊙** Operation
- **∨ ∧** B/P cuff pressure
- **⊥ T** Arterial line pressure
- **Δ** Mean arterial pressure
- **●** Pulse
- **○** Spontaneous resp
- **Ø** Assisted resp
- **⊗** Controlled resp
- **T** Tourniquet

Vent
- Tidal vol. (ml)
- Resp. rate
- Peak pres. (cm H$_2$O)
- PEEP (cm H$_2$O)
- Symbols for remarks
- Position

Anesthesia provider(s)

Remarks:

Patient's identification *(For typed or written entries give: Name–last, first, middle: ID no. (SSN or other); hospital or medical facility.)*

Helen Smith

Anesthesia
Medical record
Optional form 517 (7–95)
Prescribed by GSA/ICMR,
FPMR (41 CFR) 101–11.203(b)(10)

GODFREY REGIONAL HOSPITAL
123 Main Street • Aldon, FL 77714 • (407) 555-1234

CPT-4 Coding Steps

Procedure:	Anesthesia Anesthesia	Tympanostomy Chart Information
Step 1 Identify Range of Codes	General/ General 00100-01999 99100-99140	Regional/Spinal 00100-01999
Step 2 Determine Type/ Location	Anatomical Location Head Upper Extrem	Head
Step 3 Specific Type	Body Area Eye Thyroid	Ear
Step 4 Specific Procedure Information	Procedure Open Closed	Tympanostomy
Step 5 Extent/Specifics	Specifics Start Time: 0800 Stop Time: 0900	Age 5, no medical problems

At this point, the anesthesia section of the CPT-4 book would be used to determine the appropriate code assignment of 00120, Procedures on external, middle, or inner ear including biopsy; not otherwise specified. The only other code considerations would be 00124, otoscopy, or 00126, tympanotomy. Neither of these codes properly describes the procedure performed; therefore 00120 would be the only appropriate code for this procedure. Information regarding age, medical status, and time will be needed as the additional steps in anesthesia coding are learned.

PROVIDERS OF ANESTHESIA CARE

The administration and supervision of anesthesia services may be performed by the physician, known as an **anesthesiologist,** or by other qualified providers. The **Certified Registered Nurse Anesthetist (CRNA),** or **Anesthesia Assistant (AA),** may perform or provide anesthesia care under the medical direction of the physician provider as long as the following criteria are met:

- Not more than four anesthesia procedures are performed concurrently.
- The physician is physically present.
- The physician does not perform anesthesia care while supervising the CRNA/AA. (The physician may perform some minimal services such as

addressing an emergency for short duration, providing periodic monitoring of an obstetrics patient, checking on postanesthesia patients, and completing paperwork for discharge.)

Reimbursement may be made for the medical direction of these nonphysician individuals in these circumstances when the following guidelines are documented and performed by the physician:

- Performs the preanesthetic examination and evaluation
- Prescribes the anesthesia plan
- Personally participates in the most demanding portions of the procedure
- Remains present and available for emergencies
- Performs the postanesthesia care

TYPES OF ANESTHESIA CARE

Anesthesia may be performed and coded as follows:

- Inhalation
- Regional (administration of anesthesia to a specific region such as spinal, epidural, nerve block)
- Intravenous
- Rectal
- **Monitored Anesthesia Care (MAC)**
  MAC involves intraoperative monitoring of the patient's vital signs in anticipation of the need for administration of general anesthesia or an anesthetic agent, or the possible development of an adverse reaction during the surgical procedure. For MAC to be considered reimbursable, the provider must perform the services listed previously, including, but not limited to, pre-evaluation and postevaluation, documentation throughout monitoring, and administration of anesthetic agents should it become medically necessary. MAC services must be considered medically necessary as evidenced by documentation of the patient's condition. The medical condition must be significant enough to substantiate the need for monitored anesthesia care (e.g., present medications or patient's symptoms). A stable condition would not warrant the reimbursement of monitored anesthesia care.
  Anesthesia services that include monitored anesthesia care should always be reported with the use of an anesthetic modifier, QS, which is discussed further in this chapter.

In addition to the administration of anesthesia during a surgical procedure, the anesthesia provider may also perform pain management services, either as part of the postoperative course of treatment or for nonsurgical pain control. This therapy is typically provided by one of three methods.

- Patient Controlled Analgesia (PCA)

  PCA allows self-administration of intravenous drugs through an infusion device. When this service is performed as part of postoperative care, the initial set-up time for PCA may be included in the number of anesthesia time units only.

  No additional separate charge or code may be assigned for this service.

- Epidural Analgesia

  This method involves the administration of a narcotic drug through an epidural catheter. Insertion of the catheter is coded by an appropriate code from the Surgery/Nervous section. Daily management of the epidural drug administration is coded from the anesthesia section.

  Epidural injection of a therapeutic agent in the treatment of a nonsurgical condition, usually performed on an outpatient basis, would also be coded and reported from the Surgery/Nervous section. The use of these codes are further considered when the Surgery section of the CPT-4 manual is covered in Chapter 12.

- Nerve Blocks

  Injection of an anesthetic agent into or around a specific nerve is used when it is desirable to limit or alleviate pain of a body segment innervated by that nerve.

  Initial nerve blocks performed postoperatively may only add additional time units (as outlined for the epidural analgesic). Subsequent injections are considered part of the global anesthesia service and not codeable, billable, or reimbursable in most cases.

  Nerve blocks performed nonsurgically are assigned codes from the Surgery/Nervous System section of CPT-4.

GENERAL CODING GUIDELINES

The coding and billing of anesthesia services, unfortunately, does not conform to many of the rules learned thus far for CPT evaluation and management services. If the student approaches coding for anesthesia services in the same manner as E & M coding by following specific guidelines, anesthesia services may be coded with ease.

GLOBAL COMPONENTS

Following are guidelines for anesthesia services. For the purposes of CPT-4 coding, anesthesia services include

- **General anesthesia**
- **Regional anesthesia**
- Supplementation of local anesthesia

- Other services that may be considered appropriate by the anesthesia provider during a procedure

Anesthesia services are considered a global component, with the following services included in the anesthesia charge:

- Preoperative and postoperative services
- Anesthesia administration and care during the surgical procedure
- Administration of medically required fluids and blood
- Monitoring (e.g., ECG, temperature, blood pressure)

These services are considered "bundled" and may not be billed separately.

ANESTHESIA CODING ELEMENTS

Several components are considered in billing for anesthesia services (Tool 45). When gathering key elements for anesthesia coding, consider these components in the same manner that history, physical examination, medical decision making, and modifying circumstances were considered in the Evaluation and Management section of the book.

STEPS TO ANESTHESIA CODING

Below are guidelines for coding anesthesia services.

Step 1

Identify Key Elements That Indicate the Anesthesia Procedure or Service Provided

Identify the procedure(s) performed by the surgeon to locate the appropriate anesthesia CPT-4 code. NEVER use a code from the surgery section for the administration of anesthesia by an anesthesia provider. As mentioned earlier, using guidelines and modifiers that are specific to each section is imperative for correct CPT-4 coding. When anesthesiologists perform surgical services, such

T O O L   45

ANESTHESIA CODING ELEMENTS

1. Anesthesia Code for Specified Procedure

2. Physical Status Modifier

3. Qualifying Circumstances (when applicable)

4. Modifier Codes (when applicable)

5. Time Units/Relative Value Units

as insertion of a Swan-Ganz catheter, they may assign codes from the surgery/medicine section as appropriate. Many medical and surgical services are eligible for additional payment when furnished in conjunction with the anesthesia services or when performed separately. Some examples are the following:

- Swan-Ganz catheter
- Central venous pressure (CVP) line insertion
- Intraarterial lines
- Emergency intubation
- Critical care services
- Transesophageal echocardiogram

When these additional services are performed and codes are assigned, time units are not a consideration because they are not contained in the anesthesia section of CPT-4.

Make certain that coding from the anesthesiologist agrees with that of the surgeon, because the insurance carrier will compare this information. If there are discrepancies between the information reported by the anesthesiologist and surgeon, payment may be denied or delayed for both providers. The anesthesia practice must establish a good working relationship between the anesthesiologist and the surgeon to avoid these problems.

If the student is unsure of the appropriate anatomical section from which the procedure should be coded, the CPT-4 code of the surgeon and the anatomical portion of the surgery section can be checked as a guide.

Step 2

Assign the Appropriate Physical Status Modifier
Identify the proper **physical status modifier** that describes the patient's condition. All anesthesia services should have a physical status modifier. Some insurance carriers may not require the use of the physical status modifier because they already have included this consideration in their basic reimbursement (i.e., Medicare). Services should always be coded according to CPT-4 guidelines, however, UNLESS the carrier specifies in writing that the provider should not use this modifier code.

As with other modifier codes, physical status modifiers provide additional information regarding requests for consideration for possible additional reimbursement based on the patient's condition. There are only six appropriate physical status modifiers:

P1 Normal healthy patient with no risks
P2 Patient with mild **systemic disease**
P3 Patient with severe systemic disease
P4 Patient with severe systemic disease considered to be a constant threat to life
P5 Patient who is **moribund** (dying) and not expected to live without the surgical procedure

P6 Patient who has been declared brain-dead, organ removal for donor purposes

As discussed previously, the coder may code only for documented services and conditions. Remember that the patient with systemic disease may not be billed as such, unless documentation from the treating provider (in this case, the anesthesiologist) supports this condition. Documentation by the surgeon may be used only if it has been reviewed and validated by the anesthesiologist.

Step 3

Assign Qualifying Circumstance Codes (When Applicable)
Identify any **qualifying circumstances** for which these codes may be applicable. Not all anesthesia services have a qualifying circumstance. These are NOT modifier codes. If a qualifying circumstance is applicable, the following CPT-4 codes would be used:

99100 Anesthesia for extreme age, under 1 or over 70 years
99116 Anesthesia complicated by total body hypothermia
99135 Anesthesia complicated by controlled hypotension
99140 Anesthesia complicated by emergency conditions (must specify)

Keep in mind that "emergency" as conceptualized by the layperson does not constitute emergency in medical terms. Make certain that the procedure qualifies as a threat to life or limb when assigned code 99140. Patients scheduled for surgery and admitted on a specified date do not qualify as an emergency. Qualifying circumstances are billed in addition to the primary anesthesia services.

Step 4

Assign Modifier Codes (As Applicable)
There are only six regular modifier codes that are applicable for use with anesthesia services. These are discussed in the following paragraphs.

Modifier 22—Unusual Procedural Services
When services provided extend beyond the usual procedure, and there is no procedure code to describe the service, modifier code 22 may be appended to the procedure code to describe the complete services provided. A report documenting the additional services may be necessary for consideration of reimbursement.

Modifier 23—Unusual Anesthesia
When general anesthesia is used during procedures that typically do not require it, modifier 23 must be added to the procedure code. The procedure may usually be performed with the patient under local anesthesia or, in other circumstances, with no anesthesia.

Modifier 32—Mandated Services

Previously, modifier 32 was described in detail. It is used when services are requested by a third party or a PRO (Peer Review Organization). As with other CPT-4 modifiers, it is applicable to more than one section of CPT-4.

Modifier 51—Multiple Procedures

When multiple procedures are performed during the same anesthesia session, adding to patient risk and anesthesia time, each additional procedure should be listed using this modifier. Of note, this modifier should be listed on all subsequent procedures. The primary and most significant service should be billed, followed by subsequent procedures with the modifier 51 appended.

Reimbursement of subsequent procedures with the use of modifier 51 usually results in reduced reimbursement for these services. Because the preoperative, postoperative, and surgical procedures have been reimbursed already in the primary procedure, the reimbursement for subsequent procedures is reduced proportionately.

In the case of Medicare, reimbursement is based on the anesthesia code with the highest base unit value, and coding should include only the one procedure code with the highest base unit, with the time units combined for all procedures.

Modifier 53—Discontinued Procedure

When the anesthesiologist chooses to terminate the surgical or diagnostic procedure, the procedure code should have modifier 53 added. This modifier is NOT intended for use when the patient electively decides to terminate the procedure, nor is it appropriate for procedures that are terminated before they begin.

Modifier 59—Distinct Procedural Service

When multiple procedures are performed during the same surgical session, but are independent from one another, they should be billed using modifier 59. Modifier 51 usually indicates that multiple procedures are performed through the same approach or at the same anatomical site. The use of modifier 59 defines procedures as independent of one another.

Modifier QS—Monitored Anesthesia Care

As discussed earlier, when monitored anesthesia care is provided rather than the induction of an anesthetic agent, the use of modifier QS should be appended to the service along with any other appropriate modifier code(s). A modifier designating the provider of service should be assigned for anesthesia as follows:

AA   Performed by Anesthesiologist
AD   Medically supervised by Physician > Four Consecutive Cases

QK   Medically supervised by Physician, 2 to 4 Cases
QX   CRNA with Appropriate Physician Medical Direction
QY   Medical Direction of CRNA by Anesthesiologist
QZ   CRNA without Medical Direction by Anesthesiologist

Step 5

Calculate Anesthesia Time Units

Time is always a factor in anesthesia coding. It is imperative that the anesthesia provider always documents time accurately. An anesthesia record provided by the hospital usually allows for the recording of **anesthesia time(s).**

For purposes of coding and billing, *anesthesia time begins when the anesthesiologist or anesthesia provider begins the induction of anesthesia and ends when the provider completes the administration of anesthesia services.* As with all services provided, documentation plays a key role in coding and reimbursement for anesthesia.

Anesthesia time may be calculated in 10-minute or 15-minute increments, depending on the individual carrier. In coding for anesthesia services, one of the pieces of information to be gathered from third-party contracts is proper time increment that individual carriers use. This information may be incorporated in the Third-Party Contract Worksheets, which are discussed later. Time units are calculated as follows:

- Total minutes/10-minute or 15-minute increments (whichever is applicable) = Time Units
- Time units less than 0.5 will be rounded DOWN
- Time units greater than 0.5 or equal to will be rounded UP

In addition to the time units, the **base unit** value of each procedure is also added to the total number of units on the claim form. For instance, the time units for the service may be calculated as four, with an additional two base units assigned for the value of the CPT-4 anesthesia code, for a total of six units reported on the claim form.

Although some of the guidelines for anesthesia services are different from those applied to the rest of CPT-4 procedural coding, all necessary information for payment consideration can be successfully communicated to the insurance carrier.

Take another look at the chart for which a CPT-4 anesthesia code was assigned earlier in the chapter. Capture the additional information needed to finish the code assignment(s) for this chart.

Anesthesia CPT-4 Coding Steps

	Anesthesia	Chart Information
Step 1		
Identify	General/Regional/ Spinal	General
Range of Codes	00100-01999 99100-99140	00100-01999
Step 2		
Determine Type/ Location	Anatomical Location Head Upper Extrem	Head
Step 3		
Specific Type	Body Area Eye Thyroid	Ear
Step 4		
Specific Procedure Information	Procedure Open Closed	Tympanostomy
Step 5		
Extent/Specifics	Specifics Start Time: 0800 Stop Time: 0900	Age 5, no medical problems

It was determined that CPT-4 code 00120 would be the appropriate code assignment for this chart. Additional code assignments must be made for physical status and qualifying circumstances (when applicable), however, and a calculation of time must also be made.

Look back at the information extracted from the chart:

Step 1:   Identify Key Elements
Identify the Anesthesia Procedure or Service Provided
As determined previously, those services would be appropriately assigned code 00120.

Step 2:   Assign the Appropriate Physical Status Modifier
Because no medical conditions were documented, and, it would appear that the patient is a healthy child, a physical status modifier of "P1" would be appropriate. As indicated numerous times, when documentation does not support a higher coding level, the code with the least significance would be assigned.
Physical Status Modifier: P1

Step 3:   Assign Qualifying Circumstance Codes (when applicable)
Because the child is older than 1 and does not have any extenuating circumstances that complicate the procedure, a qualifying circumstance code in this case would not be appropriate.
Qualifying Circumstance: None

Step 4:   Assign Modifier Codes (as applicable)
None are applicable in this case, so no additional modifier codes would be applied.
Modifier Code: None

Step 5:   Calculate Time
Start Time: 0800
Stop Time: 0900
Assume that the time unit being used by the carriers for this example is a 10-minute increment. The units would be calculated by taking the total number of minutes (60) and dividing them by 10. The sample chart has 6 time units.
Time units: 6 units
Base units: Available from RBRVS
For example, use 3 base units
Total units: 9 units

CHAPTER IN REVIEW

CERTIFICATION REVIEW

The elements of anesthesia coding include the following:

- Assignment of CPT-4 codes.
- Assignment of physical status modifiers.
- Assignment of a qualifying circumstance code when appropriate.
- Assignment of modifier codes as applicable.
- Calculation of anesthesia time units.
- Physical status modifiers describe the patient's presenting condition at the time of anesthesia.
- Qualifying circumstance codes indicate additional medical risks of morbidity and mortality, such as age, hypothermia, hypotension, or emergency surgery.

STUDENT STUDY GUIDE

- Study Chapter 11.
- Review the Learning Objectives for Chapter 11.
- Review the Certification Review for Chapter 11.
- Complete the Chapter Review exercise to reinforce concepts learned in the chapter.

CHAPTER REVIEW EXERCISE

Identify the correct anesthesia CPT codes for the following:

	Anesthesia CPT Code
1. Cornea transplant	00144
2. Modified radical mastectomy	00404 pg 37
3. Cesarean section	01961
4. Total hip replacement	01214
5. Femoral artery embolectomy	01274
6. Angioplasty	01921 ?

7. Excision of cyst of humerus   _01758_
8. Knee arthroscopy   _01382_
9. TURP   _00914_
10. Repair of hiatal hernia   _00790_

Assign the correct CPT-4 codes and the other necessary modifiers and time units for the coding and billing of anesthesia.

PRACTICAL APPLICATION

11. An emergency appendectomy was performed on a 45-year-old patient with insulin-dependent diabetes that was not well controlled. The anesthesiologist began administration of general anesthesia at 10:00 AM and completed anesthesia services at 10:45 AM. Identify key elements for procedure performed.
    Anesthesia procedure code: _00810_
    Physical status modifier: _P3_
    Qualifying circumstances code(s):   _99140_
    Anesthesia modifier(s):   _none_
    Calculate time units (10-minute increments):   _5_
    (Base units assigned to the CPT-4 code are usually built into the computerized billing system.)

12. A 25-year-old patient was taken to the operating room for repair of a closed fracture to the radial shaft, which required manipulation by the orthopedic surgeon. Anesthesia administration began at 8:15 AM and was completed at 8:40 AM; surgical time was 25 minutes. Identify key elements for procedure performed.
    Anesthesia procedure code: _01820_
    Physical status modifier: _P1_
    Qualifying circumstances code(s):   _none_
    Anesthesia modifier(s):   _none_
    Calculate time units (10-minute increments):   _3_

13. A 92-year-old female with the diagnosis of small bowel obstruction and severe systemic disease was taken to the operating room for repair and resection. Before completion of the resection, the patient became unstable as a result of her heart disease, and the case had to be terminated prior to completion. The abdomen was closed, and approximately 3 days later, the patient was returned to the OR for completion of the originally planned procedure.
    Original procedure anesthesia began at 7:00 AM and was terminated at 7:45 AM on 01/01/20xx. Completion of the procedure was performed on 01/04/20xx, with anesthesia administration beginning at 7:00 AM and concluding at 8:40 PM. Identify key elements for procedures performed as follows:
    Anesthesia procedure code: _00810_
    Physical status modifier: _P3_

Qualifying circumstances code(s):   _99100_
Anesthesia modifier(s):   _53_
Calculate time units (10-minute increments):   _5_

14. An 8-month-old child presented to the OR for tonsillectomy and placement of PE tubes for tonsillitis and serous otitis media. The anesthesiologist arrived in the OR suite at 7:00 AM; administration began at 7:10 AM and concluded at 7:55 AM. Identify key elements for procedure performed as follows:
    Anesthesia procedure code: _00120_
    Physical status modifier: _P1_
    Qualifying circumstances code(s):   _none_
    Anesthesia modifier(s):   _none_
    Calculate time units (10-minute increments):   _5_

15. A 50-year-old male presented to the OR for repair of an incarcerated inguinal hernia. Induction of anesthesia began at 9:00 AM and ended at 9:45 AM. Identify key elements for procedure performed as follows:
    Anesthesia procedure code: _00830_
    Physical status modifier: _P1_
    Qualifying circumstances code(s):   _none_
    Anesthesia modifier(s):   _none_
    Calculate time units (10-minute increments):   _5_

16. A 45-year-old female presented for diagnostic arthroscopic evaluation of the shoulder. On entering the shoulder compartment, the surgeon performed an arthroscopic rotator cuff repair. Anesthesia began at 10:00 AM and ended at 11:15 AM. Identify key elements for procedure performed as follows:
    Anesthesia procedure code: _01622_
    Physical status modifier: _P1_
    Qualifying circumstances code(s):   _none_
    Anesthesia modifier(s):   _none_
    Calculate time units (10-minute increments):   _8_

17. A 75-year-old patient presented to the OR for an emergency laparoscopic cholecystectomy as a result of a ruptured gallbladder. The surgeon arrived at 8:00 AM, the anesthesiologist arrived at 8:15 AM, administration began at 8:30 AM, surgical procedure began at 8:45 AM with conclusion of both surgical and anesthetic services at 10:00 AM. Identify key elements for procedure performed as follows:
    Anesthesia procedure code: _00790_
    Physical status modifier: _P1_
    Qualifying circumstances code(s):   _99100_
    Anesthesia modifier(s):   _none_
    Calculate time units (10-minute increments):   _9_

18. A patient arrived in the OR with multiple injuries as the result of an automobile accident. An open reduction of a distal radial fracture was performed as well as open repair of a distal tibia/fibular fracture. (Patient

is NOT Medicare). Identify key elements for procedure performed as follows:

Anesthesia procedure code: 01830 01486

Physical status modifier: P1

Qualifying circumstances code(s): none

Anesthesia modifier(s): 51

Calculate time units (10-minute increments): none

19. A 79-year-old male presented to the operative suite for a cardiac catheterization with a balloon angioplasty performed. Anesthesia induction began at 7:00 AM and ended at 10:00 AM. Identify key elements for procedure performed as follows:

Anesthesia procedure code: 01920

Physical status modifier: P1

Qualifying circumstances code(s): 99100

Anesthesia modifier(s): none

Calculate time units (10-minute increments): 18

20. An 11-month-old child presented for insertion of ear tubes (tympanostomy). MAC was performed from 7:00 AM until 8:30 AM due to patient's age and history of seizures. Identify key elements for procedure performed as follows:

Anesthesia procedure code: 00120

Physical status modifier: P2

Qualifying circumstances code(s): 99100

Anesthesia modifier(s): none

Calculate time units (10-minute increments): 9

12

SURGERY SERVICES

LEARNING OBJECTIVES

Following the completion of this chapter, the student will be able to:

- Know and apply the surgery coding guidelines.
- Understand and apply the bundled services guidelines for surgery coding.
- Comprehend the components of global surgery coding.
- Understand the medical complexity of specialty surgery services.
- Follow the usage and application of modifier codes in the surgery setting.

CODING REFERENCE TOOLS

Tool 46
Basic CPT-4 Chapter Layout
Tool 47
Components of CPT Body Systems
Tool 48
Bundled Services Guidelines
Tool 49
Surgical Tray Listing
Tool 50
Surgical Global Package Definitions

KEY TERMS

Only general surgical key terms are here. Specific medical terminology needed for each anatomical section is listed at the beginning of each review of systems.

-centesis
-ectomy
-orrhaphy
-ostomy
-otomy
-pexy
-plasty

DOCUMENTATION/CODING GUIDELINES

Surgery documentation may represent the most complex part of CPT-4 coding. In determining whether the services performed are indeed surgical in nature, one must review the procedure or operative note and decide whether the procedure was invasive, definitive, or restorative in nature. Many of the procedures contained in the surgery section would not, at first glance, appear to belong in the surgery section. Laypersons would think that only procedures performed in an operating room would be included. Procedures such as laceration repairs, lesion removals, application of casts/splints, colonoscopies, and other procedures, which would not appear significant, are also contained in the surgery section. Each of these procedures is invasive, definitive, or restorative in nature. For example, the application of a cast or splint is the prescribed medical protocol for a fracture.

Documentation for surgical procedures is often lengthy and contains many medical terms that must be interpreted to assign surgical codes correctly. For this reason, background or training in medical terminology will prove beneficial in the determination of exactly what procedures were performed as described in the operative report. In addition to the length and scope of the procedure reports, physicians often dictate the procedure they plan to perform at the beginning of the operative report; however, that is not necessarily indicative of the procedure(s) performed. The physician may include additional information in the operative report that may be coded in addition to the primary procedure. Descriptors often used by the physician in the operative note may not agree with coding principles that are applied in CPT-4 code assignment.

For example, the surgeon dictates an operative report and indicates that a colonoscopy is performed. The operative note indicates that a colonoscopy was performed and two polyps were also removed by hot biopsy forceps during the procedure. Should the coder assign CPT-4 codes based on the heading, "Colonoscopy," code 45378 would be assigned. It would be more appropriate to assign 45384, colonoscopy with removal of polyp(s), and would garner additional reimbursement for the surgeon/practice.

Another example would be the operative report that indicates a "complex closure" will be performed for a laceration of the arm. The term *complex* used by the surgeon, however, is not the standard for coding guidelines, which indicate *complex* must involve "more than a layered closure." The surgeon used the term *complex* perhaps because the laceration was large and required longer to suture. The code assignment should not be complex because the repair (CPT-4 guidelines) is based on the following:

- Extent: Simple, 1 layer; Intermediate, 2 layers or 1 layer/debridement; Complex, more than a layered closure
- Anatomical location
- Size (in centimeters)

In this instance, should the coder assign CPT-4 codes based on the physician's statement of "complex," the service would be coded too high and the carrier on audit would request monies back.

Surgery coding is a perfect example of the many tasks of the office or surgical coder. As discussed in the opening chapter, the job of coder is not simply limited to reviewing reports and assigning codes. An integral part of any coder's job is education—education of the staff, including the physician or documenter(s) in the practice. Many physicians are not aware of the coding guidelines or the need for accurate and complete documentation so that appropriate codes for services may be assigned. Take the laceration example used previously; recall that one of the criteria for code assignment was size in centimeters. Note that the physician did not indicate the size in the opening header. In the event that size was not documented in the body of the operative note, the smallest size would have to be coded, thereby reducing the reimbursement significantly.

Add to the complexity of interpreting the operative report or note the fact that no physician dictates or documents the same. Even the same physician does not document identical procedures the same, so the coder must be equipped to read, interpret, query, and educate the physician, AND assign the appropriate codes for correct reimbursement. The coder is integral to practice success because he or she ensures correct reimbursement for services.

Look again at the Surgery portion of the table previously reviewed in Chapter 9 (steps and components needed for CPT-4 coding).

CPT-4 Coding Steps

Type/Service	Surgery
Step 1	
Identify Chapter	Definitive Restorative Invasive
Range of Codes	10021-69990
Step 2	
Determine Type/Location	Anatomical System Integumentary Respiratory
Step 3	
Specific Type	Anatomical Part Skin Finger

Continued

CPT-4 Coding Steps—cont'd

Step 4

Specific Procedure

Procedure Information
Excision
Incision

Step 5

Extent/Specifics

Extent
Size/cm

The student will compile an operative report by finding essential elements for coding purposes. There are a number of methods that can be used to extract the needed information from the operative report. The coder must be consistent, and consistency in processing this information will make coding operative reports much easier.

Take a look at a sample operative report and decide what key words help determine the definitive, restorative, and/or invasive procedure(s) performed.

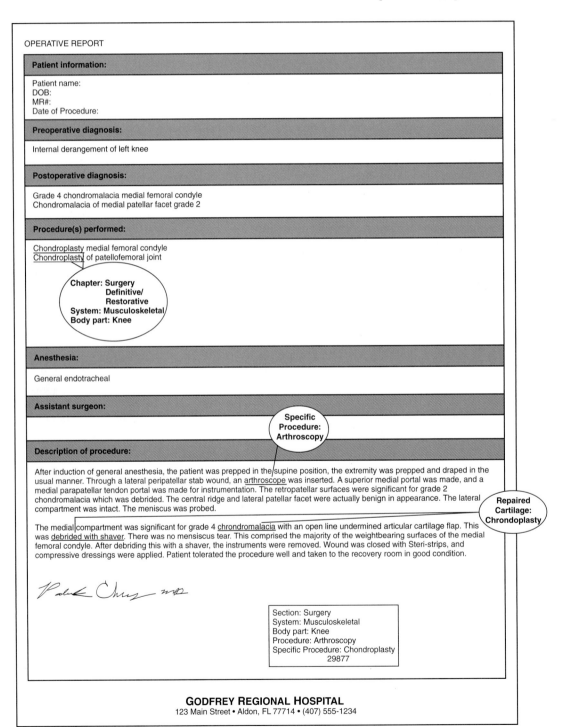

OPERATIVE REPORT

Patient information:

Patient name:
DOB:
MR#:
Date of Procedure:

Preoperative diagnosis:

Internal derangement of left knee

Postoperative diagnosis:

Grade 4 chondromalacia medial femoral condyle
Chondromalacia of medial patellar facet grade 2

Procedure(s) performed:

Chondroplasty medial femoral condyle
Chondroplasty of patellofemoral joint

Chapter: Surgery
   Definitive/
   Restorative
System: Musculoskeletal
Body part: Knee

Anesthesia:

General endotracheal

Assistant surgeon:

Specific
Procedure:
Arthroscopy

Description of procedure:

After induction of general anesthesia, the patient was prepped in the supine position, the extremity was prepped and draped in the usual manner. Through a lateral peripatellar stab wound, an arthroscope was inserted. A superior medial portal was made, and a medial parapatellar tendon portal was made for instrumentation. The retropatellar surfaces were significant for grade 2 chondromalacia which was debrided. The central ridge and lateral patellar facet were actually benign in appearance. The lateral compartment was intact. The meniscus was probed.

Repaired
Cartilage:
Chrondoplasty

The medial compartment was significant for grade 4 chrondromalacia with an open line undermined articular cartilage flap. This was debrided with shaver. There was no mensiscus tear. This comprised the majority of the weightbearing surfaces of the medial femoral condyle. After debriding this with a shaver, the instruments were removed. Wound was closed with Steri-strips, and compressive dressings were applied. Patient tolerated the procedure well and taken to the recovery room in good condition.

Section: Surgery
System: Musculoskeletal
Body part: Knee
Procedure: Arthroscopy
Specific Procedure: Chondroplasty
   29877

GODFREY REGIONAL HOSPITAL
123 Main Street • Aldon, FL 77714 • (407) 555-1234

Some key guidelines need to be remembered when extracting key terms for this chart:

- Extract the key terms for the definitive, restorative, invasive procedure only
- Only other significant procedures that represent a significant additional procedure are coded

Surgery CPT-4 Coding Steps

Type/Service	Surgery	Chart Information
Step 1		
Identify Chapter	Definitive Restorative Invasive	Definitive Procedure(s) Performed: Chondroplasty
Range of Codes	10021-69990	10021-69990
Step 2		
Determine Type/ Location	Anatomical System Integumentary Respiratory	Musculoskeletal
Step 3		
Specific Type	Anatomical Part Skin Finger	Knee
Step 4		
Specific Procedure Information	Procedure Excision Incision	Arthroscopy
Step 5		
Extent/Specifics	Extent Size/cm	Arthroscopy, Knee, Diagnostic Arthroscopy, Knee, Chondroplasty

Keep in mind that there will be many terms included in the operative report, as well as significant information regarding the planned procedure, introduction of equipment, and the conclusion of the procedure. Most of this information will not be necessary for most surgical procedure coding. Until the student is comfortable with what to extract from the operative report, more than is necessary may be extracted and eliminated during the assignment of surgical procedure code(s).

CODING GUIDELINES

GLOBAL SERVICES

The **"global"** (package) concept of surgery has been discussed previously. A review of how this concept relates to surgical services is needed. Global surgical services

represent the "package" concept wherein all preoperative, operative, and normal, uncomplicated, postoperative services are reimbursed under one CPT-4 code.

It is imperative to keep this concept in mind when reading through the operative report. Remember that codes are assigned for definitive, restorative, and invasive procedures, not for the method of approach, anatomical structures that must be moved or incised or those that must be closed when the procedure is completed. Sometimes it will help to simply think about the procedure and what normally would occur in order to accomplish it.

For example, for a lesion to be excised (Excision of lesion codes), it would be necessary to prepare the patient, cleanse the area, and make an incision (to excise the lesion). After the actual excision of the lesion, the incised area would require repair, possibly by suturing. All of these services would be included in the excision of lesion code assignment. If it were necessary to perform additional services, such as a layered closure, however, that service would be codable in addition to the excision of lesion code.

Individual guidelines for each subcategory in the surgery section are reviewed and the guidelines are applied to some actual operative reports. Keep in mind that the operative reports contained in both the workbook and additional practice exercises are actual operative reports. In many cases, complete information has not been included, ambiguous statements are made, and there are discrepancies between the procedure in the top heading and the actual report. Unfortunately, this is why surgical coding can be challenging: there are few ideal operative reports. A good coder extracts the needed information, knows when to query (question) the physician, educates the documenter about information needed, and monitors the documentation process for needed improvements. This represents the difference between a satisfactory coder and an excellent asset to the practice.

STARRED PROCEDURES

Starred procedures were eliminated from the CPT-4 guidelines in 2004. Coders who used these codes in the past need to be reminded that concept is no longer valid. All surgical procedures have a minimum follow-up of 10 days, many longer as defined by the carrier, Medicare, or RBRVS.

BASIC LAYOUT

The surgery section of CPT-4 is divided into anatomical sections in much the same way that ICD-9-CM is formatted. Within these subcategories, the procedures are listed by anatomical site and by the performed procedure.

For example, in the Integumentary subsection within the Surgery section, the integumentary system is composed of skin and subcutaneous tissue, nails, and breasts.

Different procedures within those sections may include incision, excision, introduction, repair, or reconstruction. Procedures vary from system to system. For instance, Fractures/Dislocations is a category in the Musculoskeletal System that would not be found in the Integumentary system. Tool 46 outlines a detailed breakdown of the Surgery Chapter in the CPT-4 book. The complexities of each subsection are reviewed subsequent to a review of the surgical code definitions and guidelines.

MODIFIERS

The surgery section of CPT-4 has perhaps the most comprehensive listing of modifier codes describing the circumstances that fall "outside the norm" for global procedure concepts. The complex nature of surgery coding often requires the appending of more than one modifier code to the surgical procedure. In these instances, it is important that the most significant

TOOL 46

SURGERY CODING STEPS PROCESS

1. **Identify the appropriate chapter:**

   Surgery
   (Definitive, Restorative, Invasive)

2. **Identify anatomical system:**

Integumentary	10000–19999
Musculoskeletal	20000–29999
Respiratory	30000–32999
Cardiovascular	33000–39999
Digestive disease	40000–49999
Urinary system	50000–53999
Male genital	54000–55999
Female genital	56000–59999
Endocrine	60000–60699
Nervous	61000–64999
Eye/Ocular adnexa	65000–68999
Auditory (ear)	69000–69999

3. **Identify body part:**   Code range:
   (Example: Musculoskeletal/radius)
   urinary/bladder

4. **What procedure:**   Code range:

Incision	Excision
Introduction	Fracture/dislocation
Amputation	Arthrodesis
Scopy	Repair/reconstruction

   INDENTIFY KEY WORDS:

5. **Specific information regarding procedure**   Code range:
   (Example: Musculoskeletal/radius/
   fracture/open/with/manipulation)

   INDENTIFY KEY WORDS:

   CODE ASSIGNMENT(S)/MODIFIER(S):

modifier that affects reimbursement is listed first. Some carriers will allow up to two modifiers on the claim form, but others will only allow one. In those instances, the code must assign modifier 99 with the procedure code, and then list the multiple modifiers in the correct order on the following line of the claim. A review of the modifiers applicable to the surgery section follows. These modifiers are applied to specific surgical cases throughout the chapter.

Modifier 22—Unusual Procedural Service

Modifier code 22 describes the service as greater than that usually performed for the CPT-4 code selected. A report is usually necessary to explain in detail the extensive service provided.

Modifier 26—Professional Component

Many services in the surgery, radiology, pathology, and medicine sections comprise two components for the total global procedure:

- Technical component—facility charge for equipment use, technician, supplies
- Professional component—charge for the professional interpretation and diagnosis of the service performed

When the physician supplies only the professional component of the global procedure, modifier 26 indicates that only this portion of service was provided and reimbursement is reduced. The facility providing the technical component bills for that service separately.

In the event the facility or provider codes this service incorrectly and the global component is reimbursed, the other provider receives a denial, indicating that reimbursement has already been made for this service.

In addition, coding and billing for the global component when only the professional component was performed could be interpreted as fraud because the provider has billed and been paid for a service or a portion of a service that was not provided.

A good coding and billing technique is to identify those services for which the provider does NOT have the ability to bill globally; this requires the use of modifier 26, which should be added to each of these procedure codes in the computerized billing system. This ensures that no one in the practice accidentally bills globally for professional services.

Modifier 32—Mandated Services

When surgical and diagnostic procedures listed in the surgery section are requested by a third party or a PRO (peer review organization), modifier 32 should be added.

Reimbursement may not be considered in some instances without this modifier.

Modifier 47—Anesthesia by Surgeon

When regional or general anesthesia is provided by the surgeon, and not the anesthesiologist, modifier 47 should be added to the surgical procedure performed. The surgeon should use the codes in the surgery section. The anesthesiologist would NOT use this modifier or the surgery codes; the surgeon would not use the anesthesiology codes or modifiers.

Modifier 50—Bilateral Procedure

When procedures are performed bilaterally during the same operative session, modifier 50 should be added to the listing for this service. For this modifier to be used, the same procedure must be performed on both the right and left sides. For instance, a closed fracture repair of the right distal radius is performed and an open repair of the distal radius is performed on the left. The modifier 50 would not be appropriate because the exact same procedure was NOT performed on both the left and right distal radii. Keep in mind that the use of modifier 50 would also not be appropriate if the CPT-4 descriptor is for more than one anatomical site, such as the repair of phalangeal fractures of the right and left index fingers. The CPT-4 descriptor is for phalanges and there are 10 fingers, so the use of the bilateral code would not be appropriate. In this instance, the HCPCS Level II modifiers FA to F9 would be used to identify the particular finger(s) being repaired, but only if the carrier allows for the use of HCPCS Level II modifiers.

There are two methods for attaching the modifier to this service. In the first method, the surgical procedure code is listed alone, and modifier 50 is added to the second procedure. In the second method, the code is listed only once with modifier 50 attached. The coder must determine which method is required by specific carriers for submitting claims.

Reimbursement for the second associated procedure is reduced because the preoperative and postoperative periods for both procedures have already been reimbursed in the primary procedure reimbursement.

Modifier 51—Multiple Procedures

Multiple procedures performed during the same operative session, typically through the same approach, and in the same anatomical location/general area are coded with modifier 51. Make certain these additional procedures are not "bundled" or made a part of the global component of the primary procedure.

When subsequent procedures are billed with modifier 51, reduction is made on all subsequent procedures. Typically, the second procedure is reduced by 50%, with additional procedures reduced by 75%, to a maximum of 4 to 6 procedures reimbursed. Therefore it is imperative that the CPT-4 codes not only be assigned correctly, but listed in the correct order, with the most significant code listed first.

Incorrect billing for these services results in a dramatic affect on reimbursement. Look at the following scenario, which shows the correct and incorrect use of modifier 51.

Procedure code 58260   Charge $5000
Procedure code XXXXX   Charge $1500
Procedure code YYYYY   Charge $500

Correctly billed:

Code	Charge	Reimbursement
58260	$5000	$4000
XXXXX-51	$1500	$750 (reimbursed at $\frac{1}{2}$)
YYYYY-51	$500	$125 (reimbursed at $\frac{1}{4}$)

Reimbursement amount $4875

Incorrectly billed:

XXXXX	$1500	$1500
YYYYY-51	$500	$250 (reimbursed at $\frac{1}{2}$)
58260-51	$5000 ($\frac{1}{4}$)	$1250 (reimbursed at $\frac{1}{4}$)

Reimbursement amount $3000

The total charge of the procedures is $7000. Correct coding results in a reimbursement of $4875, compared with the reimbursement of $3000 when procedures are incorrectly coded.

If multiple, independent, and distinct procedures are performed during the same operative session, they should be billed with modifier 59 instead.

Modifier 52—Reduced Services

When a portion of the usual service billed with the CPT-4 code is eliminated or reduced, the coder must modify the surgical code with modifier 52. In the event the CPT-4 descriptor is not met, it is necessary to assign an appropriate modifier to indicate why the global procedure was not performed. In some cases, the facility may have performed only the technical component (as discussed with modifier 26) or the procedure was not completed according to the CPT-4 descriptor. Modifier 52 would be appropriately appended to the CPT-4 code. Reduction in reimbursement will probably result. A report may be requested to clarify the extent of services provided.

Modifier 53—Discontinued Procedure

When the physician decides to discontinue a procedure before completion, the coder must assign modifier 53. This modifier is *not* used for procedures that are electively cancelled before they are begun or that are termi-

nated at the patient's request. Typically, this code is used for procedures that cannot be completed for medical reasons (e.g., a surgical procedure terminated because of the development of unstable blood pressure).

Make sure the physician reports all services performed, not just those completed. In the past, providers were not reimbursed for partial provision of service. Allowance is now made for that portion of the service completed before termination. Often, the most complex portion of the procedure may have been completed before termination, and the physician is reimbursed accordingly.

As has been discussed previously, a large number of the services listed in the surgical section of CPT-4 are global "package" procedures that include both postoperative and preoperative periods. Because these services may encompass an extended period, circumstances arise in which the same physician does not provide the preoperative, postoperative, and surgical care. When this occurs, the following modifiers are appropriate.

Modifier 54—Surgical Care Only

When only the surgical procedure itself is performed by the physician, that surgical procedure should be billed with modifier 54 appended. When these are global procedures, reimbursement is affected accordingly, because other physicians will code and bill independently for the postoperative and preoperative components.

Modifier 55—Postoperative Management Only

Modifier 55 is used when the physician provides only normal, uncomplicated postoperative care of the global surgical patient. This care is provided after a surgical procedure for a defined amount of time.

Modifier 56—Preoperative Management Only

Modifier 56 is used when the physician provides only preoperative care or services before the surgical procedure of the global package.

Modifier 57—Decision for Surgery

Modifier 57 is used for E & M services only, usually not for surgery services.

Modifier 58—Staged/Related Procedure or Service by Same Physician during Postoperative Global Period

For procedures to be considered as staged or related, they must meet the following criteria:

- Planned at the time of the original procedure
- More extensive than the original procedure
- Therapy following diagnostic surgical procedure

An example of this is a simple fracture repair that must be repeated on a more complex level. Keep in mind that when a surgical procedure is performed, the insurance carrier will disallow additional payment for other services if it is unable to determine whether that service is "over and above" the usual postoperative care. Remember that most insurance claims are being scanned and interpreted by computer, and computers are not programmed to interpret medical care and standards of care. Without an appropriate modifier code, services performed during the postoperative period that should be given additional consideration will be disallowed or denied.

Modifier 59—Distinct Procedural Service

When a procedure is performed on the same day as other surgical services but is independent and distinct, modifier 59 should be used. This modifier distinguishes the service as independently performed. An example is a surgical session in which repairs of a fractured wrist and fractured femur are performed. Two separate surgical approaches are necessary, requiring a complete and separate description of the medical complexity of two different operations on the same patient during a single surgical session.

Use of modifier 59 is distinct from that of modifier 51 (multiple procedures) in that the procedures are separate and are performed independently. Modifier 51 indicates multiple procedures have been performed via the same approach and in the same anatomical location. For this reason, reimbursement for services coded with modifier 59 should be similar to that given when procedures are performed independently.

Note: CPT-4 notes that modifier 59 should be used only when no other modifier is appropriate.

Modifier 62—Two Surgeons

When one specific surgical procedure requires the expertise of two skilled surgeons, modifier 62 is attached to both claims by each of the surgeons. Typically, the two physicians have different skills, which are required for completion of the surgical procedure. Reimbursement to each participating physician is affected proportionately, with the sum of the reimbursements usually not exceeding 125% of the total usual allowance for the service.

Care should be taken to include this modifier when coding for services performed in cooperation with another surgeon. Without the proper use of this modifier, one surgeon will be reimbursed 100% of the allowance for services, and the other will receive denial for services because payment has already been made to another provider. For this error to be corrected, the original submission must be amended and a refund made to the

carrier of the amount(s) paid, so that each physician can be paid correctly. The two surgeons SHOULD NOT correct this error simply by "dividing" the reimbursement from the carrier because the tax records for the original submitting physician will reflect monies paid to him or her, and he or she will be taxed accordingly. For example, for cochlear implant surgery that requires both ENT surgeon and neurosurgeon skills, both physicians must use the same cochlear implant surgical code with modifier 62 on both claims.

Modifier 66—Surgical Team

When the skills of multiple physicians (more than two) and the skills of highly technical personnel, as well as complex surgical equipment, are involved in a surgical procedure, the services should be billed with modifier 66 attached (e.g., organ transplant requiring multiple surgeons for harvesting and transplanting and a multitude of personnel making up the transplant team).

Modifier 76—Repeat Procedure, Same Physician

When procedures are repeated by the same physician, modifier 76 must be added to distinguish them from duplicate or misbilled items. For example, multiple ECGs are required for a patient with a cardiac disorder on the same day to determine the progression or resolution of the problem. If these multiple ECGs are billed without the use of modifier 76 on subsequent ECGs, they will be denied as duplicate services.

Modifier 77—Repeat Procedure, Another Physician

When procedures are repeated by another physician, subsequent services must be submitted with modifier 77 attached.

Modifier 78—Return to the Operating Room for Related Procedure during Postoperative Global Period

When it is necessary for a patient to return to surgery during the global postoperative period for a procedure related to the original procedure, those subsequent procedure(s) must be billed with modifier 78 attached. Make certain when assigning this modifier code that the original procedure was performed in the OR (operating room) and that the subsequent procedure falls within the postoperative period.

Modifier 79—Unrelated Procedure/Service, Same Physician during Global/Postoperative Period

When a patient is in the normal, uncomplicated postoperative follow-up period, and it becomes necessary to perform an additional service or procedure that is found in the surgery section of CPT-4, modifier 79 should be appended to that service. An example is the patient who has had a fracture reduction and now requires repair of a hernia. The same general surgeon performs both operations. Modifier 79 is appended to the second procedure to signify to the carrier that the two procedures are unrelated and should be considered independently. Keep in mind that the use of modifiers to indicate unrelated, related, or staged care during the postoperative period, apply only to the original surgeon and practice. Other physicians not associated with the surgeon or surgeon's practice are not excluded from payment during the postoperative period for services performed, and these modifiers should be appended for payment consideration.

When an assistant surgeon is required for the performance of a surgical service, one of the following modifiers should be attached to the assistant surgeon's service. Assistant surgeon fees are reimbursed at a significantly lower amount than those of the primary surgeon. Typically, insurance carriers reimburse this service at an average of 10% to 20% of the original allowance.

Insurance carriers differ regarding criteria for the medical necessity of an assistant surgeon in certain procedures. The coder may want to gather this information from the various carriers with whom the provider contracts and incorporate it into the Third-Party Contract Worksheet (discussed later).

Modifier 80—Assistant Surgeon

When an assistant surgeon bills for services, the same surgical procedure submitted by the primary surgeon should be used. Care should be taken to distinguish between **"two surgeons"** and **"assistant surgeons"** services. When the second surgeon provides skilled services specific to his or her specialty, these services are coded as two surgeons. A second surgeon who provides no additional skills but simply assists would be coded as an assistant surgeon.

In many instances, the second surgeon may be requested to "stand by" in the event that his or her skills are needed. If those specialty skills are not needed and that surgeon chooses or is requested to participate in the operation, the services must be coded as assistant surgeon.

There is a significant difference in the reimbursement of assistant surgeon services and two surgeon services. Typically, the reimbursement for assistant surgery codes is approximately 10% to 20% of the allowance for the primary surgical charge. Reimbursement for two surgeons is approximately 50% to 65% for each physician of the allowance for the specified surgery code.

Modifier 81—Minimum Assistant Surgeon

When minimal services are required from the assistant surgeon, the use of modifier 81 is appropriate. Many insurance carriers do not recognize modifier 81 and request that if an assistant surgeon is in fact necessary, then modifier 80 (assistant surgeon) or 82 (assistant surgeon when qualified resident surgeon not available) should be used. Each third-party carrier should have this information available. The coder may wish to incorporate this information into the Third-Party Contract Coding Worksheet.

Modifier 82—Assistant Surgeon When Qualified Resident Surgeon Is Not Available

When the participation of an assistant surgeon is necessary owing to the unavailability of a qualified resident surgeon, the use of modifier 82 is appropriate. This may occur at facilities in which residents are not available or are available only during certain hours. Because the third-party carrier is not aware of the circumstances or availability of residents at facilities, this information (lack of qualified residents) should be documented in the operative records of both the assistant surgeon and the primary surgeon.

Modifier 90—Reference (Outside Laboratory)

When laboratory procedures are billed and reported, but are actually performed by another party such as a clinical laboratory facility, the service must be coded with modifier 90 attached. Note that laboratory services may not be billed to Medicare intermediaries unless the billing entity also provides those services; therefore modifier 90 is not appropriate for any laboratory services for Medicare patients.

The purpose of this modifier is to declare that the provider is billing for services even though financial arrangement has been made with a third-party laboratory that will perform these services. In the event the third-party laboratory erroneously bills for these services as well, modifier 90 indicates what the financial arrangement is and that the provider should be paid for the services.

Modifier 99—Multiple Modifiers

When two or more modifiers are necessary to adequately describe provided services, the use of modifier 99 is attached to the billed CPT-4 code. This is followed by a list of the multiple modifiers applicable for that service. It may be accomplished on the face of the claim form or by attachment of an explanation to the claim.

Modifier 99 is frequently necessary in billing appropriately for surgical services, because many of these services require the use of multiple modifiers to describe unusual procedural circumstances. For example, a surgeon performs a secondary procedure which requires the use of modifier 51 and the surgeon discontinues it because of a problem with the stabilization of the patient, which requires modifier 53. The secondary procedure should be billed with the attachment of modifier 99 to indicate that multiple unusual circumstances occurred and must be considered for payment. These multiple circumstances may be described on an attachment as with the modifiers 51 and 53, or they may be listed on the face of the claim.

Note: Medicare allows coding with a maximum of two modifiers without the use of modifier 99. These would be listed following the CPT-4 code as follows:

CPT-4 code–Modifier #1/Modifier #2

58260-51/80

Now that the general guidelines and principles for coding surgical services have been discussed and surgical modifier codes have been reviewed, basic rules for coding the surgery section should be reviewed. These rules follow many of the same guidelines presented in previous sections, but they also encompass some specific guidelines for surgery.

Because these modifiers are so crucial to correct payment for surgical services, take a minute to identify the correct modifier code(s) needed for the following scenarios. If none are needed, indicate "None." Surgical codes at this point have not yet been reviewed, so it is not necessary to assign the appropriate CPT-4 code.

STOP AND PRACTICE

Modifier(s)

1. Patient presents for hernia repair and removal of lesion of the face — 59
2. Patient presents for knee arthroscopy and shoulder arthroscopy — 59
3. Patient presents for multiple laceration repairs — 51
4. Patient presents for EGD (esophagogastroduodenoscopy); the scope cannot be advanced to the duodenum — 52
5. Patient has repair/removal of nail due to ingrown nail — N/A
6. Patient has knee arthroscopy with: Arthroscopic lateral release Medial and lateral meniscectomy — 51
7. Patient had fracture repair with application of cast and now returns for replacement cast — N/A

8. Patient has fracture of femur with preoperative and surgical care provided by surgeon at local hospital. Returns home for postoperative care only. — 55
9. Closed reduction of tibia/fibular fracture was performed; however, it was necessary to return to the operating room and perform an additional procedure to correct the defect. — 78
10. Closed reduction of a distal radius fracture with application of cast was performed in the ED. Patient now returns for additional surgical intervention. The patient is taken to the OR where an open reduction of the same fracture is performed — 58

STEPS IN CODING FROM THE SURGERY SECTION

A basic review of the steps for coding surgical procedures is found in Tool 46. Details of these steps follow.

The coder should have the surgical (operative/procedure) report available for review. Should the physician provide vague or inaccurate information, it may be billed incorrectly and the coder, provider, and others involved may be liable for services billed and not performed. Consideration would not be given for any services that were provided but erroneously not billed.

The physician may indicate on the billing card or information sheet only those performed services that he or she thinks should be billable. When the coder reviews the surgical or operative report, he or she may often find additional billable and codable services.

Step 1

Identify the System
- Integumentary
- Musculoskeletal
- Respiratory
- Cardiovascular
- Hemic and Lymphatic
- Digestive

- Urinary
- Male Genital
- Female Genital
- Maternity Care and Delivery
- Endocrine
- Nervous
- Eye and Ocular Adnexa
- Auditory System

By identifying the appropriate system on which the procedure was performed, the coder has eliminated a large portion of codes from the Surgery Section. Background or training in medical terminology and anatomy and physiology is important in determining this information. Tool 47 addresses the basic components of each system, which may serve as an excellent reference tool.

Step 2

Identify the Anatomical Site

After identifying the anatomical system, the coder must determine what anatomical site the procedure is being performed on. Keep in mind that the coding process is a "breaking down" process. With the procedure identified as invasive, restorative, or definitive, the other chapters of the CPT-4 book have been eliminated. When the system has been identified the code has eliminated all the other subsections in the surgery section. Care should be taken so that when the correct categories or breakdowns are chosen, the codes should be found only in that section. Once the coder ventures outside the categories determined as appropriate, the codes will probably be incorrect. When using this process, the coder will often find that the breaking down process takes one and only one code—*the right code.*

Step 3

Identify the Approach/Procedure Performed

From the operative report, the coder must determine whether the definitive, restorative, or invasive procedure was incision, excision, introduction, manipulation, repair, reconstruction, fracture repair, or correction of dislocation. Just because the procedure required an incision does not mean the code will come from the Incision category. If the procedure is an excision of a lesion, for instance, the approach is the incision. The definitive procedure is "Excision," so the code is located in the Excision section.

If a scope such as an arthroscope is inserted for diagnostic purposes and before the conclusion of the surgical case, a surgical intervention is performed, and the diagnostic scope will not be assigned a code. This is discussed further, and this concept is demonstrated later in this chapter.

Step 4

Determine Extent/Specifics of Procedure

The surgical or operative report should indicate the extent of the procedure such as whether the procedure was simple, complex, closed, or open. If this is not documented, the assumption must be made of minimal service for that procedure. Consider the following example:

Laceration Repair, Thumb

If the extent is not documented, then the example would be billed as a "simple" repair, less than 2.5 cm. In fact, the services may be complex and involve a 5.0-cm laceration, a substantial difference in the amount of reimbursement.

Step 5

Select Appropriate Code(s)/Put in Appropriate Order and Make Certain the Code Used Is Inclusive of All Services Provided

Read the notes in the CPT-4 manual carefully. The most common inclusions and exclusions are listed. Coding references, such as surgery bundling books and cross-coding references, are helpful in determining whether services are considered bundled. These are available where most coding books are available. In addition, Medicare uses a list of bundled codes in the "Correct Coding Initiatives," which are published on a quarterly basis.

Step 6

Select the Appropriate Modifier Code(s) When Applicable

If the procedure code typically is not billed in addition to the global surgical code already listed, the coder must substantiate the reason for requesting reimbursement by the use of the appropriate surgery section modifier.

Operative report documentation is similar to other physician or provider documentation already reviewed. Many coders, however, find the review of operative report documentation and the coding of operative reports to be more overwhelming.

The deluge of medical terms found in medical records is not cause for alarm, because many of these have little importance in coding for services. The use of a medical dictionary may be helpful in reviewing reports if knowledge of medical terminology for a particular specialty is minimal.

As in the E & M section, successful surgical coding involves selecting only the components necessary for coding the surgical procedure(s). The important part of reading and coding the operative/surgical report is to identify and mark (circle, highlight, underline) ONLY the coding components needed. For instance, the anesthesia administered, the position of the patient, the number of

T O O L   47

COMPONENTS OF CPT BODY SYSTEMS

System	Major Components	Common Combining Form
Integumentary	Skin, Subcutaneous, Accessory Structures	dermato
	Nails	onycho/unguo
	Breast	mammo
Musculoskeletal	Bones	osteo
	Joints	arthro
	Cartilage	chrondro
	Muscles	musculo
	Fascia	fascio
	Tendons	teno/tendino
Respiratory	Nose	naso/rhino
	Sinuses	sinuso
	Larynx	laryngo
	Trachea/Bronchi	tracheo/broncho
	Lungs/Pleura	pneumo/pleuro
Cardiovascular	Heart	cardio
	Arteries	arterio
	Veins	veno/phlebo
	Blood	hemo/hemato
Digestive	Lips	cheilo
	Pharynx	pharyngo
	Adenoids/Tonsils	adenoid/tonsilo
	Mouth	oro/stomato
	Esophagus	esophago
	Stomach	gastro
	Small Intestine	entero
	Large Intestine	colo/colono
	Liver	hepato
	Pancreas	pancreato
	Appendix	appendico
	Gall Bladder	cholecysto
	Anus	ano
Urinary	Kidneys	nephro/reno
	Ureters	uretero
	Urine	urino
	Urethra	urethro
	Bladder	cysto
	Renal Pelvis	pyelo
Reproductive Male/Female	Testes	orchio/orchido
	Prostate	prostato
	Penis	balano
	Vulva	vulvo
	Vagina	colpo
	Ovary	oophoro
	Uterus	hystero
	Fallopian tubes	salpingo
Endocrine	Adrenals	adreno
	Pituitary	pituito
	Thyroid	thyroido
	Thymus	thymo
Nervous Sense Organs	Nerves	neuro
	Brain	encephalo
	Spinal Cord	myelo
	Eye	oculo/ophthalmo
	Ear	acousto/oto

sutures, and the sponge count may not be important in coding surgical services. Learn to "filter out" the nonessential components; then, the operative report will not be as complicated as it appears.

Practice coding the following surgical procedures by using the breakdown previously outlined.

STOP AND PRACTICE

Repair skin

EXAMPLE: Removal of skin foreign body by incision
SYSTEM: Integumentary System
ANATOMICAL LOCATION: Skin
PROCEDURE: Incision
SPECIFICS: Removal of Foreign Body

Code Choice(s):
10120   Incision and Removal Foreign Body, Subcutaneous Tissue, Simple
10121   Incision and Removal Foreign Body, Subcutaneous Tissue, Complicated

Because the operative report is not available and no further information is provided, documentation is not present to support the complicated code. Therefore the code assignment will be as follows:

10120   No Modifier is Necessary

Determine the appropriate code(s) for the following procedures.

1. Removal tumor, bone, finger   26210
2. Arthroscopy, knee, diagnostic   29870
3. Colonoscopy with polyp removal, 2 by snare   45385
4. Repair, laceration, arm, 3.5 cm, simple   12002
5. Full thickness skin graft, arm, 10 sq cm   15220
6. Excision malignant lesion, 4.0 cm, arm   11604
7. Cystectomy, partial   51550
8. Coronary artery bypass graft, venous, 2 grafts   33511
9. Closed reduction, distal radial fracture   25600
10. Tonsillectomy and adenoidectomy, age 10   42820
11. Abdominal hysterectomy   58150
12. Salpingectomy, unilateral   58700
13. Vasectomy   55250
14. Extracapsular cataract removal with lens implant   66984
15. Removal foreign body from the external ear   69200
16. Prostatectomy, radical, with limited pelvic lymphadenectomy   55812
17. Laparoscopic appendectomy   44970
18. Bronchoscopy with brushings   31623
19. Thoracentesis   32000
20. Closed treatment of metacarpal fracture, with manipulation   26605

Those exercises should have seemed simple if the "breaking down" method discussed earlier in the chapter was used. Apply those same principles to an actual operative report, extracting only the information that is needed for the coding assignment. If the student is not familiar with all the sections in the surgery chapter, he or she may wish to locate the general area from which the code will be obtained and identify key elements in the report. Keep in mind that some of the information will not be relevant to the assignment of CPT-4 or ICD-9-CM codes so that information may be eliminated.

OPERATIVE REPORT

Patient information:
Patient name: DOB: MR#: Date of Procedure: 01/04/XX Surgeon: Dr. Smith

Preoperative diagnosis:
Screening colonoscopy

Postoperative diagnosis:
Diverticulosis of colon Sigmoid polyp Internal hemorrhoids

Procedure(s) performed:
Colonoscopy

Anesthesia:
RN sedation

Assistant surgeon:

Description of procedure:
The patient was brought to the Endoscopy suite and placed in the left lateral position. After he was connected to the EKG, blood pressure and pulse oximeter, IV sedation was given by IV Demerol and IV Versed. After adequate sedation was obtained, Xylocaine cream was used in the perirectal area. Rectal examination was performed. **Colonoscopy** The colonoscope was introduced through the rectum and passed all of the flexures into the cecum. Position in the cecum was identified by the ileocecal valve. The scope was withdrawn, visualizing all of the sites of the colon. The patient had a few diverticulosis in the sigmoid colon. None of these were acutely inflamed. The patient had a small sessile polyp measuring 2–3 cm in the distal sigmoid. This was removed by snare technique. The scope was then retroflexed into the rectum. The patient had internal hemorrhoids and a small fibroepithelial polyp on the hemorrhoids. I did not remove it knowing that is was benign and I did not want to cause more bleeding from the hemorrhoids. The scope was withdrawn. The patient tolerated the procedure well and was transferred to the Same Day Surgery Unit in stable condition.

Section: Surgery
System: Digestive disease
Body part: Rectum
Specific procedure: Endoscopy
                   Colonoscopy
Specifics: Polypectomy by snare
       Code 45385

GODFREY REGIONAL HOSPITAL
123 Main Street • Aldon, FL 77714 • (407) 555-1234

Procedure:	Colonoscopy
Identify System:	Digestive
Anatomical Part:	Rectum
Procedure:	Scope, specifically Colonoscopy Codes start with 45378
Specifics:	Colonoscopy with removal of polyp by snare
Code(s):	45385

Surgical coding presents a challenge to many coders. Pinpointing and working with only those components that are needed significantly simplify the review of operative/surgical reports.

SEPARATE PROCEDURE

CPT-4 identifies some procedures as *separate procedure.* These codes should only be assigned when they are the only procedure (thus "separate procedure") performed on that anatomical site.

For instance, look at the operative report for the colonoscopy. Assume that both a diagnostic colonoscopy (45378/separate procedure) and a colonoscopy with removal of polyp by snare (45385) were performed. Because there is a definitive procedure performed at the anatomical site (45385), code 45378 would not be used. The only time a separate procedure may be coded is when it is the only procedure (a diagnostic colonoscopy with no definitive, invasive, or restorative procedures would be coded as 45378).

ADD-ON PROCEDURES

Add-on codes are signified in CPT-4 with the use of a (+) sign. This symbol designates procedures that are performed in conjunction with a primary procedure. An add-on code without the primary procedure code should never be used.

EACH, EACH ADDITIONAL, PER PROCEDURES

When procedures are reported in CPT-4 as "each," "each additional," or "per," multiple units of service should not be reported on several lines of the claim, but calculated in "units." For example, if a Split Thickness Skin Graft of the Arm, 200 sq cm were performed it would be coded as follows:

Code 15100	Split Graft, Trunk, Arms, Legs, First 100 sq cm or Less
+Code 15101	Split Graft, Trunk, Arms, Legs, Each Additional 100 sq cm

Note the + add-on symbol in front of 15101; this code is "each additional" and would never be used without the code for the first 100 sq cm (15100).

BUNDLED PROCEDURES

The other big challenge for surgery coders is determining whether services are included or "bundled" within the primary procedure. Those procedures that are included or bundled are often referred to as **incidental procedures.** Simply reading the complete description of the CPT-4 manual often reveals this information. Some basic rules that the coder may follow when considering whether services are bundled are shown in Tool 48.

An allowance for surgical trays is sometimes made in addition to the surgical service. Tool 49 lists those services most commonly considered for this allowance. This allowance is carrier specific and the practice must check with each carrier for additional allowances for this service.

As has been mentioned previously, many excellent reference books and tools are available for determining bundled services. Check to see what coding books are available for specific specialties or general guidelines. In addition, review each third-party contract to determine guidelines regarding bundled services.

STOP AND PRACTICE

1. Develop a matrix of what are the most commonly performed procedures, what services are considered bundled, and what follow-up days are included, so that surgical coding for services is consistent. General guidelines for bundled procedures are noted in Tool 50.
2. Develop such an outline specific to a particular practice and specialty. An example of a specialty-specific guideline is shown in Table 12-1. This information will prove helpful in the coding of services.

3. It is also imperative to track the follow-up days in the practice for these procedures. After determining the appropriate number of follow-up days, post that information in a prominent place for the practice staff.

    Many practices use a sticker on the front of the chart with the name of the procedure, the date of the procedure, and the time included for postoperative follow-up. Any procedures or services performed in this follow-up period will probably need a modifier to justify why they are NOT included in the global procedure.

BUNDLED SERVICES GUIDELINES

1. **Incidental procedures are considered BUNDLED.**
   If the procedure does not carry significant additional time, effort and risk, the procedure is considered "bundled." If the procedure does warrant additional consideration owing to unusual circumstances, the use of a modifier is necessary along with an operative report explaining the additional complexities associated with the service which modified the service for additional consideration.

2. **Surgical introduction/exploration performed in conjunction with a specified surgical procedure is considered "BUNDLED."**
   EXAMPLE:
   Laparotomy performed in conjunction with an abdominal hysterectomy.

   In this example, the laparotomy is considered only the **vehicle or approach** by which the abdominal hysterectomy was performed. Therefore, it is considered incidental or bundled, and MAY NOT be coded in addition to the primary procedure.

   However, when a laparotomy is performed independently for diagnostic purposes, the laparotomy may be coded and billed.

   There are a number of such procedures that may be coded independently, but, when utilized as the approach, they become bundled procedures.

   Before coding additional procedures through the same surgical incision, ask the question, "Is the procedure only the approach or vehicle by which the primary procedure was performed?"

   The rationale for "bundling" these services is that the third-party carrier should reimburse only once for the entire global procedure, which includes the pre-, post-, and operative procedures, that is, the preparation, incision, and repair or whatever services are performed during the operative session as a part of that reported service.

3. **Normal supplies needed to perform the given procedure are included or "BUNDLED."**
   When surgical procedures are performed in the provider's office, normal supply items are considered bundled. Hospital facilities bill according to their guidelines (discussed later).

   Surgical trays are allowed in addition to the procedure when billing certain procedures in the physician's office or outpatient setting as outlined by CMS (Centers for Medicare and Medicaid Services) several years ago. A listing of these procedures cleared for surgical tray billing follows in Tool 49.

TOOL 49

SURGICAL TRAY LISTING

An expense allowance for the following supplies that are not considered routine supplies used in a practice are sometimes considered in addition to the procedure. A separate allowance is made when these supplies are provided in the physician's office under:

A4550 Surgical Tray

in conjunction with the following procedures:

Code	Brief Description*	Code	Brief Description*
19101	Biopsy of Breast	45379	Colonoscopy
19120	Removal Breast Lesion	45380	Colonoscopy, Biopsy
19125	Excision Breast Lesion	45382	Colonoscopy, Control Bleeding
19126	Exc Breast Lesion, Ea Addtl	45383	Colonoscopy, Lesion Removal
20200	Muscle Biopsy	45384	Colonoscopy, Lesion Removal
20205	Deep Muscle Biopsy	45385	Colonoscopy, Lesion Removal
20220	Bone Biopsy, Trocar/Needle	49080	Puncture, Peritoneal, Initial
20225	Bone Biopsy, Trocar/Needle	49081	Puncture, Peritoneal, Subseq
20240	Bone Biopsy, Excisional	52005	Cystoscopy, Ureter Catheter
25111	Remove Wrist Tendon Lesion	52007	Cystoscopy, Biopsy
28290	Correction of Bunion	52010	Cystoscopy, Duct Catheter
28292	Correction of Bunion	52204	Cystoscopy and Treatment
28293	Correction of Bunion	52214	Cystoscopy and Treatment
28294	Correction of Bunion	52224	Cystoscopy and Treatment
28296	Correction of Bunion	52234	Cystoscopy and Treatment
28297	Correction of Bunion	52235	Cystoscopy and Treatment
28298	Correction of Bunion	52240	Cystoscopy and Treatment
28299	Correction of Bunion	52250	Cystoscopy, Radiotracer
32000	Drainage of Chest	52260	Cystoscopy and Treatment
36533	Insertion Access Port	52270	Cystoscopy, Revise Urethra
37609	Temporary Artery Procedure	52275	Cystoscopy, Revise Urethra
38500	Biopsy/Rem Lymph Node	52276	Cystoscopy and Treatment
43200	Esophagus Endoscopy	52277	Cystoscopy and Treatment
43202	w/biopsy	52283	Cystoscopy and Treatment
43220	w/dilation	52290	Cystoscopy and Treatment
43226	w/dilation	52300	Cystoscopy and Treatment
43234	Upper GI Endoscopy Exam	52305	Cystoscopy and Treatment
43235	Upper GI Endoscopy Diag	52310	Cystoscopy and Treatment
43239	Upper GI Endoscopy Biopsy	52315	Cystoscopy and Treatment
43245	Operative Upper GI Endo	57520	Biopsy of Cervix
43247	Operative Upper GI Endo	57522	Biopsy of Cervix
43249	Operative Upper GI Endo	58120	Dilation and Curettage
	Balloon Dilation Esophagus	62270	Spinal Fluid Tap, Diagnostic
43250	Operative Upper GI Endo	85095	Bone Marrow Aspiration Only
43251	Operative Upper GI Endo	85102	Bone Marrow Biopsy
43458	Dilation of Esophagus		
45378	Diagnostic Colonoscopy		

*Refer to CPT-4 for complete description.

T O O L 50

SURGICAL GLOBAL PACKAGE DEFINITIONS

	CPT-4		MEDICARE	
	Minor	**Major (Bundled)**	**Minor**	**Major (Bundled)**
SURGERY CATEGORY	CPT surg codes	All nonstarred CPT surg codes	CPT procedures and non-incision endoscopies	All nonstarred CPT surg codes exc non-incision endoscopies
PREOPERATIVE CARE/ SERVICES	Visit allowed for new patients on same day or if significant services unrelated to surg (use modifier[s])	Not defined	Not unless service is separately identifiable (use modifier)	Not allowed day of/ day before surg exc consultation or initial hosp care
OPERATIVE CARE/SURGERY	Included	Included	Included	Included
COMPLICATIONS DURING SURGERY	Not defined	Not defined	Not defined	Included
ANESTHETICS (Local, Topical, Digital)	Included	Included	Included	Included
POSTOPERATIVE CARE/ SERVICES	None, bill for follow-up visits	"Normal" only included	0–10 days (code-by-code basis)	90 days
TREATMENT FOR COMPLICATIONS DURING POSTOPERATIVE PERIOD	Allowed	Allowed	Not allowed if code has 10-day f/up and trmt during 10 days	Not allowed unless performed in OR
TREATMENT-UNRELATED CONDITIONS DURING POSTOPERATIVE PERIOD	Billing allowed with use of proper modifiers	Billing allowed with use of proper modifiers	Billing allowed with use of proper modifiers	Billing allowed with use of proper modifiers

Definitions specifically for physician providing surgical services or other physicians providing a portion of the surgical global package.

Although the coder cannot expect the clerical and clinical staff to become coders, the inclusion of this information on the medical chart allows personnel to make certain that the coder is alert to assign the appropriate modifier code. This is an excellent example of the staff education aspect of the coder's job.

CODING COMPLEXITIES OF INDIVIDUAL SURGICAL PROCEDURES

Within the surgery section of CPT-4 are specific rules for several anatomical sites. These are also included in the summary information of the CPT-4 manual. It is imperative to refer to the selected CPT-4 code and to review all guidelines, inclusions, and exclusions, in much the same

way as is required for ICD-9-CM diagnostic coding. Presented in this section of the book is a list of key medical terms that apply to the divisions in the CPT-4 book. This list is not inclusive nor does it replace a medical terminology or anatomy and physiology course. It should, however, assist the coder in selecting the appropriate code(s).

It is recommended that every coder possess a current CPT-4 manual. This allows for notations specific to coding guidelines, reminders, hints, and other information needed to code for specific procedures to be recorded. One suggestion would be to take each "breakdown" discussed in the individual surgical procedures section and list the bulleted items needed to code for those services.

For instance, to code for Excision of a Lesion, the student would locate the code(s) in the Integumentary Section, Skin, and Excision of Lesions. Additional

TABLE 12-1   Common Global Surgical Procedures

Obstetrical/Gynecological Procedure	Covered Assistant Surgeon Fee*		Global Follow-Up Days	
	Medicare†	Commercial	Medicare	Commercial
Laparotomy	Yes	No	90	45
Laparoscopy, diagnostic/with biopsy	Yes	Yes	10	15
Laparoscopy, other	Yes	No	90	15-45
Hysteroscopy	No	No	10	15
I/D Bartholin's	No	Yes	10	15
Excision Bartholin's cyst/gland	No	Yes	10	15
Vulvectomy	Yes	No	90	45
Colporrhaphy	Yes	No	90	15
Enterocele	Yes	No	90	15
D&C, nonobstetrical	No	Yes	10	15
Total abdominal hysterectomy	Yes	No	90	90
Total abdominal hysterectomy w/MMK	Yes	No	90	90
Vaginal hysterectomy	Yes	No	90	45
Ligation/transaction fallopian tube(s)	Yes	No	90	45
Salpingectomy	Yes	Yes	90	45
Treatment abortion	No	Yes	90	15

Intended as illustration only; verify/validate information for development of practice specific specialty form(s). Copyright 1998, MD Consultative Services; all rights reserved.
*Assistant surgeon fee may be reimbursable when no qualified resident is available (specify).
†May also apply to third-party carriers following Medicare guidelines.
D&C, Dilation and curettage; MMK, Marshall-Marchetti-Krantz; I/D, incision and drainage.

elements that are needed for this specific coding are discussed. The complete breakdown would look something like the following example. The "bulleted items" would be placed right above the lesion section and would include the following:

- Method (destruction/excision/shaving)
- Nature (malignant, benign)
- Anatomical site
- Size (in cm)
  - *NOTES:* Cannot be combined
    Simple closure included, complicated closures may be coded

From this brief bulleted format, the student can identify from the operative report that codes for lesions will be assigned. The student could turn to the integumentary section, lesions, read the list of needed information, and identify what information to gather from the operative report.

INTEGUMENTARY SYSTEM (10040-19499)

Key Medical Terms

- Lesion
- Centimeters (cm)
- Square Centimeters (sq cm)
- Debridement

- Adjacent Tissue Transfer
- Pinch Skin Graft
- Donor Site
- Recipient Site
- Split Thickness Skin Graft (STSG)
- Full Thickness Skin Graft (FTSG)
- W Plasty/X Plasty/Z Plasty
- Allograft/Homograft
- Xenograft
- Biopsy
- Mastectomy

The integumentary system subsection includes the skin and the subcutaneous and accessory structures. It consists of services such as the following:

- Incision and drainage
- Excision, debridement
- Biopsies
- Shaving of epidermal/dermal lesions
- Excision, benign lesions
- Excision, malignant lesions
- Nails
- Repairs
- Tissue transfers
- Skin grafts
- Skin flaps
- Burns, treatment
- Destruction, lesions
- Breast procedures

Specific guidelines for this subsection follow.

Lesions

This is the same section used for demonstrating the "breaking down" method to locate CPT-4 codes. A lesion is defined as any pathological change in tissue. It may be determined malignant (cancerous) or benign (non-cancerous).

These procedure codes include simple closure (the provider uses the incision as the "approach" by which the lesion excision is performed). A closure other than simple may be billed, as long as the provider has documented the reason why a more complicated closure was medically necessary.

Excision codes are assigned according to the diameter in centimeters of the excised lesion plus margins, *not* according to the size of the incision necessary to remove the lesion. In the case that an operative report indicates size in inches, the conversion is the following:

1 inch 2.54 cm

Multiple lesion removals require multiple codes and should not be combined.

Key elements would again be the following:

- Method (destruction/excision/shaving)
- Nature (malignant, benign)
- Anatomical site
- Size (in cm)
  NOTES: Cannot be combined
  Simple closure included, complicated closures may be coded

Wound/Laceration Repairs

Repair codes may be assigned for wounds repaired with surgical sutures, staples, and surgical glue (commonly referred to as *Dermabond*) only. When Steri-Strips are used for wound closure, they are not considered as repairs. An appropriate Evaluation and Management code may be necessary for the level of history, examination,, and medical decision making.

The information must be documented or the service must be coded as the smallest, simple wound repair. Significant reimbursement may be lost if needed information is missing from the documentation. Educate documenters on missing/needed information. In the event the documenter supplies the needed information, an addendum to information in the documentation must be made before coding may be revised.

Multiple wound repairs of the same anatomical grouping and extent may be combined and reported as a single code. For example, an intermediate repair of the trunk (2.5 cm) and an intermediate repair of the arm (2.5 cm) may be combined and coded as follows:

2.5 cm trunk + 2.5 cm arm = 5.0 cm intermediate repair

12032 Intermediate repair of the trunk, and/or extremities 2.6-7.5 cm

In cases in which multiple complexities or anatomical groupings are involved, the most significant service or most complicated repair would be listed first and the remainder in descending order of significance. Facial laceration repairs are considered more significant than non-facial codes due to the nature of the repair.

Repair complexities are defined as follows:

Simple   Single-layer closure, without extensive debridement
Intermediate Layered closure or single-layer closure, with extensive debridement (must be documented)
Complex   More than layered closure (e.g., scar revisions, traumatic lacerations, creation of defects, W/X/Y/Z plasty (e.g., re-shaping the wound in the shape of a "W," "X," "Y," "Z" to ensure appropriate closure).

Simple debridement is considered an integral part of wound or laceration repair. Only when the wound requires extensive cleaning or debridement may the services be coded according to a higher level of service.

The bulleted list would appear as follows:

- Extent of repair
- Anatomical site
- Size of repair (always in centimeters)
  NOTES: Can be combined when same extent/same anatomical grouping
  Not coded when performed as part of incisional repair

Skin Replacement Surgery and Skin Substitutes

To code skin grafts correctly, the coder must identify the type of graft being performed. They are categorized as follows:

- **Adjacent tissue transfers/rearrangement**
  Not a "free" skin graft, the tissue is not completely removed, but incised on two of three sides and "rotated" or "advanced" into position. The advantage of adjacent tissue transfers is that the vasculature is still attached, and the transfer stands an increased change of success.
- **Pinch skin graft**
  A small amount of tissue, a "pinch," is removed from the original location (donor site) and placed on the new site (recipient site). Codes are assigned based on the recipient site(s) only for all graft codes.
- **Split thickness graft (STSG)**
  Only the top layer of skin is obtained from the donor site and transferred to the recipient site. The recipient site may still have some viable skin tissue and only the top layer of skin is necessary for repair.

- **Full thickness graft (FTSG)**
  The full thickness of skin (all three layers) is harvested from the donor site and transferred to the recipient site. This procedure is used for more extensive wounds and burns.

A number of additional skin graft codes were added to CPT in the 2006 edition to incorporate the many new techniques for skin grafting techniques developed over the recent years. New definitions of some of these techniques are as follows:

- **Skin replacement**
  Tissue or graft that permanently replaces lost skin with healthy skin.
- **Skin substitute**
  Biomaterial, engineered tissue or materials, cells or tissue substituted for skin autograft or allograft.
- **Temporary wound covering**
  Temporary skin surface providing only temporary coverage.
- **Tissue-cultured skin**
  Small portion of tissue is taken and cultured in the laboratory to increase its size. These are typically performed when the patient does not have sufficient skin to obtain a suitable autograft.
- **Acellular dermal replacement grafts**
  These grafts involve synthetic replacement where the dermal layer is permanent, but the epidermal layer is composed of a temporary, usually silicone, substance that needs to be replaced at a later time.
- **Tissue-cultured allogeneic skin substitute**
  Skin substitute cultured in the laboratory contained both the dermal and epidermal layer.

The size of the graft is measured in square centimeters. For this measurement to be obtained, the calculation is as follows:

Width × length of graft = square centimeters

Adjacent tissue transfers/rearrangements such as rotational flaps, advancement flaps, and W/Z plasty procedures include the excision of a lesion in conjunction with advancement or rotational flap. These grafts are used to preserve the integrity of the vessels and adjoining structures.

Code 15000 may be used only when extensive preparation of the site is necessary. It may not be used for debridement or cleaning, but requires the excision of necrotic tissue to prepare the recipient site for the graft.

Grafts may be obtained from a source other than the patient, such as in the case of allografts (grafts obtained from a healthy donor [usually a cadaver]) or xenograft (biological graft or porcine [pig] graft).

Location of the appropriate code(s) from this section would be as follows:

- Type of graft (adjacent/free)
- Extent (pinch, split, full, allograft, xenograft), temporary wound covering, tissue-cultured skin, acellular dermal replacement grafts, tissue-cultured allogeneic skin substitute
- Anatomical location
- Size (sq cm)
  NOTES: Recipient site only coded
  Measurements in sq cm only
  "Each addtl" reported in "units"

Breast Procedures

Incisions, excisions, and reconstructive procedures are included within the anatomical grouping for breast procedures. When reviewing the operative report, identify the extent of the breast excision. When only a portion of a cyst or lesion is removed, the procedure is considered a *biopsy*. Removal of an entire cyst or lesion may be coded on the basis of whether the lesion or cyst is identified by a preoperative marker or clip or is simply excised. Additional codes may be assigned if the preoperative marker or clip is used to identify the cyst or lesion.

Mastectomies are classified as to the extent of the breast removal. Lumpectomies or simple mastectomies encompass removal of only part of the breast and surrounding tissue; a complete mastectomy may involve removal of the breast as well as excision of specific lymph nodes (identified with individual codes). In addition to codes for the extent of the mastectomy, additional codes may be assigned for the implantation of a breast prosthesis (either at the time of the mastectomy or later).

Categories for the breast section that the coder may wish to note in the CPT-4 manual are as follows:

- Type of procedure (incision/excision/repair/reconstruction)
- Extent/method (needle, open)
- Procedure (biopsy, removal)
- Specifics (EX: mastectomy level)
  NOTES: Watch biopsy code techniques.
  Radiological marker must be placed by surgeon for surgeon coding.

STOP AND PRACTICE

Try these integumentary coding exercises for practice in applying the coding guidelines learned in this section. Remember to assign code(s) and modifier(s), and place multiple codes in the appropriate sequence (order).

Code(s)/Modifier(s)

1. Excision malignant lesion, face, 2.0 cm — *11642*
2. Excision malignant lesion, arm, 2.0 cm — *11602*
   Excision malignant lesion, face, 2.5 cm — *11643*
3. Breast biopsy, percutaneous needle — *19100*
4. Laceration repair, 2.0 cm, face — *12011*
5. Laceration repairs as follows:
   Face, 2.0 cm, simple *12011*
   Face, 3.0 cm, intermediate *12052*
   Hand, 2.0 cm simple *12001*
   Arm, 2.0 cm simple *12001*
   Code assignment(s): _____

6. Destruction malignant lesion, 2.0 cm, face *17282* *11642* *pg 54 67*
   Excision malignant lesion, 1.5 cm, face *17282*
   Excision benign lesion, 2.5 cm, arm *11403, 403*
   Code assignment(s): _____

7. Excision malignant lesion, face, 2.0 cm with .5 cm margins — *11643*
8. Split thickness skin graft from thigh to cheek, 2 × 3 cm — *15120*
9. Repair of nail bed — *11760*
10. Adjacent tissue transfer, arm, 20 sq cm with removal of malignant lesion, arm, 16 sq cm — *14021*

MUSCULOSKELETAL SYSTEM (20000-29909)

Key Medical Terms

- Closed Treatment
- Open Treatment
- Percutaneous Skeletal Fixation
- Manipulation
- Internal/External Fixation
- Fascia
- ORIF
- Vertebral Segment
- Vertebral Interspace
- Cervical
- Thoracic
- Lumbar

This section encompasses the repair or revision of the musculoskeletal system. Keep in mind that the services in this subcategory are global and thus include both pre- and postoperative care. Subsections are anatomical sites such as the following:

- General
- Head
- Neck
- Back/flank
- Spine
- Shoulder
- Humerus, elbow
- Forearm, wrist
- Hand, fingers
- Pelvis, hip joint
- Femur, knee joint
- Leg, ankle joint
- Foot, toes
- Casts, strapping, splinting
- Endoscopy, arthroscopy

Note that the subsections of the musculoskeletal section are in anatomical progression. The anatomical sections start at the head and progress down the body to the feet and toes. This makes it simple for the coder to know not only the section (musculoskeletal) but the approximate location of the anatomical site in the section (feet at the end of the chapter, head at the beginning of the chapter). The exception to this progression is the last two subsections: cast/splints and arthroscopies. Because these two sections encompass many anatomical parts, they have been listed at the back of the musculoskeletal section for ease in locating codes specific to these techniques or procedures.

The list of anatomical sites of musculoskeletal procedures breaks down further according to the following technique or procedure performed:

- Incision
- Excision

- Repair, revision, and reconstruction
- Fracture and/or dislocation
- Manipulation (where applicable)
- Arthrodesis (when applicable)

One of the most confusing coding elements pertains to excision of lesions and biopsies. The student must determine whether the excision or biopsy is being performed on the skin (integumentary system) or within the muscles, tendons, ligaments, or bones. This must be determined before locating the appropriate code(s) because they are in different areas.

Injections (under Introduction/Removal)

Trigger point injections are included in the "General" heading of the musculoskeletal system. Because these injections could be performed at multiple sites, they have been listed in the general section instead. Note that the trigger point injection codes are assigned NOT by the number of injections but by the number of trigger points and number of muscles.

Joint injections (arthrocentesis) are also included in the general section of musculoskeletal as well. These codes are assigned on the basis of the size of the joint being injected: small (fingers, toes), medium (TMJ, wrist, elbow, ankle, olecranon bursa, acromioclavicular), and major (shoulder, hip, knee, subacromial bursa).

Removal of hardware codes are also located in this General section. When difficulties are encountered with previously placed wires, pins, or rods, and it becomes necessary to remove these devices, codes from 20670 to 20680 are used. If the removal is performed during the postoperative period of the original fracture or surgical procedure, a modifier 58 (staged or related procedure) would be appended to this secondary procedure. Most hardware removals, however, occur long after the postoperative period and do not require a modifier. Diagnostic statements would be from the V54 series, attention to surgical hardware, as the primary diagnosis.

Bone Grafts

Bone graft harvesting may be billed separately ONLY when it is not listed as part of the primary procedure already billed.

Spine (Vertebral Column) Coding Assignment

Within the spine section, bone grafting and instrumentation codes are usually assigned in addition to the main surgical procedure. Bone grafts are often necessary to replace diseased bone or bone that has been removed as part of the surgical procedure, and are reported with codes from the bone graft section (20900-20938). Note

that these codes all carry a relatively new symbol (∅) that has not been seen up to this point. This symbol indicates that modifier 51 does not need to be assigned to this series of codes even when multiple procedures are performed. CPT understands that codes from the bone graft section are often used in conjunction with other codes and does not see a need to affix the 51 modifier for these procedures.

Many of the codes in this section will require the use of multiple units for services, because a number of the codes are assigned on the basis of "each vertebral segment." For instance, 22600 is explained as "Arthrodesis, posterior or posterolateral technique, single level; cervical below C2 segment." If an arthrodesis is performed on C2/C3, C3/C4, and C4/C5 for instance, code 22614 would be assigned with multiple days/units of "2" rather than as two separate line items on the claim form for two segments. A vertebral segment is defined as "the basic constituent part into which the spine is divided." A vertebral interspace is the compartment between two adjacent vertebral bodies. One vertebral interspace (C2/C3, for example) would be described as one space, the space between the second and third vertebral segments.

Cervical vertebrae are those located in the region from the base of the skull to the top of the back. The thoracic spine includes the vertebrae from the base of the neck to just above the small of the back. The lumbar spine includes the vertebrae in the lower back and terminates just above the top of the buttocks.

For codes from the spine section to be assigned, the following breakdown should be used:

- Procedure performed (excision, fracture, manipulation)
- Anatomical site (intervertebral space or vertebral segment, cervical [C], thoracic [T], or lumbar [L] area of spine)
- Number of vertebral spaces or segments
  NOTES: Arthrodesis may be coded in addition to surgical procedure.
  Instrumental may be coded in addition to surgical procedure.
  Modifier 62 should be used when two surgeons work together, each as primary surgeon, on spinal procedures.

Fractures/Dislocations

Caution should be applied in reading the descriptions of services. Care must be taken to determine the type of procedure and extent of treatment already included in the service, such as closed, open, with or without manipulation, or with traction.

Fractures and dislocations occupy probably the largest section and number of codes of any section in the CPT-4 manual. These services are perhaps the easiest to code with the following breakdown of services performed.

- Anatomical site
- Specific site (distal, proximal, shaft)
- Open/closed
- With/without manipulation
- With/without fixation (internal/external)

    NOTES: Fracture/dislocation care includes application of initial cast
    Refractures or reductions require modifier code(s)

Keep in mind the definitions of fractures in order to assign correct code(s) for services:

Closed treatment	Surgical procedure does not involve surgically opening the site of the fracture for the purpose of repair.
Open treatment	Procedure involves surgical opening of the site and visualization of the fracture for repair and treatment. Open treatment may also include a remote opening to place an intramedullary nail or rod at the fracture site even though the fracture is not visualized.
Percutaneous skeletal fixation	Fixation device or appliance is placed across the fracture site, usually with the assistance of x-ray imaging.

Note: The type of fracture (e.g., closed or open) may have no correlation with the type of treatment performed. For example, a closed fracture may require open treatment or skeletal fixation, and it should be coded accordingly.

External Fixation

External fixation may be billed separately ONLY when it is not listed as part of the primary procedure already billed. External fixation is the use of external skeletal pins and wires to treat a fracture or other bone deformity.

Fracture Rereductions

When it is necessary to rereduce a fracture, exactly as performed previously, modifier 76 (same physician) or modifier 77 (different physician) may be used. If the fracture must be reduced by another method (e.g., closed the first time, open the second; no manipulation the first time, manipulation required the second time) modifiers 76 and 77 would not be appropriate. In this case, modifier 58 would be appropriate (if the first and second procedure were both performed outside the OR).

Application of Casts/Splints

When musculoskeletal definitive, restorative, or invasive procedures are performed to realign fractures, the application and removal of the cast or splint that immobilized that fracture/dislocation are included in the surgical code. This is considered part of the surgical procedure. If the treating provider does not provide the restorative, definitive care for the fracture or dislocation but perhaps only stabilizes the fracture until another provider gives treatment, the first provider may code for the history, examination, and medical decision making (an E & M code), and the application of the cast or splint by the provider or a licensed employee under the provider's supervision.

For example, a patient arrives at the emergency department and is given a diagnosis of misaligned fracture of the distal radius. The fracture repair will require surgical intervention, so the ED physician orders the application of a splint until the patient can see the orthopedic surgeon. Because the nursing staff at the hospital applied the splint and they are not employees under the supervision of the provider, the physician may not code for the application of the splint. In the office setting, the physician or his employed representative would apply the splint, so assignment of a code for the splint application would be appropriate.

Arthroscopic Procedures

In addition to the surgical procedures outlined in the musculoskeletal section, the last subsection is arthroscopic procedures, those performed through a scope for visualization of a joint. As with the other surgical sections, the codes are listed in anatomical order starting at the temporomandibular joint and ending at the foot.

When arthroscopic procedures are coded, the following guidelines should be applied:

1. When surgery is performed arthroscopically, the diagnostic arthroscopic procedure is included and should not be coded (term separate procedure is included).
2. Multiple arthroscopic procedures on the same anatomical site should have the modifier 51 appended to indicate multiple procedures.
3. When arthroscopic procedures are followed by a portion of the surgery performed open, both codes may be used. If no surgical intervention is performed through an arthroscopic procedure, a diagnostic arthroscopic code may be assigned in addition to the appropriate open surgical codes. A modifier 51 should be assigned to the least significant procedure(s).
4. In the case of knee arthroscopies according to CPT guidelines, the three compartments of the knee (medial, lateral, and femoropatellar) are considered distinct. When different procedures are performed on different compartments of the knee, they may be coded (e.g., if a meniscectomy is performed to the

lateral compartment and a synovectomy is performed to the femoropatellar joint, both procedures may be coded).

Codes for arthroscopic procedures would be broken down as follows:

- Technique (arthroscopic rather than open/closed)
- Anatomical site
- Procedures performed (e.g., meniscectomy, release, repair)
  - *NOTES*: Multiple procedures require the use of modifier 51 when performed in the same anatomical location.
    Procedures converted from arthroscopic to open need modifier 51.
    Anatomical modifiers RT/LT would be appropriate in many instances.

Anatomical Modifiers

Caution should be used in the musculoskeletal section because many codes will require the inclusion of a modifier code(s) to the procedure. The use of anatomical modifiers, however, is often misunderstood, and codes are assigned incorrectly. Keep in mind that the anatomical modifier(s) RT (right side of body) and LT (left side of body) should only be assigned to codes that are specific to anatomical sites that only have two sites. For instance, in the following example:

> Code 26415 Excision of extensor tendon, with implantation of synthetic rod for delayed tendon graft, hand or finger, each rod an RT/LT modifier or an FA to F9 modifier could not be appended because the code refers to both fingers and hands.
>
> In this example, though, Code 25800 Arthrodesis, wrist, complete without bone graft only the wrist is referred to; therefore because one has only a right and left wrist, the application of either an RT or an LT modifier would be appropriate.

Although the addition or omission of this anatomical modifier may not seem significant, it may result in payment denial for services, or the carrier may return the claim with a notation such as "not valid modifier for this service." Both outcomes result in nonpayment or delay in payment for services.

STOP AND PRACTICE

Try these musculoskeletal coding exercises for practice in applying the coding guidelines learned in this section.

	Code(s)/Modifier(s)
1. Removal of displaced pin from fracture site	20670
2. Closed repair, distal radius fracture	25600
3. Shoulder capsulorrhaphy	23450
4. Rotator cuff repair	23410
5. I/D, deep abscess, forearm	25035
6. Removal FB, musculature, thigh	27372
7. Right shoulder arthroscopy with claviculectomy	29824
8. Diagnostic right knee arthroscopy with medial/lateral meniscectomy	29880 29870
9. Repair of left calcaneus fracture with cast application	28400
10. Arthroscopic TMJ repair	29804

RESPIRATORY SYSTEM (30000-32999)

Key Medical Terms

- Rhino
- Septo
- Transbronchial
- Thoracentesis
- Broncho
- Atelectasis
- Hemoptysis
- Orthopnea
- Dyspnea
- URI
- COPD

This system, similar to the musculoskeletal system, follows the anatomical progression of the system. The system starts with the nose, where air is breathed, through the sinuses, the larynx, down the trachea, and into the lungs. Locating the right subsection within the respiratory system section is straightforward.

Subsections of the respiratory system section include the following:

- Nose
- Accessory sinuses
- Larynx
- Trachea, bronchi
- Lungs, pleura

Accessory Sinus Procedures

Most of these procedures are performed endoscopically (codes 31231 to 31294). In many instances, multiple procedures will be performed (modifier 51), often bilaterally (modifier 50). Keep in mind that there are three sets of sinus cavities, ethmoid, maxillary, and sphenoid, and each set has right and left sides. Once the procedure is identified as a sinus endoscopy, the following information should be gathered from the operative report:

- Sinus cavity(ies) procedures performed
- Specific procedure(s) performed
  NOTES: Watch for separate procedure code(s)
  Apply multiple modifiers appropriately (most significant to reimbursement first)

Laryngoscopy Procedures

Laryngoscopic procedures may be direct or indirect and sometimes are identified as microdirect or microindirect, indicating that some type of operating microscope may have been used to successfully complete the procedure(s). Separate codes are assigned when procedures are performed with the use of an operating microscope. Make certain that magnifying loupes are not used in these instances.

Laryngoscopies should be coded with the following information:

- Diagnostic/operative
- Direct/indirect
- With/without operating microscopy
- Specific procedure(s) performed
  NOTES: Diagnostic Laryngoscopy included in Surgical Interventions
  Modifier 51 for multiple procedures

Bronchoscopy

Bronchoscopy is performed via an endoscopic approach for the purpose of visualizing the trachea, vocal cords, and bronchi. Brushings, biopsies, and other interventional procedures may be performed at the time of a diagnostic bronchoscopy. The "separate procedure" rule applies, and diagnostic bronchoscopy would NOT be coded when a surgical bronchoscopic procedure was performed. Careful attention should be made to the biopsy codes because the approach is different (transbronchial/bronchial) as are the number of site(s). For instance, code 31628 is for a bronchoscopic transbronchial biopsy(ies) of a single lobe, without regard to the number of biopsies performed to that one lobe. Additional biopsy(ies) can only be coded in this instance when they are taken from another lobe.

Breakdown for this section would be as follows:

- Diagnostic vs surgical
- Biopsy(ies)/site(s)
- Procedure(s) performed
  NOTE: Modifier 51 when multiple procedures performed endoscopically
  Modifier RT/LT to indicate left or right bronchus

Thoracentesis and Thoracostomy

When a puncture is made for the purpose of inserting a chest tube for drainage of air or fluid from the pleural space so a collapsed lung may be expanded, the procedure is known as a tube *thoracostomy*. When a puncture is made for the sole purpose of removing fluid or air, such a procedure would be coded to the *thoracentesis* code(s).

STOP AND PRACTICE

Try these respiratory coding exercises for practice in applying coding guidelines covered in this section.

	Code(s)/Modifier(s)
1. Bronchoscopy, diagnostic	31622
2. Tracheostomy	31600
3. Tracheotomy	31502
4. Thoracentesis with tube placement	32002
5. Endoscopic ethmoidectomy, bilateral / Right maxillary antrostomy / Concha bullosa resection	31256
6. Endoscopic sphenoidotomy with tissue removal	31288
7. Laryngoscopy with FB removal	31511
8. Emergency endotracheal intubation	31500
9. Bronchoscopy with washings	31622
10. Bronchoscopic transbronchial lung biopsy, LLL / Bronchoscopic transbronchial lung biopsy, RUL	31628 / 31632

CARDIOVASCULAR SYSTEM (33010-37799)

Key Medical Terms

- Pulse generator
- Pacemaker battery
- Atrioventricular leads
- Pacemaker
- Defibrillator
- CABG (coronary artery bypass graft)
- Angioplasty
- Atherectomy
- Thrombectomy
- Thromboendarterectomy
- Aneurysm
- AAA (abdominal aortic aneurysm)
- Bypass graft
- Central venous access device
- Catheterization
- Endarterectomy
- PTCA (percutaneous transluminal coronary angioplasty)
- Anastomosis

Subcategories of the cardiovascular system section include the following:

- Heart and pericardium
- Arteries and veins

Note that heart catheterization, coronary angioplasty, stents, and atherectomies are NOT included in the cardiovascular surgery section because they are considered noninvasive in nature. They are located in the medicine section of CPT-4 and are discussed later. The cardiovascular section encompasses surgical intervention for cardiovascular disease.

Cardiovascular Guidelines

Pacemaker/Defibrillator Systems

A number of assist devices are placed in the cardiovascular system to aid in the regulation of heart rhythm. A pacemaker is implanted for the purpose of regulating an irregular heartbeat and a defibrillator is usually implanted when heart has stopped beating or the rhythm is extremely slow (bradycardia). There are a number of factors to consider when coding for pacemakers and defibrillators, and they are outlined as follows:

- Permanent/replacement/temporary/removal/repair/conversion
- Pacemaker/defibrillator
- Approach for procedure
- With/without replacement of electrodes
- Electrode(s) replaced (atrial/ventricular)

NOTES: Pulse generator is the "battery" of the pacemaker
When replacing pulse generator, code for removal and replacement
Transvenous extraction of electrode 33244
Insertion of pacing electrode 33244 or 33225

Arterial Grafting for Coronary Artery Bypass

When arterial-venous grafting associated with coronary artery bypass is reported, the following codes are appropriate:

Arterial graft 33533-33536
Combined arterial-venous graft 33517-33523

Combined Arterial-Venous Grafting for Coronary Bypass

When arterial-venous grafting for coronary bypass procedure is reported, the following services are also coded and billed:

Combined arterial-venous graft 33517-33523)
Arterial graft 33533-33536

To code coronary bypass grafts correctly, the coder must determine the following:

- Venous/arterial or venous and arterial grafting
- Number of grafts
- Procurement of grafts (upper extremity 35500; femoropopliteal 35572), separately codeable

Venous Access Devices

Venous access devices (VADs) and catheters are also included in the cardiovascular section of surgery. The coder must determine the type of device that is being placed to assign the correct codes for these procedures. A central venous catheter is placed temporarily, usually for short periods of time (10 to 14 days) to supplement IV infusion. Venous access devices involve the placement of a permanently implanted catheter under the skin, and in some cases, include an implanted reservoir. These devices are implanted for long periods of time and are completely hidden beneath the skin. For the venous access devices to be coded correctly, the following information should be extracted from the operative report:

- Introduction, removal, revision of venous catheter
- Venous versus peripheral placement
- Tunneled versus nontunneled catheter
- Age of patient
- Placement of pump or port in addition to catheter

STOP AND PRACTICE

Try these cardiovascular coding exercises for practice in applying the coding guidelines learned in this section.

Code(s)/Modifier(s)

1. Removal of pacemaker pulse generator   *33233*

2. Removal of old pacemaker pulse generator   *33233 -*
   Insertion of new pacemaker pulse generator   *33212*

3. Revision of pacemaker skin pocket   *33222*

4. CABG, venous grafting, 3 vessels   *33519 33512*

5. CABG, arterial/venous grafting, 2 vessel   *33518 - 33534*

6. Aortic peripheral atherectomy, open   *35481*

7. Thromboendarterectomy, subclavian thoracic incision   *35311*

8. Balloon angioplasty, percutaneous, iliac vessel   *35473*

9. Blood transfusion   *36430 pg 159*

10. Venipuncture, age 7   *36415*

HEMIC AND LYMPHATIC SYSTEMS (38100-38999)

Subcategories of the hemic and lymphatic systems section include the following:

- Bone marrow, stem cell transplantation
- Lymph nodes, lymphatic channels

MEDIASTINUM AND DIAPHRAGM (39000-39599)

Only two subcategories exist for this section, specifically the mediastinum and diaphragm. Procedures for these two subcategories include surgical techniques of incision, excision, repair, and endoscopy, and unlisted procedures.

DIGESTIVE SYSTEM (40490-49999)

Key Medical Terms

- Cholecysto
- Gastro
- Esophago
- Hepato
- Laparo
- Spleno
- Entero
- Fistula
- Hematemesis
- Hernia
- Snare
- Dilation
- Ablation
- Anastomosis
- EGD
- UGI

Subcategories of the digestive system section include the following:

- Lips
- Vestibule of mouth
- Tongue, floor of mouth
- Dentoalveolar structures
- Palate, uvula
- Salivary glands, ducts
- Pharynx, adenoids, tonsils
- Esophagus
- Stomach
- Intestines
- Meckel's diverticulum, mesentery
- Appendix
- Rectum
- Anus
- Liver
- Biliary tract
- Pancreas
- Abdomen, peritoneum, omentum

The subcategories by anatomical section begin with the mouth and end with the anus region, including internal organs involved in the digestive process.

General Guidelines and Definitions

Several types of endoscopic procedures are categorized within the digestive system section, including the following:

Proctosigmoidoscopy	Examination of rectum or sigmoid colon
Sigmoidoscopy	Examination of entire rectum, sigmoid colon, and possibly a portion of descending colon
Colonoscopy	Examination of entire colon, from rectum to cecum, possibly including examination of terminal ileum

Some additional coding guidelines should be applied to endoscopic procedures in the digestive disease section, including the following:

- Codes are assigned based on the technique used, not the number of lesions, tumors, or polyps removed.
- Additional procedures performed on the same anatomical site or sites are assigned modifier 51.
- When multiple anatomical sites are involved, each code for a specific separate site is assigned a modifier 59.

As with other global surgical procedures, the approach or vehicle by which a procedure is performed is considered BUNDLED. Therefore when a surgical endoscopy is performed, it includes a diagnostic endoscopy.

An appendectomy performed at the time of another major procedure is considered incidental (BUNDLED) and therefore is not coded or billed. Only when the appendectomy is performed for a specifically indicated purpose at the time of the other procedure should it be coded and considered for payment. Make certain the medical documentation clearly indicates the medical necessity for the appendectomy.

Hernia repairs included in this section are divided by the type of hernia (inguinal, femoral, incisional, ventral, epigastric, umbilical) and by the category (initial or recurrent). Other subdivisions include the presenting age of the patient and the type of hernia presentation (reducible, strangulated).

Tonsillectomies and adenoidectomies are also included in the digestive disease section. They should be assigned codes based on the age of the patient; whether the procedures are primary or secondary to another surgical procedure; and whether tonsils, adenoids, or both are involved.

Excisional codes for the appendix and gallbladder are included in the digestive disease section as well. The coder should be careful to assign codes for these procedures based on the technique used (surgical [open] versus laparoscopic).

Esophagogastroduodenoscopy

STOP AND PRACTICE

Try these digestive disease coding exercises for practice in applying the coding guidelines discussed in this section. Continue to "break down" the exercises as discussed previously.

	Code(s)/Modifier(s)
1. Exploratory laparotomy	49000
2. T & A, age 20	42821
3. EGD with polypectomy by snare *electrified wire*	43251
4. Esophagoscopy with FB removal	43215
5. Laparoscopic appendectomy	44970
6. Initial inguinal hernia repair, age 3	49500 49505 *5 years & older*
7. Cholecystectomy	47562
8. EGD with dilation of esophagus	43235
9. Colonoscopy, diagnostic with EGD with 4 biopsies	44389
10. Diagnostic anoscopy	46600

URINARY SYSTEM (50010-53899)

Key Medical Terms

- Urino
- Cysto
- Nephro
- Uretero
- Urethra
- Cystourethroscopy
- UTI

Subsections of the urinary system section include the following:

- Kidney
- Ureter
- Bladder
- Urethra

Cystoscopy, urethroscopy, and cystourethroscopy are included in this section and are broken down by the services performed. When a secondary endoscopic procedure performed at the same anatomical site constitutes more than the usual description for the service, modifier 22 should be appended. Diagnoses for both conditions should be listed, and documentation as to the performance of both procedures should be appropriately recorded in the medical record.

STOP AND PRACTICE

Try these urinary coding scenarios based on the coding guidelines from this section.

		Code(s)/Modifier(s)
1.	Diagnostic cystourethroscopy	52351
2.	Open drainage of renal abscess	50020
3.	Injection procedure for cystography	52281
4.	Needle aspiration of bladder	51060
5.	Simple cystometrogram	51725-51
	Simple uroflowmetry	51736
6.	Cysto with placement of ureteral stent	52332
7.	Urethral biopsy	50955
8.	Dilation of urethral stricture with dilator, male	53600 52281
9.	Laparoscopic radical nephrectomy	50545
10.	Partial laparoscopic nephrectomy	50543 50549 50545-52

MALE GENITAL SYSTEM (54000-55899)

Key Medical Terms

- Orchido
- Prostate
- Vasectomy
- Circumcision
- BPH

Subsections of the male genital system section include the following:

- Penis
- Testis
- Epididymis
- Tunica vaginalis
- Scrotum
- Vas deferens
- Spermatic cord
- Seminal vesicles
- Prostate

Procedures included in the male genital section include circumcision, vasectomy, and prostate procedures. Circumcision codes are assigned according to the age of the patient and the technique used. Vasectomies involve the excision or removal of the vas deferens and therefore are listed under that subsection in the male genital system. Note that prostate procedures may be listed in either the male genital system or urinary system based on the specific function of the prostate involved.

INTERSEX SURGERY (55970-55980)

Only two codes exist in this section, one for male-to-female intersex surgery, another for female-to-male. Historically, these are not services covered by third-party carriers.

LAPAROSCOPY/HYSTEROSCOPY

Because the laparoscope is the vehicle by which the laparoscopic procedure is performed in this section, the diagnostic laparoscopy should be BUNDLED in the surgical procedure. Also, laparoscopic procedures may be used for males or females, and any method may be used for the procedure (e.g., cautery, CO_2, laser).

When two or more procedures are performed laparoscopically, the subsequent procedures should be reported only when time and risk factors justify additional consideration for reimbursement.

With the printing of CPT-4 in 2000, laparoscopically performed services are now grouped within the specific anatomical area of the procedure. For that reason, they are assigned various CPT-4 codes within several areas within the surgical section of CPT-4.

FEMALE GENITAL SYSTEM (56405-58999)

Key Medical Terms

- Salpingo
- Oophoro
- Hystero
- Colpo
- Vagino
- Meno
- Vulvo
- Tubal ligation
- Laparoscopy
- Hysteroscopy
- Colpocleisis
- Colpourethrocystopexy

Subsections of the female genital system section include the following:

- Vulva, perineum, introitus
- Vagina
- Cervix uteri
- Corpus uteri
- Oviduct

- Ovary
- In vitro fertilization

Vulvectomy codes are defined as follows:

Simple	removal of skin/superficial subcutaneous tissue
Radical	removal of skin/deep subcutaneous tissue
Partial	removal of less than 80% of vulvar area
Complete	removal of more than 80% of vulvar area

Appendectomies are commonly performed at the time of hysterectomies. Remember that appendectomies performed with other intraabdominal procedures are considered incidental unless performed for a specified purpose at the time of another surgical procedure.

Tubal ligation may be performed under many circumstances. Codes are located throughout the female genital and maternity care section. This procedure may be performed laparoscopically by clamp or device, by fulguration, at the time of a C-section, or intraabdominal surgery, or during the period immediately after other delivery during the same hospitalization.

MATERNITY CARE AND DELIVERY (59000-59899)

Key Medical Terms

- Cesarean delivery (C-section)
- VBAC
- Para
- Gravida
- Incomplete abortion
- Missed abortion

The **global** maternity care package encompasses the antepartum (preoperative care), delivery (surgical care), and postpartum (postoperative) care of the patient. Because this care encompasses a 9-month period, and many patients may relocate or select another physician or provider during this time, specific CPT-4 codes are assigned for antepartum care, postpartum care, or delivery care.

General Guidelines and Definitions

The global obstetrical period encompasses the following:

Antepartum (Preop): Initial and subsequent history, physical examinations, weights, blood pressures, and other recordings

Routine urinalysis
Monthly visits (to 28 weeks)
Biweekly visits (to 36 weeks)
Weekly visits (to delivery)
Delivery (Operative): Admission to hospital
Uncomplicated labor
Vaginal delivery (with or without episiotomy; with or without forceps) OR
Cesarean delivery
Postpartum (Postop): Hospital or office visits for normal postpartum care after delivery

ALL services other than those outlined here may be coded and billed with appropriate codes from correct sections of CPT-4. A modifier code probably will be necessary to explain the unusual circumstances (complication), along with medical documentation to establish medical necessity for additional services listed outside the global component.

There is much controversy among third-party carriers regarding what services may be billed in addition to the OB package charge. If the practice provides obstetrical services regularly, the coder may wish to build these codes into the Third-Party Contract Worksheets. For instance, cephalic version (i.e., the manual "turning" of the fetus) obviously involves additional time and surgical risk. Many carriers do not reimburse for this service, with the explanation that this service is commonly provided to obstetrical patients.

The coder may wish to refer to CPT-4 and the coding guidelines established by the obstetrical/gynecological specialty organization(s) to develop a coding method for his or her practice. Keep in mind that the coder must code on the basis of these guidelines, NOT according to what the individual carrier(s) will accept, recognize, or pay.

High-risk pregnancies, which involve more than the normal number of visits or additional diagnostic or therapeutic services, should be coded with the appropriate E & M, surgical, or other CPT-4 codes. A diagnosis should be provided, indicating the reason for the additional services, including the diagnostic code for supervision of high-risk pregnancy.

Multiple deliveries that encompass the entire maternity period (antepartum, delivery, and postpartum) are coded with one code selected from the obstetrical package codes based on the delivery type (vaginal, C-section, or successful/unsuccessful vaginal after previous C-section) as well as additional codes for each additional delivery.

Because many maternity patients will not complete their full global period with one physician or group, codes are also available in this section segregated by antepartum visits only, delivery only, and postpartum only to accommodate these circumstances.

STOP AND PRACTICE

Try these exercises for the male, female, and maternity section of CPT-4 based on the coding guidelines learned in these sections.

	Code(s)/Modifier(s)
1. Vaginal delivery only	59409
2. Cesarean delivery, antepartum, delivery, and postpartum	59510
3. Incomplete abortion, completed surgically	59812
4. Amniocentesis	59000
5. Abdominal hysterectomy with oophorectomy	58150
6. Simple vulvectomy	56620 or 56625
7. Transurethral resection of prostate	52601
8. Vasectomy	55250
9. D & C	
10. Laparoscopic tubal ligation by fulguration	58670

ENDOCRINE SYSTEM (60000-60699)

Subsections of the endocrine system section include the following:

- Thyroid gland
- Parathyroid, thymus, adrenal glands, carotid body

NERVOUS SYSTEM (61000-64999)

Key Medical Terms

- Neuro
- Lamino
- Anesthesia
- Cranio
- Encephalo
- Myelo
- Neurolytic substance
- CSF
- Laminectomy
- Laminotomy

Subsections of the nervous system section include the following:

- Skull, meninges, brain
- Spine, spinal cord
- Extracranial nerves, peripheral nerves, autonomic nerves

General Guidelines and Definitions

Procedures included in this section are categorized as follows:

Approach	procedure necessary to expose the lesion
Definitive	repair, biopsy, resection, excision of lesions, and primary closure
Repair/ Reconstruction	extensive grafting or repair is required

Arthrodesis	surgical fixation of joint by fusion of joint surfaces
Corpectomy	removal of entire vertebral body or vertebral body resection
Diskectomy	excision of intervertebral disk
Laminectomy	incision of posterior arch of vertebra
Laminotomy	division of lamina of vertebra

Procedures of the nervous system involve laminectomy (surgical excision of lamina) and laminotomy (incision of lamina). Although other sections of CPT-4 have codes that bundle multiple elements necessary to most surgical protocols, the same is not true for some spinal surgery. Because of the delicate nature of surgery, the approach, definitive, and repair or reconstructive procedure are typically all billable under CPT-4 guidelines. The coder should note any exclusions; however, in this section, multiple procedures are codable or billable for these intricate and complex procedures.

The insertion of spinal catheters for pain management is also included in the nervous system surgical section. This procedure involves the placement of a permanent catheter for back pain management.

Other pain management codes are included in this section for epidural, lumbar, cervical, and thoracic injections not performed through an indwelling catheter. These are found in the Injection, Drainage, or Aspiration section of the Spine and Spinal Cord section.

EYE AND OCULAR ADNEXA (65091-68899)

Key Medical Terms

- Kerato
- Conjunctivo
- Sclero
- Blepharo
- Enucleation
- Cataract
- Phacoemulsification
- Strabismus
- Intracapsular

- Extracapsular
- EOMI
- PERRLA
- OD
- OS
- OU

Subsections of the eye and ocular adnexa sections include the following:

- Eyeball
- Anterior segment
- Posterior segment
- Ocular adnexa
- Conjunctiva

Ophthalmological examinations and refractions are NOT included in the eye and ocular adnexa section because they are not considered surgical. They are located instead in the medicine section of CPT-4, which is discussed later.

Cataract and strabismus operations are included in the eye section. When assigning codes for cataract extraction, the coder must determine whether the extraction was extracapsular or intracapsular and whether the intraocular lens prosthesis was placed at the time of the cataract extraction or later.

Strabismus procedures involve the straightening or stretching of vertical or horizontal muscles or both to correct what typically is referred to as "cross eyes" or "lazy eye." The coder must determine whether the muscles involved are horizontal or vertical, as well as the number of muscles corrected.

AUDITORY SYSTEM (69000-69990)

Key Medical Terms

- Tympano
- Myringo
- Oto

- Labyrintho
- Stapes
- Cochlear
- Cerumen
- Ventilating tube
- PE tube
- AD
- AS
- AU
- HEENT
- IOL

Subsections of the auditory system section include the following:

- External ear
- Middle ear
- Inner ear
- Temporal bone, middle fossa approach

Hearing and other diagnostic auditory evaluations are NOT included in the auditory section of the surgery section but rather in the medicine section of CPT-4, because they are not surgical in nature.

The most common procedure performed in this section would likely be the insertion of ventilating tubes into the ear (typically performed on children). Codes are assigned based on whether a myringotomy only (incision) is performed or whether a new opening is created (for placement of a tube). Codes are also assigned based on whether general or local anesthesia is used, as well as the patient's age.

STOP AND PRACTICE

Try these coding exercises for the nervous system and sense organs using the coding guidelines discussed in these sections. Remember to place the code(s) in the correct order, eliminate those procedures that are "bundled," and add modifiers accordingly.

Code(s)/Modifier(s)

1. Extracapsular cataract extraction with IOL — 66983
2. Strabismus surgery, 2 horizontal muscles, rt eye — 67312 - RT
3. Creation of subarachnoid/subdural-peritoneal shunt — 63740
4. Elevation of simple skull fracture — 62000
5. Nerve block, by anesthetic, facial nerve — 64402
6. Implantation of neurostimulator electrodes, percutaneous — 64553-64565
7. Suture 3 digital nerves of hand — 64831 + 64832x2
8. Repair of carpal tunnel nerve — 64721
9. Tympanostomy with tube placement bilateral with general anesthesia — 69436-50
10. Removal of cerumen — 69210

CHAPTER IN REVIEW

CERTIFICATION REVIEW

- Global surgical services include the preoperative care, surgery, and normal uncomplicated postoperative follow-up.
- Bundled procedures apply to those services that are considered global services.
- Incidental procedures are services considered insignificant and therefore are included in the global surgery component.
- Laceration repairs are classified as simple, intermediate, or complex.
- The antepartum period of maternity care correlates with the preoperative period for other surgical services.
- The postpartum period of maternity care correlates with the postoperative period for other surgical services.
- Fracture repairs are classified as open or closed procedures, and they do not necessarily correlate with the injury description of open or closed.
- The proper use of modifier codes for surgery services often determines whether services typically included in the global component should be considered for payment.
- When a diagnostic approach is undertaken followed by a definitive surgery procedure, the diagnostic approach is considered "incidental" or "bundled" in the major surgery procedure.
- The codes for application of casts are included in the surgery section. The initial cast is considered part of the global component when it is applied at the time of the surgical procedure and by the same physician. Additional casts, or those placed by other than the surgeon, may be coded separately.

STUDENT STUDY GUIDE

- Study Chapter 12.
- Review the Learning Objectives for Chapter 12.
- Complete the Stop and Practice exercises.
- Review the Certification Review for Chapter 12.
- Complete the Chapter Review exercise, assigning the appropriate CPT-4 codes and modifiers.

CHAPTER REVIEW EXERCISE

Review the surgical components and assign the appropriate CPT-4 codes and modifiers.

1. LEFT BREAST MASS
   Preoperative diagnosis: Rule out breast carcinoma
   Postoperative diagnosis: Same
   55-year-old female presented with a left breast mass, which was recommended for left breast biopsy. The options, risks, alternative treatments, and exact nature of the procedure were described in detail to the patient, and she seemed to understand.
   Patient was taken to the operating room; under general anesthesia, left breast was prepped and draped in a sterile fashion. Left infraareolar incision was made, mass was dissected free of surrounding tissue. Hemostasis was obtained, wound was closed with interrupted 0-Vicryl, 4-0 Vicryl subcutaneous to the skin. Patient tolerated the procedure well and was taken to the Recovery Room in stable condition.
   Adam Westgate, M.D.
   CPT-4 PROCEDURE CODE(S):   ICD-9-CM CODE(S):

   _____   _____

   _____   _____

2. CHOLECYSTECTOMY
   Preoperative diagnosis: Cholecystitis, cholelithiasis
   Postoperative diagnosis: Same
   Operation: Cholecystectomy with operative cholangiogram
   31-year-old white female presented with midepigastric and right upper quadrant pain increasing in intensity. Evaluation revealed multiple gallstones, and surgery was recommended. The options, risks, alternative treatments, and exact nature of the procedure were described in detail, and she seemed to understand well.
   Patient was taken to the operating room; under adequate general anesthesia, the abdomen was prepped and draped in a sterile fashion. The stomach and bladder were drained and supraumbilical incision was made. The Veress needle was used for institution of the pneumoperitoneum. A 10-mm port was placed, as well as the usual upper paramedian 10-mm port and lateral 5-mm ports. Gallbladder was retracted up to its bed using blunt dissection and cautery. The cystic duct was identified, and an intraoperative cholangiogram was read as normal. The cystic duct and cystic artery were ligated and divided. The gallbladder was dissected free of surrounding tissue with cautery, and was removed through the upper paramedian port. The right upper quadrant was then irrigated. After hemostasis was assured, wounds were closed with 2-0 Vicryl and 4-0 Vicryl subcuticular. Skin incisions were then infiltrated with Marcaine, at which time the patient was taken to the Recovery Room in stable condition.

Adam Westgate, M.D.
CPT-4 PROCEDURE CODE(S):   ICD-9-CM CODE(S):

_____   _____

_____   _____

3. RIGHT BREAST MASS

Preoperative diagnosis: Right breast mass

Postoperative diagnosis: Same

Operation: Right subcutaneous mastectomy

This is a 70-year-old male who presented with enlarging right breast mass, unresponsive to conservative treatment. He was recommended for mastectomy. The options, risks, alternative treatments, and exact nature of the procedure were described in detail to the patient, and he seemed to understand adequately.

The patient was taken to the operating room, where, under general anesthesia, the right breast was prepped and draped in a sterile fashion. An inferior incision was made, the large mass was dissected free of surrounding tissue, and all breast tissue was removed down to the pectoralis muscle. Clinically, it appeared to be benign. There was a fair amount of dead space following the resection; a Penrose drain was placed in the depths of the wound, brought out through the inferior wound, and sutured in place with 2-0 silk. The wound was then closed in layers with interrupted 2-0 Vicryl, and 4-0 Vicryl subcuticular on the skin. Sterile pressure dressing was applied. Patient was taken to the Recovery Room in stable condition, with drain in place and functioning well.

Rachel Perez, M.D.
CPT-4 PROCEDURE CODE(S):   ICD-9-CM CODE(S):

_____   _____

_____   _____

4. CATARACT, RIGHT EYE

Patient is a 75-year-old gentleman with a visually significant cataract of the right eye. He was seen preoperatively by his family physician and cleared for local anesthetic. Patient was brought into the outpatient surgical suite and underwent uncomplicated phacoemulsification and posterior lens implant of the right eye under local standby using topical

anesthetic. He was taken to the Recovery Room in good condition.

Linda Patrick, M.D.
CPT-4 PROCEDURE CODE(S):   ICD-9-CM CODE(S):

_____   _____

_____   _____

5. HIATAL HERNIA

Preoperative diagnosis: Dysphagia

Postoperative diagnosis: Hiatal hernia with reflux and distal esophageal stricture

Operation: Upper GI endoscopy with biopsy
Esophageal dilatation

This is an 81-year-old male who presented with increasing dysphagia and trouble swallowing. He was recommended for endoscopy after the options, risks, alternative treatments, and exact nature of the procedure were described in detail, and the patient seemed to understand. Patient was taken to the endoscopy suite, under adequate topical anesthesia; the Olympus endoscope was inserted without difficulty. The proximal and midesophagus were normal. The distal esophagus showed a circumferential stricture, which was biopsied. There was also a hiatal hernia. Upon entering the stomach, mild inflammation was noted and the antrum was biopsied for *Helicobacter*. The pyloric channel and duodenum were clean. J-maneuver revealed no fundic abnormalities. The endoscope was withdrawn. The patient tolerated the procedure well. He was then dilated to a 42-French Maloney dilator.

Rachel Perez, M.D.
CPT-4 PROCEDURE CODE(S):   ICD-9-CM CODE(S):

_____   _____

_____   _____

PRACTICAL APPLICATION

OPERATIVE REPORTS

Take the following operative reports, extract the key words, assign the appropriate CPT-4 code(s) and ICD-9-CM code(s), put them in order, adding the appropriate modifier(s).

1.

OPERATIVE REPORT

Patient information:

Patient name:
DOB:
MR#:
Date of procedure:

Preoperative diagnosis:

Lesion, left cheek

Postoperative diagnosis:

Same

Procedure(s) performed:

Excision lesion of left cheek consistent with Sebaceous cyst

Anesthesia:

IV sedation

Assistant surgeon:

Description of procedure:

Patient was brought to surgery, initially planned to do in the office but with the size, patient's excessive anxiety, we decided to do the procedure under local with monitored anesthesia. She had an IV line in place, and received IV sedation. By palpation, I was able to delineate the area in question. Making an outline of the cyst on the left cheek, the area was cleaned with Betadine and then draped. I infiltrated the site with 2% Alcohol then following the skin lines through a circular incision care dissection was initiated. The lateral margin of the mass was identified by dissection in the skin. The mass was so thin, and so attached to the skin, that we ended up entering into the mass itself yielding cheesy material consistent with sebaceous cyst. Mass was then dissected out completely with no residual and submitted for pathology. Hemostasis achieved with 6-0 Vicryl sutures and then skin closed with 6-0 Prolene sutures. Patient discharged from surgery to the Recovery Room in satisfactory condition.

Adm Westg MD

GODFREY REGIONAL HOSPITAL
123 Main Street • Aldon, FL 77714 • (407) 555-1234

CPT-4 Codes   ICD-9-CM Codes

_____   _____

_____   _____

2.

OPERATIVE REPORT

Patient information:

Patient name:
DOB:
MR#:
Date of procedure:

Preoperative diagnosis:

Question of recurrent carcinoma, right breast

Postoperative diagnosis:

Same

Procedure(s) performed:

Needle localization with excision, questionable lesion of right breast. Biopsy showed benign fibrosis secondary to radiation therapy

Anesthesia:

Assistant surgeon:

Description of procedure:

Patient admitted for repeat biopsy of the right breast. Underwent biopsy for same previously, which found carcinoma. Since then, she has had radiation therapy and follow-up mammogram recently. Area of concern was found close to the prior biopsy site. Because it could not be determined whether this was just scar tissue or not, repeat biopsy was recommended.

On admission this morning, an IV line was started. The patient was then brought to surgery. She presented to the X-ray suite, when I performed a needle localization of the area in question. IV sedation was given. Once anesthesia took, old scar was utilized to enter the area. Once the needle was appreciated, I followed it down to the hub. Since the needle was anterior to the lesion, the hub was identified, and all tissues posterior to the hub were excised completely with the needle in place. Sent to pathology which showed benign fibrosis secondary to radiation. Operation was terminated at this point. Wound edges were reapproximated in layers with 2-0 chromic for the subcutaneous and 3-0 for the skin. Appropriate dressings were applied. Patient was discharged later.

Rachel Perez MD

GODFREY REGIONAL HOSPITAL
123 Main Street • Aldon, FL 77714 • (407) 555-1234

CPT-4 Codes

ICD-9-CM Codes

_____

_____

_____

_____

3.

OPERATIVE REPORT

Patient information:

Patient name:
DOB:
MR#:
Date of procedure:

Preoperative diagnosis:

Chondromalacia patella and lateral meniscus tear, left knee

Postoperative diagnosis:

Early tricompartmental osteoarthritis, left knee and lateral meniscal tear

Procedure(s) performed:

Left knee arthroscopy, partial left arthroscopic lateral meniscectomy

Anesthesia:

Spinal

Assistant surgeon:

Description of procedure:

After suitable spinal anesthesia had been achieved, the patient's left knee was prepped and draped in the usual manner. Prior to prepping patient was given 300 mg Clindamycin because of a small area of eczema on the posterior aspect of the knee with some mild excoriation. The knee was then prepped and draped. Prior to prepping, thigh tourniquet was applied and after draping inflated to 300 mm of Mercury. After draping, the area of eczema was isolated with a Ioban drape. Anteromedial and anterolateral portals were established. Lateral compartment was examined first. Noted to be a complex tear of the lateral meniscus with a large flap portion from the inferior aspect of the middle third. The posterior horn after trimming of the flaps was slightly more mobile than normal. The articular surface revealed grade IV changes on the posterior half of the tibial plateau and grade III changes on the lateral half of the lateral femoral condyle from about 30 to 90 degrees. Examination of the medial compartment revealed intact stable meniscus. Tibial articular surfaces looked in good shape, but there was diffuse Grade II and Grade III changes with minimal articular cartilage flaps from 0 to 70 degrees on the femoral surface. Examination of the patellar femoral joint revealed diffuse Grade III changes in the trochlea and some Grade III changes of the inferior third of the lateral facet of the patella. These were smoothed with a shaver. Examination of the notch revealed the ACL that was intact but slightly lax. Knee joint was then thoroughly irrigated and the arthroscope was removed. Stab wounds were closed with 4-0 Nylon. Dressing was then applied. Tourniquet was released. Following tourniquet release, good circulation was noted to return to the foot. The patient tolerated the procedure well and the patient was returned to the Recovery Room in stable condition.

GODFREY REGIONAL HOSPITAL
123 Main Street • Aldon, FL 77714 • (407) 555-1234

CPT-4 Codes   ICD-9-CM Codes

_____   _____

_____   _____

4.

OPERATIVE REPORT

Patient information:

Patient name:
DOB:
MR#:
Date of procedure:

Preoperative diagnosis:

History of colon polyp in the past

Postoperative diagnosis:

Polyps in transverse colon, cecum
External hemorrhoids
Diverticulosis of left side

Procedure(s) performed:

Colonoscopy with polypectomy and biopsies

Anesthesia:

Conscious sedation, Versed Fentanyl

Assistant surgeon:

Description of procedure:

After obtaining informed consent, the patient was brought to the OR and put in the left lateral position. IV line was maintained. IV sedation was given. Vitals were monitored throughout the procedure, which included pulse, pulse oximetry, blood pressure, level of consciousness, and EKG monitoring. Digital rectal exam was done, which revealed external hemorrhoids, non-thrombosed, non-bleeding, and the scope was introduced into the rectum and advanced all the way up to the cecum, identified by the ileocecal valve. Right about the ileocecal valve, there was a small polyp, which was snared and sent to histopathology. Scope was further withdrawn, and, in the area of the cecum and the ascending colon, an abnormal fold was identified, which evened out with repeated washing. There is a small area that does appear abnormal, and several mucosal biopsies were taken. In the transverse colon, a large polyp was identified, 1 cm in its greatest diameter, which was snared and sent for histopathology. In the rectum, another polyp was identified which was small, and was removed with hot biopsy forceps. He has extensive left-sided diverticulosis all the way up to the transverse colon and small-size internal hemorrhoids.

Patk Adam MD

GODFREY REGIONAL HOSPITAL
123 Main Street • Aldon, FL 77714 • (407) 555-1234

CPT-4 Codes   ICD-9-CM Codes

_____   _____

_____   _____

5.

OPERATIVE REPORT

Patient information:

Patient name:
DOB:
MR#:
Date of procedure:

Preoperative diagnosis:

Chronic persistent lower back pain
Lumbar spondylosis
Facet arthropathy

Postoperative diagnosis:

Same

Procedure(s) performed:

Lumbar epidural injection of steroids and local anesthetic

Anesthesia:

Assistant surgeon:

Description of procedure:

With the patient in the prone position and adequately sedated using incremental doses of Fentanyl and Versed, external monitoring in place, the area of the back was prepared and draped in a routine sterile fashion. Using fluoroscopy in the AP projection, epidural space at the L4 level was identified and marked. After local infiltration with Lidocaine, a 17 gauge needle was inserted and advanced until the epidural space was entered using lots of resistance technique. Proper needle placement was verified by injecting 3cc of Isovue 300, demonstrating appropriate placement. Injections of Marcaine, 0.5% and Depo-Medrol 60 mg were injected into the epidural space.

The patient tolerated the procedure well. He will be discharged later today to continue reassessment and follow-up as an outpatient.

Lws Pery MD

GODFREY REGIONAL HOSPITAL
123 Main Street • Aldon, FL 77714 • (407) 555-1234

CPT-4 Codes   ICD-9-CM Codes

_____   _____

_____   _____

RADIOLOGY SERVICES

LEARNING OBJECTIVES

Following the completion of this chapter, the student will be able to:

- Understand the documentation for radiology services.
- Grasp the proper usage of modifiers for radiology services.
- Understand the appropriate application of technical/professional components.
- Identify the different types of radiological services.
- Understand coding complexities for radiological service.

KEY TERMS

CT, 304
Diagnostic, 303
Mammography, 305
MRI, 304
Nuclear Medicine, 303
Professional Component, 304
Radiation Oncology, 303
Technical Component, 304
Ultrasound, 303

RADIOLOGY DOCUMENTATION/ CODING GUIDELINES

Initial documentation for radiological services is provided in the radiology request form, in the clinical history, and information regarding the patient's clinical history. Unless the information contained in the request form is documented as reviewed, it must be incorporated in the actual radiology report to be used for coding purposes. Although the charge document or encounter form is often used for billing purposes, care should be taken to substantiate all services. This includes the correct number of views, administration of contrast, and other services, all of which must be recorded in the medical chart or medical documentation.

A written interpretive report is imperative for billing. The report should include the following:

- Symptoms
- Physical findings or clinical indication
- Procedure performed
- Final impression or diagnosis
- Number of views
- Contrast(s)

Without the radiological report, billing for the interpretation is not appropriate. In some instances, more than one physician will actually interpret the report, sometimes referred to as an "overread." Overreads occur when the ordering physician initially reads the radiology report, because of time restraints or the need to initiate treatment. Sometimes the facility where the services are performed requires the x-ray films be reviewed by a radiologist, so both the ordering physician and the radiologist interpreted the films. In these instances, Medicare and many other insurance carriers indicate that the physician who performs the interpretation independently without the need for additional interpretation or advice may code/bill for that service.

Look at the radiology column on Table 9-1 (Chapter 9) at the steps and components needed for CPT-4 coding.

CPT-4 Coding Steps

Type/Service	Radiology
Step 1	
Identify Chapter	X-rays
	MRI/CT
	Ultrasounds
	Nuclear Med
Range of Codes	70010–79999
Step 2	
Determine Type/Location	Type of Service
	Diagnostic
	Ultrasound
Step 3	
Specific Type	Anatomical Part
	Chest
	Lower Extremity
Step 4	
Specific Procedure Information	Views/Contrast
	2 Views w/contrast
Step 5	
Extent/Specifics	Additional Guidelines

Review the following radiology report and identify key words important in determining the radiological service performed.

Chapter: Radiology

RADIOLOGY REPORT

MR#:
Patient name:
DOB:
Physician:

Clinical indication:

Left knee pain

Section:
Diagnostic
X-Ray

Specifics:
AP View Standing
Both Knees

Anatomical
Part: Knees

Exam:

Left knee: Standing AP view of both knees are performed. There is asymmetric narrowing of the medial left knee joint compartment compared to the lateral joint compartment. Early bone spur formation is seen from the medial tibial plateau. There is no fracture or focal osteolytic destructive process of the left knee. Overall findings are unchanged from the previous x-ray of 04/09/200x.

Impression:

Degenerative arthritis of the medial left knee joint compartment. No acute abnormality or other remarkable change from the previous change.

Ddt/mm

D:
T:

_____
, M.D.   Date

Chapter: Radiology
Section: Dx Radiology X-Ray
Specific body part: Knee(s)
Specific procedure: AP Standing
                    Both Knees
                    73565

GODFREY REGIONAL HOSPITAL
123 Main Street • Aldon, FL 77714 • (407) 555-1234

Review the chart component listing and extract the key words needed to assign a CPT-4 code(s) for these services.

CPT-4 Coding Steps

Type/Service	Radiology	Chart Information
Step 1		
Identify Chapter	X-rays	Radiology
	MRI/CT	
	Ultrasounds	
	Nuclear Med	
Range of Codes	70010–79999	70010–79999
Step 2		
Determine Type/	Type of Service	Diagnostic
Location	X-ray	
	Diagnostic	
	Ultrasound	
Step 3		
Specific Type	Anatomical Part	Leg/Knee
	Chest	
	Lower Extremity	
Step 4		
Specific Procedure	Views/Contrast	Standing AP
Information	Both Knees	
	2 Views w/contrast	
Step 5		
Extent/Specifics	Additional	Guidelines

In summary, a CPT-4 code is required for the following:

Radiology Code:	70000–79999
Diagnostic X-ray Section:	70000–76499
Lower Extremity:	73500–73725
Knee:	73560–73580
AP Standing View(s):	73565

These categories make locating the appropriate code(s) simple.

MEDICAL NECESSITY OF RADIOLOGICAL SERVICES

Providers of radiology and other ancillary services are subject to requirements by third-party carriers for diagnostic codes that justify ancillary services performed. Because many radiology services are ordered and performed to rule out certain diagnoses, and rule-out diagnoses cannot be used for physician coding, the coder is often forced to submit signs, symptoms, and ill-defined conditions as the medical necessity for services performed.

The basis for required documentation of medical necessity for ancillary services stems from years of reimbursement by third-party carriers for services that may not have been medically necessary for a given individual. The coder must view this scenario from the carrier's perspective to appreciate the significance.

Consider a room full of 30 students, all of whom arrive at the physician's office with "chest pain." All of these patients must be examined, and, in some cases, baseline studies, such as an ECG, must be done. As the result of abnormal or questionable ECG results, a few of these "patients" need additional testing, such as an exercise stress test. Should the stress test detect an abnormality, an even smaller number of these individuals may need a thallium stress test. By requiring documented medical necessity for each level of service, the third-party carrier has authorized reimbursement of the thallium stress test in only a few individuals, thereby representing a substantial savings to the carrier.

Take a look at the previous example in dollars and cents:

30 students need ECGs ($60.00)	$1800.00
5 students with abnormal ECGs require a stress test ($200.00)	$1000.00
2 students with abnormal stress tests require thallium stress tests ($1500.00)	$3000.00
TOTAL COST	$5800.00
COMPARED WITH:	
30 students receive thallium stress tests ($1500.00)	$45,000.00

The third-party carrier wishes to make certain that all ancillary services are in fact medically necessary and that costs for these services are controlled.

CATEGORIES OF RADIOLOGICAL SERVICES

The radiology section of CPT-4 encompasses those procedures typically performed in the radiology facility of a provider's office or in an outpatient or hospital setting. These codes may be used by any physician or facility in any setting, however, as long as the definitions are met.

Radiology services include not only **diagnostic** services such as the common chest x-ray, but also diagnostic **ultrasound, radiation oncology,** and **nuclear medicine.** The radiology section of CPT-4 is divided into the following areas:

Diagnostic radiology   Encompasses the radiological imaging performed with typical x-ray equipment. This includes such services as skeletal x-rays, MRI (magnetic resonance imaging), and CT/CAT (computerized axial tomography) scans.

Diagnostic ultrasound   Sound waves produce an image. A-mode, M-mode, B-scan, or real-time scans are used for ultrasonic imaging.

Radiation oncology   Involves the services of teletherapy and brachytherapy in the provision of therapeutic radiation treatments. These treatments are typically used to treat neoplasms, most often those already diagnosed as malignant.

Nuclear medicine   Includes radiographic imaging with the injection or infusion of radio-elements for the purpose of visualizing the organ or system.

RADIOLOGY CODING GUIDELINES

GENERAL GUIDELINES

One of the distinctions of radiology services is that many of the procedures performed are provided by two individuals: the technician, who completes the **technical component,** and the individual who provides supervision and written interpretation of the result, thus fulfilling the **professional component.** The combination of technical and professional components constitutes the global component, as described in Chapter 12.

Of the procedures with both technical and professional components, many may have only one component performed, so procedures in the radiology section may be separated into these components. In those instances, it is not necessary to include a modifier indicating that only the professional component has been performed. The coder should take note that NOT all procedures in the radiology section have been divided as outlined here.

When only the radiological interpretation or professional services are performed, and the code has not been already separated by definition, modifier 26 would be appended to that service.

MODIFIERS

The following modifier codes are appropriate for use with codes in the radiology section of CPT-4:

- Modifier 22   Unusual procedural services
- Modifier 26   Professional component only
- Modifier 32   Mandated services
- Modifier 50   Bilateral procedures
- Modifier 51   Multiple procedures
- Modifier 52   Reduced services

- Modifier 53   Discontinued procedures
- Modifier 58   Related/staged procedure by same doctor during global surgical period
- Modifier 59   Distinct procedure services
- Modifier 62   Two surgeons
- Modifier 66   Surgical team
- Modifier 76   Repeat procedure by same physician
- Modifier 77   Repeat procedure by another physician
- Modifier 78   Return to OR for related procedure during global/postoperative period
- Modifier 79   Unrelated procedure/service by same doctor during global/postoperative period
- Modifier 80   Assistant surgeon
- Modifier 90   Outside/reference laboratory services
- Modifier 99   Multiple modifiers

Descriptions of these modifiers have been provided previously. Refer to the descriptions in the modifier section, the CPT-4 Coding Reference Tool in Tool 51, the complete outline of modifier codes in Figure 16-1, and the Modifier Appendix located in the CPT-4 code book.

Note: When bilateral services are performed, they should be coded with the modifier 50, bilateral procedures. If the carrier recognizes HCPCS modifier codes, use RT (right) and LT (left). HCPCS modifiers are discussed later.

When additional views not listed in CPT-4 are necessary, the appropriate CPT-4 code should be used with modifier 22. A documented explanation should be included regarding additional views and the medical necessity for such.

When fewer views than those listed in CPT-4 are performed, the appropriate CPT-4 code should be used with modifier 52. The number of views performed should be recorded in the medical documentation.

Second readings or interpretations of radiography are not reimbursable by most third-party carriers.

SUPERVISION AND INTERPRETATION CODES

Supervision and interpretation (S & I) codes are used to code the personal supervision of the radiological procedure and the interpretation. To bill for the supervision and interpretation, the physician must be present during the procedure. The interpretation itself may be performed at a later time. When the supervision (S) portion of an S & I code is performed by one entity, and the (I) portion is performed by another, both providers should bill the S & I code with modifier 52 appended to indicate they have not performed all of the services assigned to that code.

INTERPRETATION OF RADIOLOGICAL/ DIAGNOSTIC SERVICES

Generally, third-party carriers pay for only one interpretation of diagnostic services, including radiological services. Only in the case of questionable findings would an interpretation of images be paid for more than once. Any provider may code or bill for the interpretation of diagnostic results when the interpretation is made without the assistance of another provider/physician. For instance, if the emergency department (ED) physician requests or is required to seek the assistance of the radiologist in interpretation of an x-ray, the ED physician may NOT code for that service.

When third-party carriers receive two claims for the interpretive services, they typically pay for the first claim received. Should a second claim be received, the carrier will have to determine which physician's interpretation contributed to the diagnosis and treatment of that patient and pay accordingly. Another consideration would be whether the radiologist's interpretation was conveyed to the treating physician in time to contribute to the diagnosis and treatment of the patient.

CODING FOR CONTRASTS

When radiological services are performed that involve the use of contrast, only contrasts that are administered other than rectally or orally will be considered. There are a number of codes, especially for CT/MRI scans, that cover the performance of scans with, without, or without and with contrast. In the case of "with and without" contrast, the area is scanned initially without any contrast. The radiological report should indicate that contrast was administered after images without contrast were taken to establish the legitimate use of the "with and without" contrast code.

RADIOPHARMACEUTICALS

When radiopharmaceuticals (drugs for radiological imaging services over and above those incident to the imaging) are used, coding for the provision of these supplies is appropriate. Code 78990 or an appropriate HCPCS code such as A4641 should be assigned for these services.

STEPS IN CODING RADIOLOGY SERVICES

Basic steps in breaking down the coding of radiology services are the following:

Step 1   Identify the appropriate subsection in the Radiology section.
Step 2   Determine the anatomical part.
Step 3   Locate the appropriate code(s).
Step 4   Determine extent of the procedure (number of views; limited/complete; with, without, or with/without contrast).
Step 5   Assign appropriate modifier code(s).

CODING OF SPECIFIC RADIOLOGICAL CATEGORIES

DIAGNOSTIC RADIOLOGY

Procedures in the diagnostic radiology subsection are divided by anatomical site and by the number of views. Diagnostic radiology includes plain x-ray films, CAT/CT scans (computerized axial tomography), MRI (magnetic resonance imaging), MRA (magnetic resonance angiography), and angiography. Anatomical sites begin with the head, chest, and upper extremities, and progress to the lower extremities, as in other sections of CPT-4.

Radiological services may be performed with contrast, without contrast, or with and without contrast. Oral contrast given before or during a study does not constitute "with contrast" and should be assigned a "without contrast" code unless other nonoral contrast is also given.

MAMMOGRAPHY

Many states have laws that require insurance carriers to cover screening mammograms for all insured clients. The guidelines are usually modeled after federal guidelines that cover all Medicare patients or after the American Cancer Society screening guidelines.

Screening mammograms are furnished to a patient who has no signs or symptoms of breast disease or personal history/family history of breast disease. These services are typically covered for the purpose of early detection of breast cancer. A diagnostic code, such as a V76.12/Screening Mammogram, would be appropriate. Because CPT-4 code 76092 indicates bilateral screening, the use of modifier 50 would not be appropriate.

Diagnostic mammograms are performed in the presence of signs or symptoms, or a personal or family history of breast disease in male or female patients. There are two codes for diagnostic mammograms, unilateral (76090) and bilateral (76091), so it is not necessary to append modifier 50 to these codes, either.

DIAGNOSTIC ULTRASOUND

Diagnostic ultrasound involves the use of high-frequency sound waves to provide images of anatomical structures. This imagery is then used to determine the cause of specific disease or illness. There are four types of ultrasounds outlined in the CPT-4 coding manual:

Real-time scan   One-dimensional display that outlines
A-mode: the structure; the *A* is for *amplitude*

of sound waves. Ultrasound imaging relies on high-frequency sound waves that reflect off anatomical structures and return like an echo. The return time is calculated and an image created on the screen from the distances and intensities of the echoes.

M-mode: One-dimensional display of movement of anatomical structures (*M* is for *motion*).

B-scan: Two-dimensional display of tissues and organs (*B* is for *brightness*).

Real-time scan: Two-dimensional display that shows the structure and motion of tissues and organs.

Most codes in the diagnostic ultrasound section include codes for "limited" and "complete." Limited codes are typically assigned when a specific organ or body part is imaged. For instance, a kidney ultrasound would be coded as limited, because the images were of only one organ in the area. "Complete" codes are justified when all structures or organs in the specific area are imaged. Medicare guidelines differ from other carriers in that two organs or structures may be omitted and the "complete" code may still be used.

RADIATION ONCOLOGY

The Radiation Oncology section contains services performed by or under the supervision of the radiology oncologist. This physician typically provides services to patients who have already received a diagnosis of a tumor or malignant neoplasm (other diagnoses are sometimes treated). The patient who receives treatment from the radiology oncologist usually has been diagnosed at the time of the initial treatment. Patients may continue to visit the oncologist for further diagnoses, treatments, and evaluation.

The radiation oncology subsection is divided into the following groups.

Clinical Treatment Planning

Treatment planning includes test interpretation, tumor localization, volume determination, or amount of radiation to be delivered. Time and dosage determination, treatment modality, number and size of treatment ports, appropriate treatment devices, and other procedures necessary to a treatment plan are also included.

Therapeutic Radiology Simulation

This category has codes that cover the use of a simulator to determine the various treatment portal outlines and

orientation to be used in the course of radiation therapy. A simulator, which is incapable of delivering radiation therapy, can generate radiation in the diagnostic x-ray range. It permits the orientation of a radiation beam that simulates the beam(s) proposed for therapy, while at the same time providing roentgenographic visualization of the area. Therapeutic radiology simulation requires the involvement of the physician, the technician, and all equipment necessary to provide this service.

Radiation Physics

The radiation physics subcategory comprises the decisions made by the physician about the type of treatment indicated including appropriate doses, dose calculations, and the development of treatment devices.

Radiation Treatment Management

The codes in this section are used to bill for weekly management of the delivery of radiation therapy. Weekly management is defined in CPT-4 as five treatments equaling 1 week of treatment, regardless of breaks between treatment days. It is not necessary that the radiation oncologist personally examine the patient for each fraction, only that an evaluation of the patient's data be performed. Multiple fractions furnished on the same date may be counted as long as there has been a distinct break in therapy sessions and the fractions consist of services that under normal circumstances would have been performed on different days.

Clinical Brachytherapy

Placement of radioactive material into or around a tumor site is coded in the clinical brachytherapy subsection. Placement may be defined as simple, intermediate, or complex, as defined by the CPT-4 radiology guidelines.

NUCLEAR MEDICINE

The specialty of radiological nuclear medicine comprises the placement and monitoring of radioactive nuclides within the body. This section is subsectioned according to anatomical site. As with all of CPT-4, if the documentation does not substantiate multiple determinations, uptakes, or views, the coder must select a single uptake or view. Feedback should be provided to the physician regarding the possibility of documenting and coding additional items when appropriate to obtain additional reimbursement. The provision of the radiopharmaceutical should also be coded and billed with the appropriate supply or HCPCS code(s).

CHAPTER IN REVIEW

CERTIFICATION REVIEW

- All radiological services are considered global and have two components: technical and professional.
- Diagnostic radiology encompasses the radiological imaging performed with traditional x-ray equipment.
- Diagnostic ultrasound involves the use of ultrasound for imaging.
- Nuclear medicine involves use by injection or infusion of radioelements to allow visualization of a specified area.
- Modifier 50 or HCPCS modifiers RT/LT (dependent on carrier guidelines) should be used for radiological services when services are performed bilaterally.
- Radiological services must include a diagnostic statement to the highest level of specificity to justify the medical necessity of performing the requested tests.

STUDENT STUDY GUIDE

- Study Chapter 13.
- Review the Learning Objectives for Chapter 13.
- Review the Certification Review for Chapter 13.
- Complete the Chapter Review exercise to reinforce concepts learned in the chapter.

CHAPTER REVIEW EXERCISE

Assign codes for the following scenarios. Because the ICD-9-CM is imperative to denote the medical necessity for radiological services, assign both the ICD-9-CM and CPT-4 code(s) for these services. Unless otherwise specified, both the technical and professional component of these radiological services has been provided.

1. A patient visits the family physician with the complaint of cough and symptoms suggestive of upper respiratory infection. The family physician sends the patient to the radiology department and requests a PA and lateral chest x-ray to rule out pneumonia.
CPT-4 CODE: _____ ICD-9-CM CODE: _____

2. A patient arrives in the radiology department with physician orders for an x-ray of the forearm, PA, and lateral, for shaft fracture of the left radius.
CPT-4 CODE: _____ ICD-9-CM CODE: _____

3. A patient is brought to the radiology section for a two-view x-ray of the right wrist with the diagnosis of wrist fracture.
CPT-4 CODE: _____ ICD-9-CM CODE: _____

4. A patient is brought to the radiology section for multiple x-rays after an automobile accident. The patient complains of ankle pain along with pain in the clavicular area. X-rays of the right ankle and clavicle are ordered to rule out fracture.
CPT-4 CODE: _____ ICD-9-CM CODE: _____
CPT-4 CODE: _____ ICD-9-CM CODE: _____

5. A patient arrives in the radiology department with physician order to perform vaginal code irradiation, special treatment.
CPT-4 CODE: _____ ICD-9-CM CODE: _____

6. A radiologist performs an A-scan ultrasound for determination of intraocular lens power in preparation for a cataract extraction with lens implantation.
CPT-4 CODE: _____ ICD-9-CM CODE: _____

7. A patient with breast cancer who will begin radiation therapy arrives in the radiation oncology department for application of an intracavitary radioactive source.
CPT-4 CODE: _____ ICD-9-CM CODE: _____

8. A patient with a cerebral brain tumor arrives for stereotactic radiation treatment management.
CPT-4 CODE: _____ ICD-9-CM CODE: _____

9. A limited abdominal real-time echography with image documentation and interpretation is performed for an abdominal mass.
CPT-4 CODE: _____ ICD-9-CM CODE: _____

10. Radiology provides ultrasonic guidance for the performance of a needle biopsy for breast mass.
CPT-4 CODE: _____ ICD-9-CM CODE: _____

11. A pelvic ultrasound is performed for determination of fetal age because of small sizes for dates.
CPT-4 CODE: _____ ICD-9-CM CODE: _____

12. A patient arrives in the radiology department for bone imaging of the right leg for diagnosis of osteomyelitis.
CPT-4 CODE: _____ ICD-9-CM CODE: _____

13. Patient arrives for mammogram as a result of a suspected right breast mass.
CPT-4 CODE: _____ ICD-9-CM CODE: _____

14. Ultrasound of the kidney is performed to determine size and location of kidney mass.
CPT-4 CODE: _____ ICD-9-CM CODE: _____

15. Patient arrives for CT of the abdomen due to right upper quadrant pain. After several initial images are taken, contrast is introduced, and additional images are obtained.
CPT-4 CODE: _____ ICD-9-CM CODE: _____

16. Patient presents with a history of arthritis of the right wrist for bilateral wrist x-rays. Two views of the right and left wrist are performed that confirm arthritis in both joints.
CPT-4 CODE: _____ ICD-9-CM CODE: _____

17. Patient presents with a month history of low back pain for a four-view radiological exam of the

lumbosacral spine. Diagnosis is ankylosing spondylitis of L4-L6.

CPT-4 CODE: _____ ICD-9-CM CODE: _____

18. Patient with history of COPD presents with chronic cough and fever. Chest PA is performed to determine whether reoccurrence of pneumonia has occurred. No pneumonia is found, exacerbation of COPD is confirmed.

CPT-4 CODE: _____ ICD-9-CM CODE: _____

19. Radiologist performs the preoperative placement of a radiological marker for the performance of breast lesion excision by surgeon later the same day.

CPT-4 CODE: _____ ICD-9-CM CODE: _____

20. Pregnant female presents for a repeat transabdominal ultrasound to reevaluate fetal size and possible abnormality.

CPT-4 CODE: _____ ICD-9-CM CODE: _____

PRACTICAL APPLICATION

Assign the appropriate CPT-4 code(s), modifier(s), and ICD-9-CM code(s) to the following radiology reports.

1.

RADIOLOGY REPORT

MR#:
PATIENT NAME:
DOB:
PHYSICIAN: Robert Rais, MD

Clinical summary:

CLINICAL INDICATION:
OB Ultrasound

Abdomen:

IMPRESSION:
OB ULTRASOUND EXAM
Single intrauterine pregnancy with fetus in the cephalic presentation. Placenta is located posteriorly and to the right of the uterus. No evidence of placenta previa. Amniotic fluid within normal limits. Fetal anatomy appears normal on the images provided. Fetal cardiac motion observed by the technologist.

Conclusion:

Average ultrasound age estimated to be 33 weeks 2 days.

Ddt/mm

D:
T:

_____
, M.D.   Date

GODFREY REGIONAL HOSPITAL
123 Main Street • Aldon, FL 77714 • (407) 555-1234

CPT-4 CODE: _____   ICD-9-CM CODE: _____

2.

RADIOLOGY REPORT

MR#:
PATIENT NAME:
DOB:
PHYSICIAN: Robert Rais, MD

Clinical summary:

CLINICAL INDICATION:
Abdominal mass

Abdomen:

CT SCAN OF THE ABDOMEN:
Exam is made using oral and IV contrast materials. Non-contrast sections made of the liver and kidneys.

Caudad lobe of liver is quite prominent and measures at least 7 centimeters in largest diameter. However, there is no definite mass in this area with the liver parenchyma uniform in density. Recommend repeat ultrasound with special attention to the caudad lobe of the liver.
Gallbladder is generous in size. Kidneys, spleen, and abdominal aorta are negative.

Conclusion:

IMPRESSION:
Enlarged liver, no mass noted.

74160

74160

Ddt/mm

D:
T:

_____
, M.D.   Date

GODFREY REGIONAL HOSPITAL
123 Main Street • Aldon, FL 77714 • (407) 555-1234

CPT-4 CODE: _____   ICD-9-CM CODE: _____

3.

RADIOLOGY REPORT

MR#: PATIENT NAME: DOB: PHYSICIAN: Maurice Doates, MD

Clinical summary:

CLINICAL INDICATION:
Knee pain

Abdomen:

TWO VIEWS OF THE RIGHT KNEE:
Moderate degenerative changes involve the right knee with narrowing of the lateral compartment. There is mild compression of the lateral tibial plateau which probably is not due to an acute process. Degenerative changes in the patellofemoral articulation. Medial meniscus appears to be intact, however, lateral meniscus has tear around the posterior horn.

Conclusion:

IMPRESSION:
Meniscal tear, posterior horn

Ddt/mm

D:
T:

_____
, M.D.   Date

GODFREY REGIONAL HOSPITAL
123 Main Street • Aldon, FL 77714 • (407) 555-1234

CPT-4 CODE: _____   ICD-9-CM CODE: _____

4.

RADIOLOGY REPORT

MR#:
PATIENT NAME:
DOB:
PHYSICIAN: William Obert, MD

Clinical summary:

CLINICAL INDICATION:
Cough x one month

Abdomen:

CHEST PA AND LATERAL:
No evidence of infiltrates. Negative chest.

Conclusion:

IMPRESSION:
No evidence of pleural effusion or infiltrates.

71020

Ddt/mm

D:
T:

_____
, M.D.   Date

GODFREY REGIONAL HOSPITAL
123 Main Street • Aldon, FL 77714 • (407) 555-1234

CPT-4 CODE: _____   ICD-9-CM CODE: _____

5.

RADIOLOGY REPORT

MR#:
PATIENT NAME:
DOB:
PHYSICIAN: Felix Washington, MD

Clinical summary:

CLINICAL INDICATION:
R/O Foreign body, finger

Abdomen:

THREE VIEWS OF THE RIGHT MIDDLE FINGER:
Severe osteoarthritis of the distal IP joint of the finger with deviation of the distal phalanx relative to the middle phalanx. At least mild degenerative changes in the other IP joints. Small calcifications near each joint of the finger consistent with the degenerative arthritis. No foreign bodies are observed.

Conclusion:

IMPRESSION:
Osteoarthritis, distal IP joint, right middle finger

Ddt/mm

D:
T:

_____
, M.D.   Date

GODFREY REGIONAL HOSPITAL
123 Main Street • Aldon, FL 77714 • (407) 555-1234

CPT-4 CODE: _____ ICD-9-CM CODE: _____

PATHOLOGY SERVICES

LEARNING OBJECTIVES

Following the completion of this chapter, the student will be able to:

- Understand the documentation used for pathology services.
- Identify types of pathology services and explain proper application of coding rules for each category of services.
- Comprehend the various modifier codes used for coding pathology services, and use them in actual coding scenarios.
- Understand and use the basic steps for coding pathology services.

KEY TERMS

Anatomical Pathology, 317
Automated, 317
Clinical Laboratory Improvements Amendments (CLIA), 317
Dipstick, 317
Disease-Oriented Panels, 317
Evocative/Suppression Testing, 317
Manual, 317
Surgical Pathology, 317
Urinalysis, 317

PATHOLOGY DOCUMENTATION/ CODING GUIDELINES

Documentation for pathology services is provided in both the pathology request form and the actual laboratory report. Typically, the pathology laboratory or pathologist does not examine the patient and relies on information provided on the pathology order form for suspected conditions, signs, or symptoms. Pathology services typically require the use of data and statistical analysis for the determination of a diagnosis. As was the case with radiology services, for both the professional and technical components, or the global service to be coded/billed, documentation must contain both the technical performance and the professional interpretation. The interpretation may be documented on the actual laboratory slip (Figure 14-1) or dictated as part of the medical record documentation (Figure 14-2).

Review the components needed for determining the laboratory service performed. Look at the key elements in Figure 9-1, specifically pathology services.

FIGURE 14-1 Laboratory slip.

SURGICAL PATHOLOGY REPORT

Name: _____ Hosp. No.: _____ Path. No.: _____

Date: _____ Room: _____ Age: _____ Sex: _____ Surgeon: _____ M.D.

Operation: _____

Material submitted: _____

Pre-op diagnosis: _____

Post-op diagnosis: _____

Previous material: _____ Pertinent history: _____

Diagnosis:

Gross description:

Specimen consist of an elongated fragment of membranous and fatty tissue measuring approximately 17 cms in length x 3 cms at the widest part x 2 mms in average thickness. One surface is smooth and glistening and the opposite surface shows areas of hemorrhage. Representative sections are submitted.

Micro description:

Section consists of fragments of fatty tissue traversed by dense bands of connective tissue with congested capillaries. One of the fragments appears to have a lining of mesothelial cells.

Maria Callry M.D.
Pathologist

GODFREY CLINICAL LABORATORIES
465 Dogwood Court • Aldon, FL 77712 • (407) 555-9876

FIGURE 14-2 Pathology report.

Step 1
Identify Chapter
Range of Codes

Pathology
Study of Body Substances
80048-89399

Step 2
Determine Type/Location

Type of Service
Chemistry
Hematology

Step 3
Specific Type

Specific Test
Hemoglobin
Hematocrit

Step 4
Specific Procedure Information

Auto/Manual
Automated
Manual

Step 5
Extent/Additional Specifics

Additional Guidelines

OVERVIEW

The pathology section of CPT-4 comprises services performed on specimens collected by the physician or facility. The physician's office or facility may charge for the collection or preparation of the specimen based on CPT-4 guidelines in some instances.

GENERAL CODING/BILLING GUIDELINES

Automated and Manual

Pathology services may be performed by different methods, namely, automated, manual, and dipstick. Dipstick use is specific to urinalysis and involves "dipping" a chemically treated urine strip into the specimen and analyzing visual changes. Automated analysis involves the introduction of a urine specimen into a urine analysis system that provides a printout of the findings from multiple analyses for review by the physician. Manually analyzed specimens are subjected to several diagnostic protocols, each one separate, usually by a pathologist or a lab technician under the supervision of the pathologist.

When laboratory services are performed and the methods unspecified, the coder must use the least significant code. All **automated** services, with the exception of **urinalysis,** will be considered less significant because reduced provider involvement and analysis are required compared with **manual** services. With urine specimens, the **"dipstick"** method is considered the least significant.

CLIA Requirements

In 1988, the **Clinical Laboratory Improvements Amendments (CLIA)** were enacted to ensure that laboratories consistently provide accurate procedures and services. Each laboratory is assigned a CLIA certificate number or certificate of waiver number, which must be listed on the CMS-1500 claim form in Box 23.

Specimen Collection/Drawing Fee

Specific procedure codes have been established for the collection of specimens. These codes are located in the surgery and medicine sections of CPT-4 and are typically used only when the specimen is prepared to send to an outside laboratory for processing.

Specimen handling codes (99000-99002) are assigned to specimens that must be collected, prepared, and labeled. Appropriate forms must be prepared for the specimen to be forwarded to another facility for processing.

Specimen drawing fees (36400-36425) are used for venipuncture to obtain specimens. These codes are assigned based on the patient's age and how the specimen is obtained (e.g., percutaneous, cutdown). When carriers require the use of HCPCS codes, G0001, in lieu of CPT code 36415, is used for the routine venipuncture for collection of specimen(s). Code P9615 is used for catheterization for collection of specimen(s).

TYPES OF PATHOLOGY SERVICES

The pathology section of CPT-4 is divided into the following subsections:

- Organ- or **disease-oriented panels**
- Drug testing
- Therapeutic drug assays
- **Evocative/suppression testing**
- Consultations (clinical pathology)
- Urinalysis
- Chemistry
- Hematology and coagulation
- Immunology
- Transfusion medicine
- Microbiology
- **Anatomical pathology**
- **Surgical pathology**

As with the radiology section of CPT-4, diagnostic coding that identifies the medical necessity for pathology services is necessary as well. One of the most common reasons that laboratory services are not paid or are paid incorrectly by third-party carriers is that diagnosis codes do not match the pathology service. For example, if pathology service codes are for a urine specimen, a diagnosis code for blood analysis, such as anemia, would not be appropriate.

STEPS IN CODING PATHOLOGY SERVICES

The basic steps for coding pathology services include the following:

Step 1   Identify the appropriate subsection from pathology codes.

Step 2   Identify the method used (automated, manual).

Step 3   Make sure services are not bundled in "panel codes."

Step 4   Assign any necessary modifier codes.

This "narrowing down" process is important, especially in CPT-4 sections such as Pathology, because of the volume of services, and the number of subsections contained in this section.

Also, keep in mind one of the basic rules of coding: **If it is not documented, it did not happen.** When the method used for testing is not specified, the least significant method will be assigned.

REVIEW OF SUBSECTIONS

ORGAN- OR DISEASE-ORIENTED PANELS

Panel tests should not be reported separately when performed on the same day. There are 12 panels of tests commonly performed for definitive testing: basic metabolic, electrolyte, comprehensive metabolic, general health, obstetrical, hepatic function, hepatitis, lipids, arthritis, TORCH antibody, thyroid, and thyroid with TSH. Refer to the current CPT-4 manual for a list of the included procedures. Note that all tests included in a specific panel must be performed before panel codes can be assigned. If even one of these tests is not medically necessary, each test must be ordered and billed independently.

DRUG TESTING

Testing procedures from this section are usually confirmed with an additional technique using code 80102. Testing is categorized by the classification of drugs such as barbiturates and amphetamines. Testing from this section identifies only the presence or absence of drugs, not the specific drug or amount.

Code 80100 is considered a qualitative screen for multiple drug classes. In other words, the test only indicates whether drugs are present in the specimen. Code 80101 is a qualitative test as well, known as an immunoassay, wherein only one drug class is tested at a time.

THERAPEUTIC DRUG ASSAYS

Tests in this section are performed quantitatively. These codes are used when the drug identified is to be measured or quantitated. These tests are usually ordered to determine whether the patient is receiving a "therapeutic" level of a prescribed medication. Examples of the types of medications tested in this section include the following:

- Antibiotics
- Antidepressants
- Sedatives
- Anticonvulsants
- Tranquilizers
- Antiarrhythmics

EVOCATIVE/SUPPRESSION TESTING

These codes are used for procedures that measure the effects of administered drugs. CPT-4 guidelines may specify the method used with specific instructions. They are arranged in alphabetical order by name and many of the services contained in this section include multiple administrations of the identical tests. For example, the glucagon tolerance panel (Code 80422) includes three glucose tests (Code 82947) and three insulin studies (Code 83525). The service for all six tests would be coded and billed as 80422, with days/units of one (1).

CONSULTATION (CLINICAL PATHOLOGY)

Codes 80500 and 80502 are for use by the pathologist only. These codes apply to the opinion rendered by request from a pathologist concerning a pathological specimen (pathology consultation).

Evaluation and Management consultation codes may also be used when the consultation or requested opinion concerning the patient's condition requires that the pathologist consider history, examination, and medical decision making.

URINALYSIS

This section includes codes for several methods of urinalysis. When not specified in documentation, the most basic level of service is implied. In the case of pathology, the most basic service is an automated test rather than a manual one. Automated tests require less medical decision making and are less complex for the pathologist. In the urinalysis section, "dipstick" urinalysis is considered the least significant, followed by automated urinalysis.

CHEMISTRY

Performance of blood chemistry analysis is included in this section. Multiple codes may be available for testing of one agent, such as glucose. Codes are arranged in alphabetical order and can encompass multiple proce-dures. Tests are considered quantitative unless otherwise specified by the procedure definition.

HEMATOLOGY

This section encompasses hematology and coagulation studies, including blood counts. Keep in mind that ser-vices are provided only as specified. If the method for a test is not specified, the least complicated method will be assumed. In this case, automated is less significant than manual.

IMMUNOLOGY

This section identifies codes used for antibody studies and for blood bank services. Conditions of the immune system caused by the action of identified antibodies are also included.

TRANSFUSION MEDICINE

Most blood bank procedures are located in this section.

MICROBIOLOGY

This section includes bacteriology, virology, and parasi-tology assays. These codes include culture, organism identification, and sensitivity studies. When it is medi-cally necessary to perform the same test on multiple specimens or sites, modifier 59 should be appended to the subsequent codes.

ANATOMICAL PATHOLOGY

This section includes postmortem examinations, includ-ing autopsies, and cytopathological and cytogenetic studies. Codes from 88141 to 88175 are used to report cervical and vaginal tests. Codes from 88150 to 88154 should be used for Pap smears that are examined with a method other than the Bethesda method. Codes from 88164 to 88167 should be used for Pap smears with the Bethesda method. For specimens collected in fluid, com-monly known as "Thin-Prep," codes from 88142 to 88143 should be assigned.

SURGICAL PATHOLOGY

Surgical pathology involves gross and microscopic speci-mens sent to the pathology area for examination and evaluation. Each separate specimen is identified by the anatomical location from which it came, type of patho-logical examination requested, and tissue type. When multiple tissues are received together as a single speci-

men or are not individually identified, they may not be charged separately.

Services are divided into the following six levels:

Level I   Specimens that normally do not need microscopic evaluation
Level II   Tissue removed, no probability of malig-nancy
Level III   Tissue with low probability of malignancy
Level IV   Tissue with a higher probability for malig-nancy or other possible disease
Level V   Complex pathology evaluations
Level VI   Examination of neoplastic tissue or complex specimens

PATHOLOGY MODIFIERS

After **identifying services** (Step 1), **determining method** (Step 2), and **making certain no "panel" codes exist** for coded services (Step 3), the coder's last step (Step 4) of the pathology coding process involves **assigning modifier codes** when appropriate.

Many of the modifier codes for use in the pathology section have already been discussed. They are only men-tioned again for purposes of inclusion in the pathology section of this textbook.

GENERAL MODIFIERS

22   Unusual procedural services
26   Professional component only
32   Mandated services
52   Reduced services
53   Discontinued procedures
59   Distinct procedural services

SPECIFIC PATHOLOGY SECTION MODIFIERS

Modifier 90—Reference (Outside) Laboratory

This modifier is unique to the pathology section, although it is used minimally in some other sections of CPT-4 as well. When services are performed by an outside labora-tory, but the physician's office is billing the patient's third-party insurer for these services, modifier 90 should be appended. This enables the third-party insurer to recognize which provider rendered the services and which provider is authorized to bill for these services. If the laboratory also attempts to bill for these services, the third-party insurer can ascertain that the billing arrange-ment was for the physician's office to bill the insurer and the laboratory to bill the physician's office.

CMS Alert: Note that Medicare does not allow an arrangement such as this. Medicare guidelines specify that only the party providing the services may bill for those services. This applies to all services, not just pathology services, provided to Medicare recipients.

Also of note, laboratory services (all codes within the 80000 series) are reimbursed at 100% of the Medicare allowance. Make certain the practice receives the appropriate reimbursement for these services, and ensure that patients are not charged 20% coinsurance.

Modifier 91—Repeat Pathology Services

This is a relatively new modifier code specifically designed for pathology services. This modifier should be appended to pathology services only when repeat services are medically necessary. The modifier should not be used for repeat services because inadequate or insufficient specimens were submitted previously. It should be used only when the repeat pathology services are represented by the identical CPT-4 code.

CHAPTER IN REVIEW

CERTIFICATION REVIEW

- Pathology services are billed as automated (least significant) when not specified as automated or manual.
- The most commonly performed pathological services for specific diagnostic testing are "grouped" in the organ- and disease-oriented panels.
- The organ- and disease-oriented panels may be used only when all components are ordered. In the event that any of the services is not requested, the coder must code each individual test.
- Drug testing determines whether drugs are present in the patient's system.
- Drug assays determine quantity and specific drug(s) that are present.
- Surgical pathology specimens are assigned six levels of service based on the complexity of the specimen, not necessarily the size.
- When surgical pathology specimens are not received or identified separately, they may not be charged separately.
- Two specific modifiers are used in the pathology sections, namely, modifier 90, Reference (Outside) Laboratory, and modifier 91, Repeat Pathology Services.
- Medicare guidelines specify that only the provider of services may bill for those services. Arrangements with pathology laboratories for physician coding or billing of laboratory-performed testing are prohibited by federal Medicare guidelines.

STUDENT STUDY GUIDE

- Study Chapter 14.
- Review the Learning Objectives for Chapter 14.
- Review the Certification Review for Chapter 14.

- Complete the Chapter Review exercise to reinforce concepts learned in the chapter.

CHAPTER REVIEW EXERCISE

Code the following. In some instances "No code" or "Insufficient information" may be appropriate. When information is not sufficient, document the additional information required to assign an appropriate code(s).

1. Specimen received for sodium, glucose, and chloride profile
   CPT-4 CODE(S): _84295 -82947 - 82435_
2. Automated hemogram and platelet count with complete white blood cell count
   CPT-4 CODE(S): _85027_
3. Antinuclear antibody titer
   CPT-4 CODE(S): _86039_
4. ABO and RH blood typing
   CPT-4 CODE(S): _86901, 86900_
5. Prostate specimen from a transurethral resection of the prostate
   CPT-4 CODE(S): _88305_
6. Thyroid disease panel
   CPT-4 CODE(S): _not enough info_
7. Test for presence of barbiturates, opiates, amphetamines, qualitative method
   CPT-4 CODE(S): _80100_
8. Metabolic panel
   CPT-4 CODE(S): _80048_
9. Surgical pathology, appendix (not incidental)
   CPT-4 CODE(S): _88304_
10. Bacterial culture, urine
    CPT-4 CODE(S): _87086_ _need site method_
11. PSA (prostate specific antigen)
    CPT-4 CODE(S): _84152_
12. Therapeutic assay, digoxin
    CPT-4 CODE(S): _80162_
13. Carbon dioxide, chloride, potassium, sodium
    CPT-4 CODE(S): _82374, 82435, 84132_
    _84295_

14. Potassium level
    CPT-4 CODE(S): _____ 84132 _____

15. Glucose
    CPT-4 CODE(S): _____ Not enough _____

16. Bilirubin, total
    CPT-4 CODE(S): _____ 82247 _____

17. Surgical pathology, malignant neoplasm with partial mastectomy
    CPT-4 CODE(S): _____ 88307 _____

18. Surgical pathology, oophorectomy
    CPT-4 CODE(S): _____ 88307 88305 _____

19. Chemical analysis, arsenic
    CPT-4 CODE(S): _____ 82175 _____

20. Hemoglobin
    CPT-4 CODE(S): _____ 85018 _____

MEDICINE SERVICES

Following the completion of this chapter, the student will be able to:

- Understand the proper documentation for medicine services.
- Understand the proper coding guidelines for each subsection of the medicine section.
- Identify the services encompassed in the medicine section.
- Comprehend the proper usage of modifier codes for services provided in the medicine section.
- Understand how to code medicine section services in conjunction with other services provided in CPT-4, using previously acquired bundling vs. separate guidelines.

KEY TERMS

Chiropractic, 332
Infusion, 327
Injection, 327
Intramuscularly (IM), 328
Intravenously (IV), 328
Osteopathic, 332
Otorhinolaryngological, 329

DOCUMENTATION/CODING GUIDELINES

Because the services in the Medicine section of CPT-4 are varied, the documentation guidelines vary greatly as well. All services contained in the Medicine section are considered diagnostic or therapeutic in nature, and thus, a physician request or order form is required, thereby beginning the documentation process. As with other ancillary services, such as radiology and pathology, however, only documentation that is verified as reviewed may be used to determine diagnosis and procedural coding information. Many of the services contained in the Medicine section will include not only the request, but also the imaging services performed as well as a written or dictated report. In the absence of a written or dictated report, written documentation contained on the actual imaging will serve documentation purposes as long as the interpreting physician indicates the written review, date, and signature (see Chapter 1).

Because many of the services are also based on the number of units, such as extremities or hours, documentation must include information to code for the specific unit(s) of service specified in the descriptor. Keep in mind that services must coincide verbatim with the CPT-4 procedure code to justify assignment of that specific code. For example, if Code 94681, Oxygen Uptake, Expired Gas Analysis, including CO_2 output and percentage oxygen extracted, is to be assigned, the patient must have undergone a protocol that includes all of the components specified by the descriptors.

Look at the breakdown of information needed to correctly assign CPT-4 code(s) for the Medicine services.

Medicine Section

Step 1

Identify Chapter	Diagnostic Therapeutic
Range of Codes	90281-99199 99500-99600

Step 2

Determine Type/Location	Specialty Type Allergy Pulmonary

Step 3

Specific Type	Specific Test Pulmonary Function Test

Step 4

Specific Procedure Information	Tests

Step 5

Extent/Additional Specifics	Additional Guidelines

A multitude of reports will be used for these services because they vary greatly. This section is unique in that it encompasses a variety of services, rather than just E & M or surgical services. The formats in which the information will be presented will vary greatly. Figures 15-1, 15-2, and 15-3 are forms of documentation. As with radiological and pathology services, for the coding/billing entity to be coded or billed for the global service, the coding/billing provider must document both the technical and interpretive reports.

MEDICINE SECTION CATEGORIES

The subchapters in the medicine section include the following:

- Immune globulins
- Immunization/vaccination administration
- Vaccines/toxoids
- Therapeutic/diagnostic infusions
- Therapeutic/diagnostic injections
- Psychiatry
- Biofeedback
- Dialysis
- Gastroenterology
- Ophthalmology
- Special otorhinolaryngological services
- Cardiovascular medicine
- Noninvasive vascular diagnostic studies
- Pulmonary medicine
- Allergy/clinical immunology
- Neurology/neuromuscular procedures
- Central nervous system assessments
- Chemotherapy administration
- Special dermatological services
- Physical medicine and rehabilitation
- Osteopathic manipulative treatment
- Chiropractic manipulative treatment
- Special supplies and services
- Sedation with or without analgesia
- Other services
- Home health services

CODING GUIDELINES

The medicine section of CPT encompasses diverse services. Several guidelines apply specifically to each subsection of the medicine section. These are discussed later in the chapter. It is important to differentiate the services found in the Medicine section of CPT-4 from those found in the Surgery section because they are often confused. Remember from the Surgery section discussion of CPT-4 (Chapter 12) that services in the surgery section are defined as invasive, definitive, or restorative.

Place top of report No. 3 here

PULMONARY FUNCTION REPORT

Name:_____

ID #:_____

Age:_____Ht:_____Wt:____

Reason for test:_____

Smoker?_____

Dyspnea:_____

Lung surgery:_____

Frequent cough:_____

Pain breathing?_____

Heart disease?_____

Wheeze/asthma?_____

Abnormal X-ray?_____

Test	PRED	ACTL	%PRED
FVC	4.76		81%
FEV1	3.77		88%
FEV1/FVC	81%		107%
FEF 25%–75%	4.64		124%
MMET (sec.)	0.68		49%
FEF max	9.14		127%
FEF 25%	8.43		126%
FEF 50%	6.26		118%
FEF 75%	3.17		56%
ET (sec.)	—		—
Maximal FVC	4.76		81%
Maximal FEV1	3.77		88%
MVV (L/min.)	154.7		100%

BTPS factor:_____ Last cal:_____

Primary normals source: Knudson.

Base:_____

T_____

Operator:_____

Physician:_____

GODFREY CLINICAL LABORATORIES
465 Dogwood Court • Aldon, FL 77712 • (407) 555-9876

FIGURE 15-1 Pulmonary Report

ELECTROMYOGRAPHY LABORATORY REPORT

Nerve conduction studies

NR = No response
M = Motor
S = Sensory
Mx = Mixed
• = no increment after 10 sec. exercise
† = no decrement to 2/sec x3
X = Forearm median to ulnar crossover

Name: _____
Clinic number: _____ Age: _____
Birthdate: _____ Date: _____
Referring physician: _____

Nerve stimulated (Recording site)	Amplitude (Sensory = uV; Meter = mV)					Distal/peak latency (mSec)			Conduction velocity (M/sec)			F-wave latency (mSec)		
	Distal			Proximal										
	Right	Left	Normal	Rt	Lt	Rt	Lt	Normal	Rt	Lt	Normal	Rt	Lt	Normal
Lower right														
Sural (S) Pt.B ankle						NH								
Peroneal (M) knee EDB	3.0					14.8			45					
Peroneal (M) ankle EDB	3.0					4.8								
Posterior tibia (M) knee AH	1.0					14.8			41					
Posterior tibia (M) ankle AH	1.5					4.2								
H-reflex						NR	NR							
Med (s) wrist 1st	9.0					3.6								
Med (m) elbow thenar	2.8					9.6			58					
Med (m) wrist thenar	2.8					4.4								
Ulnar (s) wrist 5th	1440					2.8								

Needle examination:

Summary:

Impression:

_____ , M.D.

GODFREY CLINICAL LABORATORIES
465 Dogwood Court • Aldon, FL 77712 • (407) 555-9876

FIGURE 15-2 EMG.

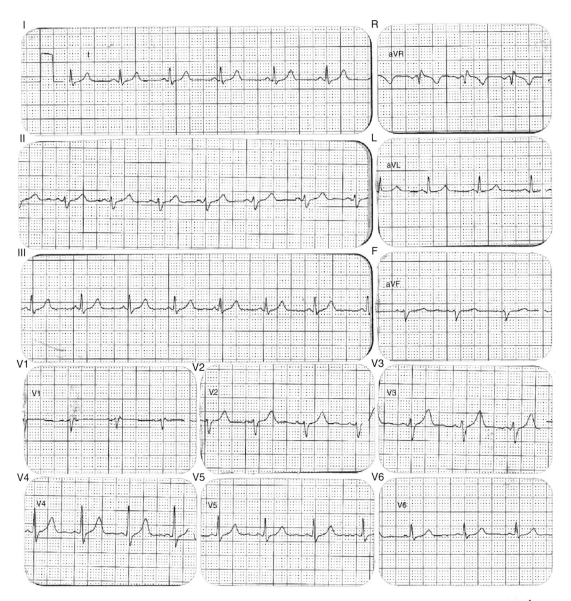

CLIN. DIAG.: Chest Pain

ECG DESCRIPTION: Stat 12 Lead

INTERPRETATION:

PATIENT: Jane Doe

DIG ( ) QUIN. ( ) AGE 29 SEX F B.P. 120/80

ECG REQUEST BY Dr. Hope U. Arewell.....
ATR. RATE ...90..... VENTR. RATE 90......
INTERVALS: P-R .12. QRS .08.. QTc........
AXIS: Left Axis shift
RHYTHM: Normal Sinus Rhythm

INTERPRETED BY: H. Arewell MD ....
DATE:

FIGURE 15-3 ECG. *(From Chester GA: Modern medical assisting, Philadelphia, 1998, WB Saunders).*

Services contained in the Medicine section, in contrast, are typically diagnostic or therapeutic or both. Most of the services contained in this section will not necessarily resolve a condition but rather diagnose or treat the problem.

MODIFIERS

Because the modifiers for the medicine section have been presented in other sections of this book, they are listed here for the convenience of the student.

Modifier 22	Unusual procedural services
Modifier 26	Professional component only
Modifier 32	Mandated services
Modifier 50	Bilateral procedures
Modifier 51	Multiple procedures
Modifier 52	Reduced services
Modifier 53	Discontinued procedures
Modifier 58	Related/staged procedure by same doctor during global surgical period
Modifier 59	Distinct procedure services
Modifier 62	Two surgeons
Modifier 66	Surgical team
Modifier 76	Repeat procedure by same physician
Modifier 77	Repeat procedure by another physician
Modifier 78	Return to OR for related procedure during global/postoperative period
Modifier 79	Unrelated procedure/service by same doctor during global/postoperative period
Modifier 80	Assistant surgeon
Modifier 90	Outside/reference laboratory services
Modifier 99	Multiple modifiers

The student may wish to refer to Chapter 16 (Modifiers) for a complete summary of codes, their definitions, and their proper usage.

STEPS IN CODING FROM THE MEDICINE SECTION

Step 1   Determine the specific subsection for Medicine services.
Step 2   Identify the procedure performed.
Step 3   Determine extent of procedure performed.
Step 4   Select appropriate code(s).
Step 5   Assign modifier code(s) when appropriate.

CODING OF SPECIFIC MEDICINE SUBSECTIONS

IMMUNE GLOBULINS

These codes identify the immune globulin product only. For administration of these products, the coder must select the appropriate injection code from codes 90765 through 90775.

IMMUNIZATION/VACCINATION ADMINISTRATION

These codes include the administration of the vaccine only, not the vaccine material for **injection**. Codes from range 90476 to 90749 should be assigned, as well as the appropriate administration code(s).

VACCINES/TOXOIDS

The codes in this section are intended for the provision of vaccine or toxoid supplies only. If the vaccine or toxoid is provided and administered, make certain to bill the appropriate administration code (90465-90474), as well as the proper vaccine or toxoid code. Note that many codes in this section are age specific, so make certain that information on patient age is taken into consideration when the code is selected.

Many of the services defined in this section are preventive in nature, so some insurance carriers will not reimburse for these services. Medicare, however, will cover the pneumococcal pneumonia vaccination and the hepatitis B vaccine in specific instances.

THERAPEUTIC/DIAGNOSTIC INFUSIONS (EXCLUDING CHEMOTHERAPY)

These codes are intended for use in prolonged intravenous **infusion.** Code 90765 should be used when the time of infusion does not exceed 1 hour. A minimum of half an hour (or half the increment) must be documented before this service can be coded; time must be documented if this service is to be billed. Additional 1-hour increments, up to eight, may be billed with code 90766. For each additional hour, an infusion requiring at least half an hour (30 minutes) must have been performed and documented. Note that when CPT-4 codes contain the term *each,* those services should NOT be billed as multiple or repeat procedures, but rather with the appropriate code and in multiple units of service (e.g., ×4, 2× in the units column of the claim form).

ADMINISTRATION/PROVISION OF DRUGS/VACCINES

	Immune globulins	Vaccine/ toxoids	Medications	Chemotherapy
ADMINISTRATION	90765–90779	90465–90474	90765–90779	96400–96542
PROVISION OF MEDICINE/AGENT	90281–90399	90476–90749	99070 or HCPCS as required by specific carrier	96545 or HCPCS as required by specific carrier

FIGURE 15-4 Administration/Provision of Drugs/Medicines/Vaccines.

THERAPEUTIC/DIAGNOSTIC INJECTIONS

When injections are performed subcutaneously, **intramuscularly (IM),** intraarterially, or **intravenously (IV),** codes from this section should be used. Make certain when coding for injection services that the name, strength, dosage, and route of medication are specified.

Figure 15-4 contains the code ranges necessary for injection services. Note that the table shows a minimum of two codes in most cases (one for the provision of the drugs and one for the administration).

PSYCHIATRY

Because many services performed by psychiatric staff may not meet the requirements for E & M services, these services are encompassed in the psychiatric subsection of the medicine section.

A word of caution when coding and billing for services provided from the psychiatric section: many insurance carriers will not pay for services provided by other than a licensed physician or credentialed provider. Make certain to incorporate this information in the Third-Party Contract Worksheet to ensure only authorized providers render these services.

Many codes listed in the psychiatry medicine section specify where the services are provided, and some may be physician specific. Make certain the services are provided only by authorized providers, and that the claim correctly reflects this information.

Psychiatric therapeutic services are categorized as insight oriented, behavior modifying, or interactive, and are divided according to location. The following steps are used to determine the correct psychiatry codes.

Step 1

Determine Whether the Service Should Be Coded from the E & M Section or from the Psychiatry/ Medicine Section

Step 2

Determine Procedure Performed
Services are divided by the following:

- Office/other outpatient
- Inpatient/partial hospital/residential care

Step 3

Determine Extent/Type of Service

- Insight oriented or behavior modifying
- Development of behavior modification and of insight and supportive therapy necessary to provide therapeutic change
- Interactive
- Use of play equipment, physical devices, or other means of nonverbal communication to effect therapeutic change

Step 4

Determine Appropriate Code(s) Based on Time
Keep in mind the "rounding" rule: half or more of a time unit must be provided before a specific code can be used. This means that all psychiatric medicine codes involving time MUST include its proper documentation.

In addition to the insight oriented and interactive psychotherapy codes, other psychotherapy codes are included in the psychiatry/medicine section; these encompass group and family therapy, and psychiatric services such as electroconvulsive therapy.

BIOFEEDBACK

Biofeedback training is encompassed in these codes; a code is included for each modality, as well as specific codes for perianal, anorectal, or urethral sphincter training.

DIALYSIS

Dialysis is not considered a surgical procedure. The coder will find dialysis codes in the medicine section. Because services for dialysis patients are typically provided on a scheduled basis in the course of a month, many of the units for these codes include months.

Patients with end-stage renal disease (ESRD) require regular dialysis and management. Codes that cover these services are assigned on the basis of the following:

1. Age of the patient (codes are specific to patient age)
2. Length of time services were performed (codes available for full or partial month)
3. The type of services (ESRD or hemodialysis)

Training and hemoperfusion codes are also included in the dialysis section. Remember that services performed, that meet criteria for codable services, should be coded and billed whether or not a given carrier provides reimbursement.

GASTROENTEROLOGY

Some gastroenterological procedures are included in the medicine section under the surgical heading because many are invasive. Keep in mind that guidelines for the medicine section should be followed for these services, but GI surgical procedures follow surgery guidelines for coding and billing. Placement of tubes (intestinal bleeding tubes, esophageal intubation) and gastrointestinal studies are included in this section. Also, those providers who are not GI physicians commonly use the gastric intubation code 91105.

OPHTHALMOLOGY

As with psychiatry, a number of services provided by ophthalmologists do not meet the E & M guidelines for physician services. Ophthalmological services are included in the medicine section of CPT-4. To code for these services, the coder must identify the following:

1. New patient/established patient status
   Keep in mind the new patient rules previously discussed. If the patient has already been seen by the physician or a member of his or her group within the last 3 years, that patient is considered an established patient.
2. Level of service provided
   Intermediate—includes history, general medical observation, external ocular and adnexal examination, and other diagnostic procedures.
   Comprehensive—includes a general evaluation of the **complete** visual system. These services constitute a single service, but they may be provided over more than one visit. These services include the following:
   - History
   - General medical observation
   - External/ophthalmoscopic examination
   - Gross visual fields
   - Basic sensorimotor examination
   Special—includes special evaluation of part of the visual system.
   In addition, special ophthalmological services are included in this section, which include the following:
   - Refractive state determination
   - Contact lens fitting
   - Visual field examination
   - Tonometry
   - Tonography
   - Ophthalmoscopy

The ophthalmology section differentiates between contact lens services provided for the patient with impaired vision, such as myopia, and those performed for the patient with aphakia. Make certain that the correct code is selected on the basis of the medical data and that these data are included in the medical record. In many instances, third-party carriers do not reimburse for contact lens services other than for the diagnosis of aphakia, so when this diagnosis is appropriate, it is important that it be included for proper reimbursement.

The codes for the fitting of eyeglasses are similarly divided into nonaphakia and aphakia diagnoses, as are the supply codes listed in this section.

SPECIAL OTORHINOLARYNGOLOGICAL SERVICES

Only those ENT services not typically included in a comprehensive E & M visit are listed in this section. These include the following:

- Treatment of speech disorders
- Vestibular function tests
- Audiological function tests (include such tests as hearing tests, hearing aid checks or testing, and other hearing-specific diagnostic testing)

CARDIOVASCULAR MEDICINE

The practice of cardiology is typically divided into at least the following three subspecialties:

1. Noninvasive cardiology
2. Cardiovascular surgery
3. Electrophysiology

Procedures typically performed by the cardiovascular surgeon have already discussed in the cardiac subsection of the surgery section. Those procedures that are noninvasive appear in the medicine section of CPT-4.

For this section, the coder may disregard the rule that includes approach for a procedure within the procedure code. When cardiac catheterization is provided in conjunction with other cardiac services listed in this section, such as balloon angioplasty, both services may be billed. Note that procedures in this section are somewhat progressive in nature. Many of the more involved cardiac procedures are inclusive of services listed elsewhere. For example, note that atherectomy includes performance with or without balloon angioplasty.

A problem encountered in coding these noninvasive procedures is that some procedures (e.g., placement of stents, balloon angioplasty, atherectomy) are coded and billed by EACH vessel treated. For purposes of coding these services, the CPT-4 and the ACC (American College of Cardiology) recognize only three main vessels and the corresponding modifiers:

LC   Left circumflex coronary artery
LD   Left anterior descending coronary artery
RC   Right coronary artery

Branch vessels from these three arteries are included in the services. For example, when two stents are placed in the same vessel (e.g., right coronary), only one code (92980) should be selected. The three vessels are identified by modifiers LC, LD, and RC to denote the specific vessel. These modifier codes represent HCPCS/National Level II modifier codes and are not recognized by all third-party carriers. Should the practice perform these services, the coder must incorporate into the submission of claims the codes for which third-party carriers wish these modifiers to be included.

As with many specialized services, there is a progression of both service level and associated medical necessity for these services. The scenario in Chapter 13 in which a few students rather than the whole group received thallium stress tests is an example. This is especially true in the cardiology section. Medicare and many other third-party carriers have specific diagnostic codes that are considered medically necessary for low-level services, such as ECGs; higher-level services require a more specific comprehensive diagnostic statement before reimbursement will be considered.

Cardiac catheterization is the medical diagnostic procedure that involves introduction, positioning, and repositioning of the catheter, in addition to recording of measurements. When angiography is performed in conjunction with a cardiac catheterization, each angiography code may be billed, in addition to the cardiac catheterization. Angiography requires dye injection. Codes for the injection, the angiography, and heart catheterization are therefore appropriate. Modifier 51 is not necessary for these services because it is assumed multiple codes or services are provided during one session.

Figure 15-5 outlines the components in assigning codes for the performance of a cardiac catheterization and associated services.

Electrophysiological procedures are also included in the noninvasive cardiology subchapter of the medicine section. Note that the procedures in this section are noninvasive, and the implantation or removal of pacemakers and stimulators is included in the cardiac surgery section. Analysis of pacemaker function is included in the "Other Vascular Studies" section of the cardiology subsection.

NONINVASIVE VASCULAR DIAGNOSTIC STUDIES

Noninvasive vascular diagnostic studies are divided into the following groups:

- Cerebrovascular arterial studies
- Extremity arterial studies
- Extremity venous studies
- Visceral and penile vascular studies
- Extremity arterial-venous studies

PULMONARY MEDICINE

The pulmonary medicine services listed in this section are diagnostic procedures and interpretations only. When E & M services are provided in addition to these services, they may be reported with the appropriate E & M code(s).

The coder must ensure that these services are performed by the billing provider. In some instances, these services may be performed in an inpatient hospital setting; in this case, the services are provided by hospital staff and are only interpreted by the medical provider. When this occurs, a code specific only to interpretation and reading should be used, or the appropriate code should have modifier 26 appended.

ALLERGY/CLINICAL IMMUNOLOGY

Allergy testing encompasses procedures performed percutaneously by scratch, puncture, or prick to determine allergy sensitivities. Allergy testing may

---

CARDIAC CATHETERIZATION CODING

1. **Access site**

Venous/right	Codes 93501/93530
Arterial/left	Codes 93510–93524
Combined left/right	Codes 93526–93533
Catheterization performed subsequent day for therapeutic services (PTCA, stent, atherectomy where left heart cath not performed	Code 93508

2. **Injection/imaging codes**

	Injection	Imaging
Arterial conduit	93539	93556
Aortocoronary venous bypass	93540	93556
Pulmonary	93541	~~93556~~
Selective right ventricular/atrial	93542	93555
Left ventricular/atrial	93543	93555
Aorta	93544	93556
Selective coronary	93545	93556

Coding guidelines:
Duplicate imaging codes should be deleted. Modifier 51 need not be assigned.

3. **Therapeutic procedures (when applicable)**

	1st vessel	Each addtl. vessel
PTCA (balloon angioplasty)	92982	92984
Intracoronary stent(s)	92980	92981
Atherectomy	92995	92996

Coding guidelines:
Definitive procedure only may be coded per vessel
Vessel modifiers:

LC	Left circumflex
LD	Left anterior descending
RC	Right coronary

FIGURE 15-5 Cardiac Catheterization Coding.

---

also be performed intracutaneously or with patch application.

The allergen immunotherapy procedure includes professional services for the administration of allergy immunotherapy, but does not include provision of the allergenic extract. Codes 95120 through 95170 include the provision of the extract, as well as administration of the allergy immunotherapy. E & M codes can be billed in addition to allergen immunotherapy codes only if other E & M services are performed.

Keep in mind that the medical documentation for these services should include a verbal or written order for all allergenic extracts, as well as documentation by the billing provider of allergen immunotherapy either provided or supervised by the billing provider.

Many patients with allergies present to their physicians for the sole purpose of receiving allergy immunotherapy.

In many instances, these patients present with their vials of allergenic extract, or that extract may be stored at the physician's office. In these instances, only the codes for administration of that extract should be charged.

NEUROLOGY AND NEUROMUSCULAR PROCEDURES

Services in this section include EEG (electroencephalogram), EMG (electromyelogram), evoked potential, and sleep services. These may be billed in addition to any E & M services provided over and above the neurological procedures.

CENTRAL NERVOUS SYSTEM ASSESSMENTS

These services, which are typically provided for testing cognitive functions, include such services as assessment of aphasia and speech, and neurobehavioral, neuro-psychological, and psychological evaluation.

CHEMOTHERAPY ADMINISTRATION

These services are separate from the patient's encounter with the physician. If chemotherapy is provided at the same encounter as the physician E & M service, both may be billed if two separate services have been provided.

Chemotherapy administration includes only the administration of the chemotherapy agent. The chemotherapy agents or drugs must be listed separately usually with an appropriate HCPCS code (discussed later).

Chemotherapy services may be provided via several routes, such as the following:

- Subcutaneous
- Intramuscular
- Intravenous
- Infusion
- Intraarterial
- Directly into the pleural cavity

Codes are also available in this section to bill for the refilling and maintenance of portable or implanted chemotherapy pumps.

Several chemotherapy administration codes are listed by the hour and, as in the diagnostic injection/infusion section, the rounding-up rule applies. Units of service are used rather than a modifier code for multiple services.

Time is important to correct coding, so documentation should include the amount of time spent performing these services. Refer to Figure 15-4 for the ranges for coding and billing chemotherapy administration and drugs.

SPECIAL DERMATOLOGICAL SERVICES

Actinotherapy and photochemotherapy services are included in this section. For the most part, the services of the dermatologist are included in the E & M section or the integumentary subsection of the surgery section.

PHYSICAL MEDICINE AND REHABILITATION

Physical therapy is provided through the following two mechanisms:

Modalities: Any physical agent applied that produces therapeutic changes in tissue. Agents include light, mechanical, electric energy, and thermal applications. They may be delivered by two methods:
Supervised—Does not require the direct supervision of the provider

Constant Attendance—Requires one-on-one contact with the provider
Therapeutic Procedures: Methods that attempt to improve functionality through the application of clinical skills. The provider is required to have one-on-one contact for the services performed in this section. Procedures such as massage, gait training, and manual therapy are included in this subsection.

Many of the codes in this section are time-driven (15-minute increment). Third party (insurance) guidelines stipulate that one-half of that time unit must be used in order to code and bill for a unit of service.

ACTIVE WOUND CARE MANAGEMENT

Codes from this section are used for the removal of devitalized or dead tissue to promote healing. These codes are intended for treatment of chronic, nonhealing wounds that require selective or nonselective debridement.

OSTEOPATHIC MANIPULATIVE TREATMENT

This section involves procedures performed by the physician who provides manual treatment to reduce, alleviate, or eliminate impairment. Codes from this section are assigned by the number of body regions involved.

CHIROPRACTIC MANIPULATIVE TREATMENT

Chiropractic treatment involves procedures designed to improve joint and neurophysiological function. These codes are assigned by the number of spinal regions including the following:

- Cervical
- Thoracic
- Lumbar
- Sacral
- Pelvic

Five extraspinal regions are also identified as the following:

- Upper extremities
- Lower extremities
- Rib cage
- Head
- Abdomen

A premanipulation assessment of the patient is included in this section and may be coded in addition to an Evaluation and Management Service, if the patient's condition requires significantly separately identifiable services above the usual work associated with the pre-manipulation assessment.

SPECIAL SUPPLIES AND SERVICES

This category represents the "miscellaneous" portion of the medicine section and those codes that do not fit in any other category in CPT-4. Many services listed in this section are coded and billed. Many insurance carriers do not reimburse for these services, which include such items as educational supplies, physician educational services, and office services provided outside normal hours or the normal confines of the office. Some of these codes are delineated in the following sections.

99000—Specimen Handling

This code should be used when a specimen must be prepared for transfer from the provider's office to a laboratory for testing. This code is discussed in the Pathology Section of the book (Chapter 14).

99024—Postoperative Follow-up Care

Normal postoperative care that is an integral part of the global surgical procedure is billed with code 99024. There is usually no charge or fee associated with this code. It serves as a "placeholder" for "counting" services provided. It also statistically tracks the average number of follow-up postoperative visits needed for specific surgical cases.

This code would NOT be used for other than normal postoperative follow-up care. Those services would be billed with the appropriate E & M service code and the appropriate modifier code(s). This is discussed in Surgery Section (Chapter 12).

99025—Code Has Been Deleted with the Deletion of the (*) Starred Concept

Most third-party carriers do not recognize this code or reimburse for these services. Carrier of workers' compen-

sation often consider this procedure code for reimbursement as defined by state rather than federal guidelines, which do not require carriers to conform to HIPAA guidelines with the current year's CPT-4 code book.

99070—Miscellaneous Supplies and Materials

This code should NOT be used for those items normally used by the physician supplying the normal E & M service. An invoice delineating the cost of the item is often requested. Make certain when using this code for medications that the name, strength, and dosage of each medication are documented on the claim.

When the provision of drugs/biologicals is coded with code 99070, it is necessary to include the name of the drug, strength, dosage, and route of administration on the second line of the CMS-1500 claim form. The use of this code is shown in Figure 15-1.

SEDATION WITH OR WITHOUT ANALGESIA (CONSCIOUS SEDATION)

This medical procedure, which induces a medically controlled state of reduced consciousness, may be performed intravenously; intramuscularly; or through inhalation, oral, rectal, and intranasal routes.

OTHER SERVICES

This category includes such services as administration of ipecac (99175), use of hyperbaric oxygen therapy or hypothermia, assembly and operation of oxygenator/heat exchanger, and phlebotomy when performed for therapeutic purposes.

HOME HEALTH SERVICES

This category, added in 2002, incorporates codes for services and visits provided by home health providers. A physician's office would not use these codes.

CHAPTER IN REVIEW

CERTIFICATION REVIEW

- Services listed in the medicine section may be coded/billed by any provider who meets the description of services outlined.
- The codes for immunization/vaccine administration are to be used for the administration only. Supply of the vaccine material is coded from 90476 through 90749.
- When code descriptions contain the word "each," the code is used for each unit of service provided. For example, when 8 hours of a particular service is provided, and the code specifies "each" hour, the service should be coded with the correct CPT-4 code once only, with the days or units of services designated as 8.
- Services outlined in the psychiatry section indicate that some specific services must be provided by physicians only.
- Many of the psychiatry codes are divided into two categories: interactive and insight oriented.
- Several codes in the dialysis subsection are billed on a monthly basis.
- Gastroenterology services in the medicine section should follow guidelines from the medicine section, but gastroenterology services from the surgical section follow surgical guidelines.
- Cardiovascular services recognize three main vessels for purposes of coding/billing: left circumflex, left anterior descending, and right coronary artery.
- In coding for allergy services, an E & M service may NOT be billed unless documentation supports a separately identifiable E & M service.
- The supply of drugs is coded/billed using 99070 from CPT-4, unless the specific carrier dictates the use of HCPCS codes for medication supplies.
- Specimen handling codes are to be used only when a specimen must be prepared for transfer from a facility to the laboratory for testing purposes.
- The postoperative follow-up care code 99024 designates those services that are an integral component of the global surgery procedure. As such, they typically hold no dollar value, but serve as a tracking mechanism for the number of postoperative follow-up visits needed for specific cases.
- When other than normal uncomplicated follow-up care is performed, the use of 99024 is NOT appropriate. Use the appropriate E & M code.

STUDENT STUDY GUIDE

- Study Chapter 15.
- Review the Learning Objectives for Chapter 15.
- Review the Certification Review for Chapter 15.
- Complete the Chapter Review exercise to reinforce concepts learned in the chapter.

CHAPTER REVIEW EXERCISE

Complete the following coding exercises using the medicine section of CPT-4.

1. Cardiac catheterization, left with stent placement to the left circumflex coronary artery
   CPT-4 CODE(S): _____
2. ECG, interpretation and report only
   CPT-4 CODE(S): _____
3. Cardiac echocardiograph with cardiac color flow Doppler imaging
   CPT-4 CODE(S): _____
4. Mumps, measles, rubella vaccine
   CPT-4 CODE(S): _____
5. Chemotherapy, infusion, IV, 2 hours
   CPT-4 CODE(S): _____
6. Dermatological ultraviolet light treatment
   CPT-4 CODE(S): _____
7. End-stage renal disease, dialysis, per month, under age 2
   CPT-4 CODE(S): _____
8. Prescription and fitting of contact lenses
   CPT-4 CODE(S): _____
9. Laryngeal function studies
   CPT-4 CODE(S): _____
10. Cardiopulmonary resuscitation
    CPT-4 CODE(S): _____
11. PTCA, left circumflex/right coronary
    CPT-4 CODE(S): _____
12. Spirometry
    CPT-4 CODE(S): _____
13. Postoperative follow-up visit
    CPT-4 CODE(S): _____
14. Intraoperative neurophysiology testing, 1 hour
    CPT-4 CODE(S): _____
15. Patch allergy test(s), 15 tests
    CPT-4 CODE(S): _____
16. Doppler study of intracranial arteries, limited, transcranial
    CPT-4 CODE(S): _____
17. Bronchospasm evaluation
    CPT-4 CODE(S): _____
18. Cardiovascular stress test, complete
    CPT-4 CODE(S): _____

19. Allergy immunotherapy, administration only
CPT-4 CODE(S): _____

20. Comprehensive ophthalmological examination, new patient
CPT-4 CODE(S): _____

PRACTICAL APPLICATION

Assign CPT-4 code(s), appropriate modifier(s), and list code(s) in the correct order for the following scenarios.

1.

OPERATIVE REPORT

Patient information:

Patient name:
DOB:
MR#:

Preoperative diagnosis:

Obstruction of right coronary and left circumflex vessels

Postoperative diagnosis:

Obstruction of right coronary and left circumflex vessels

Procedure(s) performed:

Anesthesia:

Assistant surgeon:

Description of procedure:

Access was made via the left femoral vein. Imaging was obtained of the pulmonary, coronary and left and right ventricles. Obstruction was noted in the right coronary vessels x 3 and the left circumflex x 4. PTCA was performed x 3 in the right coronary vessel, two of which required the placement of an intracoronary stent. The left circumflex required four (4) angioplasties only.

Ruth Brady Me

GODFREY REGIONAL HOSPITAL
123 Main Street • Aldon, FL 77714 • (407) 555-1234

CPT-4 CODE(S): _____

2.

OPERATIVE REPORT

Patient information:

Patient name:
DOB:
MR#:

Preoperative diagnosis:

Postoperative diagnosis:

Procedure(s) performed:

Heart catheterization with aortography, left/right ventriculogram pulmonary, and coronary vessels

Anesthesia:

Assistant surgeon:

Description of procedure:

Access was made via the left femoral artery. Imaging was obtained on the pulmonary and coronary vessels as well as the aorta and left and right ventricles. As the vessels were patent, no further procedures were necessary.

GODFREY REGIONAL HOSPITAL
123 Main Street • Aldon, FL 77714 • (407) 555-1234

CPT-4 CODE(S): _____

3.

OPERATIVE REPORT

Patient information:

Patient name:
DOB:
MR#:

Preoperative diagnosis:

Postoperative diagnosis:

Procedure(s) performed:

Left heart catheterization
Angioplasty, left circumflex with stent
Atherectomy, left circumflex
Angioplasty, left descending with stent

Anesthesia:

Assistant surgeon:

Description of procedure:

Imaging was obtained of the left and right ventricles, the aorta and coronary arteries. Obstructions were identified in the circumflex, the descending and the coronary vessel appeared clear.

Three angioplasties were performed in the left circumflex, followed by stent placement; however, neither was successful and atherectomy was necessary in the three obstructed areas of the left circumflex. Angioplasties X 2 were performed in the left descending, one followed by stent placement.

Ruth Brady Mv

GODFREY REGIONAL HOSPITAL
123 Main Street • Aldon, FL 77714 • (407) 555-1234

CPT-4 CODE(S): _____

4.

OPERATIVE REPORT

Patient information:

Patient name:
DOB:
MR#:

Preoperative diagnosis:

History and assessment
Pt admission status - elective
Atypical chest pain

Postoperative diagnosis:

Atypical chest pain
Hx Smoking 10 years ago, 1 PPD 20 years

Procedure(s) performed:

Anesthesia:

Assistant surgeon:

Description of procedure:

Pre Procedure Notes
09:42:48 Patient Assessment: Alert, oriented, calm, skin warm and dry
09:42:52 ID Band Correct. Consent signed in chart.
09:42:58 Pre-Cath Respirations: Normal - 20
09:43:12 Pre-Cath ECG Rhythm: Normal Sinus Rhythm
09:43:15 Pre-Cath Heart Rate: 55
09:43:22 Pre-Cath Distal Pulses: Bilateral DP 3+
09:43:27 Pre-Cath O2 Sat: 100%
09:45:04 IV Patent on arrival on left hand .45 NSS @20cc/hr
09:46:10 Setup complete

Diagnostic Equipment
10:09:47 Sheaths cordis standard sheath 4 Fr
10:09:57 Catheters cordis 4 Fr JL 4.0/5.0/6.0 cm catheter
10:14:12 Catheters cordis 4 Fr, straight pigtail catheter

Intra Procedure Notes
10:08:36 MD arrives
10:08:41 Lab values: Abnormal, MD notified
10:08:46 Local: Lidocaine, 2% to right groin
10:09:11 Percutaneous stick to right femoral artery
10:09:18 Arterial access: 4 Fr sheath inserted into right femoral artery
10:09:40 4 Fr JL catheter introduced
10:21:44 RCA accessed; digital angiography performed, multiple views
10:22:26 4 Fr pigtail catheter introduced
10:24:29 LV angiography, RAD 10 mg/sec
10:25:14 Aortic angiography ascending LAO 20 ml/sec
10:26:31 Aortic angiography ascending RAO 20 ml/sec
10:27:21 Procedure complete

Post Procedure
10:28:05 Post assessment, respirations, BP, ECG normal
10:28:30 IV patent on discharge
10:28:45 Sheath(s) pulled, pressure to site for 24 min
10:42:54 Patient transferred to room

GODFREY REGIONAL HOSPITAL
123 Main Street • Aldon, FL 77714 • (407) 555-1234

CPT-4 CODE(S): _____

CPT only © American Medical Association. All Rights Reserved.

5.

OPERATIVE REPORT

Patient information:
Patient name: DOB: MR#:

Preoperative diagnosis:
Indications for procedure: 52-year-old black male underwent evaluation for abnormal electrocardiogram. Noted to have multiple risk factors for coronary artery disease including hypertension, hypercholesterolemia and borderline diabetes.

Postoperative diagnosis:

Procedure(s) performed:
Left heart catheterization with coronary angiography, left ventriculography and right femoral artery, angioseal deployment.

Anesthesia:

Assistant surgeon:

Description of procedure:
After informed consent was obtained from the patient, he was taken to the cardiac catheterization lab in a fasting, mildly sedated state with peripheral IV line in place. After electrocardiographic monitoring was established, the right femoral artery was anesthetized with 1% local lidocaine. The right femoral artery was then accessed via modified Seldinger technique and a 6 French arterial sheath was placed. All subsequent catheter exchanges were performed over guidewires and under fluoroscopic monitoring. The patient underwent left heart catheterization with the use of a 6 French JL4 and JR4 catheter with multiple coronary angiograms being obtained in multiple projections. When completed, these catheters were removed and a 6 French pigtail catheter was inserted through the sheath into the left ventricle where hemodynamic data were obtained. The pigtail catheter was subsequently removed from the left ventricle, and, of note, there were no significant transvalvular gradient across the aortic valve on pullback maneuver. The pigtail catheter was then repositioned in a retrograde fashion within the right ileofemoral regional whereby hand contrast injection demonstrated appropriate vasculature for deployment of an Angioseal device. The pigtail catheter was then removed and the arterial sheath was exchanged over the guidewire for a 6 French Angioseal vascular sealing device. Complications: None Medications: Heparin 2000 units for intra-arterial injection   Nitroglycerin 200 mcg per intracavitary injections Contrast Used: 150 cc of Iso-Vue. Fluoro time 4.5 minutes

GODFREY REGIONAL HOSPITAL
123 Main Street • Aldon, FL 77714 • (407) 555-1234

CPT-4 CODE(S): _____

6.

NERVE CONDUCTION STUDIES

Median motor	R	L	NL
Amplitude			>4
Distal motor latency			<4.2
Proximal motor latency			
Conduction velocity			>50
F-Wave			<33

Ulnar motor	R	L	NL
Amplitude			>6
Distal motor latency			<3.5
Proximal motor latency			
CV below elbow to wrist			>50
CV across elbow			>50
CD above elbow to wrist			>50
Erb's to wrist			>50

Peroneal motor	R	L	NL
Amplitude			>2
Distal motor latency	3.9	5.6	<6.6
Proximal motor latency	13.9	16.4	
F-Wave			<58
Conduction velocity	44.0	41.6	>40

Tibial motor	R	L	NL
Amplitude			>4
Distal motor latency	6.0	3.5	<6.9
Proximal motor latency	16.2	14.1	
F-Wave			<58
Conduction velocity	47.0	44.3	>40
H-Reflex			<37

Median sensory	R	L	NL
Distal sensory latency			<3.5
Proximal sensory latency			
Conduction velocity			>50

Ulnar sensory	R	L	NL
Distal sensory latency			<3.5
Proximal sensory latency			
Conduction velocity			>50

Radial sensory	R	L	NL
Amplitude			>22
Distal sensory latency			<2.9

Sural sensory	R	L	NL
Amplitude			>6
Distal sensory latency			<4.5
Conduction velocity			>42

Interpretation:

Normal NCD in peroneal and tibial nerves

[signature]

GODFREY CLINICAL LABORATORIES
465 Dogwood Court • Aldon, FL 77712 • (407) 555-9876

CPT-4 CODE(S): _____

7.

ELECTROMYOGRAPHY LABORATORY REPORT

Nerve conduction studies

NR = No response
M = Motor
S = Sensory
Mx = Mixed
• = no increment after 10 sec. exercise
† = no decrement to 2/sec x3
X = Forearm median to ulnar crossover

Name: _____
Clinic number: _____ Age: ____
Birthdate: _____ Date: _____
Referring physician: _____

Nerve stimulated (Recording site)	Fib and Int												Distal/peak latency (mSec)			Conduction velocity (M/sec)			F-wave latency (mSec)		
	Insert		Fasic			Poly Pattern Amp							Rt	Lt	Normal	Rt	Lt	Normal	Rt	Lt	Normal
	L	R	L	R	L	R	L	R	L	R	L	R									
Lower right																					
Quadricep	N	N	0	0	0	0	0	0	N	N	N	N									
Tibialis Ant	N	N	0	0	0	0	0	0	N	N	N	N									
Ext Digitorum Brevis	N	N	2+	0	0	0	0	0	N	N	N	N									
Peroneus Long																					
Biceps Femoris																					
Gluteus Max																					
Gastrocnemius	N	N	3+	0	0	0	0	0	N	N	N	N									

Needle examination:

Summary:

Impression:

Interpretation:
Probable left S1 radiculopathy

_____ , M.D.

GODFREY CLINICAL LABORATORIES
465 Dogwood Court • Aldon, FL 77712 • (407) 555-9876

CPT-4 CODE(S): _____

8.

PULMONARY FUNCTION STUDY

Name:_____

ID #: _____

Age: _____Ht:_____Wt:____

Reason for test: _____

Smoker?_____

Dyspnea: _____

Lung surgery:_____

Frequent cough: _____

Pain breathing?_____

Heart disease?_____

Wheeze/asthma? _____

Abnormal X-ray?_____

Spirometry	PRED	ACTUAL	%PRED	ACTUAL	%PRED	%CHG
FVC	4.03	2.81	69	3.23	80	15
FEV1	2.89	2.07	37	1.22	42	13
FEV1/FVC	72	38		38		
FEV3/FDC	97	60	62			
FEF 25%–75%	2.91	0.27	9	0.33	11	22
FEF 50%		0.23		0.31		33
FEF 75%		0.26		0.16		0
PEF	7.66	3.05	40	4.22	55	38
						17
FET 100%		14.5		17.2		
FIVC	4.03	2.35	58	2.80	69	
FIF 50%		3.66		4.83		
PIF	3.90			5.11		
FEF 50/FIF 50	<1.00	0.06		0.06		
MVV	127	41	32	57	45	41
F		105		100		

COMMENTS:

Spirometry Pre and Post Isuprel. Pt cooperated well. ABGs done on room air. Thick to thin mucus during testing.
Blood gases, PH 7.44 PC02 39.7 PO2 81.5 HC03 27.0 B.E. 3.2

INTERPRETATION:

Forced vital capacity is mildly reduced. There is moderate reduction in forced expiratory volume in the first second.
FEV1, FEC ration maximum expiratory flow rate is markedly reduced. This is improvement following bronchodilator.

Arterial blood gases on room air are normal.

Nith Budy Mc
Pulmonologist

GODFREY CLINICAL LABORATORIES
465 Dogwood Court • Aldon, FL 77712 • (407) 555-9876

CPT-4 CODE(S): _____

9.

PROGRESS NOTE

Chief complaint: _____

Date: _____

Vital signs: BP_____ P_____ R_____

Electrocardiogram report:

This is a rhythm strip being recorded while the patient is shocked. There are bizarre, wide QRS complexes probably due to agonal rhythm. This is followed by asystole when code was called off.

Ruth Brady MD

Patient name: _____

Date of service: _____

GODFREY MEDICAL ASSOCIATES
1532 Third Avenue, Suite 120 • Aldon, FL 77713 • (407) 555-4000

CPT-4 CODE(S): _____

10.

PROGRESS NOTE

Chief complaint: _____

Date: _____

Vital signs: BP_____ P_____ R_____

Electrocardiogram report:

Chief Complaint: 62-year-old male presents to ED with chest pain off and on times one day. Nausea. NTG, Morphine and ASA given by EMS. No EMS runsheet or EKG on chart.

First ED EKG:

First EKG done at 1003 (4 min). ED physician read as Hyperacute T-Waves V1-V4. Second EKG no change. Overread: Hyperacute T waves. Borderline IV conduction delay.

Ruth Brady M

Patient name: _____

Date of service: _____

GODFREY MEDICAL ASSOCIATES
1532 Third Avenue, Suite 120 • Aldon, FL 77713 • (407) 555-4000

CPT-4 CODE(S): _____

16

MODIFIERS

LEARNING OBJECTIVES

Following the completion of this chapter, the student will be able to:

- Comprehend the rules and application of modifiers to the coding process.
- Know the proper application of each modifier.
- Understand the appropriate reason for applying modifiers to services.
- Grasp the reimbursement significance of proper modifier code(s) submission.

CODING REFERENCE TOOLS

Tool 51
CPT-4 Modifier Coding Reference Tool

KEY TERMS

Bilateral, 348
Modifier Code, 347
Professional Component, 348
Technical Component, 348

DOCUMENTATION GUIDELINES

The previous sections discussed the correct usage of **modifier codes,** perhaps the most challenging aspect of coding. It is also one of the most important aspects of medical coding because modifier use can clarify medical necessity for services in unusual circumstances. As with other services, those with an appended modifier codes must be substantiated by documentation that supports the request for payment in extenuating circumstances. For instance, the use of modifier 22, unusual procedural services, suggests that the services performed are beyond the normal scope of the CPT-4 descriptor and justifies additional reimbursement consideration. Without proper documentation or any documentation, the services will receive only the usual reimbursement for the CPT-4 code listed. Unusual circumstances that create additional complexity during the procedure, such as complications or hemorrhage, must be documented, with explanation why services more than usual were rendered and should be considered for additional payment.

Once the coder has decided that a modifier code is necessary for billed services to be considered for reimbursement, he or she must gather some additional information regarding the service.

- What type of service was provided (which chapter guidelines are appropriate)?
- Are the services listed as physician or outpatient surgery (separate modifiers for physician versus outpatient)?
- When needed, does documentation reflect the unusual circumstances (e.g., greater than usual service)?
- Does the service require a report and manual billing?

Box 16-1 illustrates why and when to use a modifier. Box 16-2 lists the rules for using modifier codes.

As with other ICD-9-CM and CPT-4 codes, the use of a modifier is supported by the documentation, whether coding/billing for more or reduced services. Typically, services coded with the use of a modifier code may be subject to manual review by the carrier, and a copy of the documentation that substantiates the request for payment may be requested. The assignment of an appropriate modifier code is essential to proper reimbursement. Documentation is even more vital to receiving reimbursement for services coded with a modifier.

TYPES OF MODIFIERS

One of the last steps in correct procedural coding is checking whether the usage of a particular modifier is

BOX 16-1 WHY and WHEN to Use a Modifier

1. Use a modifier when further explanation of performed services is necessary.
2. Use a modifier when a service typically would not be reimbursable by the carrier, but extenuating circumstances should override.
3. Remember that services usually bundled or included in the global surgical procedure are NOT typically considered without the use of a modifier.
4. Remember that insurance carrier software "blocks out" payment for ANY services performed by that provider during the global period unless a modifier is added.
5. Modifiers are assigned by section within CPT-4, and only modifiers for that specific section should be used.
6. Modifier 59 should be used when appropriate, but only when no other modifier is appropriate.
7. Multiple modifiers require the use of modifier 99 followed by a listing of the appropriate modifiers.
8. Medicare allows up to two modifiers to be used in the modifier section of the claim form before modifier 99 is required. A revision to the claim form is currently under way that will allow for the reporting of up to four modifiers without the use of modifier 99.

BOX 16-2 Rules for Using Modifier Code(s)

1. Make certain that "extenuating circumstances" billed with the modifier code selected are documented or clearly evident.
   - For example, "Significantly separately identifiable" is easier to justify if a separate surgical or procedure report is included, rather than leaving information intermingled with the visit description.
   - Services greater than usual should be explained in the medical documentation.
   - Discontinued procedures should clearly indicate what portion of the procedure was completed so that partial reimbursement for services performed can be received.
2. Reimbursement may be affected by the use of the modifier code. Depending on the modifier used, reimbursement may be increased or decreased proportionately.
3. Some third-party carriers do not recognize SOME or ANY modifiers on claims. A review process will be necessary to justify why these services are "outside the norm."
4. Carefully review the carrier's Explanation of Benefits to make certain that allowances have been made for services with modifiers, when appropriate.
5. Check the modifier list to ensure that codes used are applicable to the services billed. (Outpatient surgery modifiers are different than physician service modifiers.)
6. Check carrier specifications regarding HCPCS modifiers and those taken from CPT-4.

appropriate. Conditions that typically require a modifier are as follows:

- Services greater than or less than those usually provided
- Services provided within the global period that should be considered for reimbursement

- Repeat services
- Services provided by more than one physician
- **Professional/technical components**
- **Bilateral** procedures
- Unusual events

As discussed previously, modifier codes are typically two-digit numerical codes attached to the original CPT-4 code. They indicate a request for payment consideration because of an extenuating circumstance that required services above and beyond those ordinarily reimbursed.

This chapter gives a complete review of modifier codes so that they may be easily accessed for reference. Also included in this chapter is a CPT-4 Modifier Coding Reference Tool (Tool 51).

MODIFIER CODE LISTING

A listing of both the modifier codes and the sections of CPT for which they are applicable is found in Table 16-1. These modifiers as they applied throughout the CPT-4 chapters have been discussed.

HCPCS MODIFIER CODES

In addition to those codes listed in CPT, Level II (HCPCS/National) modifiers are available for use in coding. Before using any of these modifiers, the coder must ascertain whether specific carriers accept these codes. When the carrier accepts both CPT-4 and HCPCS codes and modifiers, the guidelines dictate that the highest level of specificity should be indicated. HCPCS codes (Level II codes) permit greater specificity than CPT-4 codes (Level I).

Common HCPCS Modifier Codes

The most common Level II HCPCS modifier codes are listed here. A complete listing is presented in Table 16-2.

LT	Left side of body
RT	Right side of body
E1	Upper left, eyelid
E2	Lower left, eyelid
E3	Upper right, eyelid
E4	Lower right, eyelid
FA	Left hand, thumb
F1	Left hand, second digit
F2	Left hand, third digit
F3	Left hand, fourth digit
F4	Left hand, fifth digit
F5	Right hand, thumb
F6	Right hand, second digit
F7	Right hand, third digit
F8	Right hand, fourth digit
F9	Right hand, fifth digit

TA	Left foot, great toe
T1	Left foot, second digit
T2	Left foot, third digit
T3	Left foot, fourth digit
T4	Left foot, fifth digit
T5	Right foot, great toe
T6	Right foot, second digit
T7	Right foot, third digit
T8	Right foot, fourth digit
T9	Right foot, fifth digit
LC	Left circumflex coronary artery
LD	Left anterior descending coronary artery
RC	Right coronary artery
QM	Ambulance service provided under arrangement with provider of services
QN	Ambulatory service provided directly by provider of services
QR	Repeat laboratory test on same day

SPECIFIC MODIFIER ISSUES

RIGHT/LEFT MODIFIER(S)

Right (RT) and left (LT) anatomical modifiers should be appended when the *CPT-4 descriptor* describes an anatomical site that ONLY has a right and left side. Consider the following examples:

Code 25600   Closed treatment of distal radial fracture

There are two radii, right and left. The anatomical RT or LT modifier should be appended for this procedure.

Code 12001   Simple repair, superficial wounds of scalp, neck, axillae, external genitalia, trunk, and /or extremities (inc hands/feet) 2.5 cm or less

There are multiple anatomical sites listed in the CPT-4 code 12001, so appending anatomical RT or LT to this procedure code would not clarify the exact location. It would NOT be appropriate to append an RT or LT for this procedure.

ANATOMICAL MODIFIERS (FA-F9, TA-T9, E1-E4)

The following modifiers are used to identify specific fingers (FA-F9), specific toes (TA-T9), or specific eyelids (E1-E4) that have been treated. As previously outlined, anatomical modifiers should only be used when the CPT-4 descriptor is specific to that body area/part.

When the CPT-4 descriptor only describes two locations, RT or LT would still be appropriate. Consider the following example:

Code 28505   Open Treatment of a great toe fracture

There is only a right (RT) great toe and a left (LT) great toe, so RT/LT modifiers would be appropriate.

Text continued on p. 356

TOOL 51

PHYSICIAN CPT-4 MODIFIER CODING REFERENCE TOOL

Modifier Code	Description	Evaluation and Management	Anesthesia	Surgery	Radiology	Pathology	Medicine	ASC/Outpatient Surgery
21	Prolonged evaluation and management service	X					X	
22	Unusual procedural services		X	X	X	X	X	
23	Unusual anesthesia services		X					
24	Unrelated evaluation and management service same physician, global/postoperative period	X						
25	Significantly separately identifiable evaluation and management service, same dr same day	X						
26	Professional component service only			X	X	X	X	
32	Mandated service	X	X	X	X	X	X	
47	Anesthesia service performed by surgeon			X				
50	Bilateral procedure			X	NO RAD			X
51	Multiple procedures performed during one operative session		X	X	X		X	
52	Reduced service	X	X	X	X	X	X	X
53	Discontinued procedure		X	X	X	X	X	
54	Surgical care of global package only performed			X			X	
55	Postop care of global package only performed			X			X	
56	Preop care of global package only performed			X				
57	Decision made during E & M for surgical service	X						
58	Related/staged procedure same dr during global surgical period			X	X		X	
59	Distinct procedure service		X	X	X	X	X	X
62	Two surgeons			X	X		X	
63	Procedures performed on infants <4 kg			X				
66	Surgical team			X			X	
73	Discontinued ASC procedure/prior to anesthesia							X
74	Discontinued ASC procedure/after anesthesia							X
76	Same physician repeats procedure			X	X		X	X
77	Different physician repeats procedure			X	X		X	X
78	Need for return to the OR for related procedure during global/postoperative period			X				
79	Need for unrelated procedure/service same dr during global/postoperative period			X	X		X	
80	Assistant surgeon services			X	X			
81	Minimum assistant surgeon services			X				
82	Assistant surgeon services provided because qualified resident not available			X				
90	Services referred to outside or reference lab			X	X	X	X	
91	Repeat pathology service same day					X		
99	Use of multiple modifiers for service billed			X	X	X	X	X

ASC = Ambulatory Surgery Center

TABLE 16-1   CPT-4 Modifier Codes

Modifier	Description and Use

21   **Prolonged Evaluation and Management Service**

Services above and beyond the scope outlined for normal E & M services
E & M Services only
Example: Services extended above and beyond the highest E & M service level, but do not qualify for critical care.

22   **Unusual Procedural Services**

Services beyond the scope of normal description provided for a service in CPT
Anesthesia, Surgery, Radiology, Pathology, Medicine
Example: Increased difficulty in performing procedural services is encountered, such as extensive lysis of adhesions during the performance of an abdominal hysterectomy.

23   **Unusual Anesthesia Services**

Services beyond the usual scope of descriptions for anesthesia services. This may indicate greater service, or general anesthesia for a procedure that typically does not require such service.
Anesthesia Services only

24   **Unrelated E & M Services by same Physician during Postoperative Period**

When E & M service is provided by a physician who has rendered a global surgical service that has a predetermined follow-up period, that E & M service must include a modifier to justify the circumstances. Further justification is typically displayed in a diagnosis code for that E & M service that is unrelated to the global service as well.
E & M Services only
Example: When a postoperative patient encounters a problem during the postoperative period such as infection, fever, or bleeding, these visits do not classify as "normal postoperative care" and may be coded and billed with modifier 24.

25   **Significantly Separately Identifiable E & M Services by Same Physician Same Day**

When an E & M service is provided in addition to a totally separate service, the E & M service must be designated with the use of this modifier.
Evaluation and Management Services only
Example: A patient arrives at the physician's office for evaluation and management of pharyngitis and repair of an open wound of the finger. The physician documentation should reflect the E & M service with a primary diagnosis of pharyngitis and, preferably, a procedure note for the finger wound repair.
Diagnosis for the two separately identifiable services is typically different; however, coding guidelines specify that this will not always be the case. Make certain the primary diagnosis for each service is in fact the primary reason for that encounter.

26   **Professional Component Only**

This modifier applies when the physician provides only a professional interpretation and report, and the technical component is provided by the facility or another entity.
Surgery, Radiology, Pathology, Medicine codes

32   **Mandated Service**

This modifier is used for any service that is required by a third party such as an insurance carrier or a PRO.
All CPT services may use this modifier.

47   **Anesthesia Service Performed by Surgeon**

When anesthesia services are provided by a surgeon rather than an anesthesiologist, the appropriate code(s) should be used. These codes are typically used by the surgeon when he or she administers a regional or general anesthesia for a surgical procedure. Only codes from the surgery section should be used for these services. No anesthesia codes should be used with this modifier.
Surgery codes only

50   **Bilateral Procedures**

For identical services performed bilaterally that are not specified as such in the CPT descriptions, modifier 50 should be used. There is some controversy regarding the correct use of this modifier code. The coder must ascertain the preferred method for each third-party carrier to ensure proper coding.
Some carriers require that the procedure be listed twice: once without the modifier and then as an additional code with modifier 50 added. Other carriers want the procedure code listed only once, with modifier 50 added to indicate that the procedure was performed bilaterally. Make certain the charge amount corresponds with the billing method the third-party carrier wishes. Obviously, if the carrier wishes the code to be listed only once, then the charge will typically be double the usual, single-procedure price.
Surgery codes, Radiology
Outpatient Surgery codes

TABLE 16-1 CPT-4 Modifier Codes—cont'd

Modifier	Description and Use

51 **Multiple Procedures during Same Operative Session**

When multiple procedures are performed during the same operative session by the same physician(s), each **subsequent** procedure must have modifier 51 added.

Consequences of multiple procedures and their effect on reimbursement were discussed. Each subsequent procedure reimbursement is dramatically reduced because the preoperative approach has already been considered in the primary procedure reimbursement. Correct order in listing the most significant primary procedure first is imperative to proper reimbursement.

Anesthesia, Surgery, Radiology, Medicine codes   *prof claims only*

52 **Reduced Services**

This modifier is used when the services provided are not those typically provided for that service. Remember that the coder should not assign a lower level of service when there is a requested decrease in charge, but should charge the correct level of service with modifier 52 and bill the appropriate charge. This modifier should also be used when the service was not completed for reasons unrelated to the physician's decision or the patient's medical condition.

Example: A colonoscopy could not be completed because of the inability of the scope to pass through the splenic flexure. The reduced service in this procedure was not due to physician decision or medical condition; therefore, the use of modifier 52 is appropriate.

All physician services may be billed with this modifier.   *facility & prof claim*
Outpatient Surgery codes

53 **Discontinued Procedure**

This modifier should be applied when a procedure is started, but at the physician's determination, the procedure is terminated before its completion. This may occur because of changes in the patient's status or an inability to complete the procedure for other reasons.

Anesthesia, Surgery, Radiology, Pathology, Medicine codes   *prof claim*
Not to be used for Ambulatory/Hospital Outpatient coding (see modifiers 73 and 74)

Example: A colonoscope cannot advance past a certain point, and the surgical procedure is halted owing to patient hypotension.

54 **Surgical Care Only**

When only the surgical component of a global surgery procedure is performed by one physician, modifier 54 should be used. This results in a significant decrease in reimbursement as the global (preoperative, postoperative, and surgical) components were not performed.

Surgery codes only

55 **Postoperative Management Only**   *post-op*

When only the postoperative care of a global procedure is performed, modifier 55 should be appended to the surgical code. This postoperative care designates only the usual uncomplicated follow-up postoperative care. In the event that the surgeon providing the postoperative management encounters complications outside the normal global concept, those services may be billed additionally.

Surgery codes only

56 **Preoperative Management Only**   *pre-op*

When only the preoperative component of a global surgery procedure is provided, modifier 56 should be added to the procedure code.

Surgery codes only

Example: Postoperative clearance visits.

57 **Decision for Surgery**

The E & M service provided to determine that surgery is necessary should have modifier 57 added. If not, the service will be considered as preoperative care within the global package.

E & M Services only

58 **Staged/Related Procedure Same Physician during the Global Operative Period**

When the physician plans to provide additional procedure(s) related to the initial procedure during the global postoperative period, or is required to perform additional, more extensive surgery than was originally performed, modifier 58 should be added to those additional procedures.

Surgery, Radiology, Medicine codes

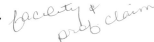

Continued

TABLE 16-1   **CPT-4 Modifier Codes—cont'd**

Modifier	Description and Use

59   Distinct Procedural Service

(handwritten: totally separate incision)

(handwritten: more than 1 procedure alone)

When procedural services are distinct from other procedures performed on the same day by the same physician, modifier 59 should be added. In some instances, this may be the result of two distinct surgical services (e.g., repair of hernia, repair of fractured humerus), different sessions/encounters such as return of the patient later in the day for an unrelated procedure (laceration repair in the morning, removal of foreign body from the eye in the evening), or different excisions/incisions as in the case of lesion removals.

This modifier should be used only if another modifier has not already been used to describe the circumstances.

Surgery, Radiology, Pathology, Medicine codes
Outpatient Surgery codes

62   Two Surgeons

When two surgeons worked together to perform one primary procedure, each physician should report the same procedural code with modifier 62. As a general rule, the third-party carrier pays approximately 125% of the total allowance, each physician receiving approximately 62.5% of the allowance.

In the event that one of the physicians bills this service incorrectly, only one physician will be paid.

63   Procedure Performed on Infants <4 kg

When procedures are performed on infants, some carriers will require the addition of this Modifier. Many carriers, however, will not require the addition of this modifier. Other modifiers that may be applicable should still be assigned in addition to this modifier code.

Surgery and Radiology codes

Example: Two surgeons are involved in a cochlear implant surgery, and each bills the same CPT-4 code with modifier 62 for services described.

66   Surgical Team

Use this modifier when the skills of more than two physicians, as well as a team of highly skilled technical employees, are required to perform a procedure.

Surgery and Radiology codes

Example: Transplant teams for kidney, heart, and lung operations.

73   Discontinued Outpatient Hospital/Ambulatory Surgery Center Procedure before Administration of Anesthesia

(handwritten: used before anesthesia)

When the procedure performed in the outpatient hospital or ambulatory surgery center setting is terminated after the preparation for surgery, but before the administration of anesthesia, modifier 73 should be appended to the surgical procedure code. These procedures may be cancelled for a number of reasons, including concern for the welfare of the patient and extenuating circumstances, but not because the patient has elected to terminate the procedure.

The facility will be reimbursed a proportionate amount for that portion of the procedure performed. It is necessary to document at what point the procedure was terminated, and why. The third-party carrier may request documentation before considering services with modifier 73 attached for reimbursement.

Outpatient Surgery codes only

74   Discontinued Outpatient Hospital/Ambulatory Surgery Center Procedure after Administration of Anesthesia

(handwritten: after anesthesia)

When a procedure scheduled in the outpatient hospital/ambulatory surgery center is terminated after the administration of anesthesia, that proportionate amount of service performed will be considered for reimbursement with the use of modifier 74. Again, documentation regarding the progression of the surgery, as well as why the procedure was terminated, is necessary for reimbursement consideration. Elective termination by the patient will not be considered.

Outpatient Surgery codes only

76   Repeat Procedure by Same Physician

This modifier is used to indicate that the same procedure was performed more than once by the same physician in a given day. Each additional repeat procedure must be listed with the addition of modifier 76.

Surgery, Radiology, Medicine codes
Outpatient Surgery codes

77   Repeat Procedure by Another Physician

When the same procedure must be performed on the same day on which it was already performed by another physician, modifier 77 should be used.

Both modifiers 76 and 77 are most commonly used for repeat procedures such as ECGs and chest x-rays, when periodic reevaluations during the course of a given day are necessary for the appropriate treatment or care of the patient.

Surgery, Radiology, Medicine codes
Outpatient Surgery codes

TABLE 16-1 CPT-4 Modifier Codes—cont'd

Modifier	Description and Use

78   **Return to the Operating Room for Related Procedure during the Postoperative Period**

When related procedures are necessary during the postoperative period of the initial procedure, the related procedure must have modifier 78 added. This is necessary only for subsequent surgical procedures that are performed in the operating suite.
Surgery, Radiology, Medicine codes *[handwritten: rush back to OR to take care of something]*

79   **Unrelated Procedure/Service by Same Physician during Postoperative Period**

When an additional surgical procedure is performed by the same physician during the postoperative period of the first procedure, the subsequent procedure must be explained with the use of modifier 79.
Surgery, Radiology, Medicine codes
Example: If a patient initially has a hernia repair performed by the surgeon on January 1 with a planned postoperative period of 30 days and returns to the general surgeon for outpatient clinic removal of a ganglion cyst during that 30-day period, the second procedure must have modifier 79 added to be considered for payment. This, of course, must be further justified by a diagnosis code unrelated to the primary diagnosis code.

80   **Assistant Surgeon**

When surgical assistant services are required to perform a given surgical procedure, the assistant surgeon should code the identical surgery code(s) as the primary surgeon, with modifier 80 added.
In the event that the second surgeon performed services in conjunction with the primary surgeon, modifier 62 would be appropriate.
Assistant surgeons not needed to perform a particular service typically are not reimbursed by third-party carriers. Third-party guidelines, as well as guidelines from the (R)esource (B)ased (R)elative (V)alue (S)tudies, assist the coder in applying for reimbursement for these services.
Surgery, Radiology codes

[handwritten: prof claims]

81   **Minimum Assistant Surgeon**

When only minimal services are required from the assistant surgeon, modifier 81 is appropriate. As the reimbursement for assistant surgeon is typically 10% to 20% of the allowance for the primary surgeon, the allowance for the minimum assistant surgeon will be even less.
Surgery codes only

82   **Assistant Surgeon (when qualified resident surgeon not available)**

When hospital guidelines require the presence of an assistant surgeon and a qualified resident is not available to provide that service because of scheduling problems, emergency services, or lack of residents within that facility, this information must be communicated to the third-party carrier with the addition of modifier 82.
Surgery codes only

90   **Reference (Outside) Laboratory**

When laboratory services are billed by the provider yet performed by an outside laboratory or other entity, these services should be listed, and modifier 90 should be added to each service. Remember that Medicare law does not allow any entity to bill for a service that it has not provided; therefore, modifier 90 should NEVER appear on a Medicare claim.
Surgery, Radiology, Pathology, Medicine codes

91   **Repeat Pathology Services Same Day**

When repeat laboratory services are designated as medically necessary on the same date as the original service, modifier 91 should be appended to subsequent listings of the same laboratory CPT code. This modifier was added in the 2000 version of CPT; it is not intended for repeat services necessary due to inadequate specimen(s).

99   **Multiple Modifiers**

When the use of multiple modifier codes is necessary to adequately explain more than one extenuating circumstance, modifier 99 must be appended to the procedure code, and a description of the multiple modifiers must be attached.
Medicare allows up to two modifiers following a procedure code before multiple modifier 99 must be attached.

TABLE 16-2 Level II HCPCS Modifiers

Modifier	Description
A1	Dressing, one wound
A2	Dressing, two wounds
A3	Dressing, three wounds
A4	Dressing, four wounds
A5	Dressing, five wounds
A6	Dressing, six wounds
A7	Dressing, seven wounds
A8	Dressing, eight wounds
A9	Dressing, nine or more wounds
AA	Anesthesia services performed personally by anesthesiologist
AB	Medical direction of own employee(s) (no more than 4) by anesthesiologist
AC	Medical direction of other than own employee(s) (no more than 4) by anesthesiologist
AD	Medical supervision by a physician: more than 4 employees concurrently
AE	Direction of residents in furnishing not more than two concurrent anesthesia services (attending physician relationship met)
AF	Anesthesia complicated by total body hypothermia
AG	Anesthesia for emergency surgery on patient who is moribund or who has an incapacitating systemic disease that is a constant threat to life
AH	Clinical psychologist
AJ	Clinical social worker
AK	Nurse practitioner, rural team member
AL	Nurse practitioner, nonrural team member
AM	Physician team member service
AN	Physician assistant services for other than assistant-at-surgery; nonteam member
AS	Physician assistant services for assistant-at-surgery
AT	Acute treatment (used with A2000 for acute treatment)
AU	Items furnished in conjunction with urological, ostomy or tracheostomy supply
AV	Items furnished in conjunction with prosthetic device, prosthetic or orthotic
AW	Items furnished in conjunction with surgical dressing
AX	Items furnished in conjunction with dialysis services
BA	Items in conjunction with parental enteral services
BO	Orally administered nutrition
BP	Beneficiary informed of purchase and rental options and has elected to purchase item (DME)
BR	Beneficiary informed of purchase and rental options and has elected to rent item (DME)
BU	Beneficiary informed of purchase and rental options, and after 30 days has not informed supplier of decision
CC	Procedure Code Change Used when procedure code submitted was changed for administrative reasons or because of filing of incorrect code
DD	Powdered enteral formula
E1	Upper left eyelid
E2	Lower left eyelid
E3	Upper right eyelid
E4	Lower right eyelid
EJ	Subsequent claim (Epoetin ALFA-EPO injection only)
EM	Emergency reserve supply (ESRD benefit only)
EP	Service provided as part of EDSDT program (Early Periodic Screening Diagnosis and Treatment)
ET	Emergency treatment (dental emergencies)
EY	No physician or licensed health care provider order
FA	Left hand, thumb
F1	Left hand, second digit
F2	Left hand, third digit
F3	Left hand, fourth digit
F4	Left hand, fifth digit
F5	Right hand, thumb
F6	Right hand, second digit
F7	Right hand, third digit
F8	Right hand, fourth digit
F9	Right hand, fifth digit
FP	Services provided by Medicaid Family Planning Program
GA	Waiver of Liability on File
GN	Service delivered under outpatient speech language pathology plan of care

TABLE 16-2   Level II HCPCS Modifiers—cont'd

Modifier	Description
GO	Service delivered under outpatient occupational therapy plan of care
GP	Service delivered under outpatient physical therapy plan of care
JW	Drug amount discarded/not administered to any patient

K Modifiers for Use with Durable Medical Equipment (DME) Claims Only

Modifier	Description
KA	Add-on option/accessory wheelchair
KB	16 square inches or less
KC	More than 16, but less than or equal to 48 square inches
KD	More than 48 square inches
KE	1 ounce
KF	1 linear yard
KG	1 cubic centimeter
KH	DMEPOS item, initial claim, purchase or first month rental
KI	DMEPOS item, second or third month rental
KJ	DMEPOS item, parenteral enteral nutrition (PEN) pump or capped rental
KK	Inhalation solution compounded for FDA-approved formulation
KL	Product characteristics defined in medical policy have been met
KO	Lower extremity prosthesis functional level 0; no ability to ambulate or transfer with or without assistance; prosthesis does not enhance quality of life or mobility
K1	Lower extremity prosthesis functional level 1
	Ability or potential to use prosthesis for transfers and/or ambulation on level surface
	Limited and unlimited household ambulator
K2	Lower extremity prosthesis functional level 2
	Ability or potential to use prosthesis for ambulation and low-level environmental barriers (curbs, stairs)
	Typical limited community ambulator
K3	Lower extremity prosthesis functional level 3
	Ability or potential to use prosthesis for ambulation and to cross most environmental barriers; may allow vocational, therapeutic, or exercise activity beyond simple locomotion
K4	Lower extremity prosthesis level 4
	Ability or potential to use prosthesis exceeding basic ambulation skills; exhibiting high impact, stress, or energy levels
	Child, active adult, athlete
LL	Lease/Rental; when DME equipment rental is applied against purchase price
LR	Laboratory round trip
LS	FDA-monitored intraocular lens implant
LT	Left side of body
MS	Six-month maintenance and service fee for parts and labor not covered under any warranty
NR	New when rented; when DME equipment, which was new at the time of rental, is subsequently purchased
NU	New equipment
PL	Progressive addition lenses
PS	Professional component charge for separate specimen
Q3	Live kidney donor surgery and related services
QB	Physician providing service in rural Health Population Service Area
QC	Single-channel monitoring
QD	Recording/storage solid-state memory by a digital recorder
QE	Prescribed amount of oxygen less than 1 liter per minute (LPM)
QF	Prescribed amount of oxygen exceeds 4 LPM and portable oxygen is prescribed
QG	Prescribed amount of oxygen exceeds 4 LPM
QH	Oxygen-conserving device being used with oxygen delivery system
QI	Deleted and replaced with modifier 57
QJ	Medically directed by physician: 2 concurrent procedures
QK	Medical direction of 2, 3, or 4 concurrent anesthesia procedures involving qualified individuals
QM	Ambulance service provided under arrangement by hospital
QN	Ambulance service furnished directly by hospital
QO	Medically directed by physician: 3 concurrent procedures
QQ	Medically directed by physician: 4 concurrent procedures
QS	Monitored anesthesia care service (can be billed by Certified Registered Nurse Anesthetist or physician)
QT	Recording and storage of tape by analog tape recorder
QU	Physician providing services in urban HPSA
QX	CRNA service: with medical direction by physician
QZ	CRNA service: without medical direction by physician
Q1	Evidence of mycosis of toenail causing marked limitation of ambulation (for podiatry codes)

Continued

TABLE 16-2 **Level II HCPCS Modifiers—cont'd**

Modifier	Description
Q2	CMS demonstration project procedure/service
Q3	Live kidney donor; services associated with postoperative complications directly related to donor
Q4	Referring/ordering physician has no financial relationship with performing/billing entity
Q5	Service furnished by substitute physician under a reciprocal agreement
Q6	Service furnished by Locum Tenens physician
Q7	One class A finding (podiatry)
Q8	Two class A findings (podiatry)
Q9	One class B and two class A findings (podiatry)
RP	Replacement and repair; may be used to indicate replacement of DME, orthotic, or prosthetic device
RR	Rental (DME)
RT	Right side of body
SF	Second opinion ordered by PRO
SG	Ambulatory surgical center (ASC) facility service
SK	Member high risk population
SL	State supplied vaccine
ST	Related to trauma/injury
SU	Procedure performed in physician's office (to denote use of facility/equipment)
TA	Left foot, great toe
T1	Left foot, second digit
T2	Left foot, third digit
T3	Left foot, fourth digit
T4	Left foot, fifth digit
T5	Right foot, great toe
T6	Right foot, second digit
T7	Right foot, third digit
T8	Right foot, fourth digit
T9	Right foot, fifth digit
TC	Technical component
TS	Follow-up service
TT	Individual services provided to more than one patient/same setting
TU	Special payment rate, overtime
UE	Used durable medical equipment rental
VP	Aphakic patient
YY	Second surgical opinion
ZZ	Third surgical opinion

CHAPTER IN REVIEW

CERTIFICATION REVIEW

Coding Concepts

- Modifier codes should be used to "explain" unusual circumstances for services.
- Modifier codes "justify" services that may not otherwise be considered for payment.
- Diagnosis codes that indicate medical necessity do not alone garner reimbursement for services typically included in the global surgical component, unless the use of a modifier code designates the need for additional consideration.
- Modifier codes that should be used with CPT-4 codes are included in the CPT-4 coding book.

- Additional modifier codes, known as HCPCS modifier codes, are used by some carriers to designate more specific information. For instance, CPT-4 modifier 50 indicates bilateral, and HCPCS modifiers RT/LT specify right versus left.

Coding Review

Many of the case exercises include the assignment of modifier code(s). Although there are no exercises specifically identified for modifier use, many of the exercises contain multiple services, or services performed during the global postoperative period, that require the assignment of modifier code(s). There is no specific section of the coding certification examination that covers modifier code use. These are included in the surgical, evaluation and management, and other services in the coding certification exam and exercises.

STUDENT STUDY GUIDE

- Study Chapter 16.
- Review the Learning Objectives for Chapter 16.
- Review the Certification Review for Chapter 16.
- Complete the Chapter Review exercise to reinforce concepts learned in this chapter.

CHAPTER REVIEW EXERCISE

Identify the correct modifier code(s) and give an example of each.

	Modifier Code	Example
1. Services greater than usually performed	21	_____
2. Services less than usually performed	52	_____
3. Office visit **for** laceration repair, 2.5 cm eyebrow	_____	_____
4. Office visit **with** laceration repair, 2.5 cm, eyebrow	25	_____
5. Office visit for postoperative follow-up	55	_____
6. Office visit for postoperative complication	55 24	_____
7. Repeat chest x-ray, same day, same physician	76	_____
8. Repeat ECG, same day, different physician	77	_____
9. Office visit during which decision for surgery is made	57	_____
10. Consult during which decision for surgery is made	57	_____
11. Hospital admission during which decision for surgery is made	_____	_____
12. Multiple procedures performed same time, same operative site	51	_____
13. Multiple procedures performed same time, different operative site	59	_____
14. Two surgeons performing same procedures	62	_____

Identify the service billed and in which section of CPT the service will be located and whether a modifier is appropriate (Y/N). It is not required to select the CPT code, only the service and appropriate chapter as well as the correct modifier code.

15. A patient with fracture repair of the clavicle performed 10 days before presents for evaluation to the same physician for a sore throat.
    Service(s): E & M
    CPT section: _____
    Modifier? Y N
    Modifier code: _____

16. A patient with a 1.2-cm laceration repair performed 3 days before presents for a "recheck" of suture repair.
    Service(s): E+M
    CPT section: 99024
    Modifier? Y (N)
    Modifier code: _____

17. A patient with fracture repair of the humerus performed 15 days earlier presents to the orthopedist for evaluation and repair of a clavicular fracture.
    Service(s): _____
    CPT section: _____
    Modifier? Y N
    Modifier code: _____

18. A laboratory service is not performed by the physician's office; however, the laboratory bills the physician's office and the physician's office bills the third-party carrier.
    Service(s): Pathology
    CPT section: 80000-89999
    Modifier? (Y) N
    Modifier code: 90

19. Two surgical procedures are provided during the same surgical session: abdominal hysterectomy and omentectomy.
    Service(s): _____
    CPT section: _____
    Modifier? Y N
    Modifier code: _____

20. Two surgical procedures are performed during the same surgical session: repair of inguinal hernia and repair of metacarpal fracture.
    Service(s): _____
    CPT section: _____
    Modifier? Y N
    Modifier code: _____

21. A patient presents to the orthopedist following open reduction and internal fixation of a humerus fracture for evaluation and treatment of an ankle sprain.
    Service(s): _____
    CPT section: _____
    Modifier? Y N
    Modifier code: _____

22. A colonoscopy scheduled to be performed is cancelled at the patient's request.
    Service(s): _____
    CPT section: _____
    Modifier? Y N
    Modifier code: _____

23. A colonoscopy that could not be completed owing to an inability to advance the scope further.
    Service(s): _____
    CPT section: _____
    Modifier? Y N
    Modifier code: _____

17

HCPCS CODES

LEARNING OBJECTIVES

Following the completion of this chapter, the student will be able to:

- Identify the differences between Level I CPT-4 modifier codes and HCPCS modifier codes.
- Understand the proper use of HCPCS modifier codes.
- Know when CPT-4 codes versus HCPCS codes should be coded and billed.
- Comprehend and apply the rules for selecting the appropriate HCPCS Level II codes.

CODING REFERENCE TOOLS

Tool 52
HCPCS Code Book Index
Tool 53
Rules for Selecting HCPCS Level II National Codes

KEY TERMS

HCPCS, 359
Level I HCPCS Codes, 359
Level II HCPCS Codes, 359
Level III HCPCS Codes, 359

In addition to the CPT-4 codes already discussed in Chapters 9 through 16, Healthcare Common Procedure Coding System **(HCPCS)** codes may be used for coding medical services. At the beginning of the CPT-4 discussion, the HCPCS system was introduced as comprising three levels:

Level I   Physicians' Current Procedural Terminology (CPT)
Level II HCPCS National Codes
Level III Local Codes

Chapters 9 through 16 discussed Level I codes found in the current CPT-4 code book. CPT-4, however, does not contain all the codes needed to report medical services and supplies. As a result, CMS developed the second level of codes to address those items not found in CPT-4.

Most entries described in the HCPCS book apply to supplies and medications. These codes are used by most Medicare and Medicaid carriers for reporting these items, rather than the codes listed under special supplies in the medicine section of CPT-4. The HCPCS codes define specific services, often identifying the name of the supply or the drug, its dosage, and its strength. Use of the HCPCS codes eliminates the need for CPT-4 codes such as 99070, which require manual listing of additional information and a manual review process by the third-party carrier. As with all services coded and billed to third-party carriers, HCPCS code assignments are driven by the documentation contained in the medical record. In some instances this information will be documented first by oral order of the physician or by medical personnel in the office. In other instances it will be contained on a separate document, such as a Medication Log. Despite where the documentation originates or who documents the original service order, the physician is still responsible for validation by signature and date so that service can be billed and reimbursed. HCPCS codes are used on a regular basis by DME (durable medical equipment) companies because they code and bill for these types of services on a regular basis.

CMS has mandated the use of HCPCS codes on Medicare claims; many Medicaid carriers require them as well. These codes obviously improve the provider's ability to effectively communicate what services have been provided, without the need for narrative descriptions and detailed attachments.

FORMAT

The HCPCS National Codes are used for reporting medical services and supplies; they use an alpha prefix followed by four numerical characters. Additional modifier codes have been included with HCPCS Level II National Codes; they appear as two-digit alpha characters, as opposed to the two-digit numerical characters of CPT-4. A complete listing of HCPCS modifiers is found in Chapter 16 (see Table 16-2) for easy reference.

HCPCS INDEX

Tool 52 outlines the contents of the HCPCS code book. As with CPT-4, the coder should select the appropriate HCPCS code, following a step-by-step process as outlined in Tool 53.

Additional information is contained in the Appendix Sections of the Level II HCPCS National Codes. These appendices provide information regarding coverage issues, specifically outlining covered and noncovered services, and describing service limitations.

T O O L 52

HCPCS CODE BOOK INDEX

A0000-A0999	Transportation Services
A4000-A8999	Medical and Surgical Supplies
A9000-A9999	Administrative, Misc/Investigational Supplies
B4000-B9999	Enteral/Parenteral Therapy
D0000-D9999	Dental Procedures
E0100-E9999	Durable Medical Equipment
G0000-G9999 (Temporary)	Procedures/Professional Services
J0000- J8999 Method	Drugs Administered by Other than Oral
J9000-J9999	Chemotherapy Drugs
K0000-K9999	Assigned by DME Regional Carriers
L0000-L4999	Orthotic Procedures
L5000-L9999	Prosthetic Procedures
M0000-M0302	Medical Services
P0000-P9999	Pathology/Laboratory Services
Q0000-Q9999	Temporary Nationally Assigned
R0000-R5999	Diagnostic Radiology Services
S0009-S9999	Temporary National Codes (Non-Medicare)
V0000-V2999	Vision Services

T O O L 53

RULES FOR SELECTING HCPCS LEVEL II NATIONAL CODES

1. Determine where services will be billed from CPT-4 or HCPCS National Codes (usually determined by carrier).

2. Consult the Index to HCPCS codes to determine the appropriate section of HCPCS codes to consult.

3. Locate the appropriate HCPCS code listed in alphabetical order with the appropriate HCPCS section.

4. Determine the appropriate number of units performed. Unlike CPT-4, the rounding rule does not apply. If any portion of the unit(s) of service is met, the code may be utilized. For example, an injection of tetracycline 150 mg would be coded as "J0120, Injection, Tetracycline" up to 250 mg. Note the description indicates "up to" and therefore the requirement has been met.

5. When multiple units of service are provided, the days or units entry should be made.
   For example: "Injection, Tetracycline, 600 mg" would be billed as: J0120, 3 units.

CHAPTER IN REVIEW

CERTIFICATION REVIEW

Coding Concepts

- HCPCS codes and HCPCS modifiers further define services that are not adequately addressed in CPT-4.
- The use of HCPCS codes and modifiers often eliminates the need for a report to specify the services or items provided.
- HCPCS codes and modifiers are accepted by specific carriers only. The coder must make certain that they are used appropriately.
- HCPCS codes are all five-digit alphanumeric codes.

Coding Review

Certification exercises are located in the Workbook as well as some additional exercises located in the Case Book and are identified as level of difficulty "Cert."

STUDENT STUDY GUIDE

- Study Chapter 17.
- Review the Learning Objectives for Chapter 17.
- Review the Certification Review for Chapter 17.
- Complete the Chapter Review exercise to reinforce concepts learned in this chapter.

CHAPTER REVIEW EXERCISE

Locate the appropriate HCPCS code(s) for the following:

	HCPCS Code
1. Prosthetic partial foot with molded socket, ankle height	L5010
2. Cervical or vaginal cancer screening	G0101
3. Commode chair, mobile, with detachable arms	E0166
4. Hospital bed, semielectric, without mattress	E0261
5. Motorized wheelchair, fixed full-length arms	K-0010
6. Injection, ceftazidime, 750 mg	J0713 2units
7. Repair to broken denture base, complete	D5510
8. Replacement batteries for medically necessary TENS unit	A4630
9. Gradient compression stocking, lymphedema	A6543
10. Breast prosthesis, mastectomy sleeve	L8010
11. Injection, cyclophosphamide, 4 g	J9091
12. Injection, methotrexate, 100 mg	J9260 2units
13. Repair of orthotic device, 30 minutes	
14. Prednisone, oral, 10 mg	J7506 or J7510 2 units
15. Drug administered through metered-dose inhaler	
16. Repair of durable medical equipment, 30 minutes	E1340 #x2
17. Crutches, underarm, pair, wood	E0112
18. Intraoral x-rays, complete	D0210
19. Injection, Rocephin, 50 mg IM	J0696
20. Injection, unlisted substance, 50 mg IM	J3490 *

* unclassified drug

PRACTICAL APPLICATION

Use the code(s) discussed in this chapter to assign the appropriate HCPCS Level II codes as well as the code(s) for other services.

1.

EMERGENCY ROOM RECORD

Name:	Age:	ER physician:
	DOB:	

Allergies/type of reaction: | **Usual medications/dosages:**

Triage/presenting complaint:

67-year-old female who yesterday afternoon noted the onset of left lower quadrant pain. She formed a stool yesterday. There was no nausea or vomiting. There is no past history of similar abdominal pain or GI problems. Two months ago she had a complete urological workup for microscopic hematuria which was normal. She has a history of coronary artery disease with an MI and angioplasty last April. She also has hypertension, and is allergic to Morphine and Codeine. She has had a cholecystectomy, appendectomy, hernia repair and right total hip replacement.

Initial assessment:

She denies chest pain or palpitations. There has been no cough or shortness of breath, no dysuria, increased urinary frequency or nocturia, with bowel function generally regular.

Time	T	P	R	BP	Other:					

Medication orders:

Lab work:

X-Ray:

Physician's report:

Reveals an alert pleasant female, afebrile, eyes clear, TM appear normal. There is no nasal congestion. Mouth is moist, throat reveals no redness or swelling, neck is supple with no adenopathy. Heart rhythm is regular with no murmur. Lungs are clear, Abdomen is soft and flat. There is left lower quadrant tenderness. There is no mass, and bowel tones are present. Genitalia are normal. No calf tenderness or ankle edema. Lab data include hemoglobin of 15.2, white count 10200, chemistry panel entirely within normal limits. Chest x-ray shows no active pulmonary disease. Abdominal series shows stool in the right colon but is otherwise unremarkable.

Given Demerol 50 mg IV.

Diagnosis:	Physician sign/date
Left lower quadrant pain probably diverticulitis. Rest, stay on clear liquids and progress diet slowly. If she develops increased pain, vomiting, fever or any other problem to return to the Emergency Room.	*Robert Rai MD*

Discharge	Transfer	Admit	Good	Satisfactory	Other:

GODFREY REGIONAL HOSPITAL
123 Main Street • Aldon, FL 77714 • (407) 555-1234

HCPCS code(s): _____

CPT code assignment(s): _____

ICD-9-CM code assignment(s): _____

2.

PROGRESS NOTE

Date:	Vital signs:	T	R
Chief complaint:		P	BP

Patient presents with complaints of left ankle pain. Reports he fell while playing basketball in his driveway. Reports ankle as tender, swelling. Denies dizziness, loss of consciousness or any other complaints

Past History: Hypertension

Examination:

Exam of the left lower extremity reveals diffuse swelling over the left lower ankle area, 2+ pitting edema. Bruising over the lateral malleolus. X-ray reveals no evidence of fracture.

Impression:

Ankle Sprain

Plan:

Prefabricated ankle splint. Wear for next 3–5 days, then wear daily for the next 10–14 days. Recheck in 3 weeks

Maurice Doater, MD

Patient name:

DOB:

MR/Chart #:

GODFREY REGIONAL OUTPATIENT CLINIC
3122 Shannon Avenue • Aldon, FL 77712 • (407) 555-7654

HCPCS code(s): _____

CPT code assignment(s): _____

ICD-9-CM code assignment(s): _____

3.

PROGRESS NOTE

Date:	Vital signs:	T	R
Chief complaint:		P	BP

This 27-year-old presents for an insect sting on her foot which occurred this evening. She reports redness and swelling. She has no history of reaction to bee stings. No allergies.

Examination:

She is afebrile, there is a sting site visible on the lateral aspect of her foot with surrounding erythema which appears to have spread significantly.

Impression:

Insect sting right foot with reaction.

Plan:

Will give SoluMedrol 40 mg IM and prescribe orally for the next 24–48 hours. She should return immediately if increased swelling, shortness of breath or any other symptoms present. She appears stable at this time.

Robert Rai MD

Patient name:

DOB:

MR/Chart #:

GODFREY REGIONAL OUTPATIENT CLINIC
3122 Shannon Avenue • Aldon, FL 77712 • (407) 555-7654

HCPCS code(s): _____

CPT code assignment(s): _____

ICD-9-CM code assignment(s): _____

4.

HISTORY AND PHYSICAL EXAMINATION

Stanley Krosette, MD

HPI: 72-year-old man with an extensive history of CAD. He has had two CABGs, a PTCA and two myocardial infarctions. He presents today with feeling of lethargy, very tired and complaints of shortness of breath and feeling nauseated. He feels as though he has heart palpitations. He was feeling fine when he went to bed; however, woke up feeling short of breath, extremely tired "wrung out", and complained of feeling dizzy when he attempted to get out of bed.

CURRENT MEDS:
Isosorbide 40 mg tid
Furosemide 100 mg bid
Diazepam 5 mg prn
Potassium chloride 8 mEq 2 tid
Metolazone 5 mg per day

Past medical history:

Family and social history:

Review of systems:

Physical exam:

Pleasant man who does not appear to be in any obvious distress. His vital signs were stable, BP 115/63, pulse 61, respirations 20. HEENT: Normocephalic, PERRLA, neck supply, heart regular rate and rhythm. Abdomen is soft and nontender without hepatosplenomegaly. Extremities: No edema.

Laboratory/radiology:

DIAGNOSTICS:
ECG, normal paced rhythm
Chemistries normal except potassium of 2.7.

X-ray:

Assessment:

Hypokalemia due to diuretics. Will give Potassium 10 mEq IV and observe patient prior to discharge. He appears stable and will have patient return in 1-2 days for follow-up. Will not increase oral potassium intake at this time, just follow-up with repeat chemistries in 24–48 hours.

Plan:

Stany Knott MD

GODFREY REGIONAL HOSPITAL
123 Main Street • Aldon, FL 77714 • (407) 555-1234

HCPCS code(s): _____

CPT code assignment(s): _____
ICD-9-CM code assignment(s): _____

CPT only © American Medical Association. All Rights Reserved.

5.

DISCHARGE SUMMARY

Discharge diagnoses:

Patient presents for discharge with diagnosis of right hip fracture femoral neck for evaluation and discharge.

History:

Patient presented approximately 5 days ago with complaint of right groin pain via ambulance. She was observed to have a right lower extremity that was externally rotated and she was unable to change the position. She reports that she tripped over something on the floor and fell.

PAST MEDICAL HISTORY:
Significant for asthma and dementia.

EXAM:
She has a healing surgical scar over the right hip with staples. Her vitals are normal, no shortness of breath, heart regular rate and rhythm.

Laboratory and radiology studies:

Hospital course:

DISCHARGE DIAGNOSIS:
Right hip fracture femoral neck

DISCHARGE INSTRUCTIONS:
We will supply with wheeled walker which she should utilize at all times. She will be transferred to an Assisted Living facility for rehab and physical therapy. She should utilize the walker for walking, transferring until her next visit in 2 weeks.

Maurice Doaters, MD

GODFREY REGIONAL HOSPITAL
123 Main Street • Aldon, FL 77714 • (407) 555-1234

HCPCS code(s): _____

CPT code assignment(s): _____

ICD-9-CM code assignment(s): _____

IV

HOSPITAL CODING AND
BILLING PROCESSES

The hospital inpatient coding process is similar to the coding processes discussed in previous sections. The hospital coder faces additional challenges, however, that physician and provider coders do not encounter. The hospital coder has an additional volume of medical records to review so that appropriate ICD-9-CM diagnostic and procedure codes may be assigned. In addition, the outpatient hospital coder must possess the skills to code ICD-9-CM diagnostic and procedural codes as well as CPT-4 codes.

Section IV discusses the hospital diagnostic coding process and DRG assignment. Chapter 18 covers the basic coding guidelines for inpatient and outpatient hospital coding; Chapter 19 details the concept of diagnosis-related groups (DRGs) and provides guidelines for DRG coding as well as Ambulatory Payment Classifications (APCs). The student will have the opportunity to identify the key components of hospital chart documentation for coding and to assign DRGs for hospitalizations. These chapters are included only as an overview to the hospital coding and billing process and are not intended to provide the level of training necessary to become a hospital coder. They also serve as a comparison of the coding duties and responsibilities of the physician coder to that of the facility coder.

HOSPITAL CODING

LEARNING OBJECTIVES

Following the completion of this chapter, the student will be able to:

- Understand the rules for selecting the appropriate diagnosis for inpatient coding.
- Describe and apply the signs and symptoms rules for coding.
- Know the do's and don'ts for inpatient coding.
- Comprehend the importance of diagnostic coding order for inpatient coding.
- Understand the importance of assigning the principal diagnosis for inpatient coding.
- Comprehend the proper use of Volume 3 ICD-9-CM procedure codes for inpatient coding.
- Assign codes for significant inpatient procedures.
- Grasp the coding nomenclature for outpatient hospital coding.
- Identify and apply the basic steps for assigning inpatient codes.
- Understand the guidelines for assigning ICD-9-CM and CPT-4 codes for outpatient facility coding.

CODING REFERENCE TOOLS

Tool 54
Rules for Selecting Appropriate Diagnoses (for Inpatient Hospital Coding)
Tool 55
Signs and Symptoms Rules (for Inpatient Hospital Coding)
Tool 56
Diagnosis Do's and Don'ts (for Inpatient Hospital Coding)
Tool 57
Diagnostic Order Rules (for Inpatient Hospital Coding)

KEY TERMS

Ambulatory Payment Classifications (APC), 385
Principal Diagnosis, 383
Query Process, 384
Significant Procedures, 384

Volume 1 (Index to Diseases), 380
Volume 3 (Index to Procedures), 380

DOCUMENTATION/CODING GUIDELINES

Although the documentation guidelines are similar to those previously discussed in the chapters about physician coding, the depth and volume of the records are much more extensive. The coder must be capable of working through a significant volume of pages for each admission in order to assign codes appropriately.

Consider a typical inpatient chart. Keep in mind that only those documents required for arriving at the appropriate diagnostic and procedural codes have been included. Because the inpatient chart is so voluminous, an outline of the components that comprise the hospital medical record may be advisable.

ADMISSION HISTORY AND PHYSICAL

Commonly referred to as an "H & P" (History and Physical), this portion of the record typically represents the initial evaluation of the patient, the plan for the admission, and the admitting diagnosis.

PROGRESS NOTES

Each day the patient is seen by the physician(s), an entry will be made in the medical record. Each date may be entered on a separate sheet or multiple entries made on the same page. Documentation may be dictated or handwritten by the physician.

NURSING NOTES

In addition to daily documentation by the physician regarding the patient's progress, the facility staff, nurses, technicians, and other staff will document care provided to the patient as well as observations regarding the patient's progress. This type of documentation can be used for assigning diagnostic or procedural codes only when the physician documents agree with the findings by other staff members. For instance, should the nurse record that "the patient appears in severe respiratory arrest," this information may be used in assigning diagnoses when documented by the physician.

The same would apply for nursing documentation of vital signs or interpretation of laboratory or other data. For example, nursing staff contact the physician because of an increase in the patient's temperature, recorded as "103.7" and documented by the nurse as "fever." The diagnosis of "fever" may not be used unless stated by the physician.

ANCILLARY RECORDS/REPORTS

Ancillary records such as radiology, laboratory, and pulmonary tests are included in the review of the hospital record. Interpretations of these data are codeable only when they are made by the physician or documented concurrence with the diagnosis is made. Many of these records may contain information that reflects additional conditions treated or considered during the course of the hospitalization. The coder may only use information documented by the physician or may "query" the physician regarding the possibility of additional diagnoses. The "query" process is discussed later in this chapter.

OPERATIVE RECORDS/REPORTS

Should the patient need surgery during the hospitalization, the operative record will reflect the procedure performed and the reason for that procedure. Keep in mind that the reason for the surgical procedure may not be the primary or principal reason for the admission. Principal diagnosis is discussed later.

MEDICATION RECORD

A record is typically kept of medications given, the route through which they are distributed, and the dosage administered during the course of the hospitalization.

DISCHARGE SUMMARY/RECORD

At the conclusion of the hospital admission, the admitting physician will report a summary of the hospitalization course, including reason for admission, progress during admission, and discharge status and instructions. The figures on the following pages represent a typical inpatient hospital record.

Text continued on p. 380

HISTORY AND PHYSICAL EXAMINATION

Admit date: 05/09/XXXX   Jay Corman, MD
Admitting Diagnoses: 1) Intrinsic Asthma - History of Steroid Requirement 2) Penicillin Sensitivity 3) Hypertension
                     4) Elevated Creatinine 5) History of Gonococcal Urethritis 6) Status Post Bilateral Inguinal Herniorrhaphies

Patient is a 56-year-old black male with a history of asthma, admitted from the Emergency Room for an exacerbation of his bronchospastic disease. The patient's history is significant for admissions relevant to asthma in: 1) 1997 patient was admitted with room air arterial blood gas of pH 7.33, pCO2 52, pO2 55. He was subsequently intubated and treated with steroids. His hospital course was complicated by hyperglycemia and hypertension. 2) Patient admitted again in 1999 and treated with steroids. 3) Patient was admitted in 2001 and treated with steroids, where his prebronchodilator pulmonary function tests revealed an FEV1 of 1.3 liters and an FVC of 3.3 liters. The patient was seen by Allergy service, and recommended the patient return for skin testing and wear a mask for his job; however, he failed to show for follow-up.

Patient now gives a history of wheezing beginning three weeks ago, after being in a fried chicken store and being irritated by the burning grease. Ten days prior to admission the patient noted swelling around his face and eyes and went to see a private allergist who diagnosed contact dermatitis of the face. The patient was skin tested and found to be positive for mites and mold. The patient was given Kenalog 20 mg IM. He was later mailed a desensitization shot to be administered at home, which he did, five days prior to admission. The patient's wheezing was exacerbated by dust at work, and, two nights prior to admission he smelled some burning bacon at home and his shortness of breath became much worse and he reported to the hospital. The patient was held in the observation unit overnight and admitted the following morning. It should be noted that the patient finished a steroid taper dose of 5 mg qid twelve days prior to admission. The patient denies any history of aspirin sensitivity. PFT in the ER were significant for an FEV1 of 900 with an FVC of 2700 cc. Room air arterial blood gas was pH 7.43, pCO2 40, pO2 73.

Past medical history:

Patient gives a history of penicillin allergy, with an episode of anaphylaxis in 1986. Hypertension following initiation of steroid therapy. Asthma, see history of present illness, herniorrhaphy times two.

Family and social history:

Works as a forklift operator at a creosote company. The patient is exposed to creosote, sawdust from oak, pine, hickory, ash and gum and a lot of dusty conditions in general. Patient denies cigarette use, use of ethanol or illegal drugs. Family history significant for patient's father who died at age 70 for unknown kidney disease, two siblings who died from sudden death and a sister who also has asthma. The patient also has two children who have asthma. He lives at home with four sons and his wife. There are no house pets. The patient has a high school education and grew up in the area.

Review of systems:

Patient has experienced a weight loss from 190 to 170 pounds during the past two months secondary to diet. The patient has a history of gonococcal urethritis times three in the past. Also has a past history of rectal bleeding in 1988 and 1989.

Physical exam:

Revealed a well-developed, well-nourished middle-aged black male in no acute distress.
Vital Signs: BP 160/120, Pulse 102 and regular, Respirations, 28, Patient afebrile.
Skin: Hyperpigmented areas around the face and eyes
Lymphatic: No adenopathy
HEENT: Benign, Tympanic membranes clear bilaterally, no sinus tenderness, mouth
                without lesions, neck supple, without thyromegaly.
Lungs: Revealed diffuse inspiratory and expiratory wheezes all lung fields
Cardiac: Carotids were 2+, no murmurs heard.
Abdomen: Benign, without bruits or hepatosplenomegaly.
GU: Normal circumcised male, rectal exam normal tone, soft prostate, no masses
Extremities: Without cyanosis, clubbing or edema
Neuro: Within normal limits

Laboratory/radiology:

Admission of SMA-6 was significant for a glucose of 227 mg/dl. Admission CBC significant for hemoglobin of 13.8 gm/dl. Admitting urinalysis was unremarkable. Admission EKG and CXR reported as normal.

X-ray:

Assessment:

Asthma, will admit and treat with steroids

Plan:

Jay Corman MD

GODFREY REGIONAL HOSPITAL
123 Main Street • Aldon, FL 77714 • (407) 555-1234

PROGRESS NOTE
_____
Date/time
05/10/XXXX

S:

56 yo BM

1) Asthma, required intubation in past
2) HTN
3) Glucose intolerance due to steroids

O:

Meds:
1) Theodur 600 bid
2) HCT 250
3) Minipress 2 tid

A:

Generally doing well. Has occasional episodes, pt dyspnea/wheezing, but overall feels good. PE 140/80, P72, reg, respirations 14. Chest, scattered expiratory wheezes.

P:

Will order respiratory therapy and IV steroids and check for improvement in the AM.

_Jay C___ MD_

PROGRESS NOTES

GODFREY REGIONAL HOSPITAL
123 Main Street • Aldon, FL 77714 • (407) 555-1234

PROGRESS NOTE
_____

Date/time
_____
05/11/XXXX

S:

56-year-old BM

1) Asthma
2) HTN
3) Glucose intolerance due to steroids

O:

A:

P:

1. Still having bilateral expiratory wheezes despite respiratory treatment 2. Will check CXR for any improvement and continue IV steroid therapy.

Jay Corn MD

PROGRESS NOTES

GODFREY REGIONAL HOSPITAL
123 Main Street • Aldon, FL 77714 • (407) 555-1234

RADIOLOGY REPORT

MR#:
DOB:
Dr. Joseph Smith

Clinical summary:

Wheezing

Abdomen:

PA AND LATERAL CHEST 05/09/XXXX

Conclusion:

Reveals infiltrates in the right and left lower lobes as well as signs of chronic pulmonary processes.

Ddt/mm

D:
T:

_____
                              , M.D.   Date

GODFREY REGIONAL HOSPITAL
123 Main Street • Aldon, FL 77714 • (407) 555-1234

RADIOLOGY REPORT

MR#:
DOB:
Dr. Jay Corman, MD

Clinical summary:

Follow up asthma

Abdomen:

PA AND LATERAL CHEST 05/11/XXXX

Conclusion:

Reveals some improvement over 05/09/XXXX x-ray. Infiltrates still present in the right and left lower lobes, however, not as prevalent as previous x-ray.

Ddt/mm

D:
T:

_____
, M.D.   Date

GODFREY REGIONAL HOSPITAL
123 Main Street • Aildon, FL 77714 • (407) 555-1234

NURSING NOTES/DISCHARGE NOTE

Date/time
05/09/XXXX

S:

Patient experiencing extreme shortness of breath. Patient states "I had an asthma attack. I was in observation last night". Patient's chief complaint shortness of breath. Lungs with crackles throughout. White frothy sputum of moderate amounts produced. IV of 500 D5W at KVO with 500 D5W with 1 gm of Aminophylline. IV patent and infusing well. IV dressing applied. CXR performed tonight. Remained at bed most of evening. Appetite fair at dinner. Up to sink with assistance. Gait steady.

O:

A:

P:

Betty Jones RN

PROGRESS NOTES

GODFREY REGIONAL HOSPITAL
123 Main Street • Aldon, FL 77714 • (407) 555-1234

PROGRESS NOTE
_____

Date/time
05/10/XXXX

S:

Alteration in oxygenation with shortness of breath.

O:

VSS afebrile. Lungs with diffuse wheezes. Received bronchosol nebulizer X2.

Cough productive, large amount of white sputum with plugs. PO intake excellent

A:

Asthmatic exacerbation

P:

Bronchodilators, steroids

Hydration

[signature] Betty Jones RN

PROGRESS NOTES

GODFREY REGIONAL HOSPITAL
123 Main Street • Aldon, FL 77714 • (407) 555-1234

NURSING NOTES

Date/time

05/11/XXXX

S:

Alteration in oxygenation, shortness of breath

O:

Afebrile, P-84, RR-18, BP 150/95, 146/80.
Resting quietly in bed most of shift.
Lungs with diffuse wheezes, productive of small amount of semi-thin, white sputum.
Continues on bronchodilator, steroids. Increased Aminophylline drip to 35 qtts.
1740 denies shortness of breath, feeling better.
Repeat CXR this PM

A:

P:

Betty Jones, RN

PROGRESS NOTES

GODFREY REGIONAL HOSPITAL
123 Main Street • Aldon, FL 77714 • (407) 555-1234

NURSING NOTES/DISCHARGE NOTE

Date/time
05/12/XXXX

S:

Patient indicates feeling much better. Scattered few wheezes heard. Patient experiencing no shortness of breath. CXR indicated clearing infiltrates.

O:

A:

P:

Discharge instructions given and discharge medications include:

1) Prednisone 60 mg po q am tapering dose thereafter 50 mg po x 2 days, 40 mg x 2 days, 30 mg x 2 days, 20 mg x 2 days until seen in clinic

2) Theodur 600 mg po bid

3) Terbutaline 5 mg po q 8 hours

Betty Jones RN

PROGRESS NOTES

GODFREY REGIONAL HOSPITAL
123 Main Street • Aldon, FL 77714 • (407) 555-1234

DISCHARGE SUMMARY

Admitted: 05/09/XXXX
Discharged: 05/12/XXXX

Discharge diagnoses:

1. Extrinsic Asthma
2. Hypertension
3. Elevated Creatinine
4. Status Post Bilateral Inguinal Herniorrhaphy

History:

Patient is a 56-year-old black male who presented with shortness of breath to the emergency room on 05/08/XXXX where he was initially treated. He was transferred to observation during the evening, and subsequently admitted on the morning of 05/09/XXXX. The patient's history of significant for previous admissions for asthma, one requiring intubation, and the other admissions requiring steroid administration.

History on admission was a three week history of wheezing, followed by increasing shortness of breath on the evening of 05/08/XXXX following the smell of burning food at home. The patient had just finished a steroid tape dose twelve days prior to admission.

Laboratory and radiology studies:

On admission, CXR indicated infiltrates in the right and lower lobes with signs of a chronic process. By 05/11/XXXX a repeat x-ray indicated improvement in infiltrates.

Hospital course:

(1) Asthma
Patient was admitted with exacerbation of asthma and treated with the usual therapy of intravenous aminophylline, intravenous steroids, bronchodilator treatments and showed rapid improvement. At the time of discharge, pulmonary function studies showed FEV1 of 2.1 liters pre-treatment, 2.5 liters post-operative, FVC 4 liters pre-treatment and 4.3 liters post-treatment.
2) Hyperglycemia: History of steroid–induced hyperglycemia. Accu-checks were followed twice per day during the patient's hospitalization and all were under 200 mg/dl.
3) Hypertension: Patient's diastolic BP were within the range of 80 to 90 mg Hg during this hospitalization on his current medications.

DISCHARGE MEDICATIONS:
Prednisone 60 mg po q am tapering dose thereafter 50 mg po x 2 days, 40 mg x 2 days, 30 mg x 2 days, 20 mg x 2 days until seen in clinic
Theodur 600 mg po bid
Terbutaline 5 mg po q 8 hours

Jay Carson MD

GODFREY REGIONAL HOSPITAL
123 Main Street • Aldon, FL 77714 • (407) 555-1234

Keep in mind that this record only encompasses information that is useful in determining diagnoses and that many other documents and papers are contained within the hospital record.

In the case of the outpatient record, the documents will usually be similar and, in both instances, when a surgical procedure is performed, an operative note would be included in the documents for documentation and coding purposes.

STEPS IN THE INPATIENT CODING PROCESS

Volume 1 (Index to Disease), Volume 2 (Tabular List of Diseases), and **Volume 3 (Index to Procedures)** of the ICD-9-CM coding book constitute the basis for inpatient hospital diagnostic coding and reimbursement. As with physician coding, the hospital coder must be accurate in order to justify medical necessity for services billed.

The process by which hospital diagnostic coding is performed is similar to that for physician diagnostic coding. Some of the guidelines differ significantly.

Step 1 Identify key elements or words for possible use as diagnoses.
Step 2 Determine which diagnostic statements are necessary for proper diagnostic coding purposes.
Step 3 Determine the appropriate diagnostic code order.
Step 4 Assign diagnostic codes to diagnoses selected from ICD-9-CM.

Review these steps in detail, noting the differences in guidelines for hospital diagnostic coding from those learned in the physician diagnostic coding section.

Step 1

Identify Key Elements or Words for Possible Use as Diagnoses
Terms such as "probable," "possible," "rule out," and "suspect" MAY be used in the inpatient hospital diagnostic coding environment, unlike with physician coding. Take a moment to review the differences between physician and hospital diagnostic coding.

	Physician Provider	**Hospital Facility**
Chief reason for encounter (WHY)	ICD-9-CM	ICD-9-CM
Procedure/service (WHAT)	CPT-4 ICD-9-CM Volume 3	ICD-9-CM/ DRG

Note that the hospital coder is also providing justification as to the medical necessity for the charges billed, typically facility charges. The use of diagnostic statements that include words such as "possible," "probable," "suspect," or "rule out" is acceptable. The facility provides the same services for the patient tested for a specific condition as it does for the patient who, at the conclusion of the physician encounter, has that specific codable diagnosis. This represents the biggest difference between physician and hospital diagnostic coding.

Step 2

Determine Which Diagnostic Statements Are Necessary for Proper Diagnostic Coding Purposes
The coder should identify those diagnostic statements in the hospital setting that may or may not be used for coding purposes. Rules for selecting appropriate diagnoses are outlined in Tool 54, as are the rules for identifying signs and symptoms in Tool 55, and the "do's" and "don'ts" for inpatient hospital coding in Tool 56. A detailed discussion regarding signs and symptoms rules was previously presented in the section on ICD-9-CM diagnostic coding. Refer to Section II for additional information.

Step 3

Determine the Appropriate Diagnostic Code Order
The diagnostic order rules for inpatient hospital coding are listed in Tool 57.

Step 4

Assign Diagnostic Codes to Diagnoses Selected from ICD-9-CM
The chart, 10 Steps to Accurate Coding from ICD-9-CM (see Tool 13), is accurate for hospital coding, as are the CMS Guidelines for ICD-9-CM Coding (see Tool 14), found in the ICD-9-CM diagnostic coding section of this book (Section II).

V codes and E codes, which have previously been discussed, are also appropriate with hospital inpatient coding. Remember that these codes do not indicate the primary or principal diagnosis; they are important in determining liability for reimbursement purposes. When conditions are stated as "history of," V codes for those conditions should be used only when they contribute additional diagnostic information or explain the complexity of the inpatient stay. Chronic conditions should be clarified so that the appropriate diagnosis may be used.

T O O L   54

RULES FOR SELECTING APPROPRIATE DIAGNOSES
(For Inpatient Hospital Coding)

1. **If it is not documented, it did not happen.**

2. The condition, problem, or other circumstance chiefly responsible for the health encounter/visit is reported. This will be referred to as:
   Chief Reason for Encounter

3. Unconfirmed diagnoses described as "possible," "probable," "questionable," "rule out," "ruled out," or "suspect(ed)" **CAN BE UTILIZED** for hospital inpatient diagnoses and coding purposes.

4. Code the condition to the **highest level of specificity.**
   In some cases, this may be the sign, symptom, abnormal test, or reason for the visit/encounter.

5. If the encounter does not identify a definite condition or problem at its conclusion, the coder should select the documented chief complaint or chief reason for the encounter.

6. Never code a diagnosis that is not listed in the diagnostic statement.

T O O L   55

SIGNS AND SYMPTOMS RULES
(For Inpatient Hospital Coding)

Signs and symptoms should be used **ONLY** when:

1. Principal diagnosis has not been established at the conclusion of the encounter.

2. No more specific diagnoses for the specific condition can be made at the end of the encounter/visit.

3. Presenting signs/symptoms are transient and no definitive diagnosis is made.

4. The symptom is treated in an outpatient setting without the additional workup necessary to arrive at a more definitive diagnosis at the conclusion of the encounter.

Signs and symptoms need NOT be used when they are an integral part of the underlying diagnosis or condition already coded.

DIAGNOSIS DO'S AND DON'TS
(For Inpatient Hospital Coding)

1. For previous conditions stated as diagnosis when previous condition has no bearing on current visit — **DO NOT CODE**
Coder may utilize a "V" Code (history of) if significant.

2. Chronic conditions not the thrust of treatment — **DO CODE**
Certain diseases such as hypertension, Parkinson's disease, diabetes, COPD are examples of systemic diseases that require continued clinical evaluation and monitoring during each visit.

   If visit does not involve evaluation/treatment of condition — **DO NOT CODE**

3. Conditions that are an integral part of the disease — **DO NOT CODE**
Example: Patient with nausea and vomiting due to infectious gastroenteritis. Nausea and vomiting are common symptoms of this disease process and need not be coded.

4. Conditions that are NOT an integral part of the disease — **DO CODE**
Example: 5-year-old with 104 fever associated with pneumonia, also experienced convulsions. Pneumonia is coded (fever usually associated with pneumonia need not be coded), convulsions are coded (not always associated with pneumonia/fever).

5. Diagnosis not listed in final diagnostic statement — **CHECK WITH MD**
If integral to correct coding, ask the physician to incorporate this information in the final diagnostic statement. This statement may appear in the discharge information or throughout the hospitalization notes.

6. Abnormal findings – **CODE WHEN NECESSARY**
Should be assigned only when physician is unable to arrive at a diagnosis prior to the conclusion of the encounter. If an abnormal finding is the only diagnostic information available, the coder should check with the physician to make certain a codeable diagnosis is not available.

DIAGNOSTIC ORDER RULES
(For Inpatient Hospital Coding)

1. Signs and symptoms codes are assigned only after diagnosis, and only when they are NOT an integral part of the diagnostic statement.

2. Acute conditions are coded as the primary diagnosis in most instances as it is assumed they are the primary reason for the encounter. The exception would be the case of a significantly more serious condition.
EXCEPTION: Myocardial Infarction not listed as Acute
                      Acute Otitis Media

   You will find that many serious conditions are "automatically" assumed as acute when coding from ICD-9-CM (the ICD-9-CM coding book lists "acute" in parentheses).

3. Chronic conditions (when coded by previous rules) are coded secondary to any acute conditions or primary reasons for the encounter. Make sure to use chronic codes.

4. The first diagnosis listed in hospital coding should be the principal or most important diagnosis, reason for encounter, or thrust of treatment.

STOP AND PRACTICE

Try coding some of the following diagnoses based on the hospital diagnostic coding rules learned thus far. Code the following diagnoses appropriately according to hospital inpatient diagnostic rules.

ICD-9-CM Code(s)

1. Abdominal pain
   Possible appendicitis _____
2. Cough _____
   Fever _____
   Probable pneumonia _____
3. Anemia, probably due to
   chronic blood loss _____
4. Angina, most likely unstable _____
5. Acute bronchitis _____
   Cough _____
   COPD _____
6. Elevated blood pressure,
   probably not hypertension _____
7. Nausea and vomiting probably
   due to either gastroenteritis or
   kidney stones _____
8. Ankle pain, ankle fracture
   ruled out _____
9. Abdominal pain, possibly due
   to ovarian cyst _____
   Pelvic inflammatory disease _____
10. Confusional state _____
    Nausea and vomiting _____
    Dehydration _____
    Alzheimer's dementia _____
11. Pneumonia _____
    Fever and cough due to
    pneumonia _____
    Hypokalemia _____
12. Cholecystitis with cholelithiasis _____
    Abdominal pain _____
    Nausea and vomiting _____
13. Abdominal pain _____
    Fever _____
    Possible appendicitis _____
14. Fever _____
    Possible influenza _____
15. Right scrotal swelling _____
    Right inguinal hernia/hydrocele _____

DEFINITIONS AND INPATIENT GUIDELINES

In addition to the steps that remain the same for hospital and physician coding, clarification needs to be made regarding some hospital-specific definitions and guidelines.

PRINCIPAL DIAGNOSIS

Principal diagnosis is defined as the condition chiefly responsible for the patient's admission to the hospital (after diagnostic/therapeutic studies). Remember that the chief reason for encounter in the case of hospital coding is the chief reason or medical necessity for the **admission.** Specific guidelines for determining principal diagnosis are as follows.

When More Than One Diagnosis Meets the Criteria for Principal Diagnosis

When more than one diagnosis meets the criteria for principal diagnosis, and ICD-9-CM guidelines do not specify the use of one code instead of the other as primary or principal, either may be sequenced first (e.g., congestive heart failure; pneumonia).

The tendency is to code the diagnosis that accounts for the majority of services provided when both codes

meet the qualifications for principal diagnosis (the more significant diagnosis).

When More Than One Condition Listed Pertains to Similar and Contrasting Conditions

In this instance, the coder selects the diagnosis, which is the condition that resulted in the admission and for which most services were provided. If during the course of the admission, one of the diagnoses possible for inclusion as the principal diagnosis is ruled out, the diagnosis not ruled out would be used.

When Symptom(s) Are Listed with Comparable Diagnosis, or When Symptoms Contrast with the Diagnosed Condition

When symptoms are NOT an integral part of one of the diagnoses, they are used in lieu of unestablished diagnoses.

Patient with abdominal pain due to either appendicitis or ovarian cyst

Because appendicitis and ovarian cyst are not confirmed diagnoses, abdominal pain should be selected as the primary diagnosis.

When Original Treatment Plan(s) Are Not Completed during the Course of the Encounter or Admission

In this case, the reason for the admission or encounter is still used as the principal or primary diagnosis. In addition to the principal and any contributing diagnoses, hospital coding requires that all significant procedures be coded. **Significant procedures** are defined as the following:

> *Surgical procedures* (including excisions, incisions, destructions, amputations, repairs, manipulations, insertions).
> *Those associated with anesthetic risk* (all procedures requiring anesthesia other than topical anesthesia).
> *Those associated with procedural risk* (all procedures that carry a risk of possible impairment, trauma, or physiological disturbance).
> *Procedures that require specialized training.*

In the case of procedural diagnostic coding, the principal diagnosis is defined as the reason for definitive treatment or for the outpatient procedure.

Review the medical chart at the beginning of the chapter and determine the appropriate diagnoses, as well as the principal diagnosis.

Although several problems were identified during the course of the hospitalization, the primary reason for the inpatient hospitalization was exacerbation of asthma. Contributing or secondary diagnosis included the following:

- Steroid-induced hyperglycemia
- Hypertension

Exacerbation of asthma was the chief reason for hospitalization, so it would be assigned as the principal diagnosis. The additional diagnoses would also be assigned appropriate ICD-9-CM codes.

USE OF VOLUME 3—PROCEDURE INDEX

When a procedure has been identified as "significant" according to the previous guidelines, the service and the reason for the procedure or encounter (diagnosis) should be coded. All procedures classified as significant based on these guidelines are coded for both outpatient and inpatient hospital services.

Layout

The layout of ICD-9-CM Volume 3—Procedure Index is identical to that used in the main sections of ICD-9-CM. Contained within Volume 3 is an Index to Procedures (alphabetical), along with a numerical index. The guidelines discussed earlier apply to selecting the appropriate code from Volume 3. If the coder uses the same guidelines that have been established for Volumes 1 and 2 of ICD-9-CM, Volume 3 (procedural coding) is not difficult to use. Remember that this section of the ICD-9-CM diagnostic coding book is used by facility and hospital coders ONLY. Physician and provider coders use the CPT-4 manual to code for services performed. Should the coder require information on provider and physician coding only, the ICD-9-CM book, Volumes 1 and 2, may be purchased.

The coder must select from the procedure index the appropriate code for the significant procedure(s) performed and must cross-reference or verify the selected code in the numerical index. The importance of this process and of the codes associated with these procedures will become apparent when DRG hospital/facility coding is discussed later in Chapter 19. In some instances, some carriers have recently discontinued the requirement of ICD-9-CM procedural codes on outpatient hospital claims.

Box 18-1 provides a list of the numerical categories for codes found in ICD-9-CM Volume 3—Procedure Codes. Note that ICD-9-CM procedural codes are based on services performed; they are indexed based on anatomical system, and procedure.

THE QUERY PROCESS

With the large volume of inpatient (and sometimes outpatient) documentation that must be reviewed, the coder will likely identify potential diagnoses and procedures that would add to the complexity of the hospital admission. Coders are not free to add these diagnostic statements, but they can "query" the physician as to whether additional diagnoses would be appropriate. The coder must be careful not to "lead" the physician to a diagnostic statement solely because that particular diagnosis would increase the reimbursement. This query process is typi-

BOX 18-1	Index to ICD-9-CM Volume 3— Procedure Codes	
Operations on the nervous system		01-05
Operations on the endocrine system		05-07
Operations on the eye		08-16
Operations on the ear		18-20
Operations on the nose, mouth, pharynx		21-29
Operations on the respiratory system		30-34
Operations on the cardiovascular system		35-39
Operations on the hemic/lymphatic system		40-41
Operations on the digestive system		42-54
Operations on the urinary system		55-59
Operations on the male genital organs		60-64
Operations on the female genital organs		65-71
Obstetrical procedures		72-75
Operations on the musculoskeletal system		76-84
Operations on the integumentary system		85-86
Miscellaneous diagnostic/therapeutic procedures		87-99

cally in place at all hospitals and facilities and is used for both inpatient and outpatient care.

OUTPATIENT HOSPITAL CODING

The outpatient hospital diagnostic coder should follow the rules for the physician/provider coder. The outpatient hospital coder may also need to include the Volume 3 Procedure Code for procedures performed when required by the carrier. Outpatient coding requires assignment of applicable CPT-4 codes, ICD-9-CM Volume 1 and 2 codes, and Volume 3 Procedure Codes, when applicable. Although the outpatient hospital coder typically is employed by the facility, the physician/provider roles for coding apply because the services are not reimbursed based on DRGs.

When the student undertakes diagnostic coding for outpatient surgery, reference should be made to the diagnostic rules presented in the section on physician coding.

STEPS IN THE OUTPATIENT HOSPITAL CODING PROCESS

The **(A)mbulatory (P)ayment (C)lassification (APC)** system of coding and reimbursement for services was implemented in August 2000 in the hospital outpatient setting. After successful implementation in this setting, the plan is to apply this same method in other settings, possibly including physician/provider services.

This system, originally based on diagnostic codes, resulting in the formulation of approximately 80 APC groups that cover every body system, was known as Ambulatory Payment Groups or APGs. After the original formulation of the APG system, CMS determined that several inconsistencies existed and therefore developed the APC system.

The primary objectives of the APC system are the following:

1. To simplify the outpatient hospital payment system
2. To ensure that payments adequately compensate hospital costs
3. To implement CMS's goals of deficit reduction

At this time, more than 700 APC groups are organized into four major categories: significant procedure APCs, surgical services APCs, ancillary services APCs, and medical visits APCs.

SIGNIFICANT PROCEDURE APCs

Procedures that are considered significant should receive separate reimbursement. Examples of these services include the following:

- Psychotherapy
- Dialysis
- Mammography
- Pulmonary tests
- Nuclear medicine
- Chemotherapy administration

SURGICAL SERVICES APCs

This category includes major surgical procedures for which multiple-procedure payment reduction applies. This is similar to the current method of "reducing" the payment for multiple procedures. Because they are considered global, only one procedure deserves global payment. Examples include the following

- Arthroplasty
- Laparoscopy
- Cardiac catheterization
- Fracture treatment
- Endoscopy
- Other surgical procedures

ANCILLARY SERVICES APCs

This group includes those ancillary services for which a separate reimbursement should be made. Examples are the following:

- Radiology
- ECG
- Immunization
- Infusion therapy (except chemotherapy)

MEDICAL VISIT APCs

The assignment of a visit APC should be based on the location of service (e.g., emergency department or outpatient clinic only). Originally, the medical visit APC was based on diagnostic information, as well as location of service. For simplicity, after the implementation of APCs in August 2000, the decision was made to assign codes based only on location and level of service.

CMS also allows for levels of service to be assigned on the basis of "acuity." These acuity levels are facility determined; therefore each facility may have different acuity levels for services performed. These levels may be assigned based on evaluation and management guidelines for levels of service, levels based on the complexity of the presenting problem or complaint, or levels designated by points assigned for the different facility resources expended in providing the visit. Currently CMS requires only that the levels are "distributive" between the five levels of services, namely 99281 to 99285 (for emergency department visits, for instance). Further, the facility must be consistent in assigning these codes. It is expected that CMS will announce a more concrete standardized method of assigning these levels of service in 2007.

Observation care under the Outpatient Perspective Payment System (OPPS) is currently not reimbursable except in three instances—congestive heart failure, asthma, and chest pain—and only then with appropriate documentation. Other observation care is considered as included in reimbursement for other ancillary, diagnostic, and surgical services performed during the same observation status admission.

NEW TECHNOLOGY AND PASS THROUGH PAYMENTS

For those new services that have not been assigned a current CPT-4 code, temporary HCPCS codes are assigned to allow for reimbursement for new biologicals, new medications, and new technology devices above and beyond the usual scope of devices or drugs used in performing an OPPS reimbursable service. These items are typically priced significantly above the usual supplies provided for a service. Following their assignment of HCPCS codes, these items are reviewed on a regular basis for the possibility of a regular HCPCS or CPT-4 code assignment.

GENERAL APC GUIDELINES

Not all services reimbursable under OPPS are reimbursable under APCs. Many services may be reimbursable only as an inpatient service under regulations other than APCs, or they may simply not be reimbursable under OPPS at all.

Payment status indicators are assigned to each CPT-4 code to indicate how and whether the procedure performed will be reimbursed under the APC system or another payment method. Keep in mind that multiple CPT-4 codes may be assigned for an encounter and may be considered reimbursable; this is not the case with inpatient hospital coding. The most common payment status indicators are listed as follows:

A Services paid under another method
C Inpatient services not payable under APC methodology
E Services not covered or allowed by Medicare program
F Acquisition of corneal tissue
G Current drug or biological pass through
H Pass through devices

J New drug or biological pass through
N Incidental services, payment packaged into another APC service
P Services paid only in partial hospitalization programs
S Significant procedures with no reduction in multiple procedures
T Surgical procedures with multiple procedure discount taken
V Medical visits
X Ancillary services payable under APCs

Coding rules differ for inpatient and outpatient coding. Inpatient and DRG coding will be further considered in the next chapter. Outpatient hospital coding uses the following systems:

- CPT-4 codes for all services rendered
- ICD-9-CM diagnostic codes to justify the medical necessity of services provided
- ICD-9-CM procedural codes for all services performed

Outpatient hospital coding is the only one that requires all three concurrent code types on all services for reimbursement. In addition, the outpatient hospital coder is limited to a smaller number of modifier codes than the physician or professional coder. The only modifier codes that are applicable to the outpatient hospital setting are listed in Tool 51 (as well as in Chapter 16). Specifically, the outpatient hospital coder does not use modifier 51 for multiple surgical procedures. This issue is addressed by the payment status indicators used in the APC reimbursement system.

Two new modifier codes, modifiers 73 and 74, used by the hospital outpatient coder are not used by the physician or professional coder. Modifier 73 is used in the outpatient hospital setting when a surgical procedure is terminated after the preparation for surgery has been completed, but before the administration of anesthesia. The facility is reimbursed proportionally for the completed part of the procedure.

Modifier 74 is used when the surgical procedure is terminated after the administration of anesthesia; with the proper documentation, the facility is reimbursed a proportionate amount for the expended resources.

Consider the following outpatient facility charts and determine the appropriate diagnosis and procedures that will be reimbursed for the encounters.

HISTORY AND PHYSICAL EXAMINATION

Rachel Perez, MD

Chief Complaint: Right scrotal swelling

25-year-old who previously underwent circumcision at birth, however, right scrotal swelling on and off since birth. Scrotal ultrasound obtained notes both testicles of normal size in the absence of solid testicular mass or testicular torsion. Right testicle displaced inferiorly secondary to 2.5–3.5 cm right hydrocele which is not septated or present internal debris noted.

Past medical history:

Noncontributory
PAST SURGICAL HISTORY: Circumcision at birth
ALLERGIES: No known drug allergies

Family and social history:

Review of systems:

Constitutional, negative for recent fever, weight loss, decreased appetite. HEENT: Positive for rhinitis. Negative for sore throat, earache. Cardiovascular: Negative for hypertension or congenital heart disease. Respiratory: Negative for asthma, bronchitis, productive cough. GI: negative for emesis, diarrhea, jaundice, constipation or melena. Hematological: Negative for bleeding disorder, bruising, anemia. Musculoskeletal: negative for congenital connective tissue disorder, recent joint swelling. Neuro: Negative for seizure disorder, meningitis, neurological disorder.

Physical exam:

In general, well developed, well nourished, 25-year-old male alert and in no acute distress:
HEENT: Normocephalic, atraumatic, EOM intact.
Neck: Supple without palpable lymphadenopathy.
Lungs: Clear to auscultation bilaterally without labored respirations or wheezing.
Heart: Regular rate and rhythm.
Abdomen: Soft, flat, nontender, nondistended, urinary bladder not palpable. No palpable abdominal organomegaly.
GU: Circumcised phallus without penile mass or lesion. Urethra meatus patent without evidence of gross blood or penile discharge. Left testicle descended and displaced laterally secondary to large right hemoscrotal mass effect due to hydrocele. Large right hydrocele present which does transilluminate for which the right testicle is not physically palpable. No scrotal fixation. No palpable inguinal adenopathy or any inguinal hernia appreciated bilaterally.
Extremities: No cyanosis, clubbing or edema.
Neuro: Alert and cooperative with no focal motor deficit

Laboratory/radiology:

White count 7.3. Hemoglobin 11.9. Platelets 323,000. PT 11.4. PTT 31.4. Urinanalysis on void; color yellow, clarity clear, no red cells, trace bacteria. Sodium 137, Potassium 4.0. BUN 14, Creatinine 0.4. Glucose 85, Calcium 9.6

X-ray:

Assessment:

IMPRESSION: Right inguinal hernia/hydrocele

Plan:

Patient scheduled for outpatient surgery consisting of right hydrocelectomy through inguinal approach with possible ligation of inguinal hernia if present under anesthesia.

Rachel Perez MD

GODFREY REGIONAL HOSPITAL
123 Main Street • Aldon, FL 77714 • (407) 555-1234

OPERATIVE REPORT

Patient information:

Patient name:
DOB:
MR#:

Preoperative diagnosis:

Right hydrocele

Postoperative diagnosis:

Right inguinal hernia/hydrocele

Procedure(s) performed:

Right inguinal hernia repair with excision of right hydrocele

Anesthesia:

General

Assistant surgeon:

Description of procedure:

After informed consent, patient was taken to the Operating Room, placed in supine position, and given general endotracheal anesthesia per protocol. The external genitalia and lower abdomen were prepped with betadine solution, draped in the usual sterile fashion. Patient did receive one dose of IV antibiotic consisting of 150 mg Ancef prior to initiation of the surgical procedure.
A left oblique incision was made approximately one finger-breadth above the right pubic tubercle in order to allow appropriate access to the right inguinal canal. The subcutaneous tissue and Scarpa's fascia were incised sharply to the level of the aponeurosis of the external oblique. Hemostasis of small perforating vessels was obtained with electrocautery. The external inguinal ring was identified where the overlying fascia of the external oblique was sharply incised in the direction of its fibers to expose and open the right inguinal canal.
The ileoinguinal nerve was identified and sharply excised from overlying tissue of the spermatic cord and retracted laterally to prevent future injury. Self-retaining retractors were placed to assist with exposure of the spermatic cord.
The spermatic cord was bluntly freed from the external oblique aponeurosis in the entire inguinal canal. A Penrose drain was placed in the area around the spermatic cord to assist with retraction.
Cremasteric fibers were sharply taken down to the level of the spermatic cord near the internal inguinal ring. The hernia sac was bluntly dissected free of the spermatic cord fascia and adjacent vascular structures.
The vas deferens was identified posterior to the hernia sac and likewise dissected free of the surface of the hernia sac. Once the vas deferens and vascular structures were dissected free of the hernia sac, a straight clamp was placed across the hernia sac and transsected distal to the clamp. The hernia sac was then dissected free of cord structures to the level of the internal inguinal ring. High ligation was performed at this level by placement of 2 silk ties of 2-0 silk. The hernia sac was excised and sent to Pathology for analysis.
The distal edges of the tunic vaginalis were grasped with mosquito clamps and subsequently opened with electrocautery where a noncommunicating hydrocele was evident. The right testicle could not be delivered into the surgical field secondary to associated hydrocele component. Aspiration of hydrocele through the scrotal sac using a 22-gauge needle was performed with the return of straw-colored fluid. Subsequent delivery of the right testicle into the surgical field was performed for which it was left attached to the gubernaculums.
Wound was then thoroughly irrigated with saline and edges of the external oblique reapproximated with a running 3-0 Vicryl suture. The Scarpa's fascia was then reapproximated with running 3-0 Vicryl. Skin edges were reapproximated with a running 4-0 Vicryl suture and Benzoin and steri-strips were applied and a sterile dressing placed.
Final needle, sponge, and instrument count were correct. The patient tolerated the procedure well.

GODFREY REGIONAL HOSPITAL
123 Main Street • Aldon, FL 77714 • (407) 555-1234

Rachel Perez MD

SURGICAL PATHOLOGY REPORT

Name: _____ Hosp. No.: _____ Path. No.: _____

Date: _____ Room: _____ Age: _____ Sex: _____ Surgeon: _____ M.D. _____

Operation: ___Excision of Hydrocele, Inguinal Hernia Repair_____

Material submitted: ___Hernia Sac, Surgical Excision_____

Pre-op diagnosis: ___Right hydrocele_____

Post-op diagnosis: ___Right inguinal hernia/hydrocele_____

Previous material: _____ Pertinent history: _____

Diagnosis:

Hernia sac, (clinically right), excision:
Benign fibroadipose tissue consistent with hernia sac

Gross description:

The specimen is labeled hernia sac. Received is a 6 mm in greatest diameter tan-grey portion of membranous-appearing tissue. The specimen is totally submitted in one cassette.

Micro description:

Slides reviewed

Maria Colley M.D.
_____
Surgical Pathologist

GODFREY CLINICAL LABORATORIES
465 Dogwood Court • Aldon, FL 77712 • (407) 555-9876

From the outpatient documentation, the following diagnoses would be appropriate, as well as the assignment of the following procedure code(s):

> Hydrocele
> Unilateral inguinal hernia
> Procedures: Repair Inguinal Hernia, Initial, Reducible
> Surgical Pathology, Level II

It would not be appropriate to assign code(s) for the surgical operating room, room, and board during the preoperative and postoperative period; these are included in the reimbursement under APCs for the procedure. It would also be inappropriate to assign code(s) for the anesthesia and any of the supplies or materials required because they are covered by reimbursement for the surgical procedure under outpatient hospital coding guidelines.

CHAPTER IN REVIEW

CERTIFICATION REVIEW

- The basis for inpatient coding assignment differs from physician coding in that the "encounter" includes everything from admission to discharge.
- Volumes 1, 2, and 3 of the ICD-9-CM diagnostic coding book are used for inpatient diagnostic coding.
- Statements such as "probable," "possible," and "rule out" are used for coding purposes with inpatient diagnostic coding.
- Principal diagnosis is defined as the condition chiefly responsible for the patient's admission to the hospital following diagnostic/therapeutic studies.
- Outpatient hospital diagnostic coding follows the rules for physician coding.
- Outpatient hospital diagnostic coding uses ICD-9-CM Volume 3 to report significant procedures when applicable.

STUDENT STUDY GUIDE

- Study Chapter 18.
- Review the Learning Objectives for Chapter 18.
- Complete the Stop and Practice exercises.
- Study the Certification Review for Chapter 18.
- Complete the Chapter Review exercise to reinforce concepts learned in this chapter.

CHAPTER REVIEW EXERCISE

Look up and code these procedures from Volume 3—Procedural Coding of the ICD-9-CM book.

Volume 3-ICD-9-CM Code

1. Exploratory laparotomy _____
2. Repair of fractured clavicle _____
3. Appendectomy _____
4. Cholecystectomy _____
5. Cystourethroscopy _____

6. Tonsillectomy with adenoidectomy _____
7. Insertion of PE tubes for otitis media _____
8. Knee arthroscopy _____
9. Blood transfusion, packed red cells _____
10. Colonoscopy with biopsy _____
11. Bone scan _____
12. Flexible sigmoidoscopy _____
13. Pacemaker implant _____
14. Cardiac catheterization _____
15. Physical therapy _____
16. Esophageal speech training _____
17. Kidney transplant _____
18. Clavicular osteotomy _____
19. Wound dressing _____
20. Amputation, below the knee _____
21. Abdominal ultrasound _____
22. CPAP ventilation _____
23. Vasectomy _____
24. Vaginal delivery with episiotomy _____
25. Corneal transplant _____

On the basis of the guidelines established for hospital inpatient diagnostic coding, and for physician coding, determine which of these diagnoses would be used for inpatient versus physician coding. Designate by indicating (I)npatient, (P)hysician, or both (IP), and assign the appropriate ICD-9-CM code. Assign ICD-9-CM codes only to those that are appropriate.

ICD-9-CM Code   (I), (P), (IP)

26. Rule out pneumonia _____ _____
27. Acute bronchitis _____ _____
28. Myocardial infarction _____ _____
29. Ruled out ankle fracture _____ _____
    Ankle pain _____ _____

30. Acute respiratory failure _____ _____
    COPD _____ _____

Given the following diagnostic information, indicate what diagnostic statement would be used for physician and inpatient purposes.

	Physician	Inpatient
31. Myocardial infarction	_____	_____
COPD	_____	_____

32. Abdominal pain _____ _____
    Rule out appendicitis _____ _____
33. Urinary tract infection, most likely streptococcal _____ _____
34. Anemia, possibly due to chronic blood loss _____ _____
35. Anemia due to GI bleed _____ _____

HOSPITAL/FACILITY BILLING PROCESS

LEARNING OBJECTIVES

Following the completion of this chapter, the student will be able to:

- Know the different methodologies for hospital inpatient/outpatient reimbursement.
- Delineate the significant differences between inpatient/outpatient and physician coding.
- Understand and apply the coding guidelines for assigning DRG/APC codes.
- Comprehend the significance of the correct assignment of principal diagnosis for the purpose of determining the correct DRG code.
- Grasp the importance of identifying the presence or absence of complications and/or comorbidities that may present additional risk consideration for inpatient hospital cases.
- Understand the grouping of DRGs into categories known as MDCs (Major Diagnostic Categories).
- Understand the assignment of Ambulatory Payment Classifications (APCs) under the Outpatient Prospective Payment System (OPPS).

CODING REFERENCE TOOLS

Tool 58
DRG Coding Guidelines
Tool 59
MDCs Listing

KEY TERMS

Ambulatory Payment Classification (APC), 400
Complications and Comorbidities, 394
Diagnosis-Related Group (DRG), 393
Fee-for-Service, 393
Major Diagnostic Category (MDC), 393
New Technology and Pass Through Services, 402
Outpatient Prospective Payment System (OPPS), 402
Payment Status Indicators, 402

Per Diem, 393
Principal Diagnosis, 394
Prospective Payment System (PPS), 393
Secondary Diagnosis, 394

DOCUMENTATION/ CODING GUIDELINES

The documentation needs for inpatient and outpatient hospital coding and billing are discussed in Chapter 18. Keep in mind that with facility coding and billing, all documentation may be reviewed and used in the assignment of codes for billing and reimbursement purposes. Also remember that the principal diagnosis for inpatient facility coding/billing is determined only at the conclusion of the encounter (admission) after the completion of all studies and ancillary services or studies.

INPATIENT BILLING/ REIMBURSEMENT METHODS

The most significant differences in hospital and physician coding involve the methods for coding the **WHAT,** or the services performed. The coder must remember that these methods differ because of the reimbursement philosophies for provider/physician compared with hospital/facility. Facility reimbursement is typically accomplished with a collection of all services required to provide care, or "facility services," rather than with individual itemization. A look at the three main methods for reimbursement of inpatient/facility care helps in understanding the coding systems for inpatient coding.

There are three basic inpatient methods used for inpatient reimbursement: fee for service, per diem, and prospective payment systems (PPS).

FEE FOR SERVICE

Fee for service coding is based on the expenses incurred by the facility in providing services to a specific patient for a specific admission. Under this method of reimbursement, all services are covered, including such items as room, meals, surgical suites, nursing care, surgical procedures, pharmaceuticals, supplies, and other items necessary for the treatment of the patient's condition or illness.

PER DIEM

Per diem charges are based on a fixed payment amount per day for all services provided by the hospital or facility. This fixed amount may vary on the basis of the type of admission or the level of service. For instance, per

diem reimbursement for a patient in a critical care bed would be greater than that for a regular medical bed.

PROSPECTIVE PAYMENT SYSTEM

The Prospective Payment System **(PPS)** of reimbursement agrees to a set amount of reimbursement according to the type of case (diagnosis, illness, symptom, or injury). The most familiar prospective payment system is the **DRG** (Diagnosis-Related Group) system used by the federal government for Medicare claims. This system is used by many other third-party carriers as well.

DRGs reimburse a set amount that is based on the patient's diagnosis and treatment during the admission. This method assumes that patients with similar illnesses or complaints undergo similar procedures and testing, and each of these illnesses or complaints is assigned a specific reimbursement as specified by the assignment of a DRG code.

Facilities are now able to formulate their reimbursement according to the DRG assignment because the dollar amount for reimbursement has *prospectively* been determined and agreed on.

The original DRG system, which was developed at Yale University, divided all principal diagnoses into similar categories, referred to as *major diagnostic categories* **(MDCs).** The primary purposes of the DRG system are reimbursement, evaluation of quality of care, and use of services. Congress mandated the use of the DRG system for all inpatient Medicare care in 1983, making it necessary for all hospitals providing care to Medicare recipients to follow this method for submitting services to Medicare Part A.

In addition to the obvious purpose of determining reimbursement, DRGs serve other important functions for hospitals because they provide a means of evaluating quality of care and use of services. Because the cases "grouped" together under one DRG assignment are similar in their treatment protocols and related conditions and treatments, the hospital has the ability to use these data for outcome analysis and quality review. In addition, the data derived from the DRG assignment are analyzed in evaluating the use of services. Each DRG represents the "average" services provided for similar patients with similar treatments, so the data give the hospital the ability to detect overuse by the facility or by a particular provider. DRGs also provide the necessary data to ensure that the quality standards of the hospital are met.

From the reimbursement perspective, each DRG is intended to represent the average resources or services necessary to treat patients placed in that group. The DRG assigned also relates to the hospital case mix and the types of patients the particular hospital treats. Each hospital calculates a hospital case mix index (CMI), which is determined by dividing all provided DRG relative weights by the total number of Medicare encounters at that particular hospital.

Reimbursement will be based on the weight assigned to that DRG multiplied by the base rate for that particular hospital. The hospital can calculate its payment based on the following formula:

$$\text{DRG Relative Weight} \times \text{Hospital Base Rate}$$
$$= \text{Hospital Payment}$$

The DRG system currently comprises approximately 499 valid groups that classify patients and correlate the services used and length-of-stay based on the following:

- Principal and secondary diagnoses
- Procedure codes
- Sex
- Age
- Discharge status
- Presence or absence of complications and comorbidities (CC)
- Birth weights for neonates

COMPONENTS OF DRG CODING

Further discussion follows regarding the components that determine the correct assignment of DRGs under this system.

PRINCIPAL AND SECONDARY DIAGNOSES

The assignment of a DRG is based primarily on the principal diagnosis and includes up to eight additional diagnoses. The DRG code is based on diagnoses and procedures designated by the use of ICD-9-CM codes. The rules for coding diagnoses from the inpatient perspective differ from those previously discussed for physician and outpatient use. Chapter 18 presents the inpatient ICD-9-CM codes.

Principal diagnosis is defined as the condition determined to have caused the hospital admission of the patient after studies were completed. After assignment of the appropriate ICD-9-CM diagnostic codes with the inpatient hospital coding rules, the coder must determine the principal diagnosis. Contributing or **secondary diagnoses** are assigned as well when they contribute to either the complexity of the case or the medical decision making process of the principal diagnosis. The assignment of principal and supporting diagnosis would be made only at the conclusion of the encounter or admission, and, only after all diagnostic studies are completed.

PROCEDURE CODES

The coder must determine whether specific surgical procedures that affect the DRG are performed during the

admission. All procedures must be coded for use in DRG assignment. The coder must also use the Volume 3—Procedure Coding section of ICD-9-CM for assignment of these codes, as discussed earlier.

SEX

There are several DRG codes that are based on the sex of the patient. Obviously, DRG assignment for prostate conditions should be assigned to male patients only, and vaginal delivery codes would be specific to female patients, classified by reproductive age only.

AGE

Following the selection of diagnostic codes, the case should be reviewed for patient age because many DRG assignments are based on age:

> Simple Pneumonia and Pleurisy Age > 17
> Simple Pneumonia and Pleurisy Age 0–17

Obviously, components such as birth weights of neonates would be appropriate only for neonates.

DISCHARGE STATUS

Some DRG codes that are assigned depend on whether the patient has been discharged alive or deceased. The coder must ascertain this information from the chart as well.

PRESENCE OR ABSENCE OF COMPLICATIONS AND COMORBIDITIES

CMS has defined a specific set of guidelines for conditions and diagnoses that present an additional risk consideration for inpatient cases. The most common categories of **complications and comorbidities** (CC) are as follows:

- Alcoholism
- Blood loss anemia
- Angina
- Atrial fibrillation
- Cardiogenic shock
- Cardiomyopathy
- Cellulitis
- Congestive heart failure
- COPD
- Decubitus ulcer
- Dehydration
- Diabetes mellitus
- Hematuria
- Hematemesis
- Hypertensive heart disease with CHF
- Hyponatremia
- Melena

- Pleural effusion
- Pneumothorax
- Renal colic
- Renal failure
- Respiratory failure
- Urinary retention
- Urinary tract infection

The complications and comorbidities listed here will not always affect the assignment of DRGs when these conditions preexist with an already diagnosed condition used for determining the DRG assignment. For example, a chronic or acute manifestation of the same condition reported with the assignment of a DRG would not be considered a complication.

BIRTH WEIGHTS FOR NEONATES

In treatment of a neonate, specific DRG assignments are made for low-birth-weight neonates. For example, DRG 386 applies to birth weights of less than 1500 g, gestation less than 28 weeks, or both.

DRG CODING PROCESS

When the coder must use a DRG coding book, he or she can refer to the steps in Tool 58 for determining DRG assignment. In most instances, the coding of DRGs is accomplished by the use of computerized or encoder software at the facility. Software has been developed that leads the coder through a series of questions; it then assigns DRGs and diagnostic code(s). Despite the convenience and ease of use of inpatient encoder systems, the hospital inpatient coder must possess the knowledge and skills to determine principal diagnosis, secondary diagnoses, and patient complications and comorbidities.

Although there are approximately 25 major diagnostic categories used for inpatient DRG assignment, the subcategory DRGs number over 499. A listing of the Major Diagnostic Categories, or MDCs, is provided in Tool 59. In addition, Box 19-1 contains a "sample" of DRG assignments for one MDC category. The listing of DRG assignments is extensive and encompasses an entire book; therefore this text has provided only sample pages as an illustration of the DRG system.

Hospital DRG coding may seem more challenging because it encompasses many records rather than just a specific visit note or operative note. The coder should remember that for coding of hospital DRG services, the "encounter" begins at admission and ends at discharge. Therefore as contrasted with physician coding, any properly documented information during the hospital encounter may be used for selecting and coding the DRG.

The coder probably will not be exposed to manual coding of DRGs; therefore this text contains only a limited number of DRG coding exercises. If necessary, use the Hospital Inpatient DRG Coding Worksheet included on page 401. Take a look at the chart example on page 398. Keep in mind that inpatient charts are usually voluminous; this example suits the student's needs for demonstrating the appropriate assignment of a DRG.

T O O L   58

DRG CODING GUIDELINES

[1] Establish principal diagnosis, secondary diagnoses.

[2] Determine all significant procedures and code accordingly.

[3] Determine whether a surgical procedure was performed.

[4] Based on the principal diagnosis, assign the correct MDC.

[5] Determine whether to utilize the medical or surgical partition.

[6] Check for contributing factors that affect DRG assignment and assign correct DRG within the appropriate MDC category:
- Age
- Sex
- Discharge status
- Presence/absence of complications or comorbidities
- Birthweight for neonates

T O O L   59

MDCs Listing

MDC	Category	DRG Range
1	Diseases/Disorders Nervous System	1-35
2	Diseases/Disorders Eye	36-48
3	Diseases/Disorders Ears, Nose, Mouth, Throat	49-74, 168-169, 185-187
4	Diseases/Disorders Respiratory System	75-102, 475
5	Diseases/Disorders Circulatory System	103-145, 478-479
6	Diseases/Disorders Digestive System	146-167, 170-184, 188-190
7	Diseases/Disorders Hepatobiliary System/Pancreas	191-208, 493-494
8	Diseases/Disorders Musculoskeletal System/Connective Tissue	209-256, 471, 491, 496-503
9	Diseases/Disorders Skin, Subcutaneous Tissue, Breast	257-284
10	Endocrine, Nutritional, Metabolic Diseases/Disorders	285-301
11	Diseases/Disorders of the Kidney/Urinary Tract	302-333
12	Diseases/Disorders Male Reproductive System	334-352
13	Diseases/Disorders Female Reproductive System	353-369
14	Pregnancy, Childbirth, Puerperium	370-384, 469
15	Newborns, Neonates with Conditions Originating in Perinatal Period	385-391, 469-470
16	Diseases/Disorders Blood, Blood-Forming Organs/Immunological Diseases	392-399
17	Myeloproliferative Diseases/Disorders and Poorly Differentiated Neoplasms	400-414, 473, 492
18	Infectious/Parasitic Diseases	415-423
19	Mental Diseases/Disorders	424-432
20	Alcohol/Drug Use/Drug-Induced Organic Mental Disorders	433-437
21	Injuries, Poisonings, Toxic Effect Drugs	439-455
22	Burns	456-460, 472
23	Factors Influencing Health Status, Other Contact Health Services	461-467
24	Multiple Significant Trauma	484-487
25	Human Immunodeficiency Virus Infections	488-490

DRGs Associated with all MDCs
468 - Extensive Operative Room Procedure Unrelated to Principal
        Diagnosis
476 - Prostatic Operating Room Procedure Unrelated to Principal Diagnosis
477 - Nonextensive Operative Room Procedure Unrelated to Principal
        Diagnosis
480 - Liver Transplant
481 - Bone Marrow Transplant
482 - Tracheostomy
483 - Tracheostomy
495 - Lung Transplant

BOX 19-1   DRG Listing (by MDC)

MDC 1—Diseases/Disorders of the Nervous System
DRG

1   Craniotomy except trauma, age 18 or older
2   Craniotomy for trauma, age 18 or older
3   Craniotomy, age 17 or younger
4   Spinal Procedures
5   Extracranial Vascular Procedures
6   Carpal Tunnel Release
7   Peripheral and Cranial Nerve and Other Nervous System Procedures with CC
8   Peripheral and Cranial Nerve and Other Nervous System Procedures without CC
9   Spinal Disorders and Injuries
10 Nervous System Neoplasms with CC
11 Nervous System Neoplasms without CC
12 Degenerative Nervous System Disorders
13 Multiple Sclerosis and Cerebellar Ataxia
14 Specific Cerebrovascular Disorders except Transient Ischemic Attack (TIA)
15 Transient Ischemic Attack (TIA) and Precerebral Occlusions
16 Nonspecific Cerebrovascular Disorders with CC
17 Nonspecific Cerebrovascular Disorders without CC
18 Cranial and Peripheral Nerve Disorders with CC
19 Cranial and Peripheral Nerve Disorders without CC
20 Nervous System Infection except Viral Meningitis
21 Viral Meningitis
22 Hypertensive Encephalopathy
23 Nontraumatic Stupor and Coma
24 Seizure and Headache, Age > 17 with CC
25 Seizure and Headache, Age > 17 without CC
26 Seizure and Headache, Ages 0–17
27 Traumatic Stupor and Coma, Coma > 1 Hour
28 Traumatic Stupor and Coma, Coma < 1 Hour, Age > 17 with CC
29 Traumatic Stupor and Coma, Coma < 1 Hour, Age > 17 without CC
30 Traumatic Stupor and Coma, Coma < 1 Hour, Ages 0–17

31 Concussion, Age > 17 with CC
32 Concussion, Age > 17, without CC
33 Concussion, Ages 0–17
34 Other Disorders of Nervous System with CC
35 Other Disorders of Nervous System without CC

MDC4—Respiratory System
DRG

075 Major Chest Procedures
076 Other Respiratory System or Procedures with CC
077 Other Respiratory System or Procedures without CC
078 Pulmonary Embolism
079 Respiratory Infections/Inflammations Age > 17 with CC
080 Respiratory Infections/Inflammations Age > 17 without CC
081 Respiratory Infections/Inflammations Ages 0–17
082 Respiratory Neoplasms
083 Major Chest Trauma with CC
084 Major Chest Trauma without CC
085 Pleural Effusion with CC
086 Pleural Effusion without CC
087 Pulmonary Edema & Respiratory Failure
088 Chronic Obstructive Pulmonary Disease
089 Simple Pneumonia/Pleurisy, Age > 17, with CC
090 Simple Pneumonia/Pleurisy, Age > 17, without CC
091 Simple Pneumonia/Pleurisy, Ages 0–17
092 Interstitial Lung Disease with CC
093 Interstitial Lung Disease without CC
094 Pneumothorax with CC
095 Pneumothorax without CC
096 Bronchitis/Asthma Age > 17, with CC
097 Bronchitis/Asthma Age > 17, without CC
098 Bronchitis/Asthma Ages 0–17
099 Respiratory Signs/Symptoms with CC
100 Respiratory Signs/Symptoms without CC
101 Other Respiratory System Diagnoses with CC
102 Other Respiratory System Diagnoses without CC
475 Respiratory System Diagnosis with Ventilator Support

HISTORY AND PHYSICAL EXAMINATION

Godfrey Regional Hospital History & Physical
Admission: 12/01/00

The patient came from a nursing home and felt weak on the right side. Workers there thought she was alert, but confused. When seen in the ER, she was able to answer questions appropriately and to follow commands but was unable to lift her right leg. She had some motion in her right arm but was unable to squeeze her right hand. When evaluated by the ER physician, she was determined to be confused, and was difficult to understand. CT was obtained, with initial impression of a large, left hemispheric bleed.

Past medical history:

Remarkable for polymyalgia, GERD, hyperthyroid, DJD of the knees. Hospitalizations for pneumonia, gout, situational depression.
CURRENT MEDICATION: Prilosec 20 mg qd, Synthroid .125 mg daily, Propulsid 10 mg bid, Prednisone 20 mg daily, Cardizem CD 120 mg daily.

Family and social history:

Unobtainable from patient.

Review of systems:

Unobtainable from patient.

Physical exam:

Patient is alert but confused. She is not dysarthric. PERRLA. Extraocular movements are normal. Sclera is clear. TMs normal. No skull lacerations noted. Slight right VII nerve weakness. Lungs clear. Abdomen is soft, nontender, without guarding or rebound. Neuro/MS: Full ROM except right arm and leg. Unable to raise her left leg or to move it at all with positive Babinski's on right. Normal labs.

Laboratory/radiology:

X-ray:

Assessment:

Intracranial bleed.

Plan:

GODFREY REGIONAL HOSPITAL
123 Main Street • Aldon, FL 77714 • (407) 555-1234

In looking at the sample chart on the previous page, consider only those components necessary for proper coding.

STEPS IN DRG ASSIGNMENT PROCESS

Step 1

Identify the Appropriate Diagnosis
First, identify the elements that make up the diagnosis:

The patient came from a nursing home and felt weak on the right side. Workers there thought she was alert, but confused. When seen in the ED, she was able to answer questions appropriately and to follow commands but was unable to lift her right leg. She had some motion in her right arm but was unable to squeeze her right hand. When evaluated by the ED physician, she was determined to be confused and was difficult to understand. CT was obtained, with initial impression of a large, left hemispheric bleed.

Current Medication:
Prilosec 20 mg qd, Synthroid 0.125 mg daily, Propulsid 10 mg bid, Prednisone 20 mg daily, Cardizem CD 120 mg daily.

Review of Systems/Family History:
Unobtainable from patient.

Medical History:
Remarkable for polymyalgia, GERD, hyperthyroidism, DJD of the knees; hospitalizations for pneumonia, gout, situational depression.

Physical Examination:
Patient is alert but confused. She is not dysarthric. PERRL. Extraocular movements are normal. Sclera is clear. TMs normal. No skull lacerations noted. Slight right VII nerve weakness. Lungs clear. Abdomen is soft, nontender, without guarding or rebound. Neuro/MSK: Full ROM except right arm and leg. Unable to raise her left leg or to move it at all with positive Babinski's on right. Normal labs.

Assessment:
Intracranial bleed.

List those components and determine which diagnosis should be included in the diagnostic statement:

1. Weak
2. Confused
3. Large, left hemispheric bleed
4. PMH polymyalgia
5. PMH GERD
6. PMH hyperthyroidism
7. PMH DJD knees
8. Intracranial bleed

"1. Weak" and "2. Confused" are signs and symptoms of: "3. Large, left hemispheric bleed" and "8. Intracranial bleed," and therefore may be eliminated. Medical histories, as long as they describe chronic continuing disorders, may be coded as existing in hospital coding, unlike physician/provider coding. Therefore the final diagnostic statement would look like the following:

1. Left hemispheric bleed, intracranial bleed
2. Polymyalgia
3. GERD
4. Hyperthyroidism
5. DJD knees

The principal diagnosis would be "the condition established after study to be chiefly responsible for admission to hospital for care." Because the four diagnoses listed as medical history were only considered for therapeutic ongoing treatment and were not the "thrust of treatment," left hemispheric bleed, intracranial bleed is considered the *principal diagnosis*.

ICD-9-CM codes would be assigned as follows:

1. Intracranial bleed	Hemorrhage, intracranial	432.9
2. Polymyalgia	Polymyalgia	725
3. GERD	Reflux, gastroesophageal	530.81
4. Hyperthyroidism	Hyperthyroidism	242.90
5. DJD knees	DJD, knees	719.96

Step 2

Determine Whether Significant Procedures Were Performed
The second step in DRG coding is to determine whether significant procedures were performed. They are not documented; therefore it must be assumed that they did not occur.

Step 3

Assign the MDC according to the Principal Diagnosis
The third step in DRG coding is to assign the MDC according to the principal diagnosis. The principal diagnosis of intracranial bleed leads to an MDC in the "nervous system" section, which narrows down selection to the DRG range of 1 through 35.

Step 4

Assign Appropriate DRG Code within Specific MDC Category
According to the MDC 1 listing included in this chapter, the assignment of DRG 14 "Specific Cerebrovascular Disorders Except Transient Ischemic Attack" would be an appropriate assignment for this chart.

Step 5

Determine Whether the Partition Should Be Medical or Surgical

The fifth step in DRG coding is to determine whether the partition should be medical or surgical. Because no surgical services were identified, the medical partition would be appropriate.

Step 6

Check for Contributing Factors

The sixth step checks for contributing factors such as the following:

- Age (0–17) (over age 17)—DRG not age specific
- Sex (diagnosis is not sex specified)
- Discharge status (patient discharged "alive"): No separate DRG in this category for alive or deceased—N/A
- Presence or absence of complications or comorbidities (None of the contributing diagnoses are considered CC)—N/A
- Birth weight of neonates (N/A)

The original assignment of DRG 14 is still appropriate. It is now apparent that the coder must use all of the skills developed in ICD-9-CM coding, procedural coding with Volume 3, ICD-9-CM (as well as Volumes 1 and 2), and DRG Inpatient Hospital Coding.

A few inpatient coding exercises have been included in the Chapter Review Exercises to allow for some assistance in working through the first inpatient exercises. If necessary, use Figure 19-1 to code step-by-step for the first DRG cases.

OUTPATIENT BILLING/ REIMBURSEMENT METHODS

Although some third party carriers continue to reimburse outpatient hospital services on a line item basis, a large number of carriers have implemented the use of **Ambulatory Payment Classification (APC)** methods for the reimbursement of outpatient hospital services.

APCs were implemented in August 2000 in the hospital outpatient setting, following the model of DRGs introduced decades before. After successful implementation in this setting, the tentative plan is to implement a similar reimbursement method in other settings, possibly including physician/provider services.

The APC system was originally based on diagnostic codes, resulting in the formulation of approximately 80 APC groups that cover every body system. After the formulation of the original ambulatory payment system, (A)mbulatory (P)ayment (G)roups, CMS determined that several inconsistencies existed within the system and therefore the APC system was developed.

The primary objectives of the APC system are the following:

1. To simplify the outpatient hospital payment system
2. To ensure that payments adequately compensate hospital costs
3. To implement CMS's goals of deficit reduction

At this time, more than 700 APC groups are organized into four major categories: significant procedure APCs, surgical services APCs, ancillary services APCs, and medical visits APCs.

SIGNIFICANT PROCEDURE APCs

These are procedures that are considered significant and therefore should receive separate reimbursement. Examples of these services include the following:

- Psychotherapy
- Dialysis
- Mammography
- Pulmonary tests
- Nuclear medicine
- Chemotherapy administration

SURGICAL SERVICES APCs

This category includes major surgical procedures for which multiple-procedure payment reduction applies. This is similar to the current method of "reducing" the payment for multiple procedures because they are considered global, and only one procedure deserves global payment. Examples include the following:

- Arthroplasty
- Laparoscopy
- Cardiac catheterization
- Fracture treatment
- Endoscopy

ANCILLARY SERVICES APCs

This group includes those ancillary services for which a separate reimbursement should be made. Examples are the following:

- Radiology
- ECG
- Immunization
- Infusion therapy (except chemotherapy)

MEDICAL VISIT APCs

The assignment of a visit APC should be based on the location of service (e.g., emergency department or outpatient clinic only). Originally, the medical visit APC was to be based on diagnostic information, as well as location of service. For simplicity, after the implementation of

HOSPITAL INPATIENT DRG CODING WORKSHEET

Chart#/Patient Name:

List Components Here	Assign Codes Here
Step 1 - Principal/Secondary Diagnosis 1A - List diagnosis 1B - Determine primary diagnosis "Condition established after study to be chiefly responsible for admission to hospital for care" Number diagnoses in appropriate order	
Step 2 - Significant Procedures	
Step 3 - Determine whether surgical procedure performed Yes/No	
Step 4 - Assign the MDC Based on principal diagnosis	
Step 5 - Determine whether medical or surgical partition Med/Surg	
Step 6 - Check for Contributing Factors Age Sex Discharge status Presence/absence of complications or comorbidities Birthweight for neonates	
ASSIGNMENT **DRG:** Principal Dx: Addtl Dx:	

FIGURE 19-1 DRG coding worksheet used for coding hospital DRG charts. (Courtesy of MD Consultative Services, Orlando, Florida. All rights reserved.)

APCs in August 2000, the decision was made to assign these codes on the basis of only location and level of service.

CMS also allows for levels of service to be assigned according to "acuity" levels. These acuity levels are facility determined; each facility may have different acuity levels for services performed. These levels may be assigned according to evaluation and management guidelines for levels of service, levels based on the complexity of the presenting problem or complaint, or levels designated that are based on points assigned for the different facility resources expended in providing the visit. Currently CMS requires only that the levels are "distributive" between the five levels of services, namely, 99281 through 99285 (for emergency department visits, for instance) and that the facility is consistent in assigning these codes. It is expected that CMS will announce a more concrete standardized method of assigning these levels of service sometime in the future.

Observation care under the **Outpatient Prospective Payment System (OPPS)** is currently not reimbursable by some carriers except in three instances: congestive heart failure, asthma, and chest pain, and only with appropriate documentation. Other observation care is considered included in reimbursement for other ancillary, diagnostic, and surgical services performed during the same observation status admission.

NEW TECHNOLOGY AND PASS THROUGH PAYMENTS

For those new services that have not been assigned a current CPT-4 code, temporary HCPCS codes are assigned to allow for reimbursement for new biologicals, new medications, and new technology devices that are above and beyond the usual scope of devices or drugs used in performing a service that is reimbursable under the OPPS reimbursement method. These items are typically priced significantly above the usual supplies required to provide a service. After their assignment of HCPCS codes, these items are reviewed on a regular basis for the possibility of a regular HCPCS or CPT-4 code assignment.

GENERAL APC GUIDELINES

Not all services reimbursable under OPPS are also reimbursable under APCs. Many services may be reimbursable only as an inpatient service under another method other than APCs, or simply not reimbursable at all.

Payment status indicators are assigned to each CPT-4 code to indicate how and whether the procedure performed will be reimbursed under the APC system of reimbursement or another payment method. Keep in mind that multiple CPT-4 codes may be assigned for an encounter and may be considered reimbursable, although this is not the case with inpatient hospital coding.

The following are the most common payment status indicators:

A   Services paid under another method
C   Inpatient services not payable under APC method
E   Services not covered or allowed by Medicare program
F   Acquisition of corneal tissue
G   Current drug or biological pass through
H   Device pass through
J   New drug or biological pass through
N   Incidental services, payment packaged into another APC service
P   Services paid only in partial hospitalization programs
S   Significant procedures with no reduction in multiple procedures
T   Surgical procedures with multiple procedure discount taken
V   Medical visits
X   Ancillary services payable under APCs

STEPS IN APC ASSIGNMENT PROCESS

Although the assignment of DRGs for inpatient and APCs for outpatient services is not made at the facility, but at the time the services are submitted for payment to the third-party carrier, it is important for the facility to determine the appropriate assignment of DRGs or APCs to determine appropriate reimbursement.

Table 19-1 contains a list of the most common APC assignments for the coding scenarios contained in this

TABLE 19-1   Common APC Assignments

	CPT	APC
Outpatient Level 1/New	99201	0600
Outpatient Level 2/New	99202	0600
Outpatient Level 1/Established	99211	0600
Outpatient Level 2/Established	99212	0600
Emergency Room Level 1 or 2	99281/2	0600
Outpatient Level 3/New	99203	0601
Outpatient Level 3/Established	99213	0601
Emergency Room Level 3	99283	0601
Outpatient Level 4/New	99204	0602
Outpatient Level 4/Established	99214	0602
Outpatient Level 5/New	99205	0602
Outpatient Level 5/Established	99215	0602
Emergency Room Level 4 or 5	99284/5	0602
X-Ray, Ankle, AP and Lateral	73600	0260
X-Ray, Chest, PA and Lat	71020	0260
X-Ray, Finger, 2 Views	73140	0260
X-Ray, Foot, AP and Lateral	73620	0260
X-Ray, Forearm, 2V	73090	0260
X-Ray, Hand, 2V	73120	0260
Electrocardiogram	93005	0366
IV Infusion	A0081	0120
Laceration Repair, Simple, Other Than Facial, <2.5 cm	12001	0024

book. This is not intended to be a complete listing because there is an APC assignment for every CPT-4 and HCPCS code and the list is extensive. The most current and complete listing of APC assignments can be found on the CMS Web site at www.cms.gov. The student may need to refer to that listing to complete some of the exercises contained in this text.

Determine appropriate coding and APC assignments for the following typical encounter in the outpatient facility.

EMERGENCY ROOM RECORD

Name:		Age:	ER physician:
		DOB:	

Allergies/type of reaction:	Usual medications/dosages:

Triage/presenting complaint:	Patient presents to the emergency room following a minor <u>automobile accident</u> in which the patient was the <u>driver</u> of a vehicle that <u>lost control</u> and hit a bridge abutment. Patient experiences an <u>open wound</u> to the <u>arm</u>, approximately <u>1.75</u> cm in length.

Initial assessment:

Time	T	P	R	BP	Other:					

Medication orders:

Lab work:

X-Ray:

Physician's report:

The patient is <u>seen by the ER physician</u> who evaluates the wound, <u>x-rays</u> the <u>forearm</u>, and <u>sutures</u> the wound and the patient is discharged for follow-up in 7–10 days.

Indicates:
<u>Procedures/Services</u>   <u>Diagnostic Statements</u>

Diagnosis:	Physician sign/date

| Discharge | Transfer | Admit | Good | Satisfactory | Other: | |

GODFREY REGIONAL HOSPITAL
123 Main Street • Aldon, FL 77714 • (407) 555-1234

From the report the following can be determined:

Services: ED visit
X-ray, forearm
Laceration repair, arm, 1.75 cm

Diagnoses: Open wound, arm
Automobile accident, driver, loss of control

Procedural: X-ray, forearm
Services: Laceration repair

Assign Codes for the Services/Diagnoses Outlined:

ICD-9-CM Diagnostic Code(s): _____
ICD-9-CM Procedure Code(s): _____
CPT-4 Code(s):   _____
APC Code(s) Assignments: _____

CHAPTER IN REVIEW

CERTIFICATION REVIEW

- Three different reimbursement methods exist for coding inpatient services.
- The fee for service reimbursement method reimburses all services necessary for treatment of the patient's condition or illness.
- The per diem method of reimbursement assigns a set rate per day for services, according to the level of service and the type of admission.
- The PPS (Prospective Payment System) reimbursement method uses the DRG (diagnosis-related group) system for determining appropriate reimbursement for services.
- The DRG method of reimbursement sets a reimbursement amount that is based on the patient's diagnosis and treatment during admission.
- Inpatient coding allows the coder to assign one principal diagnosis and additional diagnoses (up to eight).
- When significant procedures are performed during the inpatient stay, ICD-9-CM—Volume 3 is used for assigning an appropriate code.

- DRG code categories are based on patient age, sex, discharge status, presence or absence of comorbidities/complications, and birth weights of neonates.
- Outpatient reimbursement is based on Ambulatory Payment Classifications (APCs).
- Multiple APCs may be assigned per encounter in the outpatient setting.

STUDENT STUDY GUIDE

- Study Chapter 19.
- Review the Learning Objectives for Chapter 19.
- Review the Certification Review for Chapter 19.
- Complete the Chapter Review exercise to reinforce concepts learned in this chapter.
- Complete the Student Workbook exercises 1 through 30 in Chapter 19: Hospital/Facility Billing Process.

CHAPTER REVIEW EXERCISE

Using the steps for coding, apply DRG codes for the following sample charts. Keep in mind that the number of lines provided for diagnoses and procedure code(s) is not necessarily indicative of the number needed.

1.

HISTORY AND PHYSICAL EXAMINATION

Godfrey Regional Hospital History & Physical
Admission date: 02/01/20XX

CHIEF COMPLAINT: Cough and chills.

HISTORY OF PRESENT ILLNESS:
This is an 80-year-old woman who has felt poorly all week. She developed a cough 1 week ago that is productive of clear mucus, and is associated with intermittent chills. She has had essentially no appetite and reports only liquid oral intake over the past 2 to 3 days. She was noted to have rales in the right side of her chest. Chest x-ray shows pneumonia in the right base. Her white count is elevated. She has low potassium, being on Hyzaar for hypertension, and is not eating well, which is the cause of the hypokalemia. She will be admitted for treatment with IV antibiotics, oral fluids, and potassium replacement.

Past medical history:

Significant for mastectomy for breast cancer of the left breast about 2 1/2 years ago. No signs of recurrence. She did smoke for many years but quit more than 20 years ago.
CURRENT MEDICATIONS: Pravachol 20 mg PO daily, Hyzaar 100/25 one daily.

Family and social history:

Married, lives with husband, one son deceased. Patient quit smoking 20 years ago. Does not drink. FH positive for cancer of the throat in brother, diabetes in sister. She has hypertension.

Review of systems:

Unremarkable. Not having problems with ears, nose, or throat. Does not have history of heart disease. Has history of controlled hypertension. Has some aches, particularly in area of right hip. Has had no problems with edema and no neurological problems.

Physical exam:

Blood pressure: 125/65
Pulse: 87
Temperature: 98.6
Respirations: 16

Oxygen saturation on room air is 94%. No adenopathy in the neck. Lungs have some rales in the right base. Neck veins are not distended. Heart regular, no murmurs. Abdomen is soft and nontender. Extremities show no edema. She lacks her left breast, no sign of cancer recurrence on the chest wall.

Laboratory/radiology:

White count is elevated at 20.4, potassium is somewhat low.

X-ray:

Assessment:

Pneumonia Anorexia and weakness secondary to pneumonia Hypokalemia Hypertension

Plan:

Patient will be admitted for IV antibiotics. Encourage oral fluids, replace her potassium.

GODFREY REGIONAL HOSPITAL
123 Main Street • Aldon, FL 77714 • (407) 555-1234

ICD-9-CM Diagnostic Code(s): _____   MDC Assignment: _____
ICD-9-CM Procedure Code(s): _____   DRG Assignment: _____

2.

HISTORY AND PHYSICAL EXAMINATION

Godfrey Regional Hospital History & Physical
Admission Date: October 1, 20XX

CHIEF COMPLAINT: 25-year-old with pyelonephritis in early pregnancy.

HISTORY OF PRESENT ILLNESS: This 25-year-old had her last menstrual period in the middle of August. She had a home pregnancy test about 1 week ago that was positive. For approximately the past 2 weeks, she has been having dysuria, frequency, and urgency with some back pain, but then she started getting sick at work with nausea and vomiting. She had been feeling hot, was having shaking chills, and had been feeling dizzy. She was diagnosed with pyelonephritis, and inpatient versus outpatient treatment was discussed. She strongly desired to try outpatient treatment, was given Augmentin 875 mg bid, and was told to call if she was unable to keep these down, or if her symptoms worsened. She called to say she was continuing to have problems and wishes to be admitted for therapy at this time.

Past medical history:

She has a history of pyelonephritis with a previous pregnancy in 19XX and a history of frequent UTIs. She has not had any surgeries.
CURRENT MEDICATIONS: None

Family and social history:

Smokes 4 cigarettes per day, drinks occasionally.

Review of systems:

Fever and chills. HEENT no complaints. Cardiac no complaints. Respiratory no complaints. GI no diarrhea, constipation. GU—last menstrual period middle of August. Psychological—patient is quite anxious.

Physical exam:

Ill-appearing young female. Temperature is 100.2, pulse 88, respirations 28, blood pressure 126/68. HEENT examination normal. PERRLA. Pharynx remarkable for tacky mucous membranes. Neck is supple without lymphadenopathy. Heart regular rate and rhythm. Lungs clear to auscultation bilaterally. Abdomen is soft, mild tenderness in lower quadrants: Positive bowel sounds. No hepatosplenomegaly or masses palpated.

Laboratory/radiology:

X-ray:

Assessment:

Pyelonephritis and dehydration.

Plan:

Will admit; give IV fluids and antibiotics. Continue IV antibiotics until afebrile 24 to 48 hours.

GODFREY REGIONAL HOSPITAL
123 Main Street • Aldon, FL 77714 • (407) 555-1234

Note: A DRG guide or encoder is needed to code this case because it does not fall into the MDC categories listed as examples in this book.

ICD-9-CM Diagnostic Code(s): _____
ICD-9-CM Procedure Code(s): _____
MDC Assignment: _____
DRG Assignment: _____

Using the steps for coding, apply APC codes for the following sample charts.

1.

EMERGENCY ROOM RECORD

Name:		Age:	ER physician:
		DOB:	

Allergies/type of reaction: | **Usual medications/dosages:**

Triage/presenting complaint: | Food Caught in Throat.

Initial assessment:

HISTORY OF PRESENT ILLNESS:
65-year-old female presents after eating steak for supper at a restaurant and apparently choking on the steak. She now feels as though the food is stuck in her esophagus. She is unable to swallow without difficulty and cannot drink any liquids without regurgitation. No past medical history other than hypertension.

Time	T	P	R	BP	Other:					

Medication orders:

Lab work:

X-Ray:

Physician's report:

PHYSICAL EXAMINATION:
BP 140/75, Pulse 87, Temperature 98.6. Lungs are clear, heart regular without murmurs, and abdomen is soft and nontender. She appears to be gasping for air and we will have her send directly to the endoscopy suite for evaluation.

ENDOSCOPY:
Scope was inserted through the esophagus, where the food was observed and removed. Further evaluation of the esophagus, stomach and duodenum was unremarkable.

Diagnosis: | **Physician sign/date**

Discharge   Transfer   Admit   Good   Satisfactory   Other:

GODFREY REGIONAL HOSPITAL
123 Main Street • Aldon, FL 77714 • (407) 555-1234

ICD-9-CM Diagnostic Code(s): _____ CPT-4 Code(s): _____
ICD-9-CM Procedure Code(s): _____ APC(s) Assignments: _____

2.

PROGRESS NOTE

Date: 02/20/XXXX	Vital signs:	T	R
Chief complaint: Dysuria, blood in urine		P	BP

25-year-old female who presents with 2-week history of painful urination, and now reports that she observed blood in her urine this evening.

No significant past medical history.

Examination:

VS Normal, lower abdominal painful upon palpation. Urinalysis reveals urinary tract infection.

Impression:

Plan:

Patient name:

DOB:

MR/Chart #:

GODFREY REGIONAL OUTPATIENT CLINIC
3122 Shannon Avenue • Aldon, FL 77712 • (407) 555-7654

ICD-9-CM Diagnostic Code(s): _____ CPT-4 Code(s): _____

ICD-9-CM Procedure Code(s): _____ APC(s) Assignments: _____

V

PUTTING TOGETHER CODING SYSTEMS

Thus far, the student has approached each of the coding systems independently, first ICD-9-CM, then CPT-4, and finally hospital DRG coding. These coding processes were approached as a building block process, by first presenting the basics for each of these coding systems, followed by additional steps required for specialty and complex cases.

Section V serves as a culmination of that knowledge with the application of all the information learned in additional review and exercises and in the completion of coding charts for a number of scenarios. The student by now realizes the importance of reinforcement with additional practice of the many concepts presented in the text.

PUTTING TOGETHER CPT-4, ICD-9-CM, AND DRG

Following the completion of this chapter, the student will be able to:

- Know how physician coding encompasses both ICD-9-CM and CPT-4 coding, so that services to third-party carriers may be adequately described.
- Understand that hospital coding encompasses DRG coding, ICD-9-CM coding, and assignment of Volume 3 ICD-9-CM diagnostic codes when appropriate to code or bill services to third-party carriers.
- Apply the concepts previously learned by coding cases in their entirety with all appropriate codes.

OVERVIEW

On completion of the review of the ICD-9-CM diagnostic coding, procedural, and hospital coding methods, students should recap and make certain that these methods can be "put all together."

Each section of this book emphasizes the importance of "order" for services, as well as diagnosis. The likelihood of proper reimbursement is greatly influenced by the correct order for services and the correct corresponding diagnoses. This chapter focuses on the final analysis of CPT-4, ICD-9-CM, and DRG codes, and gives some additional guidelines for the correct order of the service. It is important not only that each service is placed in order, but that diagnostic information is appropriate for each service performed. Additional testing exercises are in the Chapter Review Exercise at the end of the chapter.

PHYSICIAN CODING

DIAGNOSIS

To completely report EVERY service, the coder must ensure that there is always at least one diagnosis for each service provided and vice versa. The ability to accurately report all information related to the request for payment of services rests in the accurate and complete description of WHAT services were performed (CPT-4), what alterations or modifications were made to those services (CPT-4 modifiers), and WHY those services were considered medically necessary (ICD-9-CM).

The *primary diagnosis* for each service performed is the primary reason for that service or encounter. As has been discussed previously, that diagnosis should always be assigned to the highest level of specificity, and it may differ for each service performed on a specified date or claim form. Additional diagnoses may be added for each encountered service to further justify the medical necessity, or WHY the service was performed.

PROCEDURAL SERVICES

For physician/provider services, each service performed must be reported on the CMS-1500 claim form with the use of an appropriate CPT-4 code and with the use of a modifier when necessary. Order is important in listing the services because many third-party carriers consider the first CPT-4 code listed on the claim form as the primary service. In determining what service should be billed as primary or first on the claim form, consideration should be given to which service provided on a particular date of service was the most significant. Although this service will almost always be the most significant charge,

caution should be used in selecting the primary coded service for a given date by significance, NOT by charge amount. This selection criterion will be an important factor in the event that a third-party carrier requests justification for the selection of a particular service as primary. Should the explanation be given that selection was based on the highest charge and therefore the provider wishes full reimbursement for that service, the third-party carrier may interpret this as manipulation of data to obtain payment that may not actually be due, which may also be construed as fraud.

As was explained in the CPT-4 chapters, order often determines the percentage of payment received by third-party carriers. In some cases, as with modifier 51, subsequent services are reimbursed at 50%, 25%, or sometimes not at all. In other instances, for example, when the third-party carrier considers only one line item of service per calendar date, the provider obviously will want to list the most significant service first.

HOSPITAL SERVICES

DIAGNOSIS

In the case of hospital inpatient coding, the concepts discussed in Chapters 18 and 19 are appropriate. Inpatient ICD-9-CM diagnostic coding remains the primary reason for the encounter (admission). In inpatient diagnostic terms, that primary diagnosis is referred to as *the principal diagnosis*. Any supporting diagnoses, comorbidities, or deaths should be added as subsequent diagnostic codes. With hospital outpatient coding, however, the coding rules for ICD-9-CM mirror the physician assignment of diagnostic codes.

SERVICES

From the perspective of reporting WHAT services were performed, DRG coding is used. These codes are determined by the diagnoses selected and by the following factors:

- Principal and secondary diagnoses
- Significant procedures
- Surgical procedures performed
- Contributing factors that will affect patient care such as the following:
  Age
  Sex
  Discharge status
  Presence or absence of comorbidities/deaths
  Birth weight for neonates

In the case of hospital outpatient services, CPT-4 codes are used for assigning codes for services performed. Keep in mind that some of those services will be bundled together under the APC payment method when applicable.

With a review of all the factors related to assignment of ICD-9-CM diagnostic codes, CPT-4 procedural codes, and DRG inpatient hospital assignments, this chapter serves to summarize all of the information covered thus far. Coding exercises make up most of this chapter; these will help to solidify coding skills by putting together all the coding guidelines covered.

The coder should first select the codes needed for reporting services and then establish primary and secondary diagnostic codes for each service performed. Prioritization of services should occur last, including the assignment of appropriate modifiers for CPT-4 codes.

The following, which is an example of the exercises contained in this section, illustrates "putting the coding of services together."

PROGRESS NOTE

Chief complaint: _____

Date: _____

Vital signs: BP_____ P_____ R _____

History:

The patient arrives for an established patient visit complaining of profound abdominal pain. The patient reports onset approximately 1 to 2 days ago, without relief from any over-the-counter medications, rest, or positioning. The pain has become rather intense, and is reported as a 3 on a scale of 1 to 5. Medical history is significant for hypertension and hypothyroidism. Patient indicates no allergies or significant family medical history. She currently takes only birth control pills. She is married, with one child. She reports that to her knowledge, no one in the family has experienced similar symptoms.

Exam:

Examination is unremarkable for any positive findings of HEENT, abdomen, heart, or respiratory. CBC demonstrates an elevated white count; urinalysis is positive for bacteria identified as *Escherichia coli*. The patient is instructed on the use of an antibiotic for urinary tract infection and is advised to return if symptoms persist or worsen.

Diagnosis/assessment:

E Coli Urinary Tract Infection

Stimy Kvastt MD

Patient name: _____

Date of service: _____

GODFREY MEDICAL ASSOCIATES
1532 Third Avenue, Suite 120 • Aldon, FL 77713 • (407) 555-4000

STEPS IN THE CODING PROCESS

Step 1

Select the Services Provided and Assign CPT-4/DRG Codes

Step 2

Select the Diagnosis Necessary to Describe the Medical Necessity for Each of the Services Listed in Step 1

Step 3

Determine If Services Assigned Have Been Modified or Altered in Any Way and If the Addition of a Modifier Code or CC Is Needed for Complications on Comorbidities

Assign codes to the previous exercise before attempting to complete the workbook exercises. Follow these same steps using the rules learned for applying the appropriate ICD-9-CM, DRG, and/or CPT-4 codes to the exercises listed in the Workbook. The Workbook exercises for this chapter represent a typical day in the career of a physician/provider coder or hospital coder. Remember that information may be omitted or unclear; however, these charts are intended to be representative.

In the event that difficulties are encountered, refer to the appropriate chapter(s) and review the appropriate coding guidelines, as well as those developed as **Coding Reference Tools.**

CHAPTER IN REVIEW

CERTIFICATION REVIEW

- Proper reimbursement is obtained by the correct assignment of codes listed in the correct order.
- Each service requires an explanation of medical necessity through the use of at least one diagnostic code.
- Primary diagnosis is always the chief reason for the encounter, service, or admission.
- Order of service codes for physician services is important because subsequent procedures are often disallowed or payment is reduced.
- Services are "grouped" in the form of DRGs for hospital coding.

STUDENT STUDY GUIDE

- Study Chapter 20.
- Review the Learning Objectives for Chapter 20.
- Review the Certification Review for Chapter 20.

CHAPTER REVIEW EXERCISE

Determine the correct order for service and diagnosis for the following inpatient and physician cases. For this exercise, it is not necessary to assign codes to these choices.

Physician

Services	Diagnoses
1. Office visit	Cough
Chest x-ray	Acute sinusitis
Sinus x-ray	Arm pain
Elbow x-ray	URI
2. Repair of fractured femur	Open wound, face
Repair of fractured metacarpal	Fractured metacarpal
Laceration repair, face, simple	Fractured femur
3. Laceration repair, face, simple	Open wound, face
Laceration repair, hand, intermediate	Open wound, face
Laceration repair, face, complex	Open wound, face, complicated

Inpatient

4. Admission	Pneumonia
Hernia repair	Pneumonia
Arterial blood gas	Umbilical hernia
Chest x-ray	Pneumonia
5. Admission	Pneumonia
Hospital visits	Respiratory failure
Lab/x-ray	

6. Outpatient surgery for   Umbilical hernia
   umbilical hernia
   Inpatient admission for   Cardiac arrest
   cardiac arrest during   Hypertension
   outpatient procedure   CAD
7. Admission   Fractured hip
   ORIF fractured hip   Fractured hip
   Hypotension during surgery   Hypotension
   Additional 2-day stay   Hypotension

PRACTICAL APPLICATION

The following documents from the physicians of Godfrey Regional Outpatient Clinic require assignment of the appropriate ICD-9-CM and CPT-4 codes for services. Keep in mind that only physician/professional coding is to be assigned.

1. Chart #1

HISTORY AND PHYSICAL EXAMINATION

SMITH, Edward   Stanley Krosette, MD
Admitted: 06/01/XXXX

Medical record number: 395739

This 91-year-old male recently noticed trembling and restlessness of his left leg, also had shortness of breath and was brought to the ER for evaluation. His ER evaluation was unremarkable; however, due to his complaints of dyspnea and his previous diagnoses, he was admitted for observation and further evaluation of his symptoms.

Past medical history:

He was admitted a few months ago for a ruptured appendix with extensive peritonitis. The patient has also had multiple admissions for his other health problems over the past several months.
CURRENT MEDICATIONS: Synthyroid 0.3 mg 4 times weekly, Digoxin 0.25 mg q d, Dipyridamole q d, Regland 10 mg qid, Tylenol prn

Family and social history:

Until recently, the patient and his spouse have been able to maintain their home; however, recently residing at an area assisted living center. Patient does not smoke or drink.

Review of systems:

Musculoskeletal: Patient has had numerous and gradually increasing musculoskeletal symptoms and reports many years of having a trembling or restless leg syndrome.

Physical exam:

General: Temperature 98.6, pulse 54, respirations 18, O2 room air 97%
HEENT: Pupils are equal and reactive to light and accommodation. EOMs intact.
              Tympanic membranes are dulled, pharynx not injected
Neck: No adenopathy found. Thyroid not enlaraged. No bruits or nodularity present. No carotid bruits are heard.
Chest: Mild degree of kyphosis and breath sounds are relatively distant. No dullness to percussion of the thorax
              is found. No rales or rhonchi present.
C/V: Normal heart sounds without murmurs. No dependent edema present.
Abdomen: Soft, flat and nontender. Well healed surgical scars are present. No abdominal masses are found.
Back: No point tenderness along the thoracic, lumbar or sacral regions
Extremities: Pulses are 1+ and equal bilaterally. Equal strength in all four extremities.

Laboratory/radiology:

X-ray:

Assessment:

1. Episode of dyspnea 2. Trembling/Restlessness of Leg 3. Hypothyroidism 4. Progressive arteriosclerotic vascular disease
5. Recent performated appendix with peritonitis

Plan:

Admit for further evaluation and treatment

Stony Krautt, MD

GODFREY REGIONAL HOSPITAL
123 Main Street • Aldon, FL 77714 • (407) 555-1234

ICD-9-CM code(s): _____

CPT-4 code(s): _____

2. Chart #2

PROGRESS NOTE
_____

Date/time
_____
06/XX/XXXX

S:

Recalls incident. Had right leg pain, could not get into bed. No loss of consciousness or other symptoms.

O:

Afebrile, vital signs stable

HEENT: Unshaven, oral mucosa tacky
Chest: Clear to auscultation
Abdomen: Negative
Extremities: RLE erythematous, 1–2+ edema. No knee effusion.
Neuro: Alert, oriented, speech clear, neuro check stabl

A:

RLE Cellulitis
R/O RLE DVT
R/O CVA
R/O MI
Parkinson's
Hypothyroidism

P:

Order Head CT
If negative, start Lovenox empirically

Maurice Doater, MD

PROGRESS NOTES

GODFREY REGIONAL HOSPITAL
123 Main Street • Aldon, FL 77714 • (407) 555-1234

ICD-9-CM code(s): _____

CPT-4 code(s): _____

CPT only © American Medical Association. All Rights Reserved.

3. Chart #3

STAFF NOTES   Patient name _____

Date	Time	Staff notations
03/11/XXXX	0710	Patient states feeling tired, complaining of dysuria and feeling feverish

GODFREY MEDICAL ASSOCIATES
1532 Third Avenue, Suite 120 • Aldon, FL 77713 • (407) 555-4000

PROGRESS NOTE

Date/time
03/11/XXXX

S:

Patient stated feeling tired, chills, denies cough, nausea, vomiting, diarrhea.

Does report continued dysuria.

O:

Lungs: Clear.
CV: Regular rate and rhythm.
Abdomen: Soft, nontender, positive bowel sounds.
WBC: 16.7, 85.8% seg, 8.9% lumph

A:

Fever of unknown origin, cultures pending.

Continue IV fluids and IV antibiotics.

Will repeat UA for symptoms.

P:

Stony Kractt, MD

PROGRESS NOTES

GODFREY REGIONAL HOSPITAL
123 Main Street • Aldon, FL 77714 • (407) 555-1234

ICD-9-CM code(s): _____
CPT-4 code(s): _____

4. Chart #4

PROGRESS NOTE

Date:	Vital signs:	T	R
Chief complaint: Right elbow pain		P	BP

7-year-old male in good general health who fell off a ladder onto an outstretched right hand. He complained of immediate right elbow pain and wrist pain. He was reluctant to move the elbow at first, however, on the way to the office began to move it somewhat, however still complains of elbow pain. No other injuries are reported.

Examination:

Healthy appearing white male, temperature 98.3, pulse 105, respirations 22. There appears to be no effusion of the right elbow. Starting with the shoulder, shoulder has normal range of motion. There appears to be no deformity. The patient fully extends the right elbow but has some pain with flexion at approximately the 90 degree mark. Some pain proximal to the right elbow with supination and is not able to fully extend the arm.

Wrist appears normal, neurovascularly the entire limb is intact.

Impression:

Right elbow injury, most likely soft tissue injury due to fall from ladder.

Plan:

Place in sling which can be removed when comfortable. Children's Motrin. Ice to area as needed. If no improvement or worsening symptoms should return.

Willen Obrt MD

	Patient name:
	DOB:
	MR/Chart #:

GODFREY REGIONAL OUTPATIENT CLINIC
3122 Shannon Avenue • Aldon, FL 77712 • (407) 555-7654

ICD-9-CM code(s): _____

CPT-4 code(s): _____

5. Chart #5

PROGRESS NOTE

Chief complaint: _____

Date: _____

Vital signs: BP_____ P_____ R_____

SHORT STAY SUMMARY/Observation
Admitted: 02/03/XXXX
Discharged: 02/04/XXXX

History:

Patient is a 53-year-old white female who was undergoing outpatient evaluation for possible cardiac cause of chest pain. The patient was undergoing routine outpatient adenosine-Cardiolite study when she developed significant AV block with ventricular response rate of 30–33 beats per minute. Patient became extremely lightheaded, diaphoretic, was nauseated and had emesis times two. The patient remained significantly bradycardic despite discontinuance of the adenosine drop. She required IV administration of Atropine 0.4 mg. The patient's heart rate then increased to 75–80 bpm, however, blood pressure was in the 225/103 range. Patient was then administered nitroglycerin sublingually and her blood pressure decreased over the next 20 minutes to a level of 176/92. It was felt that patient should be admitted to the observation unit for observation of her cardiac rhythm and control of her blood pressure.

Exam:

The patient continued to be monitored and developed no significant tachy/bradyarrhythmia and her blood pressure returned to a more appropriate level. Her blood pressure at this time is 145/77 with heart rate of 74. Temperature is 97.5, respirations 20. Of note, the patient's myocardiac perfusion study returned revealing a questionable ischemia on the anterior wall. Ejection fraction was noted to be 40%.

Diagnosis/assessment:

Bradycardia following adenosine-cardiolite study

Uncontrolled blood pressure

Patient will be discharged to home and follow-up as outpatient for precatheterization counseling

Ruth Brady MD
Cardiologist

Patient name: _____
Date of service: _____

GODFREY MEDICAL ASSOCIATES
1532 Third Avenue, Suite 120 • Aldon, FL 77713 • (407) 555-4000

ICD-9-CM code(s): _____

CPT-4 code(s): _____

6. Chart #6

PROGRESS NOTE

Date:	Vital signs:	T	R
Chief complaint:		P	BP

Physical examination:

Assessment:

Patient was seen today for skin testing, and all of her skin tests were negative. It is my impression, therefore, that she has intrinsic asthma.

Plan:

She is to discontinue her Theo-Dur, as she has experienced episodes of tachycardia and anxiety with the use of this medication. Prescribe Proventil 2 mg tablets 4 times daily for wheezing.

Return for further follow-up in two months.

Felix Warden M

	Patient name:
	DOB:
	MR/Chart #:

GODFREY REGIONAL OUTPATIENT CLINIC
3122 Shannon Avenue • Aldon, FL 77712 • (407) 555-7654

ICD-9-CM code(s): _____

CPT-4 code(s): _____

CPT only © American Medical Association. All Rights Reserved.

7. Chart #7

PROGRESS NOTE

Date:	Vital signs:	T	R
Chief complaint:		P	BP

28-year-old female who presents with complaints of urinary burning and frequency for approximately the last 5–7 days. She denies any other urinary problems. No chills, fever, flank pain or hematuria. She has noticed nocturia X the past 3 days but denies any abdominal pain or nausea. Otherwise, she is in good general health and denies any recent URI or the possibility of pregnancy.

Examination:

Temperature 98.6, pulse 72, BP 116/80. Patient is alert and in no distress. Skin is pale, warm and dry. Palpation of the abdomen reveals no masses or organomegaly. Bladder is not palpable or tender. On pelvic exam, no evidence of vulvar edema or erythema and no discharge. Cervix is clean, and she had a negative Pap smear approximately 8 months ago.

Clean-voided urine shows 15–20 white blood cells per high power field, 8–10 red blood cells, 4+ occult blood, 1+ protein.

Impression:

Acute cystitis

Plan:

Septra DS one bid X 5 days
Pyridium 200 mg 1 4–6 hours prn burning
Increase oral fluids
If the patient has persisting symptoms over the next 2–3 days she is to return to our office.

Stony Knott, MD

	Patient name:
	DOB:
	MR/Chart #:

GODFREY REGIONAL OUTPATIENT CLINIC
3122 Shannon Avenue • Aldon, FL 77712 • (407) 555-7654

ICD-9-CM code(s): _____

CPT-4 code(s): _____

8. Chart #8

PROGRESS NOTE

Chief complaint: _Abdominal Pain_

Date: _04/XX/XXXX_

Vital signs: BP_____ P_____ R_____

History:

The patient has been previously diagnosed with biliary cirrhosis. She continues to complain of abdominal pain. I gave her a trial of Reglan 20 mg po qid and also scheduled an upper GI with small bowel follow-through. The series was interpreted as normal.

Exam:

Today the patient continues to complain of abdominal pain. Her friend had just died of colon cancer. She complained of fatigue and malaise as well as new symptoms of reflux and heartburn.

Upon examination, her abdomen was soft with slight lower quadrant tenderness. PERRLA, neck, supple. Lungs are clear to auscultation and heart is regular rate and rhythm. Extremities show no cyanosis, clubbing or edema. The patient appears neurologically intact.

Diagnosis/assessment:

My impression is she has irritable bowel syndrome as well as esophageal reflux. I prescribed Sinequan 25 mg qid and Tagamet 400 mg bid.

She will call us if her symptoms do not improve over the next 3–5 days.

Maurice Doates, MD

Patient name: _____

Date of service: _____

GODFREY MEDICAL ASSOCIATES
1532 Third Avenue, Suite 120 • Aldon, FL 77713 • (407) 555-4000

ICD-9-CM code(s): _____

CPT-4 code(s): _____

9. Chart #9

PROGRESS NOTE

Date:	Vital signs:	T	R
Chief complaint:		P	BP

Symptoms of recurrent episodes of coughing and wheezing. She has never been hospitalized, but her asthma requires daily therapy with an inhaled bronchodilator. She has done much better with Pulmo-Aide with inhalations of Alupent and Atropine than she has done on handheld nebulizers.

Examination:

Impression:

Plan:

She should continue her current treatment regimen and return in 3 months unless she develops worsening symptoms prior to that time.

Felix Wander M

Patient name:

DOB:

MR/Chart #:

GODFREY REGIONAL OUTPATIENT CLINIC
3122 Shannon Avenue • Aldon, FL 77712 • (407) 555-7654

ICD-9-CM code(s): _____

CPT-4 code(s): _____

10. Chart #10

PROGRESS NOTE

Date:	Vital signs:	T	R
Chief complaint:		P	BP

Patient has been seen in my office on several occasions for intrinsic asthma. She has been on long-term steroids as she prefers this medication in an attempt to lower her medication costs.

Examination:

She appears to be doing well, taking her prednisone 10 mg every other day. She will continue with her present regimen. I reluctantly will agree to this regimen for a short period of time until she has remained stable for six months. At that time, we will discuss other options.

Impression:

Plan:

At the present time she is on Theo-Dur 750 mg per day, Ventolin 2 mg tid, prednisone 10 mg every other day, Azmacort and Vancenase. If she has increasing symptoms, she is to return immediately for further evaluation.

Felix Wander M

Patient name:

DOB:

MR/Chart #:

GODFREY REGIONAL OUTPATIENT CLINIC
3122 Shannon Avenue • Aldon, FL 77712 • (407) 555-7654

ICD-9-CM code(s): _____

CPT-4 code(s): _____

11. Chart #11

PROGRESS NOTE

Chief complaint: Parkinson's

Date: 04/XX/XXXX

Vital signs: BP_____ P_____ R _____

History:

This pleasant 85-year-old male presents with rather advanced parkinsonism which has been present for a number of years. It is affecting his daily living at this point. He has difficulty dressing, has frequent falls which occur without any apparent cause. He has marked hesitancy on changing direction and unsteadiness with fatigue. He also has problems with eating and swallowing. He now shows symptoms of depression along with his Parkinson disease.

Exam:

On neurological exam he had mild to moderate impairment in cognition and short-term memory. He is oriented X 3. He has a mild tremor, worse in the left arm than the right. He has rigidity in the upper extremity. He has marked poverty of movement, with long delays in initiating movement and frequent freezing. His speech is mildly dysarthric and has paucity of spontaneous facial expression. Can arise from a chair with multiple attempts, deep tendon reflexes are symmetrical and toes are downgoing. Cranial nerves are unremarkable.

Diagnosis/assessment:

He has been on Sinemet 25/100 tid for past several years. He is going on vacation soon, so I will not attempt to add a second antiparkinsonian medication at this time. However, will increase the Sinemet to qid for now and introduce bromocriptine 1 mg per day upon his return.

Patient name: _____

Date of service: _____

GODFREY MEDICAL ASSOCIATES
1532 Third Avenue, Suite 120 • Aldon, FL 77713 • (407) 555-4000

ICD-9-CM code(s): _____
CPT-4 code(s): _____

12. Chart #12

OPERATIVE REPORT

Patient information:

Patient name:
DOB:
MR#:

Preoperative diagnosis:

Chronic adenotonsillitis

Postoperative diagnosis:

Chronic adenotonsillitis

Procedure(s) performed:

Adenotonsillectomy

Anesthesia:

General endotracheal

Assistant surgeon:

Description of procedure:

Patient was brought to the OR and general endotracheal anesthesia was induced. Patient was placed in the Rose position and the McIvor mouth gag inserted in routine fashion.

Red rubber catheter was passed transnasally and adenoid bed inspected with mirror. Using adenoid curets, the adenoid bed was curetted. Adenoid packs were placed and attention turned to the right tonsil.

Right tonsil was grasped with tonsil tenaculum, and, using electrocautery, incision was created. Using scissors and sharp and blunt dissection, the tonsillar capsule was entered. Electrocautery was utilized to free the mucosal and fibrotic attachments of the right tonsil. Right tonsil was then snared without difficulty and tonsil packs were placed. An identical procedure was carried out on the left side. The tonsillar beds were then dried up using suction cautery.

Adenoid bed was then inspected and suction cautery was used on the adenoid bed as well until cessation of any further bleeding.

Wounds were inspected and there was no further bleeding. Mouth gag was removed and patient was transferred to the recovery room with all vital signs being stable.

Rachel Perez MD

GODFREY REGIONAL HOSPITAL
123 Main Street • Aldon, FL 77714 • (407) 555-1234

ICD-9-CM code(s): _____

CPT-4 code(s): _____

13. Chart #13

PROGRESS NOTE

| Date: | Vital signs: | T | R |
| Chief complaint: | | P | BP |

The patient comes in stating he has some irritation in his left ear. He also describes a musty smell in his nose when he inhales. He has been using some nasal spray, name unknown, for some time.

Physical examination:

PE: General appearance of well-developed 76-year-old male in no distress.

Ears: Right ear, external canal is slightly irritated. Tympanic membrane is intact and not inflamed. Left ear is clear. No cerumen in either ear.

Nose: Airway is adequate. Septum slightly deviated to right. No evidence of polyps, abnormal discharge.

Throat: Normal mucous membrane, no evidence of inflammation.

Neck: No adenopathy.

Assessment:

IMPRESSION:
Mild right external otitis

Plan:

Recommend 0.5% hydrocortisone cream in the outer ear and a couple drops of alcohol in ear at night before he goes to bed. Nasal irrigation using a normal saline solution. If symptoms progress, we will get sinus x-rays.

Willen Obot MD

	Patient name:
	DOB:
	MR/Chart #:

GODFREY REGIONAL OUTPATIENT CLINIC
3122 Shannon Avenue • Aldon, FL 77712 • (407) 555-7654

ICD-9-CM code(s): _____

CPT-4 code(s): _____

14. Chart #14

EMERGENCY ROOM RECORD

Name:		Age:	ER physician:
		DOB:	

Allergies/type of reaction: | **Usual medications/dosages:**

Triage/presenting complaint: Cough, Congested X 5 days

Initial assessment: Alert child in mild respiratory distress

Time	T	P	R	BP	Other:					

Medication orders:

Lab work:

X-Ray:

Physician's report:

HISTORY OF PRESENT ILLNESS:
2-year-old male who has been congested for almost a week. Child has sounded hoarse, with croupy cough and was seen 2 days ago by his Pediatrician. He has been treated with Alupent, Amoxicillin, Ventolin, cough syrup, and Slo-bid 100 mg bid with no improvement. Child is not taking any food or fluids, has been unable to rest and no struggling with breathing.
PHYSICAL EXAMINATION:
General: Exam showed an alert child in moderate respiratory distress
 Vital signs, temperature 99.6, pulse 120, respiratory rate 40
HEENT: Within normal limits
Neck: Positive for mild to moderate stridor
Chest: Chest shows diffuse inspiratory and expiratory wheezing. No rales noted
Heart: Regular rate and rhythm without murmur, gallop or rub
Abdomen: Soft and nontender
Extremities: Within normal limits

In examination of the chest wall, the child has subcostal and intercostal retractions. PA and lateral x-ray was performed which did not show pneumonia. Patient's parents agreed to admission to the pediatric unit for further respiratory treatment.

Diagnosis:	Physician sign/date
Acute layngotracheal bronchitis Bronchial asthma	*Nancy Conolly* MD

Discharge	Transfer	Admit	Good	Satisfactory	Other:

GODFREY REGIONAL HOSPITAL
123 Main Street • Aldon, FL 77714 • (407) 555-1234

ICD-9-CM code(s): _____

CPT-4 code(s): _____

15. Chart #15

DISCHARGE SUMMARY

Admitted: 06/10/XXXX
Discharged: 06/13/XXXX

Discharge diagnoses:

1. Left lower leg cellulitis
2. Left lower leg ulceration
3. Diabetes Mellitus

History:

41-year-old white male with obesity and diabetes who has had a smoldering left lower extremity cellulitis for the past 2–3 months. He has been treated with Coumadin and IV antibiotics. On the day of admission, presented to the office with worsening of cellulitis and a new 2-cm ulceration and was therefore admitted for IV antibiotics and further evaluation.

Extremities:
Revealed bilateral edema 1–2+ to the knees, with erythema and diffuse excoriations with erythema from the ankle to the midshin on the left lower extremity. Had a 2 x 2 cm superficial ulcer on the lateral aspect of the ankle.

Laboratory and radiology studies:

On admission, revealed sodium was 138. Electrolytes were normal. BUN and creatinine were normal. PT was slightly elevated at 15.6, PPT normal. CBC revealed a white blood cell count of 6,000, hemoglobin 12, hematocrit 35, with 345,000 platelets.

Hospital course:

Patient was seen in consultation with dermatology who confirmed cellulitis. Placed in IV Kefzol for 48 hours with marked improvement. His coumadin was not continued as he had no venogram or Doppler evidence of deep venous thrombosis in the past.

On discharge, Glyburide 2.5 mg qd, Keflex 500 mg po qid, Lasix 20 mg qd, Mellaril 50 mg qhs.

Jay Carson MD

GODFREY REGIONAL HOSPITAL
123 Main Street • Aldon, FL 77714 • (407) 555-1234

ICD-9-CM code(s): _____

CPT-4 code(s): _____

VI

THE REIMBURSEMENT PERSPECTIVE

Up to this point, the student has learned the various coding methods and the guidelines needed to perform correct coding. As mentioned at the beginning of this text, the coding process is a continual building process of rules and guidelines.

These guidelines do not end at the conclusion of the discussion on coding. Although understanding and implementing the guidelines covered thus far are crucial to successful coding, additional guidelines provided by third-party carriers may change, eliminate, or deviate somewhat from these guidelines. Therefore Section VI consists of a discussion of the idiosyncrasies of third-party carriers with respect to coding systems.

The student will have the opportunity to review several documents outside the realm of the medical record documentation, such as claim forms and third-party explanations of benefits, to achieve a thorough understanding of the impact of coding on all aspects of the reimbursement process.

21

CODING FROM A REIMBURSEMENT PERSPECTIVE

LEARNING OBJECTIVES

Following the completion of this chapter, the student will be able to:

- Identify the different reimbursement methods.
- Comprehend the purpose of third-party contracts and their effect on coding.
- Grasp coding from the perspective of receiving proper reimbursement.
- Understand the forms used for coding and billing provider services compared with facility services.
- Know the areas in which third-party reimbursement differs.
- Describe the clean claim process.

CODING REFERENCE TOOLS

Tool 60
Third-Party Contract Worksheet
Tool 61
Third-Party Contract Review Outline

KEY TERMS

Charge Ticket, 435
Clean Claim, 435
CMS-1500, 433
Explanation of Benefits (EOB), 437
Resource-Based Relative Value Study (RBRVS), 434
Superbill, 435
UB-92, 433
Usual, Customary, and Reasonable (UCR), 434

OVERVIEW

Thus far, coding has been discussed from a coding perspective, following the rules and guidelines outlined in CPT, ICD-9-CM, and other supporting coding books. In this chapter, the "real world" of coding is discussed—what gets paid and what does not, how to code to carrier specifications, and the compilation of this information into a Third-Party Contract Worksheet.

First and foremost, the coder must understand that third-party carriers are not required to strictly follow CPT-4, ICD-9-CM, HCPCS, DRG, or other coding guidelines as outlined in the universal coding books. Their only requirement is to accept these coding systems on claim forms (**CMS-1500** or **HCFA-1500** claim form for physician/provider and **UB-92** form for hospital inpatient). Also, remember that inclusion of codes in any of these coding books does not imply coverage by third-party carriers; it only serves as a uniform mechanism for describing WHAT services were performed and WHY. Deviations and variations in the interpretation of the guidelines in these coding structures may be seen, as deemed appropriate by the individual third-party carrier. In this light, it is imperative that the coder/biller for the facility be aware of these idiosyncrasies in coding for individual third-party carriers.

THIRD-PARTY CONTRACTS

The best place to clarify the variances imposed by individual third-party carriers is in the contracts between the facility or provider and the individual third-party carrier. It is essential to review and keep these documents on hand and to make certain that the practice or facility needs are addressed in the third-party contract. The third-party contract should serve as the "mutual understanding" of how codes should be used for reimbursement and, if used correctly, what reimbursement will occur and when.

DEFINITIONS

Third-party contracts are an agreement between the third-party carrier (typically an insurance carrier) and the provider (e.g., physician, physician group, supplier, facility) and should represent the terms of both parties, not just the third-party carrier. For instance, many third-party contracts outline the maximum time limits for a clean claim to be submitted. This period may vary from 15 days to 90 days, or it may last up to a year. After that time, the third-party carrier will not consider charges except possibly by an appeal process. The facility, however, also has the right to request imposition of some type of time frame for response of submitted claims and

some type of penalty to the carrier for not upholding these guidelines.

GUIDELINES

This chapter discusses the most common and sometimes controversial interpretations of third-party contracts. With this information, a customized contract grid for use in the practice to convey this information to all appropriate staff may be developed. This can be used as guidelines, as well as for the development of future contracts from this standardized format.

The coder should always keep in mind that coding must be accomplished according to guidelines from the appropriate coding sources (e.g., CPT, ICD-9-CM, HCPCS). Whether the carrier reimburses for a specific service, the service should be coded according to the appropriate guidelines. By coding and billing for all services, even though reimbursement may not be expected, the practice will be able to track services performed. In the event that the carrier determines that these services should have been paid during a specific period, the practice will possess the historical data necessary to refile for reimbursement.

If the practice thinks that a specific service should be paid by the third-party carrier, denial by the carrier is not always the "last word." The coder must establish the premise of why reimbursement should be made, using guidelines from the appropriate CPT-4, ICD-9-CM, DRG, or HCPCS coding book(s). For specialty services, the coder may also be guided by the coding guidelines recommended by the specialty organization (e.g., emergency department services based on ACEP [American College of Emergency Physicians]). Care should be taken to use these resources in justifying request for reimbursement. Make certain not to use conference or seminar notes, or guideline books other than those accepted by the third-party carrier.

Most third-party carriers have an appeals process established within their organizations. Appeals are best presented when a certified coder as the "expert" cites those references described earlier. If the initial decision of the third-party carrier is upheld, additional appeals may be made by the practice, perhaps with the physician involved through the third-party carrier's medical director. Medicare and other governmental third parties have an elaborate appeals process that involves an initial appeal and a hearing process, as well as an administrative judge to hear appeals by both the provider of service and the third-party carrier.

Remember that despite correct coding, not all services described with the use of proper codes will be reimbursed by all carriers. These coding books serve only as the mechanism to describe WHAT services were provided and WHY they were performed, and to list all services that may be considered for reimbursement. The contract or regulations of the specific carrier determine whether a provider will be compensated for a specific service.

REIMBURSEMENT METHOD

It is important for the coder and biller of the practice to understand the reimbursement process and to know what reimbursement should be expected. This means the coder must understand some of the terminology of the reimbursement process to determine whether the coded services will be reimbursed and at what amount.

One of the most important factors to take into consideration is whether the practice *participates* with the third-party carrier. When a practice or facility participates, that entity agrees to accept the amount contractually agreed on as payment in full. In some instances, the third-party carrier will pay only a portion of the contracted amount, leaving the rest as patient responsibility. Should the facility not participate, it is under no contractual obligation to accept as payment in full the amount determined by the third-party carrier to be the allowed amount. This is important when services are coded according to appropriate guidelines yet the carrier elects to deny or reduce payment for these services.

When the facility participates with the third-party carrier and specific codes are not covered, the contract specifies whether the facility is required to write off these services, or if it may bill the patient. If the facility does not participate, it may bill the patient for these services after the appeals process has been exhausted. In these instances, the facility or practice must document the "reasonable" attempts made to receive payment from the carrier before patient billing.

Once the carrier makes a determination regarding payment for services, it is also important to make certain that services are paid according to the third-party contract.

UCR (USUAL, CUSTOMARY, AND REASONABLE)

Most third-party carriers use one of two methods for determining the appropriate amount of reimbursement for physician services. The first of these reimbursement methods, the **(U)sual, (C)ustomary, and (R)easonable** method, has been around for many years. This method is based on the following components:

Usual　The facility/practice/provider's usual charge for the service performed.

Customary　The amount usually charged by all providers/facilities for the service. An "average" or "mean" is then calculated, which represents the customary reimbursement for that service.

Reasonable　Amount determined by the third party to represent data gathered on usual and customary fees and the assignment of a "reasonable" percentile of these data. For example, the "reasonable" allowance may be 80% of the customary fee.

Consider the importance of modifiers as they relate to the correct calculation of the previous numbers. When services are billed with modifiers because these modifiers signify "unusual circumstances," they are not calculated in the UCR reimbursement method. Omission of the appropriate modifiers with varying charge amounts, however, has a significant effect on the calculation of these UCR reimbursements. The following example demonstrates this concept.

CPT code 99213   Usual charge for practice is $75.00

During a specified period, the practice submitted the charge a total of 50 times as follows:

99213   Office Visit Established, Level 3

30 times @ $75.00 (usual charge) = $2,250
20 times @ $60.00 (usual charge) = $1,200

(Reduced charge for reduced service without modifier 52)

TOTAL CHARGES = $3,450

Total charges $3,450/50 patients = average charge of $69

On the basis of these submissions by this provider, the customary reimbursement for this service would now be $69.00, rather than the $75.00 charge.

In some cases, the coder or biller may notice a significantly reduced reimbursement compared with the charge amount because other providers are submitting charges at lesser amounts or without modifiers when appropriate.

In addition, third-party carriers often use data that have been compiled some time in the past, in some cases more than a year earlier. When this occurs, the customary calculation will reflect the providers' charges from previous years, and reimbursement will be substantially less than the current charge information.

RBRVS (RESOURCE-BASED RELATIVE VALUE STUDY)

Another reimbursement method used by third-party carriers for provider reimbursement is referred to as **Resource-Based Relative Value Study (RBRVS).** Because of the growing number of complaints from providers and facilities regarding the "flaws" of the UCR method, the federal government commissioned Harvard University to develop this new method of reimbursement calculation. The RBRVS method takes into account the following components:

Geographical allowance	Consists of an index called the Geographical Practice Cost Index (GPCI). These GPCIs measure the differences in physician costs for practice expenses and malpractice expenses in different geographical areas, compared with the national average.
Work units	A value assigned to each CPT-4 code that reflects the physician's or provider's work value.
Practice expense	The cost to the practice of providing the service based on geographical adjustment by area.
Malpractice expense	An assigned value based on the malpractice history and records on morbidity and mortality for the service.

PRACTICE REIMBURSEMENT MECHANISMS

The immediate job of the coder is to review or assign appropriate codes to the services provided. The long-term job of the coder encompasses a number of duties within the medical practice.

Obviously, coding is an integral part of the reimbursement process; however, this process extends from the time the patient schedules an appointment to the time the patient checks in and out for the appointment. The codes are then entered into the computerized or manual billing system.

It is imperative that the coder be involved in these processes. Coding correctly on the initial attempt is vital for prompt turnaround on claims submitted. Initial claims processing usually averages 30 to 60 days. Some states have passed legislation specifying the amount of time each carrier is allowed to process a "clean claim." The term **clean claim,** however, can be ambiguous, and insurance carriers identify any minor problems with claims to avert processing and avoid paying claims within the defined period if possible. The goal of the practice should be that all initial claims are clean claims. This would afford prompt and accurate reimbursement without the need for additional work and intervention on the part of the practice.

Should the initial claim not be processed as the result of error or should additional information be needed, either a corrected claim form or additional information must be forwarded to the carrier for consideration. Most states have not legislated time limits for processing these claims; therefore carriers may delay processing of these claims as long as possible. Some of the large carriers may take an average of an additional 6 to 12 weeks to process the resubmitted claim.

Discussion follows on medical office processes and the effect of coder involvement in these processes.

FILE MAINTENANCE AND COMPUTER SETUP OF CODING NOMENCLATURE

This is an area in which errors can multiply quickly. When an erroneous code or amount is entered into the computer system, the error will multiply each time that code is used by the practice.

The addition of new procedure and diagnosis codes, as well as the review of previously entered codes, should be accomplished by an established coder. Once these codes are verified, data entry personnel with little coding knowledge will enter the correct codes. Access to adding, editing, or deleting these codes should be restricted to the coder and a limited number of administrative staff members.

CHARGE TICKET AND HOSPITAL CHARGE DOCUMENT

In addition to verifying information entered into the computerized or manual billing system, the design of the practice **charge ticket** or **superbill** and the development of a hospital charge document aid greatly in ensuring that correct codes are being used for coding and billing the practice's services.

The coder should be involved with this process, which should occur at least biannually. Service analyses or productivity reports available from the computerized billing system identify the most frequent procedures and diagnosis codes to be included on the charge documents. Other information needed to code appropriately, such as the following, should be preprinted on the charge ticket or hospital document:

- Referring physician (consultation codes)
- Modifier codes (those used for specific codes [e.g., E & M modifiers listed in the E & M section of the charge document])
- A mechanism to "match" diagnosis codes and procedure codes for medical necessity (when multiple services are performed, which specific diagnoses match specified procedures)

The review and updating of charge documents should correlate with the yearly publication of CPT-4 and ICD-9-CM/ICD-10-CM, and with the time the practice updates most of its third-party contracts and the contract worksheet information. Figure 21-1 demonstrates a sample hospital charge document intended to capture all necessary charge information for the practice.

HOSPITAL CHARGE WORKSHEET

Date Received: _____ Info Taken By: _____

PROCEDURE(S): CARDIAC CATHETERIZATIONS/INJECTIONS/IMAGING

HEART	CATHS
93510-26	Left, Percutaneous
93511-26	Left, By Cutdown
93524-26	Left, Combined
	Transep/ Retrograde
93526-26	Combined Rt/Lt

INJECTION PROC	
93539-26	Arterial Conduits, Sel Opacification
93540-26	Aortocoronary Venous Bypass Grafts, Sel Opacification
93541-26	Pulmonary Angiography
93542-26	Rt Ventricular/Right Atrial Angiography
93543-26	Lt Ventricular/Left Atrial Angiography
93544-26	Aortography
93545-26	Selective Coronary Angiography

OTHER	
93503	Swan-Ganz
93536	Insert Intra-Aortic
	Balloon Catheter

IMAGING PROCEDURE	
93555	Ventricular/Atrial Angiography
93556	Pulm Angiography, Aortography and/or Sel Coronary Angio

DETERMINATION OF APPROPRIATE CODING:

Choose Approp Injection/Imaging Codes

VALID DIAGNOSIS CODE(S): FOR CATHS ONLY/OTHER PROCEDURES ON REVERSE

MITRAL VALVE					
394.0	Stenosis	410.3*	Inferopost Wall	414.01	Native Coronary
394.1	Rheum Insuff	410.4*	Oth Inferior Wall	414.02	Auto Biol Bypass Gr
394.2	Stenosis w/Insuff	410.5*	Other Lat Wall	414.03	NonAuto Bypass Gr
394.9	Other Diseases	410.6*	True Post Wall	414.04	Artery Bypass Graft
AORTIC VALVE		410.7*	Subendocardial	414.05	Unspec Byp Graft
395.0	Rheum Stenosis	410.8*	Other Spec Sites	414.10	Aneurysm Hrt Wall
395.1	Rheum Insuff	410.9*	Unspec Site	414.11	Aneurysm Cor Vess
395.2	Rheum Stenosis	*5th digit for episode of care		414.19	Aneurysm Other
	w/Insuff	0-episode unspec		421.0	Bact Endocarditis
395.9	Other Rheum Dz	1-initial	2-subsequent	421.1	In Dz Stated Else
MITRAL AND AORTIC VALVES				421.9	Unspecified
396.0	Stenosis	411.0	Post MI Syndrome	424.0	Mitral Valve Dis
396.1	Mitral Stenosis with	411.1	Inter Coronary Sny	424.1	Aortic Valve Dis
	Aortic Insuff		Unstable Angina	424.90	Endocarditis, Valve
396.2	Mitral Insuff w/		Impending MI	424.99	Other Endocarditis
	Aortic Stenosis	411.81	Coronary Occlus	429.71	Acq Card Septal Def
396.3	Mitral/Aortic Insuff		w/o MI		Seq to MI
396.8	Multiple Involve	411.89	Other Isch Hrt Dz	**CONGENITAL DEFECTS**	
396.9	Unspecified	412	Old MI	746.3	Stenosis Aortic Valv
MYOCARDIAL INFARCTION		413.0	Angina Decubitus	746.4	Insuff Aortic Valve
410.0*	Anterolateral Wall	413.1	Prinzmetal Angina	746.5	Mitral Stenosis
410.1*	Oth Anterior Wall	413.9	Unspec Angina	746.6	Mitral Insuff
410.2*	Inferolateral Wall	**CORONARY ATHEROSCH**		746.7	Hypoplastic Lt Hrt
		414.00	Unspec Type Vess		Syndrome

CHARGE ENTRY INFORMATION:

Patient Name: _____ Hospital: _____ Inpt _____ Outpt _____ Other: _____

Date of Current Service: _____ Admit Date: _____ Other: _____

Referring Phy Info: _____

Attending Physician: _____

CPT	Mod	Dx #1	Dx #2	Dx #3	Dx #4	Other (Specify):
1-						
2-						
3-						
4-						
5-						

Date Entered: _____ Initials: _____

Comments: _____

FIGURE 21-1 A hospital charge ticket sample for a cardiology practice. Be sure to include all information from a coding perspective so that the physician and coder may accurately reflect services provided. *(Courtesy of MD Consultative Services, Orlando, Florida. All rights reserved.)*

ANCILLARY SERVICE REQUEST FORMS

Ancillary services require the diagnosis to justify medical necessity of providing those services. If the facility provides ancillary services for outside facilities or providers (such as stress treadmills or radiology), the appropriate diagnostic information must be obtained from the ordering physician. Because the requesting physician is not a part of the practice, it is imperative to provide ordering physicians with the information needed to order, perform, code, and receive reimbursement for this service. Many practices provide ancillary services to outside providers as a supplement to their practice income. Many do not realize that a large percentage of these services may in fact not be paid because of insufficient diagnostic information from the ordering physician. For instance, highly comprehensive cardiac testing, such as thallium stress tests, may not be reimbursed for the diagnosis of "chest pain," but may be reimbursed for "angina" or "abnormal ECG."

It is imperative that the practice provides ordering physicians with the information needed to correctly code and bill for services performed. The practice may wish to design an ancillary request sheet with the needed information and the most common diagnosis codes, excluding diagnoses that are not covered by most insurance carriers. For Medicare patients, the performing provider must inform the patient in advance that the service may not be covered and must obtain a signed waiver form from the patient. If the diagnostic information provided by the ordering/referring physician is not sufficient for reimbursement, the patient should be informed before his or her arrival at the facility. If the diagnosis is not covered, the ordering/referring physician can explain this to the patient in advance, thus avoiding an uncomfortable situation for all involved. The practice may wish to market ancillary services that it provides; an ancillary request form provides a convenient mechanism for referring patients, and it offers assistance in selecting the most appropriate diagnostic information and the most appropriate test for the presenting complaint. A sample of an ancillary request form is shown in Figure 21-2.

THE CODER AS OFFICE CODING OR REIMBURSEMENT EDUCATOR

Another crucial job of the coder in the medical practice is the job of educator. The business office/billing department may possess the expertise to bill the services for reimbursement; however, the coder has the knowledge to select the proper codes to place on the billing form to obtain appropriate reimbursement. Without that knowledge and the correct code on the claim form, the practice or facility will not be reimbursed appropriately. The billing staff may produce and file claims or UB-92s efficiently. If coding is not correct and if it does not completely describe the services and justify why they were performed, the practice or facility may not get paid.

As the coding expert in the facility, the coder must create mechanisms to spread coding information to other personnel who, at a minimum, need to understand the selection of codes, the purpose of justifying medical necessity, and the use of modifier codes. This does not mean that the practice or facility should expect all personnel to become proficient coders, but all should recognize inconsistencies and triggers that will result in denial or nonpayment of claims.

In the process of choosing procedure codes or modifier codes that a specific carrier does or does not recognize, information can be automatically loaded into the computerized billing system, thus guiding the practice or facility staff to select the correct code(s). For instance, a specific carrier does not use the preventive medicine codes for "well woman visits" but has developed a set code "99999" for this purpose. The computerized billing system can be programmed so that anytime that particular carrier code is entered and a preventive medicine code is entered by data entry personnel, the system should convert that code to "99999." This eliminates the need for data entry personnel to manually override the billing system and avoids the opportunity for error.

When specific diagnosis codes are required in conjunction with certain procedure codes, the system can be programmed to reject other code combinations or to alert the data entry personnel of a potential error. For instance, when preventive medicine codes for a specific carrier require that all such services must be billed with diagnosis code "general medical examination," the system can be triggered to alert personnel when this combination is not used.

Review of the charge entry process also aids the billing office in the submission of payable claims. The best-spent 15 to 30 minutes of time during the coder's workday (or that of another trained individual) is used to review the charge tickets or charge entry documents before charge entry for incompleteness, coding deficiencies, or missing information such as modifiers and medical necessity diagnoses. An additional 15 to 30 minutes is well spent reviewing the paper claims and electronic claims register of claims prepared for transmittal. Despite the review of the charge document before data entry, errors are made, omissions do happen, and a "clean claim" may no longer be "clean." The practice must now wait an additional 6 to 12 weeks for payment after initial rejection, and additional work must be done by staff to resubmit.

In addition, a review of the **Explanation of Benefits (EOB)** received from insurance carriers is imperative to identify those claims that, despite programming of the computerized billing system and review of the charge document and claim, still did not receive proper reimbursement. Improperly paid or denied claims should not

DIAGNOSTIC CARDIOLOGY ORDER FORM

Practice Name/Address:
Practice Phone/Fax:

ECHOCARDIOGRAPHY (Please mark applicable diagnosis)

☐	Angina	413.9
☐	Aortic Valve Disorder	424.1
☐	Atrial Fibrillation	427.31
☐	ASHD	414.00
☐	Cardiomegaly	429.3
☐	Cardiomyopathy	425.4
☐	Chest Pain Unspec	786.50
☐	Chest Pain,Tightness	786.59
☐	Congenital Heart Dz	746.9
☐	Coronary Artery Dz	414.00

☐	Heart Murmur	785.2
☐	Mitral Valve Prolapse	424.0
☐	Mitral Stenosis	394.0
☐	Myocardial Infarc Old	412
☐	Pulmonary HTN	426.0
☐	Pulmonary Valve Disorder	424.3
☐	Syncope	780.2
☐	Tachycardia	427.2
☐	Tricuspid Valve Disorder	424.2
☐	Ventricular Fibrillation	427.41
☐	Other: CONTACT PRACTICE FOR ASSISTANCE	

HOLTER MONITORING (Please mark applicable diagnosis)

☐	Angina, Unspecified	413.9
☐	Angina, Unstable	411.1
☐	ASHD	414.00
☐	Atrial Fibrillation	427.31
☐	Atrial Flutter	427.32
☐	Arrhythmia, Unspec	427.9
☐	Bradycardia	427.89
☐	Cardiomegaly	429.3
☐	Cardiomyopathy	425.4

☐	Mitral Valve Disorders	424.0
☐	Palpitations	785.1
☐	PVCs	427.69
☐	Premature Beats	427.61
☐	Syncope	780.2
☐	Tachycardia	427.81
☐	Ventricular Fibrillation	427.41
☐	Ventricular Flutter	427.42
☐	Other: CONTACT PRACTICE FOR ASSISTANCE	

THALLIUM STRESS TEST (Please mark applicable diagnosis)

☐	Atherosclerosis/Arteries	414.00
☐	Atherosclerosis/Unspec	440.20
☐	Atherosclerosis/Inter Claudification	440.21
☐	Abnormal EKG	794.31
☐	Angina, Unstable	411.1
☐	Angina, Unspecified	413.9
☐	Atrial Fibrillation	427.31
☐	Congestive Heart Failure	428.0
☐	Coronary Artery Disease	414.9

☐	Heart Blocks:	426.3
☐	Left Bundle Branch	426.4
☐	Right Bundle Branch	426.10
☐	Unspecified	428.9
☐	Heart Failure Unspec	414.9
☐	Ischemic Heart Disease	424.0
☐	Mitral Valve Disorders	V67.0
☐	Postsurgical F/Up	
☐	Other: CONTACT PRACTICE FOR ASSISTANCE	

Patient Name: _____	DOB: _____
Insurance Type: _____	Auth #: _____
Ordering/Referring Physician: _____	Phone: _____

In the event one of the above diagnoses is not applicable for the service requested, contact THE PRACTICE for assistance in selecting the correct test/diagnosis for the patient's condition.

FIGURE 21-2 An ancillary request form. This may be used to help referring physicians supply adequate information for coding and billing of services requested by outside physicians. *(Courtesy of MD Consultative Services, Orlando, Florida. All rights reserved.)*

be dealt with on a one-on-one basis, but on the basis of how the error occurred and how the correction is made. For instance, suppose that multiple units were placed on the charge document for medication, were entered into the system, and appeared to have been successfully printed on the claim, yet the carrier paid for only one unit. A review of the EOB indicates how the practice received the claim (paper/electronic), how many units were received on the claim, and so forth. Appropriate action can then be taken to correct this problem in the future.

If modifier codes are missing on the EOB, isolate the source of this error (e.g., charge ticket completion, data entry), educate staff, and correct the problem. Use the computerized billing system whenever possible to "fool-proof" this system. When this is not possible, make sure staff members are aware of the problem and know how to address it.

GENERAL THIRD-PARTY CODING AND REIMBURSEMENT GUIDELINES

Although third-party carriers have specific guidelines that they follow regarding coding, many follow CPT-4, ICD-

9-CM, and DRG guidelines along with general guidelines that are published and are available to facilities and providers. Some of these common guidelines are the following:

Correct Coding Initiative	Indicates those CPT-4 code combinations that are considered bundled
Surgical Cross-Reference Unbundling Books	List each surgical code contained in CPT with those CPT codes considered "bundled" or "included" in the global package for that specific surgical code. Remember that extenuating circumstances may allow coding of these services with the appropriate modifier for reimbursement consideration.
Coders' Desk Reference	Lists each procedure (CPT-4) and gives a detailed description about what the procedure is, what is included, and what may be coded separately.

SPECIFIC THIRD-PARTY CODING/ REIMBURSEMENT GUIDELINES

In addition to general guidelines regarding coding and reimbursement, most carriers have specific guidelines that they use for reviewing and determining reimbursement for coded services. Along with general guidelines and principles, these specific third-party guidelines should be incorporated into the Third-Party Contract Worksheet (see Tool 60). Areas that should be delineated include the following.

TIME LIMITS

Determine the time limit established by each third-party carrier for submission of claims, as well as appeal and resubmission time limits. Make certain that claims are submitted within these guidelines. In some cases, this means follow-up, not only for status, but for receipt of claim during the specified time limits.

Even though the practice has sent a claim during the specified time limits, this does not mean that the third party will acknowledge receipt within that same time frame. Dating the receipt of claims after the time limit is a common practice among third-party carriers for not paying claims. Claims that are just "lost" and never received will also exceed time limits if they are not followed up expediently.

HCPCS COMPARED WITH CPT-4 CODES

Make certain the contract worksheet encompasses the coding nomenclature(s) used by each carrier. In some

cases, carriers will not accept HCPCS procedure or modifier codes. In other instances, third-party carriers insist on the use of these codes when appropriate. Denial or payment sometimes rests on the appropriate use of these codes along carrier-specific guidelines. Third-party guidelines indicate that when both CPT-4 and HCPCS codes are acceptable, the codes with the highest level of specificity (HCPCS) should be assigned.

CODING/BILLING FOR NONPHYSICIAN SERVICES (MODIFIER FOR PHYSICIAN ASSISTANT/OTHER PHYSICIAN EXTENDERS)

Make certain the practice determines whether services are reimbursable when they are provided by health professionals other than physicians. Determine not only whether the carrier recognizes these "nonphysician" entities, but also what services and providers they recognize.

Physician assistants and nurse practitioners typically may provide services under the direction of the physician. Some carriers allow these services to be billed under the name of the provider; others require that these services be billed only under the name of the supervising physician.

Make certain that services requiring the supervision of a licensed physician are documented as such with the appropriate physician countersignatures for overseeing the care and concurring with the assessment and treatment plan. This typically requires a minimum notation of "Reviewed and Concur," the date, and the physician's "mark" of authentication.

In many instances, the third-party carrier will require the use of a modifier code to indicate that services were performed with the use of a physician extender. Many carriers reimburse these services at a reduced rate from when the physician provides the services.

Specific HCPCS modifiers designate that services have been performed by a physician extender or in connection with a physician extender. These modifiers are located in the HCPCS modifier section on CPT-4 coding.

EVALUATION AND MANAGEMENT SERVICES GUIDELINES (DOWNCODING)

Many third-party carriers have instituted coding software that "downcodes" services that are based on diagnostic coding provided on the claim form. The only information used for paying a large volume of services is the ICD-9-CM diagnostic code(s) and CPT-4 procedure code(s). Often, however, these codes do not take into consideration the large number of diagnostic options and other factors used in determining level of service. As a cost-saving measure, many third-party carriers have instituted the use of software that determines the level of service based simply on the diagnostic code(s) provided. If the provider has coded the service at a higher level, the claim will automatically be downcoded and the reimbursement will be significantly less than the original level submitted.

Medical service providers should watch for these downcoding practices on their Explanation of Benefits. The medical practice reserves the right to appeal the third-party decision, usually by submitting a copy of the physician documentation used to determine the correct level of service. Once again, the physician documentation will determine the proper reimbursement. Many medical practices and several medical societies representing physicians have begun to challenge this practice in the court system.

PREVENTIVE MEDICINE VISITS

Many insurance carriers still do not recognize the need for preventive medicine services and therefore do not reimburse for these services. Make certain the services are, in fact, "preventive," meaning no treatment of complaints is provided during the visit; the diagnosis would be a "well" diagnosis such as "well woman" or "well baby."

Other third-party carriers do reimburse for these well visits but do not recognize the use of preventive medicine codes. Make sure to capture this information on the Third-Party Contracts Worksheet as well.

Despite the fact that CPT-4 guidelines indicate a preventive medicine visit, as well as a regular level of service (with modifier 25), there may be instances where the patient presents for a well visit but with a number of problems; few carriers reimburse for more than one E & M service per day. If these two "significantly separately identifiable" E & M services do take place, they should be billed accordingly. The practice will want to code the most significant service (usually the preventive medicine service) first, followed by the level of office visit with modifier 25. If the third party disallows one of these services, it typically would be the second service; therefore the least significant service may not be reimbursed.

MODIFIERS (GENERAL)

CPT-4 defines the modifier codes and their usage, and explains which sections of CPT these modifiers are used for; however, many third-party carriers interpret these guidelines differently. Some carriers do not recognize any modifier codes; others recognize certain modifier codes only in specific instances. For instance, Medicare's interpretation is that all surgical services have a minimum follow-up period of 10 days. Medicare may not recognize the use of modifier 57 (decision for surgery) for reimbursement of any E & M services. This can differ

with each Medicare carrier or Fiscal Intermediary (FI) as well.

Check each of the practice's or facility's third-party carrier contracts, making sure the use of these modifiers is specifically spelled out. If this is not specified in the contract, third-party carriers are free to interpret these guidelines in whatever manner they wish. In most cases, their interpretation will NOT be to the practice's or facility's advantage.

GLOBAL (BUNDLED) SERVICES

Although CPT-4 and several coding bundling/unbundling books specify those services covered under the "global" concept, many third-party carriers interpret these guidelines differently. If the practice or facility provides specialty services that include global surgical services, make certain these guidelines are clarified in each carrier contract. For instance, if the practice provides global maternity care services, make certain guidelines for services outside the global package, such as "high-risk" pregnancies, and additional services over and above the global guidelines in CPT and provided by the American College of Obstetrics/Gynecology (ACOG), are outlined by each carrier. Significant reimbursement may be lost if this information is not specified in the third-party contract.

COSURGEON/TWO SURGEONS

Carriers usually have specific guidelines pertaining to cosurgeons that include whether these services will be reimbursed and what the effect is on reimbursement. The practice will want to make certain that their providers always include such information in the operative report because many third-party carriers request this information as proof that both surgeons were involved.

Reimbursement for cosurgeons or "two surgeons" is typically around 125% of the regular allowance for the service, with each provider receiving approximately 62.5%. This may vary from carrier to carrier, so the practice will need to determine the correct reimbursement for each carrier for these services.

ASSISTANT SURGEONS

Many hospital and outpatient facilities have specific bylaws that detail when the use of an assistant surgeon is required; however, third-party carrier guidelines will not necessarily coincide with these facility requirements.

The practice must determine both the surgical codes that will be reimbursable by each carrier for assistant surgeons, and the reimbursable amount, which will dramatically differ from the primary surgeon fee. Some carriers reimburse as little as 10% to 20% of the surgery allowance for the assistant surgeon.

As a result, many assistant surgeons may request that the primary surgeon list them, or allow them to bill as cosurgeons. Not only is this practice illegal and unethical, but it meets the definition of "fraud" for all parties involved. In addition, the primary surgeon would be paid only approximately 62.5% of the allowance for the service, rather than the 100% allowance for services coded and billed correctly.

MULTIPLE PROCEDURES

Reimbursement for multiple surgical procedures, with or without the proper use of modifier 51, may differ from carrier to carrier. The practice must make certain that the specific carrier's interpretation is included in the contract with each carrier. Significant differences in ultimate reimbursement may result from differences in interpretation.

DEVELOPMENT OF THIRD-PARTY CONTRACT WORKSHEETS

Perhaps the best tool for the coder to introduce into the practice is a Third-Party Contract Worksheet. Development of this involves review of each of the third-party contracts for specific requirements regarding codes, such as the following:

- Services the practice is contracted to perform
- Services the practice may or may NOT perform
- Locations where services may be referred or rendered
- Services requiring preauthorization
- Acceptable/unacceptable modifier codes
- Acceptable/unacceptable procedure codes
- Special carrier-specific procedure codes

After acquiring this information, the coder, with the assistance of the billing or business office, can develop information sheets for use by the staff. At an easy glance, the scheduler and the data entry, clinical, and professional staff members can determine whether a service can be provided and whether the practice will be reimbursed.

This information will serve as a helpful tool to all practice employees for obtaining appropriate authorizations and using specific CPT codes, modifiers, or guidelines. A blank form of the Third-Party Contract Worksheet is included as Tool 60. Figure 21-3 is a sample of such a worksheet. In development of this Third-Party Contract Worksheet, it will be necessary for the practice to read carefully through each contract, gather the needed information, and request clarification or modification of the contract when information is missing or ambiguous. This is the time for clarification, rather than when claims are denied or are not reimbursed to the practice's or facility's expectations because of a misunderstanding on contract issue(s).

Most third-party contracts include a fee schedule; however, they often include only the most frequently used CPT-4 codes. Make certain the carrier clearly spells out reimbursement protocol (e.g., Medicare fee schedule, percent of charges) for all services not specified in the fee schedule provided.

Gather the information needed for the Third-Party Contract Worksheet by using an outline such as Tool 61. This same type of information can be gathered for hospital services as well. Hospitals may need to employ an individual or a group of individuals to research, update, and disburse this information to all employees, and to present educational materials regarding this information to other employees.

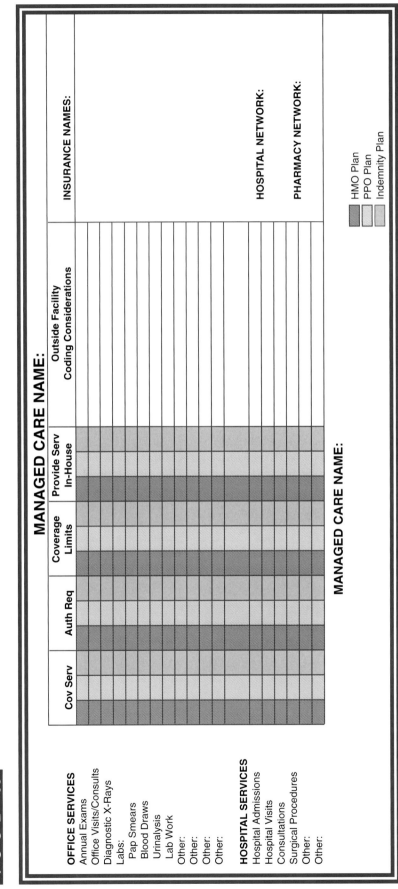

MANAGED CARE NAME:

OFFICE SERVICES	Cov Serv		Auth Req		Coverage Limits			Provide Serv In-House		Outside Facility Coding Considerations
Annual Well-Woman Exams	Y	Y	Y	N	1 YR	1 YR	1 YR	Y	Y	Must use Preventive Med Codes, Dx V72.3 only
Office Visits/Consults	Y	Y	Y	N	N	N		Y	Y	Do not use Confirm Consult Codes
Diagnostic X-Rays	Y	Y	Y	N	N	N		Y	Y	Dx Rad Only/All Others Outside
Labs:										
Pap Smears	Y	Y	N	N	N	N		N	N	SKL
Blood Draws	Y	Y	N	N	N	N		Y	Y	Use Code 99000 (No Modifier 90)
Urinalysis	Y	Y	N	N	N	N		Y	Y	Urinalysis 81000 In-House Only/All Others Out SKL
Lab Work	N	N	N	N	N	N		N	N	Blood Draws In-House Only/All Others Out SKL
Other:										
Other:										
Other:										
Other:										
HOSPITAL SERVICES			All inpatient services require preauthorizations							
Hospital Admissions	Y	Y	Y	Y	N	N		N	N	
Hospital Visits	Y	Y	Y	Y	N	N		N	N	
Consultations	Y	Y	Y	Y	N	N		N	N	
Surgical Procedures	Y	Y	Y	Y	N	N		N	N	
Other:										
Other:										

INSURANCE NAMES:

DDD Insurance
AAA Employers Group
Rad Centers:
  XYZ Radiology (407) 888-8888
  ABC Radiology (407) 777-7777

HOSPITAL NETWORK:

EEE Hospital
FFF Hospital

PHARMACY NETWORK:

Pharmacies Are Us (407) 222-2222

- HMO Plan
- PPO Plan
- Indemnity Plan

MANAGED CARE NAME:

FIGURE 21-3 Sample contract worksheet. This worksheet shows the information included in the contract to which other office staff must have access on a daily basis. (Courtesy of MD Consultative Services, Orlando, Florida. All rights reserved.)

T O O L   61

MANAGED CARE CONTRACT REVIEW

Managed Care Plan: _____

Plan #s:_____

(List)

HMO: _____ PPO: _____ Cap: _____ Other: _____

Original Contract Date: _____

Last Date Reviewed:_____ By: _____

CONTRACT BENEFITS:

Termination Clause: _____

Claims Filing Deadline: _____

Covered Services:	Y	N	Comments	Other :
EKG				
Lab				
X-ray				
Diag				
Other:				
Other:				

Authorizations:	Y	N	Comments	Other :
EKG				
Lab				
X-ray				
Diag				
Hosp:				
Hosp Proc				
Other:				
Other:				

Plan Limitations:	Y	N	Comments	Other :
EKG				
Lab				
X-ray				
Diag				
Hosp:				
Hosp Proc:				
Other:				

Bill Aboves:	Y	N	Comments	Other :
(List)				

Modifiers:	Y	N	Comments	Other :

Fee Schedule: _____

Last Date Reviewed: _____ By _____

In Computer: Y___ N___ Reviewed Date _____

Adj Code: _____   Payment Code: _____   Reviewed Date _____

CHAPTER IN REVIEW

CERTIFICATION REVIEW

- Third-party carriers are not required to follow guidelines outlined in CPT-4, ICD-9-CM, and other coding books.
- Provider/physician services are reported on the CMS/HCFA-1500.
- Facility/hospital services are reported on the UB-92.
- The third-party contract should serve as a "mutual understanding" of how codes should be used for reimbursement.
- The third-party contract should represent the terms of both parties: third party and provider of service.
- Participation with a third-party carrier means the provider agrees to accept as payment in full the amount contractually allowed.
- The Usual, Customary, and Reasonable (UCR) method involves the usual charge, the customary charge, and the amount considered reasonable by the carrier.
- The RBRVS methodology is based on geographical allowance, work units, practice expense, and malpractice expense.
- The coder serves as the office reimbursement educator.
- Third-party contracts should delineate such items as the following:
  Time limits
  HCPCS and CPT-4 codes
  Reimbursement for nonphysician services
  E & M service guidelines
  Preventive medicine guidelines
  Modifiers
  Global services
  Cosurgeons/assistant surgeons
  Multiple procedures
- Third-party contract worksheets should be developed by the practice to educate and inform office personnel of the specifics of each third-party contract.

STUDENT STUDY GUIDE

- Study Chapter 21.
- Review the Learning Objectives for Chapter 21.
- Review the Certification Review for Chapter 21.
- Complete the Chapter Review exercise to reinforce concepts learned in this chapter.
- Complete the Claims Review exercises 1 through 20, found in Chapter 21: Coding from a Reimbursement Perspective, in the Workbook.
- Complete Explanation of Benefits exercises 1 through 20: Coding from a Reimbursement Perspective, in the Workbook.

CHAPTER REVIEW EXERCISE

Obtain a third-party contract from a practice or facility. Review the contract, identifying the key elements to incorporate into the Third-Party Contract Worksheet, as well as any clarification, or missing information needed from the third-party carrier. Enter this information on the outline form before incorporating it into the actual Third-Party Contract Worksheet.

Remember that third-party contracts may be renegotiated, and addendums for clarification can be made at any time. The practice does not have to accept a third-party contract as presented. Approach the third-party carrier from the perspective of clarification rather than confrontation. The third-party carrier usually will be willing to clarify or provide any missing information.

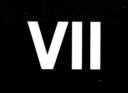

MONITORING/COMPLIANCE AND CERTIFICATION REVIEW

Monitoring and compliance of the coding process is perhaps the culmination of successful coding. Coding begins and ends with documentation, so it is appropriate to conclude this book with a reemphasis on the importance of documentation in the coding process. The coder must understand the coding systems and their differences from a third-party carrier perspective and must ensure that all coding processes have been completely successful. A comprehensive monitoring process ensures compliance and decreases the risk to a facility for accusations of fraudulent activity.

Section VII encompasses the legislation regarding fraud and abuse, as well as processes that ensure compliance. The student will have the opportunity to complete a chart audit and prepare a report of those findings. This section also includes review information for the coding certification examination. Medical terminology and coding examinations provide the opportunity for certification preparation.

22

MONITORING AND COMPLIANCE PROCESS

Following the completion of this chapter, the student will be able to:

- Define and identify fraud, abuse, and their differences.
- Know the implications of fraudulent or abusive activities.
- Understand the mechanisms of the practice monitoring process.
- Describe the steps to follow in completing a chart audit.
- Comprehend the importance of a compliance program.
- Identify the events that typically trigger a third-party audit.

CODING REFERENCE TOOLS

Tool 62
Data Entry Review Form
Tool 63
Claims Review Process
Tool 64
Chart Audit Logsheet
Tool 65
Chart Audit-E & M Worksheet
Tool 66
Practice Protocol Logsheet

KEY TERMS

Abuse, 450
Compliance Programs, 463
False Claims Act, 449
Fraud, 450
HIPAA (Health Insurance Portability and Accountability Act), 463
JCAHO (Joint Commission on the Accreditation of Hospital
  Organizations), 463
Line Item, 452
Manual Review/Flag, 453
OIG (Office of Inspector General), 449
Qui Tam Act, 450
Whistleblower Act, 450

FRAUD AND ABUSE LEGISLATION

Many practices do not employ a full-time coder. Instead, they rely on office staff or the provider(s) to determine levels of services provided. Not only does this typically subject the practice to reduced reimbursement, but the potential for fraud and abuse is substantially higher in this setting as well.

A number of years ago, the federal government investigated only a small number of these practices and facilities for potential fraud and abuse. In most cases, the practice or facility was unaware of potentially fraudulent activity, either owing to ignorance or as a result of inadequate involvement in the billing/coding process.

Increased legislation over the past few years, however, has made all individuals who are involved in the coding and billing process potentially liable for fraudulent billing activity. In addition, the "ignorance" excuse is no longer a defense with federal or third-party carriers. Fraud and abuse are widespread in the health care industry today, and virtually all third-party carriers have increased resources devoted to recovering monies paid for fraudulent claims.

Fines, penalties, and potential imprisonment are the effects of fraudulent activity in the health care industry today. These may be imposed on any individual involved in the fraudulent activity and any individual who is aware of a potentially fraudulent activity but does not take action. This could include even the office receptionist, if he or she were aware of inappropriate billing practices.

CMS (formerly known as HCFA) and the **OIG (Office of the Inspector General)** have the authority to suspend, exclude, terminate, and impose fines and penalties on providers, practitioners, and suppliers who commit acts in direct violation of one of the many antifraud and antiabuse amendments enacted since the mid-1970s. Penalties may involve fines, imprisonment, and exclusion from the Medicare program on a permanent basis.

The OIG publishes and distributes annually a "Work Plan for the Fiscal Year," with 100 items targeted for review for potential fraud and abuse. Many of the items discussed in this text have been targeted on an annual basis since the inception of this "Work List" because of the inability of providers to comply with government regulations for documentation and coding guidelines. Both E & M levels of service and documented medical necessity have remained top items on this list as a direct result of completed audits in which physicians have been unable to comply with E & M guidelines, as well as physician charts lacking diagnostic documentation to substantiate services performed and billed.

There have been many newspaper articles regarding large facilities that were fined millions of dollars for services billed and not provided. In reality, many of these services were performed. Documentation did not, however, substantiate services billed. In these circumstances, the government had the authority to penalize the facility with fines; penalties; and, in some cases, imprisonment of high-level officials for those organizations.

The following are some of the major legislative actions and amendments passed in response to the rising practice of fraud and abuse in the United States.

MEDICARE/MEDICAID ANTI-FRAUD AND ABUSE AMENDMENT (1977)

Anyone who knowingly and willfully makes or causes another to make false statements regarding services performed is guilty of a felony and may be fined not more than $25,000 or may be imprisoned for not longer than 5 years, or both. This same amendment applies to beneficiaries who commit such an act, punishable by a fine of no more than $20,000, imprisonment for not longer than 1 year, or both.

AMENDMENT TO MEDICARE/ MEDICAID ANTI-FRAUD AND ABUSE AMENDMENT (1980)

This addition to the amendment states that any person who knowingly and willfully solicits or receives payment or remuneration, such as kickback, bribe, or rebate, is guilty of a felony with fines not more than $25,000, imprisonment of up to 5 years, or both.

MEDICARE/MEDICAID PATIENT AND PROGRAM PROTECTION ACT OF 1987 AND FALSE CLAIMS ACT

This act provides authority to impose civil monetary penalties under Section 1128A of the Social Security Act for the following:

- Fraudulent or false claims are presented for payment
- Fraudulent or false records are used to file claim
- False or fraudulent claims are paid as a result of conspiracy to defraud the government

The penalties under the **False Claims Act** call for not less than $5,000 or more than $10,000 per false claim, plus damages up to three times the total amount of false payments. Under this act, the government is not required to prove specific intent to defraud. The civil standard of proof under this act is "by the preponderance of evidence," not the criminal criterion of "beyond a reasonable doubt." Actions under the False Claims Act may be taken within 6 years of the violation or within 3 years of the date when material facts are known. The time may not extend past a 10-year period following the violation.

False Claim Act cases may be initiated either by the Department of Justice or under the **Whistleblower Act,** wherein private citizens under the **Qui Tam** provision are entitled to a percentage of monies recovered from the fraudulent activities.

STARKE ANTI-KICKBACK AND SELF-REFERRAL ACTS OF 1995, 1998, AND 2002

Under more recent legislation, the federal government has dictated that it is illegal to knowingly and willfully solicit payment in return for referrals, purchasing, leasing, or arranging for the purchasing of referrals, purchasing, or leasing. A physician or other entity may not refer to an individual in which the physician or any immediate member of his family has a financial relationship. There is an extensive list of exceptions. Some common areas that are included under the antikickback and self-referral mandate include such services as clinical laboratory services, occupational and physical therapy, radiological services, durable medical equipment, and home health services. Under the self-referral guidelines of Starke I and Starke II legislation, the physician who has a financial relationship with an entity may only refer to that entity with the express permission and consent of the patient.

There are many other legislative amendments and orders that perpetuate the prosecution of fraudulent activities. The coder must remain current at all times on legislative amendments and proposals in this arena. The coder must understand not only what constitutes fraud and abuse, but also what can be done to comply with governmental and third-party guidelines.

As a result of the increased investigative efforts of governmental and third-party agencies against potential fraud and abuse, the field of compliance within the health care industry has grown immensely. The coder must be aware of the need for compliance and must ensure that processes are put into place to ensure it at his or her practice or facility.

The coder and other office staff should understand the definitions of fraud and abuse. They also must be aware of the consequences when such activities take place within the practice.

FRAUD AND ABUSE

Specific federal guidelines exist regarding the definition(s) for both **fraud** and **abuse.** As was mentioned earlier, ignorance that such activities are taking place in a particular practice or facility is no longer defensible. Most practices at first insist that no such procedures occur within their organizations; however, after review, they realize that fraud and abuse may be taking place. Keep in mind that the definitions of fraud and abuse may differ

from one third-party carrier to another. Therefore the practice or facility will want to gather such information for each contract in which it participates.

FRAUD

Fraud is a FELONY that is punishable by imprisonment, fines, and interest for all parties involved or for those who have knowledge that such acts have taken place. Fraud is defined as follows:

MAKING FALSE STATEMENTS OR MISREPRESENTATION OF FACTS ON CLAIMS. This may occur in the form of incorrect information submitted on the claim form or submission to the carrier in error of services that were not performed (e.g., urinalysis ordered by physician, unable to be completed, yet billed to third-party carrier).

HAVING KNOWLEDGE THAT FALSE STATEMENTS OR REPRESENTATION WAS MADE WITH THE INTENT EITHER TO GAIN A GREATER AMOUNT THAN DUE OR TO RECEIVE PAYMENT WHEN NONE IS DUE. This involves filing claims for services that are noncovered in a manner that may make them payable or submitting a diagnosis code in such a way as to make a noncovered service a payable service. Whether this practice is initiated by the provider or at a patient's request (e.g., having knowledge that the practice or facility changes diagnoses or dates of services at the request of patients so charges will be covered by their carriers) does not change the fact that it constitutes fraud.

RECEIVING BENEFITS ON BEHALF OF ONE PERSON AND PUTTING THEM TO USE OTHER THAN FOR THE BENEFIT OF THAT PERSON. Providing a prescription for a DME item or another item for the Medicare recipient when that item will be used by the spouse, who may not be covered, constitutes fraud whether it is an oversight by the provider or is at the patient's request.

PRESENTING A BILL FOR MEDICAL ITEMS OR SERVICES WHILE KNOWING OR HAVING REASON TO KNOW THAT THE CLAIM IS FALSE OR FRAUDULENT. Because ignorance is no longer a defense, should the individual have reason to know that the claim is false, such as the facility does not provide the service or medical item, and perhaps, in fact, does not stock a specific item that is being billed, the individual involved in the billing and the others who had knowledge that this item could not be billed are liable.

PRESENTING A CLAIM ON BEHALF OF A PERSON EXCLUDED FROM THE MEDICARE/MEDICAID PROGRAM. It is the responsibility of the billing entity to know those providers or facilities that have been excluded from the Medicare program and to submit no billing on their behalf. This information is readily available on the Medicare Internet site.

PRESENTING CLAIMS OF PHYSICIAN SERVICES UNDER A PROVIDER NUMBER OTHER THAN EITHER THAT PHYSICIAN'S PROVIDER NUMBER OR AN APPROPRIATE GROUP PROVIDER NUMBER. If a practice bills for services NOT provided by that specific practice, then this act is also fraud. In the past, it was acceptable for a practice to enter into arrangements whereby it would bill for the services of another provider in exchange for a billing fee. Federal laws have been passed since that time to prohibit billing for ANY services not provided by the billing entity.

PRESENTING A CLAIM FOR PHYSICIAN SERVICES WHEN THE PERSON WHO PROVIDED OR SUPERVISED THE SERVICES WAS NOT AN APPROPRIATELY LICENSED PHYSICIAN OR WHEN THE PHYSICIAN WAS MISREPRESENTED AS BEING SPECIALTY CERTIFIED WHEN HE OR SHE WAS NOT. This most commonly occurs when a physician extender (nurse practitioner/physician assistant) provides a service without meeting the guidelines under the Medicare program for proper supervision by the supervising physician.

PROVIDING ITEMS OR SERVICES AND SOLICITING, OFFERING, OR RECEIVING KICKBACKS, BRIBES, OR REBATES OF A FEE. An entity receiving any financial incentive for services referred or received meets the definition of fraud as defined by federal guidelines.

ABUSE

Abuse is a misdemeanor, punishable by fines, interest, jail term, or all three. Abuse is defined as follows.

OVERUSE OF MEDICAL AND HEALTH SERVICES. This occurs when more than the services usually necessary are ordered, such as unnecessary "rechecks." Again, the coder sees the need for medical documentation of the medical necessity. If this documentation is included, the definition of abuse has not been met.

BILLING EXCESSIVE CHARGES FOR SERVICES OR SUPPLIES. This refers to billing for services or supplies in excess of fair market value plus the cost of administration. The practice should establish a practice charge formula for supplies and medications that is part of the compliance manual, as well as the policies and procedures manual for the practice. This formula should establish the method used for determining both practice or facility fees for these services and the percentage of increase justified by the practice or facility costs for stocking supplies, spoilage, and so forth.

FILING CLAIMS FOR SERVICES DEEMED "NOT MEDICALLY NECESSARY," OR IF MEDICALLY NECESSARY, NOT TO THE EXTENT RENDERED. This includes excessive office visits or ancillary services not justified by medical documentation as medically necessary and repeat procedures for which no justification or documentation exists regarding the need to repeat.

BREACHING ASSIGNMENT AGREEMENTS, RESULTING IN THE BENEFICIARY BEING BILLED FOR AMOUNTS DISALLOWED BY THE CARRIER ON THE BASIS THAT SUCH CHARGES EXCEED "REASONABLE CHARGE" CRITERIA. This may occur as the result of contractuals not being properly taken at the time the Medicare Explanation of Benefits is received. This may be an oversight; however, as has been discussed previously, ignorance is not a defense in fraud and abuse cases. There is an obvious need for the individual responsible for posting payments to understand the coding concepts and the contractual obligations of the third party and the practice, so that a breach of assignment agreement does not take place.

USING A SEPARATE SCHEDULE OF CHARGES FOR MEDICARE CHARGES THAT IS HIGHER THAN NON-MEDICARE CHARGES. Medicare legislation prohibits the use of a multiple-tier fee schedule for the practice. In other words, Medicare law prohibits non-Medicare patients from receiving services for less than a Medicare patient. The practice should make certain not to offer self-pay discounts to patients at the time of service that are lower than those allowed by Medicare. Practice policy and procedure should dictate that no discounts can be quoted or given at the time of service; however, any discounts to be offered should be given after the patient's financial agreement is completed (i.e., the patient pays the agreed-on portion).

EXCEEDING THE LIMITING CHARGE IMPOSED ON NONPARTICIPATING PROVIDERS FOR SPECIFIC SERVICES. In the event the practice is "nonparticipating" with Medicare, it may not collect from a patient more than 115% of the limiting nonparticipating allowance. (This is stated in the yearly Medicare Fee Allowance information, which is available from the carrier or on its Web site.)

USING IMPROPER BILLING PRACTICES, INCLUDING SUBMISSION OF BILLS TO MEDICARE INSTEAD OF THIRD-PARTY PAYORS THAT ARE PRIMARY INSURERS FOR MEDICARE BENEFICIARIES. When Medicare beneficiaries have other primary insurance or insurance that is responsible for services (such as workers' compensation, liability or auto insurance, or other primary insurance under the "Working Aged"), the provider or practice must bill that insurance carrier/payor first. The practice or provider is expected to make the determination regarding other third-party coverage and bill the appropriate primary insurance carrier for services. Attempting to bill or collect from Medicare when other coverage should be primary is considered abuse.

ORDERING PROCEDURES OR SERVICES MORE FREQUENTLY THAN GOOD STANDARD MEDICAL PRACTICE ALLOWS. Documentation of medical necessity would eliminate any accusations of abuse because the services would be documented as justified. All ancillary services ordered should include documentation of both an ordering physician and medical necessity.

ORDERING A BATTERY OF DIAGNOSTIC TESTS WHEN DIAGNOSIS INDICATES THE NEED FOR ONLY A FEW TESTS. When medical documentation supports the need for a specific test as opposed to the number of ancillary tests performed, investigation of abuse would be appropriate. This definition of abuse came about as the result of physicians and providers who would automatically order specific "screening" tests on the basis of a patient's age, sex, and presenting complaint without determining which tests were in fact medically necessary for that particular patient. Many times these tests were ordered and performed before the patient was even seen by the physician or provider. As long as the medical necessity for each ordered test can be substantiated from the medical documentation, this will not be an issue for the practice.

Some additional facts about determination and prosecution of fraudulent or abusive practices should be considered, as discussed in the following paragraphs.

IMPORTANT CONSIDERATIONS REGARDING FRAUD AND ABUSE

FRAUD AND ABUSE ARE PUNISHABLE REGARDLESS OF INTENT. Even when a provider or practice commits fraudulent acts in error, charges may still result. In most instances, when a practice or provider has been found responsible for fraudulent billing, the OIG, as part of the audit process, requires that entity to implement a compliance program in the event that one has not already been put into place. Compliance programs are discussed later.

IGNORANCE IS NO LONGER A DEFENSE FOR FRAUD OR ABUSE. Ignorance, or the lack of knowing what constitutes fraud or abuse, or the oversight that fraudulent or abusive activities are taking place in the practice is no longer a defense.

ALL PARTIES WHO HAVE KNOWLEDGE OF FRAUDULENT OR ABUSIVE ACTIVITY ARE PUNISHABLE. This includes any staff member that is party to, participates

in, or should be aware of the occurrence or potential occurrence of fraudulent or abusive activity. Billers, coders, clerical and administrative staff, physicians, and owners can all be liable. No one is exempt if his or her responsibilities involve the billing/coding and reimbursement process within the practice. For this reason, liability insurance is now available for these individuals. Certified coders are particularly vulnerable in a fraudulent situation, because they are considered experts. The coder should be involved in the reimbursement and coding process and should be able to determine whether these types of activities are taking place.

FRAUD AND ABUSE ARE CHARGED BY THE LINE ITEM. The assessment for fraudulent and abusive activity is charged on the basis of each line item, averaging between $3,000 and $10,000 per line. The third party auditing the practice has the right to perform an audit of additional items and to determine percentage of error based on the sampling. The number of fraudulent or abusive claims will be determined according to the error percentage. This number will be charged the $3,000 to $10,000 line item fine.

A **line item** represents one "line" of the claim form. For instance, if the claim form lists five "lines" or five CPT-4 codes on a given claim, this represents five line items, and each fraudulent line item would be assessed.

THE PRACTICE/PROVIDER/FACILITY HAS THE RESPONSIBILITY OF CHALLENGING AND DISPROVING ANY ERROR PERCENTAGE OF FRAUDULENT OR ABUSIVE ACTIVITY THROUGH THE APPEAL AND LEGAL PROCESSES. If the practice thinks that the "representative" sampling chosen by the third-party carrier is erroneous, it has the responsibility to gather the data to disprove this finding. This typically will involve much research on the part of the practice, often requiring the employment of a consulting firm to gather the facts. In addition, the practice may need to employ legal representation to contest the charges. Even in the event that no fraud or abuse is proven, the financial effect of challenging these charges is astronomical.

MEDICARE AND OTHER THIRD-PARTY CARRIERS HAVE THE RIGHT TO EXCLUDE PHYSICIANS OR PROVIDERS FROM THEIR PROGRAMS AS THE RESULT OF FRAUDULENT OR ABUSIVE ACTIVITY. When fraudulent activity is confirmed, the third-party carrier may exclude the billing entity, which may be the physician, the group provider, or the facility. This means the practice or facility must notify many of its patients that it no longer participates and cannot continue to treat them. This, of course, will have a significant financial impact on the entity as well. In addition, many third-party carriers now communicate this information through a network to other third-party carriers who may choose to disqualify the provider or practice from their programs.

THE THIRD-PARTY CARRIER MAY PLACE THE PRACTICE OR PROVIDER ON "MANUAL REVIEW" OR "FLAG" FOR AN INDETERMINATE AMOUNT OF TIME.

Medicare refers to this process as "flagging" the physician. Third-party carriers often require that all claims for a provider or practice found guilty of fraudulent or abusive activity must undergo a **manual review/flag** process. This includes all claims, even those that typically would be processed automatically. Unfortunately, most third-party carriers do not set a time limit for this process, and it is left to the third-party carrier to make the determination when the provider or practice will be reviewed and possibly removed from this flag.

Providers or practices have sometimes stayed in this flag status for years before the carrier returned them to their previous status. Obviously, the financial impact of this status is overwhelming, because no claims will be paid for approximately 60 to 90 days, the time required to manually review all claims. If the third-party carrier represents a large portion of the practice's patient population, the loss of revenue for this carrier for a 90-day period will be significant.

FINANCIAL IMPACT TO THE PRACTICE OR PROVIDER IS SIGNIFICANT REGARDLESS OF THE FINDINGS.

The financial impact from a fraud or abuse investigation is monumental, even to the large practice. In addition to the potential loss from fines, penalties, and possible imprisonment, the practice typically must hire legal representation and health care consultants to assist in defense of the allegations. Should the practice or provider survive the financial penalties imposed, additional financial impact will result should the carrier make the decision to impose the manual review process on all claims submitted by the practice or provider.

Therefore it is in the best interest of the practice to identify any activities that might be construed as fraudulent and to act on them immediately. The coder is probably vulnerable and is in a good position to identify any such activity.

STEPS FOR REPORTING FRAUD AND ABUSE

In the event the coder identifies activities he or she believes to be fraudulent, the following steps should be taken.

REPORT THE INFORMATION TO THE DIRECT SUPERVISOR.
Initially, this may be done verbally; however, if no action seems forthcoming, the coder should document his or her concern in writing.

NOTIFY THE CARRIER ABOUT ANY ERROR AND BE WILLING TO CORRECT THE ERROR.
Determine the extent of the error and the financial impact. Prepare a response to the carrier, including identification of the error(s), the explanation of benefits for each error, and a check in the total amount of the error(s) made. Send the detailed information to the carrier, certified return receipt.

In many instances, the carrier will respond by returning the check; however, in the event the carrier wishes to prosecute at a later time, the legal system probably will not find the practice or provider guilty of any intent, and the financial impact will be significantly less.

Keep in mind that if the carrier identifies the potential fraud or abuse before the practice or provider does, the practice and anyone who was aware of the issues can be held accountable.

REQUEST A RESPONSE IN WRITING FROM THE SUPERVISOR.
Indicate willingness to assist in preparing a response to the carrier. Insist on receiving a written response from the supervisor. If the immediate supervisor does not respond, put any concerns in writing to the Administrator, CEO, or CFO, and ask to receive a response in writing.

CONTACT THE COMPLIANCE OFFICER OR DIRECTOR.
If the practice has a Compliance Officer, make certain that the individual is informed. Do not rely on the direct supervisor or the administrator to inform the Compliance Officer.

MAKE CERTAIN THE PRACTICE OWNERS OR PHYSICIANS ARE AWARE OF THE INFORMATION.
Do not rely on others to inform all responsible parties.

CONTACT THE PRACTICE ATTORNEY OR LEGAL REPRESENTATIVE IF NO ACTION IS TAKEN BY THOSE PREVIOUSLY CONTACTED.
Document all contacts concerning the issue, requests for response, and subsequent findings. In the event the practice is investigated for fraud or abuse, any actions that have been taken in notifying the practice of the situation will need to be defended.

USE THE "WHISTLEBLOWER" PROGRAM TO ANONYMOUSLY REPORT FRAUD AND ABUSE.
Most third-party carriers have a program for surrendering information regarding suspected fraud and abuse activities. Many of these programs offer an incentive to the individual who reports the activity in an effort to encourage reporting.

IF CODING ETHICS ARE SIGNIFICANTLY COMPROMISED, DISCUSS WHETHER RESIGNATION IS NECESSARY.
Make certain that all entities that have been contacted previously are informed by YOU, THE CODER,

about the decision. Address why it is necessary to consider resignation and what actions should be taken to correct the problems within the practice.

The coder will want to maintain copies of all correspondence sent to practice supervisors, administrators, legal representatives, and any other individuals. In the event the carrier decides to prosecute the practice or provider, the coder may need the written documentation to prove to the carrier that he or she attempted to resolve the problem without success. Fraudulent and abusive activities will have a profound effect not only on the coder, but on the provider and the practice as well.

The remainder of this chapter is dedicated to monitoring processes that may identify or eliminate any fraudulent or abusive activity, or accusations thereof. The implementation of these processes may save the practice from such fraudulent and abusive activities. Alternatively, the use of such processes may prove to the third-party carrier that the errors were without intent, and the resulting penalties may be less extensive. In addition, these monitoring processes ensure maximum revenue coding and ensure that the practice is cognizant of reimbursement for all services rendered. This is extremely important in the health care industry because third-party carriers continue to reimburse less and less.

MONITORING PROCESSES

In the section on coding from a reimbursement perspective, the importance of monitoring is briefly discussed. The coder will find that his or her involvement in the monitoring process is imperative to ensuring the correctness of documents and their appropriate preparation for third-party carriers.

Many coders believe their responsibilities begin at the point at which codes are assigned to services and diagnoses; however, the importance of everyone's participation in the coding process has been demonstrated. Also demonstrated is the importance of the physician's documentation and of the information gathered from the charge documents by other clerical and clinical staff in the office. The monitoring process for the coder involves the following elements.

DATA ENTRY PROCESS AND MONITORING TECHNIQUES

From the moment the data enter the practice's computerized billing system, the accuracy of information determines the number of clean claims the practice will send to third-party carriers. The clean claim process has already been discussed, along with the delays or denials that occur as a result of what might seem small and insignificant oversights.

The data entry personnel in the practice typically are not educated as coders, so the coding staff will need to teach data entry personnel and provide them with educational reference tools for correctly entering data. Many of these "tools" can be built into the computerized billing system by means of programming; other issues must be manually identified by data entry personnel.

Most computerized billing systems have much potential for gathering the correct information for specific services. Critical data, such as referring physician names and UPINs (universal physician identifier numbers) for consultations, may be preloaded into the computer. The billing system may then be programmed to require a referring physician name when any CPT-4 code identified as a "consultation" is entered. Many such "safety catches" can be preprogrammed into the computer system to assist data entry and other personnel in successfully entering data for a clean claim.

The coder should work with the systems administrator or information specialist in the practice and identify which of the following options are available for use in the practice's computerized billing system. Use as many of these as possible; they will prevent unneeded errors and delays in reimbursement.

"Macro Codes" for Multiple Services Performed Together

When the provision of a surgical service always allows for a special supply item to be billed in addition to the service, these may be entered into many billing systems with one code, which will actually print the two or more codes necessary to completely describe and bill the services performed. For example, when performing colonoscopy, the physician may bill the services for the colonoscopy, as well as the provision of a surgical tray. Rather than leaving the entry of two procedure codes to data entry personnel, allowing the possibility that one will be overlooked, most billing systems are capable of building a "macro" code. This is similar to the mechanism in word processing software whereby one word or phrase is entered, and a standardized group of words appears (used for documentation/transcription purposes). In this instance, for the colonoscopy service and surgical tray, the macro will be entitled COLON. When the data entry personnel enter the procedure code COLON, the system will automatically enter two charges, one for the colonoscopy and one for the surgical tray, thus eliminating the possibility of oversight.

Macro codes may also be useful for injections that require a code for the administration, as well as for the medication itself.

Multiple Units

Another error that commonly occurs when data entry personnel enter charges is multiple units of service.

Typically, either the computerized billing system does not ask for number of units, or the data entry operator is not familiar with the service and does not realize that multiple units of service may occur for a particular code.

Modifier Code Usage

When modifier codes are necessary for certain procedures, the computerized billing system can be used to enter these codes with their respective modifier codes; it can also enable them to be offered as a selection on charge documents.

A frequent review of the charges entered into the computerized billing system will reflect whether services are being entered into the system as intended, or if errors are being made that may implicate the practice for fraud or abuse.

A data entry audit process should be a part of the facility or practice review plan for compliance. Tool 62 provides guidelines for completing a data entry audit. Specified guidelines for performing this data entry audit process should be incorporated into the policy and procedure manual or compliance plan. Set time intervals for performing this review should be defined in this documentation as well, along with a log recording the performance of this function.

CLAIMS REVIEW PROCESS

The coder should also be directly involved in the claims review process. After completion of the charge document and data entry, **all claims should be reviewed, electronically and on paper before they are forwarded to the third-party carrier(s).**

The "clean claim" process and its importance in receiving proper reimbursement on a timely basis have been discussed. Errors that have occurred up to the point the claim is generated should be detected before mailing. Keep in mind that many of the staff involved in the recording of these charges and subsequent claims are not coders and, therefore may not realize that coding errors have occurred.

Electronic claims may also be reviewed before transmission by means of an audit trail programmed into the computerized billing system, or by the generation of a "claims worksheet," or similar report of each claim as it will be transmitted to the carrier.

Claims may be reviewed by noncoding personnel for the most common errors, such as incomplete insurance information, incorrect identification numbers, and relationship discrepancies.

Coding information that should be reviewed includes such items as the following:

- CPT-4 codes that require a modifier
- ICD-9-CM codes matched correctly to the appropriate CPT-4 codes
- CPT-4 codes requiring specific ICD-9-CM diagnostic codes
- High-level procedures requiring specialized diagnostic codes

The practice may wish to develop some type of "model claim" for use when reviewing claim forms. If the practice deals with a carrier that has unusual guidelines specific to that carrier only, it may wish to develop a separate "model claim" for that carrier.

One suggestion for doing this is to make an overhead transparency of a blank CMS insurance claim form and mark those fields that must be completed by highlighting or other designation. Mark those fields requiring specialized information, using notations such as "correct number of digits" or "leave blank." This transparency may then be overlaid on paper claims for this specific carrier for review of completeness.

When errors are encountered, the problem can be identified and the root corrected, not just for that specific claim. For instance, if a specific diagnosis code requires five digits and the claim has a code with only four, identify the origin of the problem in the computerized billing system and correct it, but NOT just for that specific claim. This will eliminate the error in the future and prevent the chance that the error will not be captured on subsequent claims.

If errors occur as the result of data entry mistakes, the individual responsible for those errors should be notified and retrained appropriately, so the errors do not occur in the future.

Errors may also occur as the result of misprints or mistakes on the charge documents. These must be corrected immediately by reprinting the document or, if necessary, making a temporary correction in the computerized billing system that takes out the wrong code and directs the system to print the correct code, until reprinting of the charge document occurs.

Most important, when errors are encountered during the claims review process, these errors should be recorded over time for review. During the month end process, these categorizations of errors can be totaled and reviewed, and the appropriate action taken to avoid them in the future. This process should be incorporated into the policy and procedure manual or compliance plan, and set time intervals for performance established. Tool 63 includes a Claims Review form.

CODING/CHART REVIEW PROCESS

Whether charges are coded by a practice coder or a physician, or are determined by other office staff, all coding should be reviewed on a regular basis. Many practices or facilities, especially the smaller ones, do not

TOOL 62

DATA ENTRY REVIEW FORM

Date: _____

Practice Name: _____

Operator	Date of Service	Physician/ Provider	Patient Name	Cht# Pt#	Line Item Submitted	Line Item Keyed	EXPLANATION	Calculation +/-
							TOTAL	

Page ____ of ____

TOOL 63

Date:	CLAIMS REVIEW PROCESS		
CLAIMS PROCESSED	**# Claims**	**$ Billed**	**COMMENTS**
ELECTRONIC			
Medicare			
Commercial			
TOTALS			
PAPER			
Medicare			
Medicaid			
Commercial			
TOTALS			
GRAND TOTAL			

BILLING ERRORS	**# Claims**	**$ Billed**	**COMMENTS**
REGISTRATION			
- ID#			
- Wrong Insur			
- Other			
TOTALS			
CHARGE DOCUMENT			
- Referring Phy			
- Other			
- Auth #			
TOTALS			
CODING			
- Diagnosis			
- Procedure Code			
- Place of Service			
- Other			
TOTALS			
OTHER (Specify):			
TOTALS			
GRAND TOTAL			

Completed by: _____   Date: _____

employ a full-time coder and instead depend on other office staff or the physician(s) to select the proper codes for billing and reimbursement. It is imperative that coding be reviewed on a regular basis by the practice coder or an outside coder or coding group. Chart audits, or chart reviews, should be conducted by the practice, both internally and by an external source, to ascertain whether appropriate coding protocols are being followed. If a compliance program is in place for the practice, the chart audit should also determine whether compliance guidelines are being followed. In the event of a third-party audit, if the practice has a compliance program in place, the third party will want to determine whether that com-

pliance plan is being followed (see discussion later in chapter).

Tools 64 and 65 show examples of typical chart audit forms. These forms may vary on the basis of the services typically performed in the practice but should include evaluation and management, surgical procedure review, and medical documentation review.

The need for the chart review process has already been discussed. The primary purpose is to review and recommend enhancements to medical record documentation to prevent third-party audit; to identify undercoding and overcoding; and to detect documentation deficiencies that may result in third-party targeting for audit, disciplinary action by third parties, or legal action from a fraud, abuse, or liability standpoint.

The following is an overview of the chart audit process.

T O O L   64

CHART AUDIT LOGSHEET

Date: _____   Practice: _____

Date of Service	Physician/ Provider	Pt Name	Chart# Pt#	Code Submitted	Coder Review	Change		REASON	Calculation +/-
						Up	Down		
									TOTAL

Page _____ of _____

T O O L   65

CHART AUDIT - E & M WORKSHEET

Patient: _____   Date of Service: _____

Location of Service: Off/Output ☐   Off/Consult ☐   ER ☐   Prev Med ☐
                       Init/Hosp ☐   Sub Hosp ☐   Discharge ☐
                       Init NH ☐   Sub NH ☐
Patient Status: New Patient ☐   Established Pt ☐
Referring Physician: Yes ☐   No ☐

HISTORY
Problem Focused   ☐ Chief complaint;Brief history of problem
Expanded Problem Focused   ☐   + Problem Pertinent System Review
Detailed   ☐ CC;Extended History;Extended ROS;Pertinent PMH/FH/SH
Comprehensive   ☐ CC;Extended History;Complete ROS;Complete PMH/FH/SH

EXAM
Problem Focused   ☐ Affected body area or organ system
Expanded Problem Focused   ☐   + other related systems
Detailed   ☐ Extended exam of affected/extended body area/organ system
Comprehensive   ☐ Complete single system specialty exam/complete multisystem exam

MEDICAL DECISION MAKING

Elements	A	B	C	D
Number of Diagnosis and Management Options	Minimal	Limited	Multiple	Extensive
Amount/Complexity of Data Reviewed	Minimal	Limited	Multiple	Extensive
Risk Complications/Morbidity/Mortality	Minimal	Low	Moderate	High

Straightforward   ☐ 2/3 Column A Elements Met
Low Complexity   ☐ 2/3 Column B Elements Met
Moderate Complexity   ☐ 2/3 Column C Elements Met
High Complexity   ☐ 2/3 Column D Elements Met

TIME   Only if >50% of face-to-face time with patient in counseling/coordination of care
            Total Time Documented: _____

E & M Code Assigned: _____   ICD-9-CM Code Assigned: _____
Recommendations: _____
_____

Reviewer: _____   Date: _____

What Should Be Included in the Chart Audit

A representative sampling of the chart activity for the practice should be included in the audit. If multiple physicians belong to the practice, a representative sampling for each provider, including any physician extenders (e.g., physician assistants, nurse practitioners), should be completed. There is no specific formula for identifying the number of charts that should be reviewed; however, the volume for each provider should be proportionate to the volume or percentage of patients each provider sees. At a minimum, the number of patients seen in a typical day per physician should be pulled; the same protocol should be followed for surgical procedures.

Although the number of charts pulled would be equal to one day's service by each provider, the charts typically should be pulled from different dates and months to make certain that results are based on a true random sampling. In addition, the chart audit or review may be extended to a billing audit or review as well. This would involve reviewing not only the medical record documentation process, but also the charge documentation process. In this process, charges are reviewed as they are submitted from the provider or the charge document, to charge entry, to billing and final adjudication of the claim. Hospitals and other facilities are required to perform such audits for their services as the result of **Joint Commission on the Accreditation of Hospital Organizations (JCAHO)** standards. JCAHO requires that these types of activities be performed and recorded on a regular basis.

Preparing Charts for the Audit

Typically, the auditing entity (e.g., the practice or outside auditor) is responsible for randomly pulling the medical charts necessary for the chart audit. The practice or facility, however, may pull the charts for the audit, making certain the charts remain a random sample for accurate auditing. A small number of charts may be pulled from medical records at one time, or all charts may be pulled at one time. Keep in mind, however, that typically the practice continues to see patients during the audit. Some of the charts pulled for the random sampling may in fact be pulled back in the event the patient(s) selected must be seen during the audit period. In the event this occurs, it is necessary to replace each of these charts with an additional randomly sampled chart. The audit process should occur with as little disruption to the practice as possible. For this reason, many chart audits are performed in increments.

Tools Needed for the Chart Audit or Review Process

In addition to the current CPT-4 and ICD-9-CM or current coding books, the chart auditor must use the appropriate forms to complete the audit. The forms differ according to the type and extent of the review. Samples of the most common review documents are included in this chapter discussion. Worksheets similar to those used for initial coding of CPT-4 and DRG services may also be helpful in this process.

What Is Reviewed in the Chart Audit

Because each chart audit may be performed for various reasons, the chart auditor should meet with the requesting party of the audit to determine if there are specific concerns or areas of concentration. Some of the most common reasons the chart audit is performed are as follows.

Undercodes/Overcodes
When medical record documentation substantiates a higher or lower level of service than that reported, these services are termed "overcoded" or "undercoded." Many practices undercode to be "safe" from fraud and abuse. Significant revenue is lost as the result of this unnecessary undercoding practice.

Obviously, overcoding may result in third-party audit and the possibility of fraud and abuse allegations. The goal of the practice should be to code and bill services at the level they are performed. When overcoding or undercoding occurs, the chart auditor determines the significance and identity of medical documentation that may be missing or deficient in maximizing the coding level.

Missing Documentation or Signatures
As discussed in the physician documentation section, if it is not documented it did not happen. In many instances, the service provided probably achieves the level of service billed. If the documentation to substantiate that level of service, ancillary service, or procedure is not present, however, it should not be coded or billed. This includes the completion of the medical documentation by acknowledging that statements are complete and accurate with a signature or authentication "mark," as well as a date.

In the event that physician extenders are responsible for providing services, or portions of service, the attending or overseeing physician must review and document the report with a signature or "mark" and the date.

Levels of Service Distribution
For the practice to determine whether the volume of each level of service is "within the norm" for its specialty, level of service distribution is determined by the volume of each level of service calculated as a percentage to the total number of visits. The practice may monitor its percentage level of service distributions before a chart audit by contacting any of the medical management associations it belongs to. This information is gathered for the past year through a process of practice surveys by specialty.

Ancillary Service Documentation and Signature Requirements
Each and every service that requires a physician order MUST have certain information documented for that service to be coded and billed. The required documentation includes the following:

- Physician order to provide the service
- Documentation of service provided
- Interpretation of test by physician
- Signature/countersignature of physician when services are provided by nursing or physician extender staff

The inclusion of laboratory slips or ECG printouts, for instance, does not constitute proof that the service was completed unless the physician has read, interpreted, and documented the interpretation of results by signing and dating the results. Services such as medications, injections, and immunizations require documentation of the order for services, as well as review by the ordering physician that they were completed as ordered, and confirmation of physician review by signature and date.

Compliance with Practice or Facility Chart Protocol
If practice protocols call for charts to be dictated, filed in a certain order, signed, and dated in specific locations, these procedures should be reviewed in relation to compliance with practice or facility protocols. In the event

the practice has adopted a compliance program, this portion of the review should encompass whether the guidelines of the practice compliance program are being adhered to as well. Tool 66 shows the types of issues the practice should review.

Documenting Chart Deficiencies

When deficiencies are noted in the elements discussed, the chart auditor should make note of those deficiencies. Additional notations can also be made of enhancements that might be made to achieve compliance. Documentation of the following deficiencies should be noted with details:

- Changes in level of service
- Documentation deficiencies
- Signature deficiencies

Compiling Audit Data

On completion of the actual chart review, a compilation of results is necessary, along with a report back to the requesting party. For the financial impact of the results to be calculated, pricing information should be obtained for services audited from the office. With the use of the Chart Audit Logsheet, overcoded or undercoded items should be recorded. The auditor will then need to calculate the difference between actual reimbursement and the correct reimbursement for services as documented. Services that have been coded and billed, but were audited as not documented sufficiently to warrant coding, should be entered on the Chart Audit Logsheet as well. If the chart audit extends into a billing audit as well, a Charge Capturing Review should also be completed.

The Charge Capturing Review requires several randomly sampled day schedules or appointment logs from the practice or facility. A review of coding/billing records should be conducted to determine whether the patients seen were billed and if other procedures performed were coded as well.

Preparation of the Audit Report

When the results of the chart audit are prepared, the report must not sound offensive to the practice. The auditor should keep in mind that the practice apparently identified the need for the audit and therefore has taken the first step in determining the extent of discrepancies and correcting them. For this reason, the auditor should eliminate the use of words such as "errors" and replace them with words such as "recommendations." The auditor will also want to assure the practice that the purposes of the audit are to prevent third-party audit, to enhance

documentation, and to work with the practice toward that end. The chart auditor should make certain that the chart audit is not construed as an attempt to find all the "errors" or "mistakes" made by the practice staff. The auditor must make sure to include positives along with the negatives. For instance, if practice coding is deficient, but charts are all dictated, well written, signed, and efficiently organized, the auditor must be sure to mention the positive findings as well. Even if the extensive effort made by staff to achieve chart or documentation completion falls short of the needs as evidenced by the chart audit, their efforts should be praised.

The chart auditor should prepare written documentation of findings, referencing documentation from the coding reference books (CPT-4 and ICD-9-CM).

Level of Service Deficiencies

The level of service distribution curve for the practice's particular specialty should be stated. The practice's level of service curve based on the charts audited must be calculated and compared with that standard.

Remember that the level of service curve for the audited practice may, in fact, be different from the norm, even if the levels of services are documented and coded correctly. Thus, the practice has the opportunity and should be prepared to substantiate that its levels of service have been coded correctly. At a minimum, the practice can be confident in the event of an audit that their levels of service distribution have already been substantiated.

Documentation Deficiencies

Any and all documentation deficiencies relating to the practice should be identified and information provided on how these deficiencies may be corrected easily and efficiently without a great deal of additional work on the part of the practice. The need for complete documentation should be emphasized from both a fraud and an abuse perspective, as well as from a liability standpoint.

Calculation of Deficiencies

After each deficiency and the resultant increase or decrease in reimbursement has been documented, this increase or decrease should be calculated on a monthly and annualized basis for the practice.

One of the most common complaints from coders is that the staff and physicians do not seem to comprehend the extent of their documentation/coding deficiencies. Communicating to the physician on a daily basis that a $100 discrepancy exists would seem nominal and of little consequence. Taking that $100 discrepancy times 22 working days, however, means a $2,200 loss per month, and times 12 months it means an annual loss of $26,400. Deficiencies must be put in terms that will draw needed attention and result in a simple resolution. Providers are more willing to make simple adjustments

TOOL 66

PRACTICE PROTOCOL LOGSHEET

Date: _____

Practice Name: _____

Patient Name	DOS	MR/Cht#	Documentation Style				Chart Contents			Documentation of Review				
			Dictated	Written	SOAP	Narrative	Dated	Signed	Legible	Vital Signs	Pt Hx	Labs	X-Ray	Other Ancill
TOTALS — No.														
GRAND TOTALS														
% ERROR														

Y = Yes   N = No

Page _____ of _____

to documentation deficiencies rather than major changes in order to maximize levels of all services performed.

Summarizing Audit Findings

The auditor should make sure to reinforce the purpose of the audit, address concerns discussed with the practice before the audit, follow up on results, and determine how the practice can implement any needed corrections. It should be emphasized that the auditor will be available to assist in making the changes necessary to achieve maximum documentation and coding.

Every type of deficiency should be identified, as well as the extent of these deficiencies and the corrective steps needed. The impact on the practice, uncorrected and corrected, should be explained. Define step-by-step processes to correct the problems, as well as prioritize a list of deficiencies to address first. Priorities should be based not just on the cost to the practice in increased or decreased reimbursement, but on the potential risks for fraud and abuse and the calculated financial impact.

Both an in-depth detailed analysis of the audit and a "quick reference" one-page summary should be prepared so that individuals who tend to lack the time to read the details can, at a minimum, "read the bottom line." The financial impact of each error and the total impact of all items identified should be given, including the annualized numbers. This often encourages review of the more detailed information.

COMPLIANCE PROGRAMS

Compliance programs are well-defined written policies and procedures outlining a specific set of guidelines to ensure that the practice adheres to third-party standards. These standards may involve such areas as medical documentation, coding, billing, or other defined processes.

At this time, there are no legal requirements for physicians to implement compliance programs. Should a provider be audited by the federal government, however, the government reserves the right to mandate that a compliance plan be put into place within a set period if it believes that this step is appropriate.

Even though a corporate or practice compliance plan is not required, federal regulations mandate that Health Insurance Portability and Accountability Act (HIPAA) guidelines be monitored and followed.

HIPAA REQUIREMENTS

Under **HIPAA,** which was enacted in 1996, set standards are required for the confidentiality of patient records and the processing of health care claims, including but not limited to such areas as the following:

- Standards for electronic claims transactions such as common codes, identifiers, and security methods to ensure consumer records are protected from inappropriate use and disclosure. This affects health plans, health care clearinghouses, and health care providers conducting financial and administrative transactions electronically.
- Creating privacy standards for patient records such as limiting the use and release of medical records and other personal health insurance information, and patients' access to their records.
- Establishing an employer identification number that will be effective no later than July 30, 2004. (This has been put on hold.)
- Establishing common code sets to be used for assigning codes to all claim forms. These common code sets were established as ICD-9-CM and CPT-4.

Additional or up-to-date progress on HIPAA legislation is available from the CMS Web site at www.cms.gov/hipaa.

JCAHO ACCREDITATION REQUIREMENTS

As was discussed previously, hospitals are mandated by such organizations as JCAHO to comply with standards to receive and maintain accreditation. This accreditation process is necessary for the following reasons:

- Requirement for reimbursement by many third-party carriers
- Validates quality of care
- Provides a competitive edge over facilities that are not accredited

At a minimum, JCAHO (and other accrediting authorities) requires the following review criteria:

- Each department must have a quality assessment plan.
- Results of documentation monitoring or clinical pertinence reviews must be reviewed in the appropriate committees with interdisciplinary input.
- Qualified personnel must perform all tasks of documentation and all documentation reviews.
- Overall content of the medical record must be sufficient to provide continuity of care.
- Basic documentation elements must be present, such as the following:
Patient informed consent
Patient education
Diagnoses and procedures
Pertinent history
Observations, assessments, plans
Diagnostic data
Therapeutic data

- Reviews must focus on the following:
  Problem cases
  High-volume cases
  Sampling across cases
- Departments responsible for entries into the record must have written policies on timeliness and data distribution.
- Evidence of morbidity/mortality measurements/ indicators HIM/transcription/QA must show pertinent policies and examples of documentation reviews.
- There must be evidence of policies relating to data correction, revisions, and editing.

Policies and procedures are maintained in the hospital facility that outline exactly how all of the previous guidelines will be implemented, monitored, and maintained. These documents are reviewed at the time the facility is reviewed for accreditation.

Practice compliance programs are not right for all providers and practices. Most important, should the practice decide to implement such a program, it will be obligated to enforce the guidelines outlined in the compliance program.

The following should be taken into consideration when determining whether a practice should institute a compliance program.

DETERMINING PRACTICE NEED FOR A COMPLIANCE PROGRAM

The practice's vulnerability for fraud and audit is based on the following elements:

Coding Practices/ Practice size	The third party performing the audit is interested in identifying some of the largest offenders and those that, owing to their size, will press smaller practices into compliance.
Specialty	Certain specialties may be more prone to investigation because of past audits in such practices that revealed a high degree of fraudulent activity.
E & M Levels of Distribution	Levels of service distribution and volume of high-ticket items are identified for potential fraud investigation.

ELEMENTS THAT TRIGGER AN INVESTIGATION/AUDIT

Keep in mind the three main reasons practices or facilities are investigated for fraud and abuse the following:

1. Patient complaint
2. Employee complaint
3. Level of service distribution inconsistencies

In addition to the previous components, the following reasons can be added:

4. Information from other investigations (referral patterns, other services already under investigation)
5. Data gathered from processed claims:
   Abnormal distribution of levels of service
   Billing errors
   Repetitive care protocols
   Copay/deductible violations

The implementation of a practice compliance program is time-consuming and detail oriented. The compliance program ensures quality of care, documentation, coding, and other services provided by the practice in much the same way that the accreditation of hospitals attempts to ensure quality of care for patients in those facilities. Having a written, enforced compliance program in place has a number of advantages; however, a compliance plan that has no follow-up or is not enforced may actually be more of a threat to the practice than no compliance plan at all. Box 22-1 lists seven federal guidelines for compliance programs.

ADVANTAGES TO HAVING A COMPLIANCE PROGRAM IN PLACE

The advantages to implementing a compliance program proactively are the following:

BOX 22-1 Seven Federal Guidelines for Compliance Programs

For a compliance program to be implemented, several elements must be present so that it conforms to federal guidelines. The seven main components required for a federally approved compliance program are the following:

1. The organization has established compliance standards reasonably capable of reducing the prospect of criminal conduct.
2. High-level personnel have overall responsibility to oversee compliance.
3. Substantial discretionary authority is not delegated to individuals with a propensity to engage in illegal activities.
4. The organization has communicated standards and procedures to employees and agents.
5. The organization has taken reasonable steps to achieve compliance with its standards and to publicize a reporting system for employees without fear of retribution.
6. Standards are consistently enforced through appropriate disciplinary measures.
7. The organization takes all reasonable steps to respond appropriately to offenses and to prevent recurrences.

- Identification of potential problems within the practice before those outside the practice investigate and possibly prosecute.
- Ability to show consistency in coding protocols (Consistently wrong is better than no consistency. Consistency shows effort and eliminates the possibilities of intent to defraud.)
- Consistency of data for statistical purposes within the practice. These data may be used for contract-ing, as well as in revenue projections and budgeting for the practice.
- Ability to deal consistently with patient inquiries and complaints regarding level of service questions. All personnel can interpret how the levels of service were determined and can explain in a consistent manner to the satisfaction of the patient or third party inquiry.

CHAPTER IN REVIEW

CERTIFICATION REVIEW

- CMS and OIG have the authority to suspend, exclude, terminate, and impose fines and penalties on providers, practitioners, and suppliers who commit acts in direct violation of antifraud and antiabuse legislation.
- Fines and penalties for fraud and abuse are imposed by line item charged, rather than by claim form.
- Fraud is defined as requesting payment for services that should not be paid according to third-party guidelines.
- Abuse is defined as provision of excessive services that are not medically necessary.
- Variations on the definitions of fraud and abuse exist with each third-party carrier.
- Fraud and abuse are punishable regardless of intent.
- All parties who are involved, or who had knowledge of fraudulent activity, are liable for fraud and abuse charges.
- The financial impact to the practice from fraud and abuse charges is significant, regardless of the findings.
- All suspected fraudulent and abusive activities should be reported in writing.
- Data entry personnel should be monitored for efficiency, as well as for errors in data entry of codes.
- Claims should be reviewed by an individual knowledgeable in coding to determine whether the claims are clean and the codes are appropriately indicated.

- Coding/chart reviews should take place in the practice on a regularly scheduled basis. Coding trends or problems can be identified internally before third-party carriers identify, audit, and impose fines and penalties.
- Compliance programs are important for assuring consistency in coding and billing.
- The three main reasons providers are investigated for fraud and abuse are patient complaints, employee complaints, and level of service distribution inconsistencies.

STUDENT STUDY GUIDE

- Study Chapter 22.
- Review the Learning Objectives for Chapter 22.
- Review the Certification Review for Chapter 22.
- Complete the Chapter Review exercise to reinforce concepts learned in this chapter.

CHAPTER REVIEW EXERCISE

Complete the following exercises:
1. Give examples of fraud.
2. Give examples of abuse.
3. Outline the proper steps in reporting fraud and abuse.
4. Identify and explain what elements should be identified in a chart audit process.
5. Define the seven components that make up a Compliance Program.

23

THE CERTIFICATION PROCESS

CONGRATULATIONS on your decision to take one of the coding certification examinations. Coding certifications are designed to recognize and reward mastery in clinical coding, as well as provide a first-line defense against fraud and abuse. Certified coders are recognized and acknowledged across the country as a valuable source of professional expertise.

The demand for credentialed coders continues to skyrocket as physicians and facilities continue to experience increased fraud and abuse investigation by third-party carriers and the Office of the Inspector General. The inability to find qualified coders, unacceptable chart audit error rates, and an increased focus on coding compliance have resulted in an increased demand for certified coders.

Now that the learning process has been completed, it is time to consider the different organizations that certify coders and the types of certification that are possible. Consideration should be given to all organizations and the tests they offer that best meet the needs of the coder. Obviously, the decision to become a physician/professional coder instead of a facility coder (inpatient or outpatient) will assist in making that decision. A comparison of the different coding certification examinations offered by AAPC and AHIMA are outlined in Table 23-1. Please note that all certification examinations require registration some time in advance, so register early!

Preparing for the certification examination should not be taken lightly. It involves significant preparation time, practice, practice, and more practice! Use materials in the workbook or case study book for additional review and coding practice. Mock examinations have been included in the workbook in the event the following suggested study schedule listed is used.

As the student prepares to study for the certification examination, the following are some suggested strategies:

- Set a specific study schedule. If not preparing for the certification examinations as part of an academic program, set aside time a minimum of 4 to 6 weeks in advance of the actual examination for reviewing materials, practice coding and additional review. A sample 6-week schedule is outlined in Figure 23-1.
- Remember that examinations are time restricted so make certain when taking practice examinations/exercises to set the specific time allotted for the number of exercises that have been chosen. Keep in mind the following:
  Do not spend a great deal of time on any one question.
  Each question, regardless of length or complexity, is worth the same credit.
  Try "skipping" an extremely time-consuming or complex question to answer other questions that may be easier to correctly answer.
- Review practice examination materials, including the correct answer(s) and the rationale for successfully reaching the correct answer. If a key coding concept was missed, check the CPT-4, ICD-9-CM, or HCPCS Level II manual to make certain note(s) are sufficient to bring to mind the key concept during the actual examination.
- Only CPT-4, ICD-9-CM, and HCPCS books are allowed in the examination. Note that the AAPC examinations require the use of the AMA (American Medical Association) edition of the CPT-4 manual only. The AHIMA examinations DO allow for the use of a medical dictionary for a portion of the examination; the AAPC examinations do not. It is imperative that THE STUDENT'S additional notes for coding guidelines/tips be appropriately marked/entered in these code books. If a coding program has just been completed, it is hoped that the instructor has stressed the need for the student's own notes in these books throughout the program. In the event that notes are contained in other textbooks, personal notes, or other locations, the student may want to incorporate those notes that are unfamiliar with the student's coding books now. This will allow the student to "test" the successfulness of this material as the student prepares, takes mock examinations, and practices exercises. The student should know where to locate appropriate information needed during the actual certification examination.

The following are some additional suggestions regarding notes in code books:

Items may not be taped, glued, or pasted into coding reference books, so now is the time to remove those inserts; copy needed information into the texts to test its effectiveness.

If the student has made voluminous notes during the course of the coding program and a number of those guidelines are now imbedded in the student's mind and simply "clutter" the needed notes, the student should use a colored marker to specifically mark those notes that are needed for the test so they will stand out when the student is focusing on guidelines during the test.

Keep notes brief, perhaps in bullet format, rather than in narrative format, so they are easy to find and reference. Remember that time is an element in successfully completing the examination. These summaries needed for coding are included in the text.

Insert tabs for frequently referenced information. The professional editions of the coding books typically are already tabbed; however, additional tabs may be added to areas the coder cannot locate easily.

TABLE 23-1	Coding Certification Examinations						
Certification	Certifying Body	Exam Type	Schedule	Books Required	# Questions/ Time-5 hr	Format	Competencies Evaluated
Certified professional coder hospital (CPC-H)	AAPC	Hospital Outpatient	Quarterly by local AAPC	CPT-4 ICD-9, volume 1-3 HCPCS II	150 total	Multiple choice	Medical terminology ASC facility CPT/ICD-9 guidelines HCPCS II Human anatomy UB-92 claims Medicare guidelines APCs Revenue codes
Certified coding specialist (CCS)	AHIMA	Hospital Inpatient Ambulatory Care	Twice yearly	CPT-4 ICD-9 volume 1-3 Medical dictionary (optional) (Books used for section II only)	102 total	Multiple choice/ coding	Health info Documentation ICD-9-CM guidelines Procedure guidelines Inpatient hospital Guidelines Outpatient hospital Data quality Data management
Certified professional coder (CPC)	AAPC	Physician- based office Group practice Multispecialty specialty	Quarterly by local AAPC	CPT-4 ICD-9 volume 1-3 HCPCS II	150 total	Multiple choice	Medical Human anatomy CPT coding guidelines ICD-9 coding guidelines HCPCS level II Evaluation/ management Anesthesia Surgery Modifier use
Certified coding specialist physician (CCS-P)	AHIMA	Physician setting		CPT-4 ICD-9 volume 1-3 Medical dictionary (optional) All books for section II only	81 total	Multiple choice/ coding	Health info documentation Coding Reimbursement methods Regulatory guidelines Data quality

- Keep in mind that examinations are based on the student's comprehension of coding rules and concepts and that many of the correct answers on the examinations are based on the student's comprehension and application of coding guidelines.
- Additional study materials are available in the workbook and case studies of this test. Additional outside materials are available for preparation for the certification examination from a number of organizations. Assess whether these materials are necessary or whether the current textbook, workbook, and the additional case studies are sufficient.
- Several short mock examinations are located in the workbook with time specifications indicated for completion. Also included is a final examination that tests comprehension of all examination sections. Do not attempt the practice examinations or final practice examination until a review has been completed. Make notations in the code books and be sure to be prepared for the tests.
- All examinations require knowledge of medical terminology, anatomy, and physiology. This material

Suggested Six-Week Study Schedule

Week	Number of Hours	Concentration
1	2 hours 3 hours 2 hours 4 hours 2 hours	• Prepare medical terminology cards • Review medical terminology • Review ICD-9-CM guidelines • ICD-9-CM practice exercises • Mock exam (available in workbook) composed of medical terminology/A & P ICD-9-CM coding
Total	13 hours	
2	2 hours 2 hours 1 hour 6 hours	• Review medical terminology cards • Review general surgery guidelines integumentary, musculoskeletal, respiratory, cardiovascular, digestive systems guidelines • Addition of coding notes to book • Surgery practice exercises integumentary, musculoskeletal, respiratory, cardiovascular, digestive systems
Total	11 hours	
3	1 hour 2 hours 1 hour 6 hours	• Review medical terminology • Review surgery guidelines urinary/male/female • Addition of coding notes to book • Surgery practice exercises urinary/male/female
Total	10 hours	
4	1 hour 2 hours 1 hour 6 hours	• Review medical terminology • Review surgery guidelines nervous/eye/ear • Addition of coding notes to book • Surgery practice exercises nervous/eye/ear
Total	10 hours	
5	1 hour 1 hour 2 hours 1 hour 2 hours 1 hour	• Review medical terminology • Review surgery guidelines • Mock surgery exam (all sections) available in workbook • Review/addition of coding notes • Review radiology, pathology, medicine, HCPCS guidelines • Addition of coding notes to book
Total	8 hours	
6	2 hours 1 hour 2 hours 1 hour 5 hours 2 hours	• Mock exam radiology, pathology, medicine, HCPCS sections • Exam review/addition of notes • Mock exam (all sections) available in workbook • Exam review/addition of notes • 5 hour complete mock exam • Exam review/additional review
Total	13 hours	
Grand total:	65 hours	

FIGURE 23-1 Suggested 6-Week Study Schedule.

is tested either through specific examinations on these categories or in the student's application of this knowledge in reading and extrapolating information from operative reports and other medical record notes. Do not forget to review combining forms, suffixes, pre-

fixes, and abbreviations in preparation for the examination, as well as coding principles. If the student has not used this text as part of a medical coding program and therefore has not studied medical terminology, the student may want to purchase a medical terminology review book for this purpose. Also note that if the student possesses the professional edition of CPT-4, the introduction includes some medical terms and medical illustrations that may be modified as necessary for key words lists.

Each student should evaluate his or her knowledge level so that the student can prepare for the amount of time necessary for preparation of the certification examination.

Following are two short medical terminology examinations with 25 questions each and a 25-question coding examination to help the student determine his or her knowledge base.

Take time to evaluate the performances on the practice examinations. Determine those areas that need additional study. When coding concepts were missed, resulting in an incorrect answer, make certain the appropriate notes are outlined clearly in the CPT-4, ICD-9-CM, or HCPCS book(s).

Additional review and practice exercises are available in the workbook and case studies that accompany this book.

Study hard, review coding concepts, take the mock examinations, practice, practice, practice and you, too, can become a professional certified coder. Good Luck!!

MEDICAL TERMINOLOGY PRACTICE EXAMINATION 1

1. Histo is defined as
   a. fat
   b. nucleus
   c. organ
   d. tissue
2. Onco is defined as
   a. cancer
   b. disease
   c. tumor
   d. organ
3. The term lateral describes movement toward the
   a. front
   b. side
   c. top
   d. back
4. The outer layer of skin is called the
   a. dermis
   b. corium
   c. epidermis
   d. keratin
5. The combining form that means nail is
   a. unguo
   b. onycho
   c. tricho
   d. a and b
6. The combining form that means hidden is
   a. conio
   b. rhytido
   c. xero
   d. crypto
7. Ortho is defined as
   a. straight
   b. oxygen
   c. incomplete
   d. breathe
8. The word root that means kidney is
   a. nephro
   b. vesico
   c. reno
   d. a and c
9. The combining form pyelo is defined as
   a. bladder
   b. renal pelvis
   c. urethral meatus
   d. ureter
10. Tomo is defined as
    a. cut, section
    b. sound
    c. scanty
    d. night

11. The combining form meaning sugar is
    a. glycoso
    b. hydro
    c. glycol
    d. a and c
12. The definition of trans is
    a. around
    b. before
    c. through
    d. after
13. To give birth is denoted by the word part
    a. paro
    b. nato
    c. parto
    d. either a or c
14. The upper chambers of the heart are the
    a. atrium
    b. ventricles
    c. pericardium
    d. epicardium
15. The function of the ear is
    a. hearing
    b. equilibrium
    c. speech
    d. a and b
16. The combining form acouo means
    a. balance
    b. ear
    c. hearing
    d. a and b
17. The set of vertebrae that forms the inward curve of the spine
    a. thoracic
    b. sacral
    c. lumbar
    d. b and c
18. The first vertebra in the neck is abbreviated as
    a. C1
    b. T1
    c. L1
    d. S1
19. The upper jawbone is called the
    a. maxilla
    b. mandible
    c. clavicle
    d. ulna
20. The combining form myelo is defined as
    a. spinal cord
    b. gray matter
    c. brain
    d. nerve root
21. The combining form encephalo is defined as
    a. spinal cord
    b. brain

c. nerve root

d. cerebellum

22. The combining form phaso means

a. one

b. mind

c. speech

d. sensation

23. The combining form that means mind is

a. mento

b. phreno

c. psycho

d. all of the above

24. The combining form that means grey matter is

a. polio

b. myelo

c. meningo

d. rhizo

25. The suffix paresis is defined as

a. slight paralysis

b. sensitivity

c. seizure

d. softening

MEDICAL TERMINOLOGY PRACTICE EXAMINATION 2

1. The suffix that means control, stop, standing
   a. osis
   b. plasm
   c. genesis
   d. stasis
2. The term meaning pertaining to below is
   a. posterior
   b. dorsal
   c. inferior
   d. distal
3. The combining form myco is defined as
   a. fungus
   b. muscle
   c. oil
   d. dust
4. Adeno means
   a. wrinkles
   b. life
   c. gland
   d. scaly
5. Ostomy is a suffix that means
   a. creation of an artificial opening
   b. cut into, incision
   c. for visual examination
   d. stretching out, dilatation, expansion
6. The suffix that means surgical puncture to aspirate fluid is
   a. capnia
   b. centesis
   c. otomy
   d. either b or c
7. The prefix poly is defined as
   a. many
   b. without
   c. through
   d. few
8. The suffix that means suturing, repairing is
   a. megaly
   b. trophy
   c. orrhaphy
   d. esis
9. The term cystocele is defined as
   a. stone in the bladder
   b. drooping in the bladder
   c. protrusion of the bladder
   d. inflammation of the bladder
10. Orchidopexy is defined as
   a. surgical fixation of a testicle
   b. excision of the seminal vesicles
   c. incision into a testis
   d. surgical repair of the glans penis

11. Painful menstrual discharge is the definition of
   a. metrorrhea
   b. amenorrhea
   c. dysmenorrheal
   d. metrorrhagia
12. The prefix ante means
   a. against
   b. after
   c. before
   d. without
13. The suffix meaning hardening is
   a. malacia
   b. sclerosis
   c. penia
   d. crit
14. Cholecystectomy refers to:
   a. excision of bile
   b. excision of gallbladder
   c. excision of stones from gallbladder
   d. repair of gallbladder
15. The suffix pepsia means
   a. opening
   b. small growth
   c. tumor
   d. digestion
16. The term rectocele is defined as
   a. inflammation of the uvula
   b. prolapse of the rectum
   c. protrusion of the rectum
   d. disturbance of bowel function
17. The combining form for cornea is
   a. kerato
   b. corneo
   c. core
   d. a and b
18. The combining form cryo is
   a. cold
   b. light
   c. vision
   d. cornea
19. The wrist bone is called the
   a. radius
   b. phalange
   c. carpal
   d. calcaneus
20. The foot bones are called the
   a. phalanges
   b. metacarpals
   c. tarsals
   d. metatarsals
21. When one is lying flat on his or her back, face up, the position is known as
   a. supination

b. extension

c. inversion

d. pronation

22. The combining form that means rib is

    a. chrondro

    b. clavico

    c. claviculo

    d. costo

23. Inflammation of the membranous coverings of the brain/spinal cord

    a. duritis

    b. poliomyelitis

    c. polyneuritis

    d. meningitis

24. The term that means blood tumor below the dura mater

    a. neuroblast

    b. neuroma

    c. cerebral thrombosis

    d. subdural hematoma

25. Spondylo is defined as

    a. scapula

    b. vertebra

    c. cranium

    d. symphysis pubis

CODING PRACTICE EXAMINATION

1. Pelvic mass, rule out cervical neoplasm
   a. Cervical neoplasm
   b. 789.3
   c. 789.30
   d. 199.1
2. Viral illness with exposure to strep throat
   a. 079.00
   b. V01.8
   c. 079.99, V02.52
   d. 079.99
3. Fracture distal radius following fall from steps of bus
   a. 813.42
   b. 813.44
   c. E817.1
   d. 813.42, E817.1
4. Blood pressure reading of 220/150
   a. 401.1
   b. 401.9
   c. 796.2
   d. 401.0
5. Uncontrolled hypertension
   a. 401.9
   b. 401.1
   c. 401.0
   d. 796.2
6. Expressive aphasia
   History of cerebrovascular accident
   a. 784.3
   b. 784.30
   c. 784.30, V12.59
   d. 315.31, V12.59
7. COPD with bronchitis
   a. 491.20
   b. 491.21
   c. 496, 490
   d. 496
8. Gastritis as a result of erythromycin
   a. 535.50
   b. 535.50, 995.2, E930.3
   c. 535.50, E930.3
   d. 995.2, E930.3
9. Patient arrives at the physician's office for exacerbation of asthma. During the wait to see the physician, the patient experiences extreme difficulty in breathing. The patient is seen immediately, IV medications are started, and the physician continues to treat the patient until the patient becomes stable and the ambulance arrives, approximately 45 minutes.

   a. 99215-21
   b. 99215
   c. 99291
   d. none of the above
10. Patient is readmitted to the skilled nursing facility after recent hospitalization. Readmission required comprehensive reassessment and establishment of a new treatment plan as the result of her recent stroke. Additional medications, physical therapy, and changes in her daily treatment protocol are established by the physician with moderate MDM.
    a. 99303
    b. 99313
    c. 99238
    d. 99310
11. Patient schedules an appointment for an annual examination. A comprehensive history and examination are performed on this 62-year-old male during which time a gastrointestinal ulcer is discovered as well as the diagnosis of hypertension. The patient is requested to return in 1 week for further evaluation and treatment of these two problems.
    a. 99213
    b. 99396
    c. 99396, 99212-25
    d. 99396, 99212
12. Patient is admitted to observation care at 11:00 PM for chest pain, presumably cardiac in origin. A detailed history, comprehensive examination, and low MDM complexity are performed. The patient is discharged at 11:00 AM the following day after reevaluation by the physician. Discharge diagnosis is musculoskeletal chest pain.
    a. 99218
    b. 99219, 99217
    c. 99218, 99217
    d. 99238
13. Anesthesia should be coded with the codes from the surgery section of the CPT-4 code book.
    a. true
    b. false
14. P1 indicates
    a. Patient in otherwise good health
    b. Patient has other chronic health problems
    c. The patient successfully passes anesthesia screening with a score of "P1"
    d. None of the above
15. Chest x-ray, PA only is performed at the hospital. The hospital will bill
    a. 71020
    b. 71010
    c. 71010-TC
    d. None of the above

16. X-rays taken and interpreted on Bilateral Standing Knees, AP; code as:
    a. 73560-RT, 73560-LT
    b. 73560, 73560-50
    c. 73565
    d. None of the above

17. Pathologists would use what codes for consultations?
    a. E & M consultation codes only
    b. E & M codes when an evaluation and management are performed; clinical path consultations when no patient E & M is performed
    c. Clinical path consults only
    d. Whichever the pathologists choose to use as long as they are consistent

18. Arthroscope was inserted into the shoulder and the surfaces of the humeral head and glenoid were intact without evidence of cracking or tears. The rotator cuff showed fraying, and the decision was made to perform an arthroscopic acromioplasty. A rotary shaver was used to perform a bursectomy with debris removed via shaver. A rotary burr was then used to perform an anterior inferior acromioplasty with debris produced removed via suction. Because of the location of the tear, the decision was made to repair the rotator cuff through a miniarthrotomy. This was accomplished and the procedure was completed.
    a. 29826
    b. 23410, 29826-51
    c. 23412
    d. 23415

19. Left knee arthroscopy is done under four portals, anterolateral, anteromedial, superolateral, and posteromedial. The diagnostic arthroscopy was started placing the arthroscope in the anterolateral portal. There is severe fibrosis and hypertrophy of the fat pad and Grade 2 and 3 chondromalacia of the femoral condyle. A partial medial meniscectomy is performed as well as a partial lateral meniscectomy, after which a chondroplasty of the patellofemoral joint was performed.
    a. 29880-LT
    b. 29880-LT, 29877-59-LT, 29870-50-LT
    c. 29880-LT, 29877-59-LT
    d. 29881-LT

20. Patient was prepped in usual manner, and the scope was advanced through the cecum. There was an area that appeared to be flat and had an almost flat lesion, where I took a few biopsy specimens. The rest of the colon appeared normal. In the sigmoid colon two polyps were identified and both were snared in toto and retrieved.
    a. 45385, 45380-51, 45378-51
    b. 45385

c. 45385, 45378-51
d. 45385, 45380-51

21. Chronic wound of the left thigh. FTSG was obtained from the right thigh and placed on a 4 × 4-cm chronic wound on the left thigh after appropriate flushing and irrigation.
    a. 15100, 15000
    b. 15000
    c. 15200
    d. 15100

22. Closed reduction with manipulation of a metacarpal fracture of the thumb and index finger. With the patient under general anesthesia, the patient was placed in position, and a lateral incision was made distal to the fractures. Guidewires, pins, and screws were inserted to percutaneous fixate the fractures. Closure performed with 2-0 and 3-0 Dexon and a short arm splint applied.
    a. 26605 X2
    b. 26608 X2
    c. 26608
    d. 26650

23. A 2-cm infraumbilical incision was performed, peritoneum was insufflated, trocar was introduced, and scope was introduced. Liver, bowel, appendix, bladder, and uterus appeared normal. There were multiple cysts on the left ovary consistent with benign follicular cysts, which were aspirated. Chromotubation was then performed and bilateral tubal patency was documented.
    a. 49322
    b. 58350
    c. 49322, 58350-51
    d. 58679

24. Patient with Serous Otitis Media presents for replacement of right ventilation tube and placement of left myringotomy tube. After the administration of general anesthesia, the right tube was examined and determined to need removal. A replacement tube was placed in the right ear. A myringotomy was performed and fluid was aspirated. A modified T-grommet tube was placed in the right ear.
    a. 69436-LT, 39436-76-52-RT
    b. 69436-50
    c. 69421-50
    d. 69436-LT, 69424-RT

25. Patient presents with left axillary swelling. Left axilla was prepped and incision was made. Axillary contents were removed and there were some enlarged lymph nodes.
    a. 38530
    b. 38500
    c. 38520
    d. 38525

ICD-9-CM OFFICIAL GUIDELINES FOR CODING AND REPORTING

Effective December 1, 2005

The Centers for Medicare and Medicaid Services (CMS) and the National Center for Health Statistics (NCHS), two departments within the U. S. Federal Government's Department of Health and Human Services (DHHS) provide the following guidelines for coding and reporting using the International Classification of Diseases, 9th Revision, Clinical Modification (ICD-9-CM). These guidelines should be used as a companion document to the official version of the ICD-9-CM as published on CD-ROM by the U.S. Government Printing Office (GPO).

These guidelines have been approved by the four organizations that make up the Cooperating Parties for the ICD-9-CM: the American Hospital Association (AHA), the American Health Information Management Association (AHIMA), CMS, and NCHS. These guidelines are included on the official government version of the ICD-9-CM, and also appear in *"Coding Clinic for ICD-9-CM"* published by the AHA.

These guidelines are a set of rules that have been developed to accompany and complement the official conventions and instructions provided within the ICD-9-CM itself. These guidelines are based on the coding and sequencing instructions in Volumes I, II and III of ICD-9-CM, but provide additional instruction. Adherence to these guidelines when assigning ICD-9-CM diagnosis and procedure codes is required under the Health Insurance Portability and Accountability Act (HIPAA). The diagnosis codes (Volumes 1-2) have been adopted under HIPAA for all healthcare settings. Volume 3 procedure codes have been adopted for inpatient procedures reported by hospitals. A joint effort between the healthcare provider and the coder is essential to achieve complete and accurate documentation, code assignment, and reporting of diagnoses and procedures. These guidelines have been developed to assist both the healthcare provider and the coder in identifying those diagnoses and procedures that

Source: Centers for Medicare and Medicaid Services and National Center for Health Statistics.

are to be reported. The importance of consistent, complete documentation in the medical record cannot be overemphasized. Without such documentation accurate coding cannot be achieved. The entire record should be reviewed to determine the specific reason for the encounter and the conditions treated.

The term encounter is used for all settings, including hospital admissions. In the context of these guidelines, the term provider is used throughout the guidelines to mean physician or any qualified health care practitioner who is legally accountable for establishing the patient's diagnosis. Only this set of guidelines, approved by the Cooperating Parties, is official.

The guidelines are organized into sections. Section I includes the structure and conventions of the classification and general guidelines that apply to the entire classification, and chapter-specific guidelines that correspond to the chapters as they are arranged in the classification. Section II includes guidelines for selection of principal diagnosis for non-outpatient settings. Section III includes guidelines for reporting additional diagnoses in non-outpatient settings. Section IV is for outpatient coding and reporting.

ICD-9-CM OFFICIAL GUIDELINES FOR CODING AND REPORTING

Section I. Conventions, general coding guidelines and chapter specific guidelines
  A. Conventions for the ICD-9-CM
    1. Format
    2. Abbreviations
      a. Index abbreviations
      b. Tabular abbreviations
    3. Punctuation
    4. Includes and Excludes Notes and Inclusion terms
    5. Other and Unspecified codes
      a. "Other" codes
      b. "Unspecified" codes

6. Etiology/manifestation convention ("code first," "use additional code" and "in diseases classified elsewhere" notes)
7. "And"
8. "With"
9. "See" and "See Also"
B. General Coding Guidelines
   1. Use of Both Alphabetic Index and Tabular List
   2. Locate each term in the Alphabetic Index
   3. Level of Detail in Coding
   4. Code or codes from 001.0 through V84.8
   5. Selection of codes 001.0 through 999.9
   6. Signs and symptoms
   7. Conditions that are an integral part of a disease process
   8. Conditions that are not an integral part of a disease process
   9. Multiple coding for a single condition
   10. Acute and Chronic Conditions
   11. Combination Code
   12. Late Effects
   13. Impending or Threatened Condition
C. Chapter-Specific Coding Guidelines
   1. Chapter 1: Infectious and Parasitic Diseases (001-139)
      a. Human Immunodeficiency Virus (HIV) Infections
      b. Septicemia, Systemic Inflammatory Response Syndrome (SIRS), Sepsis, Severe Sepsis, and Septic Shock
   2. Chapter 2: Neoplasms (140-239)
      a. Treatment directed at the malignancy
      b. Treatment of secondary site
      c. Coding and sequencing of complications
      d. Primary malignancy previously excised
      e. Admissions/Encounters involving chemotherapy, immunotherapy and radiation therapy
      f. Admission/encounter to determine extent of malignancy
      g. Symptoms, signs, and ill-defined conditions listed in Chapter 16
   3. Chapter 3: Endocrine, Nutritional, and Metabolic Diseases and Immunity Disorders (240-279)
      a. Diabetes mellitus

4. Chapter 4: Diseases of Blood and Blood Forming Organs (280-289)
   a. Anemia of chronic disease
5. Chapter 5: Mental Disorders (290-319)
   Reserved for future guideline expansion
6. Chapter 6: Diseases of Nervous System and Sense Organs (320-389)
   Reserved for future guideline expansion
7. Chapter 7: Diseases of Circulatory System (390-459)
   a. Hypertension
   b. Cerebral infarction/stroke/cerebrovascular accident (CVA)
   c. Postoperative cerebrovascular accident
   d. Late Effects of Cerebrovascular Disease
   e. Acute myocardial infarction (AMI)
8. Chapter 8: Diseases of Respiratory System (460-519)
   a. Chronic Obstructive Pulmonary Disease [COPD] and Asthma
   b. Chronic Obstructive Pulmonary Disease [COPD] and Bronchitis
9. Chapter 9: Diseases of Digestive System (520-579)
   Reserved for future guideline expansion
10. Chapter 10: Diseases of Genitourinary System (580-629)
   a. Chronic kidney disease
11. Chapter 11: Complications of Pregnancy, Childbirth, and the Puerperium (630-677)
   a. General Rules for Obstetric Cases
   b. Selection of OB Principal or First-listed Diagnosis
   c. Fetal Conditions Affecting the Management of the Mother
   d. HIV Infection in Pregnancy, Childbirth and the Puerperium
   e. Current Conditions Complicating Pregnancy
   f. Diabetes mellitus in pregnancy
   g. Gestational diabetes
   h. Normal Delivery, Code 650
   i. The Postpartum and Peripartum Periods
   j. Code 677, Late effect of complication of pregnancy
   k. Abortions
12. Chapter 12: Diseases Skin and Subcutaneous Tissue (680-709)

Reserved for future guideline expansion

13. Chapter 13: Diseases of Musculoskeletal and Connective Tissue (710-739)
    Reserved for future guideline expansion

14. Chapter 14: Congenital Anomalies (740-759)
    a. Codes in categories 740-759, Congenital Anomalies

15. Chapter 15: Newborn (Perinatal) Guidelines (760-779)
    a. General Perinatal Rules
    b. Use of codes V30-V39
    c. Newborn transfers
    d. Use of category V29
    e. Use of other V codes on perinatal records
    f. Maternal Causes of Perinatal Morbidity
    g. Congenital Anomalies in Newborns
    h. Coding Additional Perinatal Diagnoses
    i. Prematurity and Fetal Growth Retardation
    j. Newborn sepsis

16. Chapter 16: Signs, Symptoms and Ill-Defined Conditions (780-799)
    Reserved for future guideline expansion

17. Chapter 17: Injury and Poisoning (800-999)
    a. Coding of Injuries
    b. Coding of Fractures
    c. Coding of Burns
    d. Coding of Debridement of Wound, Infection, or Burn
    e. Adverse Effects, Poisoning and Toxic Effects
    f. Complications of care

18. Classification of Factors Influencing Health Status and Contact with Health Service (Supplemental V01-V84)
    a. Introduction
    b. V codes use in any healthcare setting
    c. V Codes indicate a reason for an encounter
    d. Categories of V Codes
    e. V Code Table

19. Supplemental Classification of External Causes of Injury and Poisoning (E-codes, E800-E999)

    a. General E Code Coding Guidelines
    b. Place of Occurrence Guideline
    c. Adverse Effects of Drugs, Medicinal and Biological Substances Guidelines
    d. Multiple Cause E Code Coding Guidelines
    e. Child and Adult Abuse Guideline
    f. Unknown or Suspected Intent Guideline
    g. Undetermined Cause
    h. Late Effects of External Cause Guidelines
    i. Misadventures and Complications of Care Guidelines
    j. Terrorism Guidelines

Section II.   Selection of Principal Diagnosis
    A. Codes for symptoms, signs, and ill-defined conditions
    B. Two or more interrelated conditions, each potentially meeting the definition for principal Diagnosis
    C. Two or more diagnoses that equally meet the definition for principal diagnosis
    D. Two or more comparative or contrasting conditions
    E. A symptom(s) followed by contrasting/comparative diagnoses
    F. Original treatment plan not carried out
    G. Complications of surgery and other medical care
    H. Uncertain Diagnosis
    I. Admission from Observation Unit
        1. Admission Following Medical Observation
        2. Admission Following Post-Operative Observation
    J. Admission from Outpatient Surgery

Section III.   Reporting Additional Diagnoses
    A. Previous conditions
    B. Abnormal findings
    C. Uncertain Diagnosis

Section IV.   Diagnostic Coding and Reporting Guidelines for Outpatient Services
    A. Selection of first-listed condition
        1. Outpatient Surgery
        2. Observation Stay
    B. Codes from 001.0 through V84.8
    C. Accurate reporting of ICD-9-CM diagnosis codes
    D. Selection of codes 001.0 through 999.9
    E. Codes that describe symptoms and signs

F. Encounters for circumstances other than a disease or injury

G. Level of Detail in Coding
 1. ICD-9-CM codes with 3, 4, or 5 digits
 2. Use of full number of digits required for a code

H. ICD-9-CM code for the diagnosis, condition, problem, or other reason for encounter/visit

I. "Probable," "suspected," "questionable," "rule out," or "working diagnosis"

J. Chronic diseases

K. Code all documented conditions that coexist

L. Patients receiving diagnostic services only

M. Patients receiving therapeutic services only

N. Patients receiving preoperative evaluations only

O. Ambulatory surgery

P. Routine outpatient prenatal visits

SECTION I. CONVENTIONS, GENERAL CODING GUIDELINES AND CHAPTER SPECIFIC GUIDELINES

The conventions, general guidelines and chapter-specific guidelines are applicable to all health care settings unless otherwise indicated.

A. Conventions for the ICD-9-CM

The conventions for the ICD-9-CM are the general rules for use of the classification independent of the guidelines. These conventions are incorporated within the index and tabular of the ICD-9-CM as instructional notes. The conventions are as follows:

1. Format:
 The ICD-9-CM uses an indented format for ease in reference

2. Abbreviations
 a. Index abbreviations
  NEC "Not elsewhere classifiable"
  This abbreviation in the index represents "other specified" when a specific code is not available for a condition the index directs the coder to the "other specified" code in the tabular.
 b. Tabular abbreviations
  NEC "Not elsewhere classifiable"
  This abbreviation in the tabular represents "other specified." When a specific code is not available for a condition the tabular includes an NEC entry under a code to identify the

code as the "other specified" code (See Section I.A.5.a. "Other" codes).
  NOS "Not otherwise specified"
  This abbreviation is the equivalent of unspecified. (See Section I.A.5.b., "Unspecified" codes)

3. Punctuation
 [ ] Brackets are used in the tabular list to enclose synonyms, alternative wording or explanatory phrases. Brackets are used in the index to identify manifestation codes. (See Section I.A.6. "Etiology/manifestations")
 ( ) Parentheses are used in both the index and tabular to enclose supplementary words that may be present or absent in the statement of a disease or procedure without affecting the code number to which it is assigned. The terms within the parentheses are referred to as nonessential modifiers.
 : Colons are used in the Tabular list after an incomplete term which needs one or more of the modifiers following the colon to make it assignable to a given category.

4. Includes and Excludes Notes and Inclusion terms
 Includes: This note appears immediately under a three-digit code title to further define, or give examples of, the content of the category.
 Excludes: An excludes note under a code indicates that the terms excluded from the code are to be coded elsewhere. In some cases the codes for the excluded terms should not be used in conjunction with the code from which it is excluded. An example of this is a congenital condition excluded from an acquired form of the same condition. The congenital and acquired codes should not be used together. In other cases, the excluded terms may be used together with an excluded code. An example of this is when fractures of different bones are coded to different codes. Both codes may be used together if both types of fractures are present.
 Inclusion terms: List of terms is included under certain four and five digit codes. These terms are the conditions for which that code number is to be used. The terms may be synonyms of the code title, or, in the case of "other specified" codes, the terms are a list of the various conditions assigned to that code. The inclusion terms are not necessarily exhaustive. Additional terms found only in the index may also be assigned to a code.

5. Other and Unspecified codes
   a. "Other" codes
      Codes titled "other" or "other specified" (usually a code with a 4th digit 8 or fifth-digit 9 for diagnosis codes) are for use when the information in the medical record provides detail for which a specific code does not exist. Index entries with NEC in the line designate "other" codes in the tabular. These index entries represent specific disease entities for which no specific code exists so the term is included within an "other" code.
   b. "Unspecified" codes
      Codes (usually a code with a 4th digit 9 or 5th digit 0 for diagnosis codes) titled "unspecified" are for use when the information in the medical record is insufficient to assign a more specific code.

6. Etiology/manifestation convention ("code first," "use additional code" and "in diseases classified elsewhere" notes)
   Certain conditions have both an underlying etiology and multiple body system manifestations due to the underlying etiology. For such conditions, the ICD-9-CM has a coding convention that requires the underlying condition be sequenced first followed by the manifestation. Wherever such a combination exists, there is a "use additional code" note at the etiology code, and a "code first" note at the manifestation code. These instructional notes indicate the proper sequencing order of the codes, etiology followed by manifestation.

   In most cases the manifestation codes will have in the code title, "in diseases classified elsewhere." Codes with this title are a component of the etiology/manifestation convention. The code title indicates that it is a manifestation code. "In diseases classified elsewhere" codes are never permitted to be used as first listed or principal diagnosis codes. They must be used in conjunction with an underlying condition code and they must be listed following the underlying condition.

   There are manifestation codes that do not have "in diseases classified elsewhere" in the title. For such codes a "use additional code" note will still be present and the rules for sequencing apply.

   In addition to the notes in the tabular, these conditions also have a specific index entry structure. In the index both conditions are listed together with the etiology code first followed by the manifestation codes in brackets. The code in brackets is always to be sequenced second.

   The most commonly used etiology/manifestation combinations are the codes for Diabetes mellitus, category 250. For each code under category 250 there is a use additional code note for the manifestation that is specific for that particular diabetic manifestation. Should a patient have more than one manifestation of diabetes, more than one code from category 250 may be used with as many manifestation codes as are needed to fully describe the patient's complete diabetic condition. The category 250 diabetes codes should be sequenced first, followed by the manifestation codes.

   "Code first" and "Use additional code" notes are also used as sequencing rules in the classification for certain codes that are not part of an etiology/manifestation combination. See—Section I.B.9. "Multiple coding for a single condition."

7. "And"
   The word "and" should be interpreted to mean either "and" or "or" when it appears in a title.

8. "With"
   The word "with" in the alphabetic index is sequenced immediately following the main term, not in alphabetical order.

9. "See" and "See Also"
   The "see" instruction following a main term in the index indicates that another term should be referenced. It is necessary to go to the main term referenced with the "see" note to locate the correct code.

   A "see also" instruction following a main term in the index instructs that there is another main term that may also be referenced that may provide additional index entries that may be useful. It is not necessary to follow the "see also" note when the original main term provides the necessary code.

B. General Coding Guidelines
   1. Use of Both Alphabetic Index and Tabular List
      Use both the Alphabetic Index and the Tabular List when locating and assigning a code. Reliance on only the Alphabetic Index or the Tabular List leads to errors in code assignments and less specificity in code selection.
   2. Locate each term in the Alphabetic Index
      Locate each term in the Alphabetic Index and verify the code selected in the Tabular List. Read and be guided by instructional notations that appear in both the Alphabetic Index and the Tabular List.
   3. Level of Detail in Coding
      Diagnosis and procedure codes are to be used at their highest number of digits available.

      ICD-9-CM diagnosis codes are composed of codes with either 3, 4, or 5 digits. Codes with three digits are included in ICD-9-CM as the heading of a category of codes that may be further subdivided by the use of fourth and/or fifth digits, which provide greater detail.

      A three-digit code is to be used only if it is not further subdivided. Where fourth-digit subcategories and/or fifth-digit subclassifications are provided, they must be assigned. A code is invalid if it has not been coded to the full number of digits required for that code. For example, Acute myocardial infarction, code 410, has fourth digits that describe the location of the infarction (e.g., 410.2, Of inferolateral wall), and fifth digits that identify the episode of care. It would be incorrect to report a code in category 410 without a fourth and fifth digit.

ICD-9-CM Volume 3 procedure codes are composed of codes with either 3 or 4 digits. Codes with two digits are included in ICD-9-CM as the heading of a category of codes that may be further subdivided by the use of third and/or fourth digits, which provide greater detail.

4. Code or codes from 001.0 through V84.8
The appropriate code or codes from 001.0 through V84.8 must be used to identify diagnoses, symptoms, conditions, problems, complaints or other reason(s) for the encounter/visit.

5. Selection of codes 001.0 through 999.9
The selection of codes 001.0 through 999.9 will frequently be used to describe the reason for the admission/encounter. These codes are from the section of ICD-9-CM for the classification of diseases and injuries (e.g., infectious and parasitic diseases; neoplasms; symptoms, signs, and ill-defined conditions, etc.).

6. Signs and symptoms
Codes that describe symptoms and signs, as opposed to diagnoses, are acceptable for reporting purposes when a related definitive diagnosis has not been established (confirmed) by the provider. Chapter 16 of ICD-9-CM, Symptoms, Signs, and Ill-defined conditions (codes 780.0–799.9) contain many, but not all codes for symptoms.

7. Conditions that are an integral part of a disease process
Signs and symptoms that are integral to the disease process should not be assigned as additional codes.

8. Conditions that are not an integral part of a disease process
Additional signs and symptoms that may not be associated routinely with a disease process should be coded when present.

9. Multiple coding for a single condition
In addition to the etiology/manifestation convention that requires two codes to fully describe a single condition that affects multiple body systems, there are other single conditions that also require more than one code. "Use additional code" notes are found in the tabular at codes that are not part of an etiology/manifestation pair where a secondary code is useful to fully describe a condition. The sequencing rule is the same as the etiology/manifestation pair - , "use additional code" indicates that a secondary code should be added.

For example, for infections that are not included in chapter 1, a secondary code from category 041, Bacterial infection in conditions classified elsewhere and of unspecified site, may be required to identify the bacterial organism causing the infection. A "use additional code" note will normally be found at the infectious disease code, indicating a need for the organism code to be added as a secondary code.

"Code first" notes are also under certain codes that are not specifically manifestation codes but may be due to an underlying cause. When a "code first" note is present and an underlying condition is present the underlying condition should be sequenced first.

"Code, if applicable, any causal condition first," notes indicate that this code may be assigned as a principal diagnosis when the causal condition is unknown or not applicable. If a causal condition is known, then the code for that condition should be sequenced as the principal or first-listed diagnosis.

Multiple codes may be needed for late effects, complication codes and obstetric codes to more fully describe a condition. See the specific guidelines for these conditions for further instruction.

10. Acute and Chronic Conditions
If the same condition is described as both acute (subacute) and chronic, and separate subentries exist in the Alphabetic Index at the same indentation level, code both and sequence the acute (subacute) code first.

11. Combination Code
A combination code is a single code used to classify:
Two diagnoses, or
A diagnosis with an associated secondary process (manifestation)
A diagnosis with an associated complication
Combination codes are identified by referring to subterm entries in the Alphabetic Index and by reading the inclusion and exclusion notes in the Tabular List.

Assign only the combination code when that code fully identifies the diagnostic conditions involved or when the Alphabetic Index so directs. Multiple coding should not be used when the classification provides a combination code that clearly identifies all of the elements documented in the diagnosis. When the combination code lacks necessary specificity in describing the manifestation or complication, an additional code should be used as a secondary code.

12. Late Effects
A late effect is the residual effect (condition produced) after the acute phase of an illness or injury has terminated. There is no time limit on when a late effect code can be used. The residual may

be apparent early, such as in cerebrovascular accident cases, or it may occur months or years later, such as that due to a previous injury. Coding of late effects generally requires two codes sequenced in the following order: The condition or nature of the late effect is sequenced first. The late effect code is sequenced second.

An exception to the above guidelines are those instances where the code for late effect is followed by a manifestation code identified in the Tabular List and title, or the late effect code has been expanded (at the fourth and fifth-digit levels) to include the manifestation(s). The code for the acute phase of an illness or injury that led to the late effect is never used with a code for the late effect.

13. Impending or Threatened Condition

Code any condition described at the time of discharge as "impending" or "threatened" as follows:

If it did occur, code as confirmed diagnosis.

If it did not occur, reference the Alphabetic Index to determine if the condition has a subentry term for "impending" or "threatened" and also reference main term entries for "Impending" and for "Threatened."

If the subterms are listed, assign the given code.

If the subterms are not listed, code the existing underlying condition(s) and not the condition described as impending or threatened.

C. Chapter-Specific Coding Guidelines

In addition to general coding guidelines, there are guidelines for specific diagnoses and/or conditions in the classification. Unless otherwise indicated, these guidelines apply to all health care settings. Please refer to Section II for guidelines on the selection of principal diagnosis.

1. Chapter 1: Infectious and Parasitic Diseases (001-139)

a. Human Immunodeficiency Virus (HIV) Infections

1) Code only confirmed cases

Code only confirmed cases of HIV infection/illness. This is an exception to the hospital inpatient guideline Section II, H.

In this context, "confirmation" does not require documentation of positive serology or culture for HIV; the provider's diagnostic statement that the patient is HIV positive, or has an HIV-related illness is sufficient.

2) Selection and sequencing of HIV codes

(a) Patient admitted for HIV-related condition

If a patient is admitted for an HIV-related condition, the principal diagnosis should be 042, followed by additional diagnosis codes for all reported HIV-related conditions.

(b) Patient with HIV disease admitted for unrelated condition

If a patient with HIV disease is admitted for an unrelated condition (such as a traumatic injury), the code for the unrelated condition (e.g., the nature of injury code) should be the principal diagnosis. Other diagnoses would be 042 followed by additional diagnosis codes for all reported HIV-related conditions.

(c) Whether the patient is newly diagnosed

Whether the patient is newly diagnosed or has had previous admissions/encounters for HIV conditions is irrelevant to the sequencing decision.

(d) Asymptomatic human immunodeficiency virus

V08 Asymptomatic human immunodeficiency virus [HIV] infection, is to be applied when the patient without any documentation of symptoms is listed as being "HIV positive," "known HIV," "HIV test positive," or similar terminology. Do not use this code if the term "AIDS" is used or if the patient is treated for any HIV-related illness or is described as having any condition(s) resulting from his/her HIV positive status; use 042 in these cases.

(e) Patients with inconclusive HIV serology

Patients with inconclusive HIV serology, but no definitive diagnosis or manifestations of the illness, may be assigned code 795.71, Inconclusive serologic test for Human Immunodeficiency Virus [HIV].

(f) Previously diagnosed HIV-related illness

Patients with any known prior diagnosis of an HIV-related illness should be coded to 042. Once a patient has developed an HIV-related illness, the patient should always be assigned code 042 on every subsequent admission/encounter. Patients previously diagnosed with any HIV illness (042) should never be assigned to 795.71 or V08.

(g) HIV Infection in Pregnancy, Childbirth and the Puerperium

During pregnancy, childbirth or the puerperium, a patient admitted (or presenting for a health care encounter) because of an HIV-related illness should receive a principal diagnosis code of 647.6X, Other specified infectious and parasitic diseases in the mother classifiable elsewhere, but complicating the pregnancy, childbirth or the puerperium, followed by 042 and the code(s) for the HIV-related illness(es). Codes from Chapter 15 always take sequencing priority.

Patients with asymptomatic HIV infection status admitted (or presenting for a health care encounter) during pregnancy, childbirth, or the puerperium should receive codes of 647.6X and V08.

(h) Encounters for testing for HIV

If a patient is being seen to determine his/her HIV status, use code V73.89, Screening for other specified viral disease. Use code V69.8, Other problems related to lifestyle, as a secondary code if an asymptomatic patient is in a known high risk group for HIV. Should a patient with signs or symptoms or illness, or a confirmed HIV related diagnosis be tested for HIV, code the signs and symptoms or the diagnosis. An additional counseling code V65.44 may be used if counseling is provided during the encounter for the test.

When a patient returns to be informed of his/her HIV test results use code V65.44, HIV counseling, if the results of the test are negative.

If the results are positive but the patient is asymptomatic use code V08, Asymptomatic HIV infection. If the results are positive and the patient is symptomatic use code 042, HIV infection, with codes for the HIV related symptoms or diagnosis. The HIV counseling code may also be used if counseling is provided for patients with positive test results.

b. Septicemia, Systemic Inflammatory Response Syndrome (SIRS), Sepsis, Severe Sepsis, and Septic Shock

1) Sepsis as principal diagnosis or secondary diagnosis

(a) Sepsis as principal diagnosis

If sepsis is present on admission, and meets the definition of principal diagnosis, the underlying systemic infection code (e.g., 038.xx, 112.5, etc) should be assigned as the principal diagnosis, followed by code 995.91, Systemic inflammatory response syndrome due to infectious process without organ dysfunction, as required by the sequencing rules in the Tabular List. Codes from

subcategory 995.9 can never be assigned as a principal diagnosis.

(b) Sepsis as secondary diagnoses

When sepsis develops during the encounter (it was not present on admission), the sepsis codes may be assigned as secondary diagnoses, following the sequencing rules provided in the Tabular List.

(c) Documentation unclear as to whether sepsis present on admission

If the documentation is not clear whether the sepsis was present on admission, the provider should be queried. After provider query, if sepsis is determined at that point to have met the definition of principal diagnosis, the underlying systemic infection (038.xx, 112.5, etc) may be used as principal diagnosis along with code 995.91, Systemic inflammatory response syndrome due to infectious process without organ dysfunction.

2) Septicemia/Sepsis

In most cases, it will be a code from category 038, Septicemia, that will be used in conjunction with a code from subcategory 995.9 such as the following:

(a) Streptococcal sepsis

If the documentation in the record states streptococcal sepsis, codes 038.0 and code 995.91 should be used, in that sequence.

(b) Streptococcal septicemia

If the documentation states streptococcal septicemia, only code 038.0 should be assigned, however, the provider should be queried whether the patient has sepsis, an infection with SIRS.

(c) Sepsis or SIRS must be documented

Either the term sepsis or SIRS must be documented, to assign a code from subcategory 995.9.

3) Terms sepsis, severe sepsis, or SIRS

If the terms sepsis, severe sepsis, or SIRS are used with an underlying infection other than septicemia, such as pneumonia, cellulitis or a nonspecified urinary tract infection, a code from category 038 should be assigned first, then code 995.91, followed by the code for the initial infection. The use of the terms sepsis or SIRS indicates that the patient's infection has advanced to the point of a systemic infection so the systemic infection should be sequenced before the localized infection.

The instructional note under subcategory 995.9 instructs to assign the underlying systemic infection first.

Note: The term urosepsis is a nonspecific term. If that is the only term documented then only code 599.0 should be assigned based on the default for the term in the ICD-9-CM index, in addition to the code for the causal organism if known.

4) Severe sepsis

For patients with severe sepsis, the code for the systemic infection (e.g., 038.xx, 112.5, etc) or trauma should be sequenced first, followed by either code 995.92, Systemic inflammatory response syndrome due to infectious process with organ dysfunction, or code 995.94, Systemic inflammatory response syndrome due to noninfectious process with organ dysfunction. Codes for the specific organ dysfunctions should also be assigned.

5) Septic shock

(a) Sequencing of septic shock

Septic shock is a form of organ dysfunction associated with severe sepsis. A code for the initiating underlying systemic infection followed by a code for SIRS (code 995.92) must be assigned before the code for septic shock. As noted in the sequencing instructions in the Tabular List, the code for septic shock cannot be assigned as a principal diagnosis.

(b) Septic Shock without documentation of severe sepsis

Septic shock cannot occur in the absence of severe sepsis. A code from subcategory 995.9 must be sequenced before the code for septic shock. The use additional code notes and the code first note provide sequencing instructions.

6) Sepsis and septic shock associated with abortion

Sepsis and septic shock associated with abortion, ectopic pregnancy, and molar pregnancy are classified to category codes in Chapter 11 (630-639).

7) Negative or inconclusive blood cultures

Negative or inconclusive blood cultures do not preclude a diagnosis of septicemia or sepsis in patients with clinical evidence of the condition, however, the provider should be queried.

8) Newborn sepsis

See Section I.C.15.j for information on the coding of newborn sepsis.

9) Sepsis due to a Postprocedural Infection

Sepsis resulting from a postprocedural infection is a complication of care. For such cases code 998.59, Other postoperative infections, should be coded first followed by the appropriate codes for the sepsis. The other guidelines for coding sepsis should then be followed for the assignment of additional codes.

10) External cause of injury codes with SIRS

An external cause code is not needed with codes 995.91, Systemic inflammatory response syndrome due to infectious process without organ dysfunction, or code 995.92, Systemic inflammatory response syndrome due to infectious process with organ dysfunction.

Refer to Section I.C.19.a.7 for instruction on the use of external cause of injury codes with codes for SIRS resulting from trauma.

2. Chapter 2: Neoplasms (140-239)

General guidelines

Chapter 2 of the ICD-9-CM contains the codes for most benign and all malignant neoplasms. Certain benign neoplasms, such as prostatic adenomas, may be found in the specific body system chapters. To properly code a neoplasm it is necessary to determine from the record if the neoplasm is benign, in-situ, malignant, or of uncertain histologic behavior. If malignant, any secondary (metastatic) sites should also be determined.

The neoplasm table in the Alphabetic Index should be referenced first. However, if the histological term is documented, that term should be referenced first, rather than going immediately to the Neoplasm Table, in order to determine which column in the Neoplasm Table is appropriate. For example, if the documentation indicates "adenoma," refer to the term in the Alphabetic Index to review the entries under this term and the instructional note to "see also neoplasm, by site, benign." The table provides the proper code based on the type of neoplasm and the site. It is important to select the proper column in the table that corresponds to the type of neoplasm. The tabular should then be referenced to verify that the correct code has been selected from the table and that a more specific site code does not exist.

See Section I. C. 18.d.4. for information regarding V codes for genetic susceptibility to cancer.

a. Treatment directed at the malignancy

If the treatment is directed at the malignancy, designate the malignancy as the principal diagnosis.

b. Treatment of secondary site

When a patient is admitted because of a primary neoplasm with metastasis and treatment is directed toward the secondary site only, the secondary neoplasm is designated as the principal diagnosis even though the primary malignancy is still present.

c. Coding and sequencing of complications

Coding and sequencing of complications associated with the malignancies or with the therapy thereof are subject to the following guidelines:

1) Anemia associated with malignancy

When admission/encounter is for management of an anemia associated with the malignancy, and the treatment is only for anemia, the appropriate anemia code (such as code 285.22, Anemia in neoplastic disease) is designated as the principal diagnosis and is followed by the appropriate code(s) for the malignancy.

Code 285.22 may also be used as a secondary code if the patient suffers from anemia and is being treated for the malignancy.

2) Anemia associated with chemotherapy, immunotherapy and radiation therapy

When the admission/encounter is for management of an anemia associated with chemotherapy, immunotherapy or radiotherapy and the only treatment is for the anemia, the anemia is sequenced first followed by code E933.1. The appropriate neoplasm code should be assigned as an additional code.

3) Management of dehydration due to the malignancy

When the admission/encounter is for management of dehydration due to the malignancy or the therapy, or a combination of both, and only the dehydration is being treated (intravenous rehydration), the dehydration is sequenced first, followed by the code(s) for the malignancy.

4) Treatment of a complication resulting from a surgical procedure

When the admission/encounter is for treatment of a complication resulting from a surgical procedure, designate the complication as the principal or first-listed diagnosis if treatment is directed at resolving the complication.

d. Primary malignancy previously excised

When a primary malignancy has been previously excised or eradicated from its site and there is no further treatment directed to that site and there is no evidence of any existing primary malignancy, a code from category V10, Personal history of malignant neoplasm, should be used to indicate the former site of the malignancy. Any mention of extension, invasion, or metastasis to another site is coded as a secondary malignant neoplasm to that site. The secondary site may be the principal or first-listed with the V10 code used as a secondary code.

e. Admissions/Encounters involving chemotherapy, immunotherapy and radiation therapy

1) Episode of care involves surgical removal of neoplasm

When an episode of care involves the surgical removal of a neoplasm, primary or secondary site, followed by adjunct chemotherapy or radiation treatment during the same episode of care, the neoplasm code should be assigned as principal or first-listed diagnosis, using codes in the 140-198 series or where appropriate in the 200-203 series.

2) Patient admission/encounter solely for administration of chemotherapy, immunotherapy and radiation therapy

If a patient admission/encounter is solely for the administration of chemotherapy, V58.11, Encounter for antineoplastic chemotherapy, or V58.12, Encounter for antineoplastic immunotherapy as the first-listed or principal diagnosis. If a patient receives more than one of these therapies during the same admission more than one of these codes may be assigned, in any sequence.

3) Patient admitted for radiotherapy/chemotherapy and immunotherapy and develops complications

When a patient is admitted for the purpose of radiotherapy, immunotherapy or chemotherapy and develops complications such as uncontrolled nausea and vomiting or dehydration, the principal or first-listed diagnosis is V58.0, Encounter for radiotherapy, or V58.11, Encounter for antineoplastic chemotherapy, or V58.12, Encounter for antineoplastic immunotherapy followed by any codes for the complications.

See Section I.C.18.d.7. for additional information regarding aftercare V codes.

f. Admission/encounter to determine extent of malignancy

When the reason for admission/encounter is to determine the extent of the malignancy, or for a procedure such as paracentesis or thoracentesis, the primary malignancy or appropriate metastatic site is designated as the principal or first-listed diagnosis, even though chemotherapy or radiotherapy is administered.

g. Symptoms, signs, and ill-defined conditions listed in Chapter 16

Symptoms, signs, and ill-defined conditions listed in Chapter 16 characteristic of, or associated with, an existing primary or secondary site malignancy cannot be used to replace the malignancy as principal or first-listed diagnosis, regardless of the number of admissions or encounters for treatment and care of the neoplasm.

See section I.C.18.d.14, Encounter for prophylactic organ removal

3. Chapter 3: Endocrine, Nutritional, and Metabolic Diseases and Immunity Disorders (240-279)

a. Diabetes mellitus

Codes under category 250, Diabetes mellitus, identify complications/manifestations associated with diabetes mellitus. A fifth-digit is required for all category 250 codes to identify the type of diabetes mellitus and whether the diabetes is controlled or uncontrolled.

1) Fifth-digits for category 250:

The following are the fifth-digits for the codes under category 250:

0 type II or unspecified type, not stated as uncontrolled

1 type I, [juvenile type], not stated as uncontrolled

2 type II or unspecified type, uncontrolled

3 type I, [juvenile type], uncontrolled

The age of a patient is not the sole determining factor, though most type I diabetics develop the condition before reaching puberty. For this reason type I diabetes mellitus is also referred to as juvenile diabetes.

2) Type of diabetes mellitus not documented

If the type of diabetes mellitus is not documented in the medical record the default is type II.

3) Diabetes mellitus and the use of insulin

All type I diabetics must use insulin to replace what their bodies do not produce. However, the use of insulin does not mean that a patient is a type I diabetic. Some patients with type II diabetes mellitus are unable to control their blood sugar through diet and oral medication alone and do require insulin. If the documentation in a medical record does not indicate the type of diabetes but does indicate that the patient uses insulin, the appropriate fifth-digit for type II must be used. For type II patients who routinely use insulin, code V58.67, Long-term (current) use of insulin, should also be assigned to indicate that the patient uses insulin. Code V58.67 should not be assigned if insulin is given temporarily to bring a type II patient's blood sugar under control during an encounter.

4) Assigning and sequencing diabetes codes and associated conditions

When assigning codes for diabetes and its associated conditions, the code(s) from category 250 must be sequenced before the codes for the associated conditions. The diabetes codes and the secondary codes that correspond to them are paired codes that follow the etiology/manifestation convention of the classification (See Section I.A.6., Etiology/manifestation convention). Assign as many codes from category 250 as needed to identify all of the associated conditions that the patient has. The corresponding secondary codes are listed under each of the diabetes codes.

(a) Diabetic retinopathy/diabetic macular edema

Diabetic macular edema, code 362.07, is only present with diabetic retinopathy. Another code from subcategory 362.0, Diabetic retinopathy, must be used with code 362.07. Codes under subcategory 362.0 are diabetes manifestation codes, so they must be used following the appropriate diabetes code.

5) Diabetes mellitus in pregnancy and gestational diabetes

(a) For diabetes mellitus complicating pregnancy, see Section I.C.11.f., Diabetes mellitus in pregnancy.

(b) For gestational diabetes, see Section I.C.11, g., Gestational diabetes.

6) Insulin pump malfunction

(a) Underdose of insulin due insulin pump failure

An underdose of insulin due to an insulin pump failure should be assigned 996.57, Mechanical complication due to insulin pump, as the principal or first listed code, followed by the appropriate diabetes mellitus code based on documentation.

(b) Overdose of insulin due to insulin pump failure

The principal or first listed code for an encounter due to an insulin pump malfunction resulting in an overdose of insulin, should also be 996.57, Mechanical complication due to insulin pump, followed by code 962.3, Poisoning by insulins and antidiabetic agents, and the appropriate diabetes mellitus code based on documentation.

4. Chapter 4: Diseases of Blood and Blood Forming Organs (280-289)

a. Anemia of chronic disease
   Subcategory 285.2, Anemia in chronic illness, has codes for anemia in chronic kidney disease, code 285.21; anemia in neoplastic disease, code 285.22; and anemia in other chronic illness, code 285.29. These codes can be used as the principal/first listed code if the reason for the encounter is to treat the anemia. They may also be used as secondary codes if treatment of the anemia is a component of an encounter, but not the primary reason for the encounter. When using a code from subcategory 285 it is also necessary to use the code for the chronic condition causing the anemia.
   1) Anemia in chronic kidney disease
      When assigning code 285.21, Anemia in chronic kidney disease. It is also necessary to assign a code from category 585, Chronic kidney disease, to indicate the stage of chronic kidney disease. See I.C.10.a. Chronic kidney disease (CKD)
   2) Anemia in neoplastic disease
      When assigning code 285.22, Anemia in neoplastic disease, it is also necessary to assign the neoplasm code that is responsible for the anemia. Code 285.22 is for use for anemia that is due to the malignancy, not for anemia due to antineoplastic chemotherapy drugs, which is an adverse effect.
         See I.C.2.c.1 Anemia associated with malignancy
         See I.C.2.c.2 Anemia associated with chemotherapy, immunotherapy and radiation therapy
         See I.C.17.e.1. Adverse effects
5. Chapter 5: Mental Disorders (290-319)
   Reserved for future guideline expansion
6. Chapter 6: Diseases of Nervous System and Sense Organs (320-389)
   Reserved for future guideline expansion
7. Chapter 7: Diseases of Circulatory System (390-459)
   a. Hypertension
      Hypertension Table
         The Hypertension Table, found under the main term, "Hypertension," in the Alphabetic Index, contains a complete listing of all conditions due to or associated with hypertension and classifies them according to malignant, benign, and unspecified.
         1) Hypertension, Essential, or NOS
            Assign hypertension (arterial) (essential) (primary) (systemic) (NOS) to category code 401 with the appropriate fourth digit to indicate malignant (.0), benign (.1), or unspecified (.9). Do not use either .0

malignant or .1 benign unless medical record documentation supports such a designation.
   2) Hypertension with Heart Disease
      Heart conditions (425.8, 429.0-429.3, 429.8, 429.9) are assigned to a code from category 402 when a causal relationship is stated (due to hypertension) or implied (hypertensive). Use an additional code from category 428 to identify the type of heart failure in those patients with heart failure. More than one code from category 428 may be assigned if the patient has systolic or diastolic failure and congestive heart failure.
         The same heart conditions (425.8, 429.0-429.3, 429.8, 429.9) with hypertension, but without a stated causal relationship, are coded separately. Sequence according to the circumstances of the admission/encounter.
   3) Hypertensive Kidney Disease
      Assign codes from category 403, Hypertensive kidney disease, when conditions classified to categories 585-587 are present. Unlike hypertension with heart disease, ICD-9-CM presumes a cause-and-effect relationship and classifies renal failure with hypertension as hypertensive kidney disease.
   4) Hypertensive Heart and Kidney Disease
      Assign codes from combination category 404, Hypertensive heart and kidney disease, when both hypertensive kidney disease and hypertensive heart disease are stated in the diagnosis. Assume a relationship between the hypertension and the kidney disease, whether or not the condition is so designated. Assign an additional code from category 428, to identify the type of heart failure. More than one code from category 428 may be assigned if the patient has systolic or diastolic failure and congestive heart failure.
   5) Hypertensive Cerebrovascular Disease
      First assign codes from 430-438, Cerebrovascular disease, then the appropriate hypertension code from categories 401-405.
   6) Hypertensive Retinopathy
      Two codes are necessary to identify the condition. First assign the code from subcategory 362.11, Hypertensive retinopathy, then the appropriate code from categories 401-405 to indicate the type of hypertension.
   7) Hypertension, Secondary

Two codes are required: one to identify the underlying etiology and one from category 405 to identify the hypertension. Sequencing of codes is determined by the reason for admission/encounter.

8) Hypertension, Transient
Assign code 796.2, Elevated blood pressure reading without diagnosis of hypertension, unless patient has an established diagnosis of hypertension. Assign code 642.3x for transient hypertension of pregnancy.

9) Hypertension, Controlled
Assign appropriate code from categories 401-405. This diagnostic statement usually refers to an existing state of hypertension under control by therapy.

10) Hypertension, Uncontrolled
Uncontrolled hypertension may refer to untreated hypertension or hypertension not responding to current therapeutic regimen. In either case, assign the appropriate code from categories 401-405 to designate the stage and type of hypertension. Code to the type of hypertension.

11) Elevated Blood Pressure
For a statement of elevated blood pressure without further specificity, assign code 796.2, Elevated blood pressure reading without diagnosis of hypertension, rather than a code from category 401.

b. Cerebral infarction/stroke/cerebrovascular accident (CVA)
The terms stroke and CVA are often used interchangeably to refer to a cerebral infarction. The terms stroke, CVA, and cerebral infarction NOS are all indexed to the default code 434.91, cerebral artery occlusion, unspecified, with infarction. Code 436, Acute, but ill-defined, cerebrovascular disease, should not be used when the documentation states stroke or CVA.

c. Postoperative cerebrovascular accident
A cerebrovascular hemorrhage or infarction that occurs as a result of medical intervention is coded to 997.02, Iatrogenic cerebrovascular infarction or hemorrhage. Medical record documentation should clearly specify the cause-and-effect relationship between the medical intervention and the cerebrovascular accident in order to assign this code. A secondary code from the code range 430-432 or from a code from subcategories 433 or 434 with a fifth digit of "1" should also be used to identify the type of hemorrhage or infarct.

This guideline conforms to the use additional code note instruction at category 997. Code 436, Acute, but ill-defined, cerebrovascular disease, should not be used as a secondary code with code 997.02.

d. Late Effects of Cerebrovascular Disease
1) Category 438, Late Effects of Cerebrovascular disease
Category 438 is used to indicate conditions classifiable to categories 430-437 as the causes of late effects (neurologic deficits), themselves classified elsewhere. These "late effects" include neurologic deficits that persist after initial onset of conditions classifiable to 430-437. The neurologic deficits caused by cerebrovascular disease may be present from the onset or may arise at any time after the onset of the condition classifiable to 430-437.

2) Codes from category 438 with codes from 430-437
Codes from category 438 may be assigned on a health care record with codes from 430-437, if the patient has a current cerebrovascular accident (CVA) and deficits from an old CVA.

3) Code V12.59
Assign code V12.59 (and not a code from category 438) as an additional code for history of cerebrovascular disease when no neurologic deficits are present.

e. Acute myocardial infarction (AMI)
1) ST elevation myocardial infarction (STEMI) and non ST elevation myocardial infarction (NSTEMI)
The ICD-9-CM codes for acute myocardial infarction (AMI) identify the site, such as anterolateral wall or true posterior wall. Subcategories 410.0-410.6 and 410.8 are used for ST elevation myocardial infarction (STEMI). Subcategory 410.7, Subendocardial infarction, is used for non ST elevation myocardial infarction (NSTEMI) and nontransmural MIs.

2) Acute myocardial infarction, unspecified
Subcategory 410.9 is the default for the unspecified term acute myocardial infarction. If only STEMI or transmural MI without the site is documented, query the provider as to the site, or assign a code from subcategory 410.9.

3) AMI documented as nontransmural or subendocardial but site provided
If an AMI is documented as nontransmural or subendocardial, but the site is provided, it is still coded as a subendocardial AMI. If NSTEMI evolves to STEMI, assign the STEMI code. If STEMI converts to NSTEMI due to thrombolytic therapy, it is still coded as STEMI.

8. Chapter 8: Diseases of Respiratory System (460-519)
   a. Chronic Obstructive Pulmonary Disease [COPD] and Asthma
      1) Conditions that comprise COPD and Asthma
      The conditions that comprise COPD are obstructive chronic bronchitis, subcategory 491.2, and emphysema, category 492. All asthma codes are under category 493, Asthma. Code 496, Chronic airway obstruction, not elsewhere classified, is a nonspecific code that should only be used when the documentation in a medical record does not specify the type of COPD being treated.
      2) Acute exacerbation of chronic obstructive bronchitis and asthma
      The codes for chronic obstructive bronchitis and asthma distinguish between uncomplicated cases and those in acute exacerbation. An acute exacerbation is a worsening or a decompensation of a chronic condition. An acute exacerbation is not equivalent to an infection superimposed on a chronic condition, though an exacerbation may be triggered by an infection.
      3) Overlapping nature of the conditions that comprise COPD and asthma
      Due to the overlapping nature of the conditions that make up COPD and asthma, there are many variations in the way these conditions are documented. Code selection must be based on the terms as documented. When selecting the correct code for the documented type of COPD and asthma, it is essential to first review the index, and then verify the code in the tabular list. There are many instructional notes under the different COPD subcategories and codes. It is important that all such notes be reviewed to assure correct code assignment.
      4) Acute exacerbation of asthma and status asthmaticus
      An acute exacerbation of asthma is an increased severity of the asthma symptoms, such as wheezing and shortness of breath. Status asthmaticus refers to a patient's failure to respond to therapy administered during an asthmatic episode and is a life threatening complication that requires emergency care. If status asthmaticus is documented by the provider with any type of COPD or with acute bronchitis, the status asthmaticus should be sequenced first. It supersedes any type of COPD including that with acute

exacerbation or acute bronchitis. It is inappropriate to assign an asthma code with 5th digit 2, with acute exacerbation, together with an asthma code with 5th digit 1, with status asthmatics. Only the 5th digit 1 should be assigned.
   b. Chronic Obstructive Pulmonary Disease [COPD] and Bronchitis
      1) Acute bronchitis with COPD
      Acute bronchitis, code 466.0, is due to an infectious organism. When acute bronchitis is documented with COPD, code 491.22, Obstructive chronic bronchitis with acute bronchitis, should be assigned. It is not necessary to also assign code 466.0. If a medical record documents acute bronchitis with COPD with acute exacerbation, only code 491.22 should be assigned. The acute bronchitis included in code 491.22 supersedes the acute exacerbation. If a medical record documents COPD with acute exacerbation without mention of acute bronchitis, only code 491.21 should be assigned.
9. Chapter 9: Diseases of Digestive System (520-579)
   Reserved for future guideline expansion
10. Chapter 10: Diseases of Genitourinary System (580-629)
   a. Chronic kidney disease
      1) Stages of chronic kidney disease (CKD)
      The ICD-9-CM classifies CKD based on severity. The severity of CKD is designated by stages I-V. Stage II, code 585.2, equates to mild CKD; stage III, code 585.3, equates to moderate CKD; and stage IV, code 585.4, equates to severe CKD. Code 585.6, End stage renal disease (ESRD), is assigned when the provider has documented end-stage-renal disease (ESRD).
         If both a stage of CKD and ESRD are documented, assign code 585.6 only.
      2) Chronic kidney disease and kidney transplant status
      Patients who have undergone kidney transplant may still have some form of CKD because the kidney transplant may not fully restore kidney function. Code V42.0 may be assigned with the appropriate CKD code for patients who are status post kidney transplant, based on the patient's post-transplant stage. The use additional code note under category 585 provides this instruction.
         Use of a 585 code with V42.0 does not necessarily indicate transplant rejection or failure. Patients with mild or moderate CKD following a transplant should not be coded as having transplant failure, unless it is doc-

umented in the medical record. For patients with severe CKD or ESRD it is appropriate to assign code 996.81, Complications of transplanted organ, kidney transplant, when kidney transplant failure is documented. If a post kidney transplant patient has CKD and it is unclear from the documentation whether there is transplant failure or rejection it is necessary to query the provider.

3) Chronic kidney disease with other conditions

Patients with CKD may also suffer from other serious conditions, most commonly diabetes mellitus and hypertension. The sequencing of the CKD code in relationship to codes for other contributing conditions is based on the conventions in the tabular list.

See I.C.3.a.4 for sequencing instructions for diabetes.

See I.C.4.a.1. for anemia in CKD.

See I.C.7.a.3 for hypertensive kidney disease.

See I.C.17.f.1.b. Transplant complications, for instructions on coding of documented rejection or failure.

11. Chapter 11: Complications of Pregnancy, Childbirth, and the Puerperium (630-677)

a. General Rules for Obstetric Cases

1) Codes from chapter 11 and sequencing priority

Obstetric cases require codes from chapter 11, codes in the range 630-677, Complications of Pregnancy, Childbirth, and the Puerperium. Chapter 11 codes have sequencing priority over codes from other chapters. Additional codes from other chapters may be used in conjunction with chapter 11 codes to further specify conditions. Should the provider document that the pregnancy is incidental to the encounter, then code V22.2 should be used in place of any chapter 11 codes. It is the provider's responsibility to state that the condition being treated is not affecting the pregnancy.

2) Chapter 11 codes used only on the maternal record

Chapter 11 codes are to be used only on the maternal record, never on the record of the newborn.

3) Chapter 11 fifth-digits

Categories 640-648, 651-676 have required fifth-digits, which indicate whether the encounter is antepartum, postpartum and whether a delivery has also occurred.

4) Fifth-digits, appropriate for each code

The fifth-digits, which are appropriate for each code number, are listed in brackets under each code. The fifth-digits on each code should all be consistent with each other. That is, should a delivery occur all of the fifth-digits should indicate the delivery.

b. Selection of OB Principal or First-listed Diagnosis

1) Routine outpatient prenatal visits

For routine outpatient prenatal visits when no complications are present codes V22.0, Supervision of normal first pregnancy, and V22.1, Supervision of other normal pregnancy, should be used as the first-listed diagnoses. These codes should not be used in conjunction with chapter 11 codes.

2) Prenatal outpatient visits for high-risk patients

For prenatal outpatient visits for patients with high-risk pregnancies, a code from category V23, Supervision of high-risk pregnancy, should be used as the principal or first-listed diagnosis. Secondary chapter 11 codes may be used in conjunction with these codes if appropriate.

3) Episodes when no delivery occurs

In episodes when no delivery occurs, the principal diagnosis should correspond to the principal complication of the pregnancy, which necessitated the encounter. Should more than one complication exist, all of which are treated or monitored, any of the complications codes may be sequenced first.

4) When a delivery occurs

When a delivery occurs, the principal diagnosis should correspond to the main circumstances or complication of the delivery. In cases of cesarean delivery, the selection of the principal diagnosis should correspond to the reason the cesarean delivery was performed unless the reason for admission/encounter was unrelated to the condition resulting in the cesarean delivery.

5) Outcome of delivery

An outcome of delivery code, V27.0-V27.9, should be included on every maternal record when a delivery has occurred. These codes are not to be used on subsequent records or on the newborn record.

c. Fetal Conditions Affecting the Management of the Mother

1) Codes from category 655

Known or suspected fetal abnormality affecting management of the mother, and category 656, Other fetal and placental problems affecting the management of the mother, are assigned only when the fetal condition is actually responsible for modifying the management of the mother, i.e., by requiring diagnostic studies, additional observation, special care, or termination of pregnancy. The fact that the fetal condition exists does not justify assigning a code from this series to the mother's record.

2) In utero surgery

In cases when surgery is performed on the fetus, a diagnosis code from category 655, Known or suspected fetal abnormalities affecting management of the mother, should be assigned identifying the fetal condition. Procedure code 75.36, Correction of fetal defect, should be assigned on the hospital inpatient record.

No code from Chapter 15, the perinatal codes, should be used on the mother's record to identify fetal conditions. Surgery performed in utero on a fetus is still to be coded as an obstetric encounter.

d. HIV Infection in Pregnancy, Childbirth and the Puerperium

During pregnancy, childbirth or the puerperium, a patient admitted because of an HIV-related illness should receive a principal diagnosis of 647.6X, Other specified infectious and parasitic diseases in the mother classifiable elsewhere, but complicating the pregnancy, childbirth or the puerperium, followed by 042 and the code(s) for the HIV-related illness(es).

Patients with asymptomatic HIV infection status admitted during pregnancy, childbirth, or the puerperium should receive codes of 647.6X and V08.

e. Current Conditions Complicating Pregnancy

Assign a code from subcategory 648.x for patients that have current conditions when the condition affects the management of the pregnancy, childbirth, or the puerperium. Use additional secondary codes from other chapters to identify the conditions, as appropriate.

f. Diabetes mellitus in pregnancy

Diabetes mellitus is a significant complicating factor in pregnancy. Pregnant women who are diabetic should be assigned code 648.0x, Diabetes mellitus complicating pregnancy, and a secondary code from category 250, Diabetes mellitus, to identify the type of diabetes.

Code V58.67, Long-term (current) use of insulin, should also be assigned if the diabetes mellitus is being treated with insulin.

g. Gestational diabetes

Gestational diabetes can occur during the second and third trimester of pregnancy in women who were not diabetic prior to preg-

nancy. Gestational diabetes can cause complications in the pregnancy similar to those of pre-existing diabetes mellitus. It also puts the woman at greater risk of developing diabetes after the pregnancy. Gestational diabetes is coded to 648.8x, Abnormal glucose tolerance. Codes 648.0x and 648.8x should never be used together on the same record.

Code V58.67, Long-term (current) use of insulin, should also be assigned if the gestational diabetes is being treated with insulin.

h. Normal Delivery, Code 650

1) Normal delivery

Code 650 is for use in cases when a woman is admitted for a full-term normal delivery and delivers a single, healthy infant without any complications antepartum, during the delivery, or postpartum during the delivery episode. Code 650 is always a principal diagnosis. It is not to be used if any other code from chapter 11 is needed to describe a current complication of the antenatal, delivery, or perinatal period. Additional codes from other chapters may be used with code 650 if they are not related to or are in any way complicating the pregnancy.

2) Normal delivery with resolved antepartum complication

Code 650 may be used if the patient had a complication at some point during her pregnancy, but the complication is not present at the time of the admission for delivery.

3) V27.0, Single liveborn, outcome of delivery

V27.0, Single liveborn, is the only outcome of delivery code appropriate for use with 650.

i. The Postpartum and Peripartum Periods

1) Postpartum and peripartum periods

The postpartum period begins immediately after delivery and continues for six weeks following delivery. The peripartum period is defined as the last month of pregnancy to five months postpartum.

2) Postpartum complication

A postpartum complication is any complication occurring within the six-week period.

3) Pregnancy-related complications after 6 week period

Chapter 11 codes may also be used to describe pregnancy-related complications after the six-week period should the provider document that a condition is pregnancy related.

4) Postpartum complications occurring during the same admission as delivery

Postpartum complications that occur during the same admission as the delivery are identified with a fifth digit of "2." Subsequent admissions/encounters for postpartum complications should be identified with a fifth digit of "4."

5) Admission for routine postpartum care following delivery outside hospital

When the mother delivers outside the hospital prior to admission and is admitted for routine postpartum care and no complications are noted, code V24.0, Postpartum care and examination immediately after delivery, should be assigned as the principal diagnosis.

6) Admission following delivery outside hospital with postpartum conditions

A delivery diagnosis code should not be used for a woman who has delivered prior to admission to the hospital. Any postpartum conditions and/or postpartum procedures should be coded.

j. Code 677, Late effect of complication of pregnancy

1) Code 677

Code 677, Late effect of complication of pregnancy, childbirth, and the puerperium is for use in those cases when an initial complication of a pregnancy develops a sequelae requiring care or treatment at a future date.

2) After the initial postpartum period

This code may be used at any time after the initial postpartum period.

3) Sequencing of Code 677

This code, like all late effect codes, is to be sequenced following the code describing the sequelae of the complication.

k. Abortions

1) Fifth-digits required for abortion categories

Fifth-digits are required for abortion categories 634-637. Fifth-digit 1, incomplete, indicates that all of the products of conception have not been expelled from the uterus. Fifth-digit 2, complete, indicates that all products of conception have been expelled from the uterus prior to the episode of care.

2) Code from categories 640-648 and 651-659

A code from categories 640-648 and 651-659 may be used as additional codes with an abortion code to indicate the complication leading to the abortion.

Fifth digit 3 is assigned with codes from these categories when used with an abortion code because the other fifth digits will not apply. Codes from the 660-669 series are not to be used for complications of abortion.

3) Code 639 for complications

Code 639 is to be used for all complications following abortion. Code 639 cannot be assigned with codes from categories 634-638.

4) Abortion with Liveborn Fetus

When an attempted termination of pregnancy results in a liveborn fetus assign code 644.21, Early onset of delivery, with an appropriate code from category V27, Outcome of Delivery. The procedure code for the attempted termination of pregnancy should also be assigned.

5) Retained Products of Conception following an abortion

Subsequent admissions for retained products of conception following a spontaneous or legally induced abortion are assigned the appropriate code from category 634, Spontaneous abortion, or 635 Legally induced abortion, with a fifth digit of "1" (incomplete). This advice is appropriate even when the patient was discharged previously with a discharge diagnosis of complete abortion.

12. Chapter 12: Diseases Skin and Subcutaneous Tissue (680-709)

Reserved for future guideline expansion

13. Chapter 13: Diseases of Musculoskeletal and Connective Tissue (710-739)

Reserved for future guideline expansion

14. Chapter 14: Congenital Anomalies (740-759)

a. Codes in categories 740-759, Congenital Anomalies

Assign an appropriate code(s) from categories 740-759, Congenital Anomalies, when an anomaly is documented. A congenital anomaly may be the principal/first listed diagnosis on a record or a secondary diagnosis.

When a congenital anomaly does not have a unique code assignment, assign additional code(s) for any manifestations that may be present.

When the code assignment specifically identifies the congenital anomaly, manifestations that are an inherent component of the anomaly should not be coded separately. Additional codes should be assigned for manifestations that are not an inherent component.

Codes from Chapter 14 may be used throughout the life of the patient. If a congenital anomaly has been corrected, a personal history code should be used to identify the history of the anomaly. Although present at birth, a congenital anomaly may not be identified until later in life. Whenever the condition is diagnosed by the physician, it is appropriate to assign a code from codes 740-759.

For the birth admission, the appropriate code from category V30, Liveborn infants, according to type of birth should be sequenced as the principal diagnosis, followed by any congenital anomaly codes, 740759.

15. Chapter 15: Newborn (Perinatal) Guidelines (760-779)

For coding and reporting purposes the perinatal period is defined as before birth through the 28th day following birth. The following guidelines are provided for reporting purposes. Hospitals may record other diagnoses as needed for internal data use.

a. General Perinatal Rules

1) Chapter 15 Codes

They are never for use on the maternal record. Codes from Chapter 11, the obstetric chapter, are never permitted on the newborn record. Chapter 15 code may be used throughout the life of the patient if the condition is still present.

2) Sequencing of perinatal codes

Generally, codes from Chapter 15 should be sequenced as the principal/first-listed diagnosis on the newborn record, with the exception of the appropriate V30 code for the birth episode, followed by codes from any other chapter that provide additional detail. The "use additional code" note at the beginning of the chapter supports this guideline. If the index does not provide a specific code for a perinatal condition, assign code 779.89, Other specified conditions originating in the perinatal period, followed by the code from another chapter that specifies the condition. Codes for signs and symptoms may be assigned when a definitive diagnosis has not been established.

3) Birth process or community acquired conditions

If a newborn has a condition that may be either due to the birth process or community acquired and the documentation does not indicate which it is, the default is due to the birth process and the code from Chapter 15 should be used. If the condition is community-acquired, a code from Chapter 15 should not be assigned.

4) Code all clinically significant conditions

All clinically significant conditions noted on routine newborn examination should be coded. A condition is clinically significant if it requires:

- clinical evaluation; or
- therapeutic treatment; or
- diagnostic procedures; or
- extended length of hospital stay; or

- increased nursing care and/or monitoring; or
- has implications for future health care needs

Note: The perinatal guidelines listed above are the same as the general coding guidelines for "additional diagnoses," except for the final point regarding implications for future health care needs. Codes should be assigned for conditions that have been specified by the provider as having implications for future health care needs. Codes from the perinatal chapter should not be assigned unless the provider has established a definitive diagnosis.

b. Use of codes V30-V39

When coding the birth of an infant, assign a code from categories V30-V39, according to the type of birth. A code from this series is assigned as a principal diagnosis, and assigned only once to a newborn at the time of birth.

c. Newborn transfers

If the newborn is transferred to another institution, the V30 series is not used at the receiving hospital.

d. Use of category V29

1) Assigning a code from category V29

Assign a code from category V29, Observation and evaluation of newborns and infants for suspected conditions not found, to identify those instances when a healthy newborn is evaluated for a suspected condition that is determined after study not to be present. Do not use a code from category V29 when the patient has identified signs or symptoms of a suspected problem; in such cases, code the sign or symptom.

A code from category V29 may also be assigned as a principal code for readmissions or encounters when the V30 code no longer applies. Codes from category V29 are for use only for healthy newborns and infants for which no condition after study is found to be present.

2) V29 code on a birth record

A V29 code is to be used as a secondary code after the V30, Outcome of delivery, code.

e. Use of other V codes on perinatal records

V codes other than V30 and V29 may be assigned on a perinatal or newborn record code. The codes may be used as a principal or first-listed diagnosis for specific types of encounters or for readmissions or encounters when the V30 code no longer applies.

See Section I.C.18 for information regarding the assignment of V codes.

f. Maternal Causes of Perinatal Morbidity
Codes from categories 760-763, Maternal causes of perinatal morbidity and mortality, are assigned only when the maternal condition has actually affected the fetus or newborn. The fact that the mother has an associated medical condition or experiences some complication of pregnancy, labor or delivery does not justify the routine assignment of codes from these categories to the newborn record.

g. Congenital Anomalies in Newborns
For the birth admission, the appropriate code from category V30, Liveborn infants according to type of birth, should be used, followed by any congenital anomaly codes, categories 740-759. Use additional secondary codes from other chapters to specify conditions associated with the anomaly, if applicable.

Also, see Section I.C.14 for information on the coding of congenital anomalies.

h. Coding Additional Perinatal Diagnoses
1) Assigning codes for conditions that require treatment
Assign codes for conditions that require treatment or further investigation, prolong the length of stay, or require resource utilization.
2) Codes for conditions specified as having implications for future health care needs
Assign codes for conditions that have been specified by the provider as having implications for future health care needs.
Note: This guideline should not be used for adult patients.
3) Codes for newborn conditions originating in the perinatal period
Assign a code for newborn conditions originating in the perinatal period (categories 760-779), as well as complications arising during the current episode of care classified in other chapters, only if the diagnoses have been documented by the responsible provider at the time of transfer or discharge as having affected the fetus or newborn.

i. Prematurity and Fetal Growth Retardation
Providers utilize different criteria in determining prematurity. A code for prematurity should not be assigned unless it is documented. The 5th digit assignment for codes from category 764 and subcategories 765.0 and 765.1 should be based on the recorded birth weight and estimated gestational age.

A code from subcategory 765.2, Weeks of gestation, should be assigned as an additional code with category 764 and codes from 765.0 and 765.1 to specify weeks of gestation as documented by the provider in the record.

j. Newborn sepsis
Code 771.81, Septicemia [sepsis] of newborn, should be assigned with a secondary code from category 041, Bacterial infections in conditions classified elsewhere and of unspecified site, to identify the organism. It is not necessary to use a code from subcategory 995.9, Systemic inflammatory response syndrome (SIRS), on a newborn record. A code from category 038, Septicemia, should not be used on a newborn record. Code 771.81 describes the sepsis.

16. Chapter 16: Signs, Symptoms and Ill-Defined Conditions (780-799)
Reserved for future guideline expansion

17. Chapter 17: Injury and Poisoning (800-999)
a. Coding of Injuries
When coding injuries, assign separate codes for each injury unless a combination code is provided, in which case the combination code is assigned. Multiple injury codes are provided in ICD-9-CM, but should not be assigned unless information for a more specific code is not available. These codes are not to be used for normal, healing surgical wounds or to identify complications of surgical wounds.

The code for the most serious injury, as determined by the provider and the focus of treatment, is sequenced first.
1) Superficial injuries
Superficial injuries such as abrasions or contusions are not coded when associated with more severe injuries of the same site.
2) Primary injury with damage to nerves/blood vessels
When a primary injury results in minor damage to peripheral nerves or blood vessels, the primary injury is sequenced first with additional code(s) from categories 950-957, Injury to nerves and spinal cord, and/or 900-904, Injury to blood vessels. When the primary injury is to the blood vessels or nerves, that injury should be sequenced first.

b. Coding of Fractures
The principles of multiple coding of injuries should be followed in coding fractures. Fractures of specified sites are coded individually by site in accordance with both the provisions within categories 800-829 and the level of detail furnished by medical record content. Combination categories for multiple fractures are provided for use when there is insufficient detail in the medical record (such as trauma cases transferred to another hospital), when the reporting form limits the number of codes that can be used in reporting pertinent clinical data, or when there is insufficient specificity at

the fourth-digit or fifth-digit level. More specific guidelines are as follows:

1) Multiple fractures of same limb
   Multiple fractures of same limb classifiable to the same three-digit or four-digit category are coded to that category.

2) Multiple unilateral or bilateral fractures of same bone
   Multiple unilateral or bilateral fractures of same bone(s) but classified to different fourth-digit subdivisions (bone part) within the same three-digit category are coded individually by site.

3) Multiple fracture categories 819 and 828
   Multiple fracture categories 819 and 828 classify bilateral fractures of both upper limbs (819) and both lower limbs (828), but without any detail at the fourth-digit level other than open and closed type of fractures.

4) Multiple fractures sequencing
   Multiple fractures are sequenced in accordance with the severity of the fracture. The provider should be asked to list the fracture diagnoses in the order of severity.

c. Coding of Burns
   Current burns (940–948) are classified by depth, extent and by agent (E code). Burns are classified by depth as first degree (erythema), second degree (blistering), and third degree (full-thickness involvement).

   1) Sequencing of burn and related condition codes
      Sequence first the code that reflects the highest degree of burn when more than one burn is present.
      a. When the reason for the admission or encounter is for treatment of external multiple burns, sequence first the code that reflects the burn of the highest degree.
      b. When a patient has both internal and external burns, the circumstances of admission govern the selection of the principal diagnosis or first-listed diagnosis.
      c. When a patient is admitted for burn injuries and other related conditions such as smoke inhalation and/or respiratory failure, the circumstances of admission govern the selection of the principal or first-listed diagnosis.

   2) Burns of the same local site
      Classify burns of the same local site (three-digit category level, 940–947) but of different degrees to the subcategory identifying the highest degree recorded in the diagnosis.

3) Non-healing burns
   Non-healing burns are coded as acute burns.
   Necrosis of burned skin should be coded as a non-healed burn.

4) Code 958.3, Posttraumatic wound infection
   Assign code 958.3, Posttraumatic wound infection, not elsewhere classified, as an additional code for any documented infected burn site.

5) Assign separate codes for each burn site
   When coding burns, assign separate codes for each burn site.
   Category 946 Burns of Multiple specified sites, should only be used if the location of the burns are not documented.
   Category 949, Burn, unspecified, is extremely vague and should rarely be used.

6) Assign codes from category 948, Burns
   Burns classified according to extent of body surface involved, when the site of the burn is not specified or when there is a need for additional data. It is advisable to use category 948 as additional coding when needed to provide data for evaluating burn mortality, such as that needed by burn units. It is also advisable to use category 948 as an additional code for reporting purposes when there is mention of a third-degree burn involving 20 percent or more of the body surface.
   In assigning a code from category 948:
   Fourth-digit codes are used to identify the percentage of total body surface involved in a burn (all degree).
   Fifth-digits are assigned to identify the percentage of body surface involved in third-degree burn.
   Fifth-digit zero (0) is assigned when less than 10 percent or when no body surface is involved in a third-degree burn.
   Category 948 is based on the classic "rule of nines" in estimating body surface involved: head and neck are assigned nine percent, each arm nine percent, each leg 18 percent, the anterior trunk 18 percent, posterior trunk 18 percent, and genitalia one percent. Providers may change these percentage assignments where necessary to accommodate infants and children who have proportionately larger heads than adults and patients who have large buttocks, thighs, or abdomen that involve burns.

7) Encounters for treatment of late effects of burns

Encounters for the treatment of the late effects of burns (i.e., scars or joint contractures) should be coded to the residual condition (sequelae) followed by the appropriate late effect code (906.5-906.9). A late effect E code may also be used, if desired.

8) Sequelae with a late effect code and current burn

When appropriate, both a sequelae with a late effect code, and a current burn code may be assigned on the same record (when both a current burn and sequelae of an old burn exist).

d. Coding of Debridement of Wound, Infection, or Burn

Excisional debridement involves surgical removal or cutting away, as opposed to a mechanical (brushing, scrubbing, washing) debridement.

For coding purposes, excisional debridement is assigned to code 86.22.

Nonexcisional debridement is assigned to code 86.28.

e. Adverse Effects, Poisoning and Toxic Effects

The properties of certain drugs, medicinal and biological substances or combinations of such substances, may cause toxic reactions. The occurrence of drug toxicity is classified in ICD-9-CM as follows:

1) Adverse Effect

When the drug was correctly prescribed and properly administered, code the reaction plus the appropriate code from the E930-E949 series. Codes from the E930-E949 series must be used to identify the causative substance for an adverse effect of drug, medicinal and biological substances, correctly prescribed and properly administered. The effect, such as tachycardia, delirium, gastrointestinal hemorrhaging, vomiting, hypokalemia, hepatitis, renal failure, or respiratory failure, is coded and followed by the appropriate code from the E930-E949 series.

Adverse effects of therapeutic substances correctly prescribed and properly administered (toxicity, synergistic reaction, side effect, and idiosyncratic reaction) may be due to (1) differences among patients, such as age, sex, disease, and genetic factors, and (2) drug-related factors, such as type of drug, route of administration, duration of therapy, dosage, and bioavailability.

2) Poisoning

(a) Error was made in drug prescription

Errors made in drug prescription or in the administration of the drug by pro-vider, nurse, patient, or other person, use the appropriate poisoning code from the 960-979 series.

(b) Overdose of a drug intentionally taken

If an overdose of a drug was intentionally taken or administered and resulted in drug toxicity, it would be coded as a poisoning (960-979 series).

(c) Nonprescribed drug taken with correctly prescribed and properly administered drug

If a nonprescribed drug or medicinal agent was taken in combination with a correctly prescribed and properly administered drug, any drug toxicity or other reaction resulting from the interaction of the two drugs would be classified as a poisoning.

(d) Sequencing of poisoning

When coding a poisoning or reaction to the improper use of a medication (e.g., wrong dose, wrong substance, wrong route of administration) the poisoning code is sequenced first, followed by a code for the manifestation. If there is also a diagnosis of drug abuse or dependence to the substance, the abuse or dependence is coded as an additional code.

See Section I.C.3.a.6.b. if poisoning is the result of insulin pump malfunctions and Section I.C.19 for general use of E-codes.

3) Toxic Effects

(a) Toxic effect codes

When a harmful substance is ingested or comes in contact with a person, this is classified as a toxic effect. The toxic effect codes are in categories 980-989.

(b) Sequencing toxic effect codes

A toxic effect code should be sequenced first, followed by the code(s) that identify the result of the toxic effect.

(c) External cause codes for toxic effects

An external cause code from categories E860-E869 for accidental exposure, codes E950.6 or E950.7 for intentional self-harm, category E962 for assault, or categories E980-E982, for undetermined, should also be assigned to indicate intent.

f. Complications of care

1) Transplant complications

(a) Transplant complications other than kidney

Codes under subcategory 996.8, Complications of transplanted organ, are for use for both complications and rejection of transplanted organs. A transplant complication code is only assigned if the complication affects the function of the transplanted organ. Two codes are required to fully describe a transplant complication, the appropriate code from subcategory 996.8 and a secondary code that identifies the complication.

Pre-existing conditions or conditions that develop after the transplant are not coded as complications unless they affect the function of the transplanted organs.

Post-transplants surgical complications that do not relate to the function of the transplanted organ are classified to the specific complication. For example, a surgical wound dehiscence would be coded to the wound dehiscence, not as a transplant complication.

Post-transplant patients who are seen for treatment unrelated to the transplanted organ should be assigned a code from category V42, Organ or tissue replaced by transplant, to identify the transplant status of the patient. A code from category V42 should never be used with a code from subcategory 996.8.

(b) Kidney transplant and chronic kidney disease

Patients with chronic kidney disease (CKD) following a transplant should not be assumed to have transplant failure or rejection unless it is documented by the provider. If documentation supports the presence of failure or rejection, then it is appropriate to assign code 996.81, Complications of transplanted organs, kidney followed by the appropriate CKD code.

18. Classification of Factors Influencing Health Status and Contact with Health Service (Supplemental V01-V84)

Note: The chapter specific guidelines provide additional information about the use of V codes for specified encounters.

a. Introduction

ICD-9-CM provides codes to deal with encounters for circumstances other than a disease or injury. The Supplementary Classification of Factors Influencing Health Status and Contact with Health Services (V01.0-V84.8) is provided to deal with occasions when circumstances other than a disease or injury (codes 001-999) are recorded as a diagnosis or problem.

There are four primary circumstances for the use of V codes:

1) A person who is not currently sick encounters the health services for some specific reason, such as to act as an organ donor, to receive prophylactic care, such as inoculations or health screenings, or to receive counseling on health related issues.

2) A person with a resolving disease or injury, or a chronic, long-term condition requiring continuous care, encounters the health care system for specific aftercare of that disease or injury (e.g., dialysis for renal disease; chemotherapy for malignancy; cast change). A diagnosis/symptom code should be used whenever a current, acute, diagnosis is being treated or a sign or symptom is being studied.

3) Circumstances or problems influence a person's health status but are not in themselves a current illness or injury.

4) Newborns, to indicate birth status

b. V codes use in any healthcare setting

V codes are for use in any healthcare setting. V codes may be used as either a first listed (principal diagnosis code in the inpatient setting) or secondary code, depending on the circumstances of the encounter. Certain V codes may only be used as first listed, others only as secondary codes. See Section I.C.18.e, V Code Table.

c. V Codes indicate a reason for an encounter

They are not procedure codes. A corresponding procedure code must accompany a V code to describe the procedure performed.

d. Categories of V Codes

1) Contact/Exposure

Category V01 indicates contact with or exposure to communicable diseases. These codes are for patients who do not show any sign or symptom of a disease but have been exposed to it by close personal contact with an infected individual or are in an area where a disease is epidemic. These codes may be used as a first listed code to explain an encounter for testing, or, more commonly, as a secondary code to identify a potential risk.

2) Inoculations and vaccinations

Categories V03-V06 are for encounters for inoculations and vaccinations. They indicate that a patient is being seen to receive a prophylactic inoculation against a disease. The injection itself must be represented by the appropriate procedure code. A code from V03-V06 may be used as a secondary code if the inoculation is given as a routine part of preventive health care, such as a well-baby visit.

3) Status

Status codes indicate that a patient is either a carrier of a disease or has the sequelae or residual of a past disease or condition. This includes such things as the presence of prosthetic or mechanical devices resulting from past treatment. A status code is informative, because the status may affect the course of treatment and its outcome. A status code is distinct from a history code. The history code indicates that the patient no longer has the condition.

A status code should not be used with a diagnosis code from one of the body system chapters, if the diagnosis code includes the information provided by the status code. For example, code V42.1, Heart transplant status, should not be used with code 996.83, Complications of transplanted heart. The status code does not provide additional information. The complication code indicates that the patient is a heart transplant patient.

The status V codes/categories are:

V02   Carrier or suspected carrier of infectious diseases

       Carrier status indicates that a person harbors the specific organisms of a disease without manifest symptoms and is capable of transmitting the infection.

V08   Asymptomatic HIV infection status

       This code indicates that a patient has tested positive for HIV but has manifested no signs or symptoms of the disease.

V09   Infection with drug-resistant microorganisms

       This category indicates that a patient has an infection that is resistant to drug treatment. Sequence the infection code first.

V21   Constitutional states in development

V22.2   Pregnant state, incidental

       This code is a secondary code only for use when the pregnancy is in no way complicating the reason for visit.

Otherwise, a code from the obstetric chapter is required.

V26.5x   Sterilization status

V42   Organ or tissue replaced by transplant

V43   Organ or tissue replaced by other means

V44   Artificial opening status

V45   Other postsurgical states

V46   Other dependence on machines

V49.6   Upper limb amputation status

V49.7   Lower limb amputation status

V49.81   Postmenopausal status

V49.82   Dental sealant status

V49.83   Awaiting organ transplant status

V58.6   Long-term (current) drug use

       This subcategory indicates a patient's continuous use of a prescribed drug (including such things as aspirin therapy) for the long-term treatment of a condition or for prophylactic use. It is not for use for patients who have addictions to drugs.

       Assign a code from subcategory V58.6, Long-term (current) drug use, if the patient is receiving a medication for an extended period as a prophylactic measure (such as for the prevention of deep vein thrombosis) or as treatment of a chronic condition (such as arthritis) or a disease requiring a lengthy course of treatment (such as cancer). Do not assign a code from subcategory V58.6 for medication being administered for a brief period of time to treat an acute illness or injury (such as a course of antibiotics to treat acute bronchitis).

V83   Genetic carrier status

       Genetic carrier status indicates that a person carries a gene, associated with a particular disease, which may be passed to offspring who may develop that disease. The person does not have the disease and is not at risk of developing the disease.

V84   Genetic susceptibility status

       Genetic susceptibility indicates that a person has a gene that increases the risk of that person developing the disease.

Codes from category V84, Genetic susceptibility to disease, should not be used as principal or first-listed codes. If the patient has the condition to which he/she is susceptible, and that condition is the reason for the encounter, the code for the current condition should be sequenced first. If the patient is being seen for follow-up after completed treatment for this condition, and the condition no longer exists, a follow-up code should be sequenced first, followed by the appropriate personal history and genetic susceptibility codes. If the purpose of the encounter is genetic counseling associated with procreative management, a code from subcategory V26.3, Genetic counseling and testing, should be assigned as the first-listed code, followed by a code from category V84. Additional codes should be assigned for any applicable family or personal history. See Section I.C. 18.d.14 for information on prophylactic organ removal due to a genetic susceptibility.

Note: Categories V42-V46, and subcategories V49.6, V49.7 are for use only if there are no complications or malfunctions of the organ or tissue replaced, the amputation site or the equipment on which the patient is dependent. These are always secondary codes.

4) History (of)
There are two types of history V codes, personal and family. Personal history codes explain a patient's past medical condition that no longer exists and is not receiving any treatment, but that has the potential for recurrence, and therefore may require continued monitoring. The exceptions to this general rule are category V14, Personal history of allergy to medicinal agents, and subcategory V15.0, Allergy, other than to medicinal agents. A person who has had an allergic episode to a substance or food in the past should always be considered allergic to the substance.

Family history codes are for use when a patient has a family member(s) who has had a particular disease that causes the patient to be at higher risk of also contracting the disease.

Personal history codes may be used in conjunction with follow-up codes and family history codes may be used in conjunction with screening codes to explain the need for a test or procedure. History codes are also acceptable on any medical record regardless of the reason for visit. A history of an illness, even if no longer present, is important information that may alter the type of treatment ordered.

The history V code categories are:
V10   Personal history of malignant neoplasm
V12   Personal history of certain other diseases
V13   Personal history of other diseases
       Except: V13.4, Personal history of arthritis, and V13.6, Personal history of congenital malformations. These conditions are life-long so are not true history codes.
V14   Personal history of allergy to medicinal agents
V15   Other personal history presenting hazards to health
       Except: V15.7, Personal history of contraception.
V16   Family history of malignant neoplasm
V17   Family history of certain chronic disabling diseases
V18   Family history of certain other specific diseases
V19   Family history of other conditions

5) Screening
Screening is the testing for disease or disease precursors in seemingly well individuals so that early detection and treatment can be provided for those who test positive for the disease. Screenings that are recommended for many subgroups in a population include: routine mammograms for women over 40, a fecal occult blood test for everyone over 50, an amniocentesis to rule out a fetal anomaly for pregnant women over 35, because the incidence of breast cancer and colon cancer in these subgroups is higher than in the general population, as is the incidence of Down's syndrome in older mothers.

The testing of a person to rule out or confirm a suspected diagnosis because the patient has some sign or symptom is a diagnostic examination, not a screening.

In these cases, the sign or symptom is used to explain the reason for the test. A screening code may be a first listed code if the reason for the visit is specifically the screening exam. It may also be used as an additional code if the screening is done during an office visit for other health problems. A screening code is not necessary if the screening is inherent to a routine examination, such as a pap smear done during a routine pelvic examination.

Should a condition be discovered during the screening then the code for the condition may be assigned as an additional diagnosis.

The V code indicates that a screening exam is planned. A procedure code is required to confirm that the screening was performed.

The screening V code categories:

V28   Antenatal screening
V73-V82   Special screening examinations

6) Observation

There are two observation V code categories. They are for use in very limited circumstances when a person is being observed for a suspected condition that is ruled out. The observation codes are not for use if an injury or illness or any signs or symptoms related to the suspected condition are present. In such cases the diagnosis/symptom code is used with the corresponding E code to identify any external cause.

The observation codes are to be used as principal diagnosis only. The only exception to this is when the principal diagnosis is required to be a code from the V30, Live born infant, category. Then the V29 observation code is sequenced after the V30 code. Additional codes may be used in addition to the observation code but only if they are unrelated to the suspected condition being observed.

The observation V code categories:

V29   Observation and evaluation of newborns for suspected condition not found

For the birth encounter, a code from category V30 should be sequenced before the V29 code.

V71   Observation and evaluation for suspected condition not found

7) Aftercare

Aftercare visit codes cover situations when the initial treatment of a disease or injury has been performed and the patient requires continued care during the healing or recovery phase, or for the long-term consequences of the disease. The aftercare V code should not be used if treatment is directed at a current, acute disease or injury. The diagnosis code is to be used in these cases. Exceptions to this rule are codes V58.0, Radiotherapy, and codes from subcategory V58.1, Encounter for chemotherapy and immunotherapy for neoplastic conditions. These codes are to be first listed, followed by the diagnosis code when a patient's encounter is solely to receive radiation therapy or chemotherapy for the treatment of a neoplasm. Should a patient receive both chemotherapy and radiation therapy during the same encounter code V58.0 and V58.1 may be used together on a record with either one being sequenced first.

The aftercare codes are generally first listed to explain the specific reason for the encounter. An aftercare code may be used as an additional code when some type of aftercare is provided in addition to the reason for admission and no diagnosis code is applicable. An example of this would be the closure of a colostomy during an encounter for treatment of another condition.

Certain aftercare V code categories need a secondary diagnosis code to describe the resolving condition or sequelae, for others, the condition is inherent in the code title.

Additional V code aftercare category terms include, fitting and adjustment, and attention to artificial openings.

Status V codes may be used with aftercare V codes to indicate the nature of the aftercare. For example code V45.81, Aortocoronary bypass status, may be used with code V58.73, Aftercare following surgery of the circulatory system, NEC, to indicate the surgery for which the aftercare is being performed. Also, a transplant status code may be used following code V58.44, Aftercare following organ transplant, to identify the organ transplanted. A status code should not be used when the aftercare code indicates the type of status, such as using V55.0, Attention to tracheostomy with V44.0, Tracheostomy status.

The aftercare V category/codes:

V52   Fitting and adjustment of prosthetic device and implant
V53   Fitting and adjustment of other device

V54   Other orthopedic aftercare

V55   Attention to artificial openings

V56   Encounter for dialysis and dialysis catheter care

V57   Care involving the use of rehabilitation procedures

V58.0   Radiotherapy

V58.11   Encounter for antineoplastic chemotherapy

V58.12   Encounter for antineoplastic immunotherapy

V58.3   Attention to surgical dressings and sutures

V58.41   Encounter for planned postoperative wound closure

V58.42   Aftercare, surgery, neoplasm

V58.43   Aftercare, surgery, trauma

V58.44   Aftercare involving organ transplant

V58.49   Other specified aftercare following surgery

V58.7x   Aftercare following surgery

V58.81   Fitting and adjustment of vascular catheter

V58.82   Fitting and adjustment of non-vascular catheter

V58.83   Monitoring therapeutic drug

V58.89   Other specified aftercare

8) Follow-up

The follow-up codes are used to explain continuing surveillance following completed disease, condition, or injury. They imply that the condition has been fully treated and no longer exists. They should not be confused with aftercare codes that explain current treatment for a healing condition or its sequelae. Follow-up codes may be used in conjunction with history codes to provide the full picture of the healed condition and its treatment. The follow-up code is sequenced first, followed by the history code.

A follow-up code may be used to explain repeated visits. Should a condition be found to have recurred on the follow-up visit, then the diagnosis code should be used in place of the follow-up code.

The follow-up V code categories:

V24   Postpartum care and evaluation

V67   Follow-up examination

9) Donor

Category V59 is the donor codes. They are used for living individuals who are donating blood or other body tissue. These codes are only for individuals donating for others, not for self donations. They are not for use to identify cadaveric donations.

10) Counseling

Counseling V codes are used when a patient or family member receives assistance in the aftermath of an illness or injury, or when support is required in coping with family or social problems. They are not necessary for use in conjunction with a diagnosis code when the counseling component of care is considered integral to standard treatment.

The counseling V categories/codes:

V25.0   General counseling and advice for contraceptive management

V26.3   Genetic counseling

V26.4   General counseling and advice for procreative management

V61   Other family circumstances

V65.1   Person consulted on behalf of another person

V65.3   Dietary surveillance and counseling

V65.4   Other counseling, not elsewhere classified

11) Obstetrics and related conditions

See Section I.C.11., the Obstetrics guidelines for further instruction on the use of these codes.

V codes for pregnancy are for use in those circumstances when none of the problems or complications included in the codes from the Obstetrics chapter exist (a routine prenatal visit or postpartum care). Codes V22.0, Supervision of normal first pregnancy, and V22.1, Supervision of other normal pregnancy, are always first listed and are not to be used with any other code from the OB chapter.

The outcome of delivery, category V27, should be included on all maternal delivery records. It is always a secondary code.

V codes for family planning (contraceptive) or procreative management and counseling should be included on an obstetric record either during the pregnancy or the postpartum stage, if applicable.

Obstetrics and related conditions V code categories:

V22   Normal pregnancy

V23   Supervision of high-risk pregnancy
   Except: V23.2, Pregnancy with history of abortion.
      Code 646.3, Habitual aborter, from the OB chapter is required to indicate a history of abortion during a pregnancy.

V24   Postpartum care and evaluation

V25 Encounter for contraceptive management

Except V25.0x (See Section I.C.18.d.11, Counseling)

V26 Procreative management

Except V26.5x, Sterilization status, V26.3 and V26.4 (See Section I.C.18.d.11., Counseling)

V27 Outcome of delivery

V28 Antenatal screening

(See Section I.C.18.d.6., Screening)

12) Newborn, infant and child

See Section I.C.15, the Newborn guidelines for further instruction on the use of these codes.

Newborn V code categories:

V20 Health supervision of infant or child

V29 Observation and evaluation of newborns for suspected condition not found (See Section I.C.18.d.7, Observation).

V30-V39 Liveborn infant according to type of birth

13) Routine and administrative examinations

The V codes allow for the description of encounters for routine examinations, such as, a general check-up, or, examinations for administrative purposes, such as, a pre-employment physical. The codes are for use as first listed codes only, and are not to be used if the examination is for diagnosis of a suspected condition or for treatment purposes. In such cases the diagnosis code is used. During a routine exam, should a diagnosis or condition be discovered, it should be coded as an additional code. Pre-existing and chronic conditions and history codes may also be included as additional codes as long as the examination is for administrative purposes and not focused on any particular condition.

Pre-operative examination V codes are for use only in those situations when a patient is being cleared for surgery and no treatment is given.

The V codes categories/code for routine and administrative examinations:

V20.2 Routine infant or child health check

Any injections given should have a corresponding procedure code.

V70 General medical examination

V72 Special investigations and examinations

Except V72.5 and V72.6

14) Miscellaneous V codes

The miscellaneous V codes capture a number of other health care encounters that do not fall into one of the other categories. Certain of these codes identify the reason for the encounter, others are for use as additional codes that provide useful information on circumstances that may affect a patient's care and treatment.

Prophylactic Organ Removal

For encounters specifically for prophylactic removal of breasts, ovaries, or another organ due to a genetic susceptibility to cancer or a family history of cancer, the principal or first listed code should be a code from subcategory V50.4, Prophylactic organ removal, followed by the appropriate genetic susceptibility code and the appropriate family history code.

If the patient has a malignancy of one site and is having prophylactic removal at another site to prevent either a new primary malignancy or metastatic disease, a code for the malignancy should also be assigned in addition to a code from subcategory V50.4. A V50.4 code should not be assigned if the patient is having organ removal for treatment of a malignancy, such as the removal of the testes for the treatment of prostate cancer.

Miscellaneous V code categories/codes:

V07 Need for isolation and other prophylactic measures

V50 Elective surgery for purposes other than remedying health states

V58.5 Orthodontics

V60 Housing, household, and economic circumstances

V62 Other psychosocial circumstances

V63 Unavailability of other medical facilities for care

V64 Persons encountering health services for specific procedures, not carried out

V66 Convalescence and Palliative Care

V68 Encounters for administrative purposes

V69 Problems related to lifestyle

15) Nonspecific V codes

Certain V codes are so non-specific, or potentially redundant with other codes in the classification, that there can be little justification for their use in the inpatient setting. Their use in the outpatient setting should be limited to those instances when there is no further documentation to permit more precise coding. Otherwise, any sign or symptom or any other reason for visit that is captured in another code should be used.

Nonspecific V code categories/codes:

V11 Personal history of mental disorder

A code from the mental disorders chapter, with an in remission fifth-digit, should be used.

V13.4 Personal history of arthritis

V13.6 Personal history of congenital malformations

V15.7 Personal history of contraception

V23.2 Pregnancy with history of abortion

V40 Mental and behavioral problems

V41 Problems with special senses and other special functions

V47 Other problems with internal organs

V48 Problems with head, neck, and trunk

V49 Problems with limbs and other problems

Exceptions:

V49.6 Upper limb amputation status

V49.7 Lower limb amputation status

V49.81 Postmenopausal status

V49.82 Dental sealant status

V49.83 Awaiting organ transplant status

V51 Aftercare involving the use of plastic surgery

V58.2 Blood transfusion, without reported diagnosis

V58.9 Unspecified aftercare

V72.5 Radiological examination, NEC

V72.6 Laboratory examination

Codes V72.5 and V72.6 are not to be used if any sign or symptoms, or reason for a test is documented. See Section IV.K. and Section IV.L. of the Outpatient guidelines.

V CODE TABLE

FIRST LISTED: V codes/categories/subcategories which are only acceptable as principal/first listed.

Codes:

V22.0 Supervision of normal first pregnancy

V22.1 Supervision of other normal pregnancy

V46.12 Encounter for respirator dependence during power failure

V46.13 Encounter for weaning from respirator [ventilator]

V56.0 Extracorporeal dialysis

V58.0 Radiotherapy

V58.0 and V58.11 may be used together on a record with either one being sequenced first, when a patient receives both chemotherapy and radiation therapy during the same encounter code.

V58.11 Encounter for antineoplastic chemotherapy

V58.0 and V58.11 may be used together on a record with either one being sequenced first, when a patient receives both chemotherapy and radiation therapy during the same encounter code.

V58.12 Encounter for antineoplastic immunotherapy

Categories/Subcategories:

V20 Health supervision of infant or child

V24 Postpartum care and examination

V29 Observation and evaluation of newborns for suspected condition not found

Exception: A code from the V30-V39 may be sequenced before the V29 if it is the newborn record.

V30-V39 Liveborn infants according to type of birth

V57 Care involving use of rehabilitation procedures

V59 Donors

V66 Convalescence and palliative care

Exception: V66.7 Palliative care

V68 Encounters for administrative purposes

V70 General medical examination

Exception: V70.7 Examination of participant in clinical trial

V71 Observation and evaluation for suspected conditions not found

V72 Special investigations and examinations

Exceptions:

V72.4 Pregnancy examination or test

V72.5 Radiological examination, NEC

V72.6 Laboratory examination

V72.86 Encounter for blood typing

FIRST OR ADDITIONAL: V code categories/subcategories which may be either principal/first listed or additional codes

Codes:

V15.88 History of fall

V43.22 Fully implantable artificial heart status

V46.14 Mechanical complication of respirator [ventilator]

V49.81 Asymptomatic postmenopausal status (age-related) (natural)

V49.84 Bed confinement status

V49.89 Other specified conditions influencing health status

V70.7 Examination of participant in clinical trial

V72.5 Radiological examination, NEC

V72.6 Laboratory examination

V72.86 Encounter for blood typing

Categories/Subcategories:

V01	Contact with or exposure to communicable diseases
V02	Carrier or suspected carrier of infectious diseases
V03-06	Need for prophylactic vaccination and inoculations
V07	Need for isolation and other prophylactic measures
V08	Asymptomatic HIV infection status
V10	Personal history of malignant neoplasm
V12	Personal history of certain other diseases
V13	Personal history of other diseases
	Exception:
	V13.4 Personal history of arthritis
	V13.69 Personal history of other congenital malformations
V16-V19	Family history of disease
V23	Supervision of high-risk pregnancy
V25	Encounter for contraceptive management
V26	Procreative management
	Exception: V26.5 Sterilization status
V28	Antenatal screening
V45.7	Acquired absence of organ
V49.6x	Upper limb amputation status
V49.7x	Lower limb amputation status
V50	Elective surgery for purposes other than remedying health states
V52	Fitting and adjustment of prosthetic device and implant
V53	Fitting and adjustment of other device
V54	Other orthopedic aftercare
V55	Attention to artificial openings
V56	Encounter for dialysis and dialysis catheter care
	Exception: V56.0 Extracorporeal dialysis
V58.3	Attention to surgical dressings and sutures
V58.4	Other aftercare following surgery
V58.7	Aftercare following surgery to specified body systems, not elsewhere classified
V58.8	Other specified procedures and aftercare
V61	Other family circumstances
V63	Unavailability of other medical facilities for care
V65	Other persons seeking consultation without complaint or sickness
V67	Follow-up examination
V69	Problems related to lifestyle
V72.4	Pregnancy examination or test
V73-V82	Special screening examinations
V83	Genetic carrier status

ADDITIONAL ONLY: V code categories/subcategories which may only be used as additional codes, not principal/first listed

Codes:

V13.61	Personal history of hypospadias
V22.2	Pregnancy state, incidental
V46.11	Dependence on respirator, status
V49.82	Dental sealant status
V49.83	Awaiting organ transplant status
V66.7	Palliative care

Categories/Subcategories:

V09	Infection with drug-resistant microorganisms
V14	Personal history of allergy to medicinal agents
V15	Other personal history presenting hazards to health
	Exception:
	V15.7 Personal history of contraception
	V15.88 History of fall
V21	Constitutional states in development
V26.5	Sterilization status
V27	Outcome of delivery
V42	Organ or tissue replaced by transplant
V43	Organ or tissue replaced by other means
	Exception: V43.22 Fully implantable artificial heart status
V44	Artificial opening status
V45	Other postsurgical states
	Exception: Subcategory V45.7 Acquired absence of organ
V46	Other dependence on machines
	Exception: V46.12 Encounter for respirator dependence during power failure
	V46.13 Encounter for weaning from respirator [ventilator]
V49.6x	Upper limb amputation status
V49.7x	Lower limb amputation status
V58.6	Long-term current drug use
V60	Housing, household, and economic circumstances
V62	Other psychosocial circumstances
V64	Persons encountering health services for specified procedure, not carried out
V84	Genetic susceptibility to disease
V85	Body Mass Index

NONSPECIFIC CODES AND CATEGORIES:

V11	Personal history of mental disorder
V13.4	Personal history of arthritis
V13.69	Personal history of congenital malformations
V15.7	Personal history of contraception
V40	Mental and behavioral problems
V41	Problems with special senses and other special functions
V47	Other problems with internal organs
V48	Problems with head, neck, and trunk
V49.0	Deficiencies of limbs
V49.1	Mechanical problems with limbs
V49.2	Motor problems with limbs
V49.3	Sensory problems with limbs
V49.4	Disfigurements in limbs
V49.5	Other problems with limbs
V49.9	Unspecified condition influencing health status

V51   Aftercare involving the use of plastic surgery
V58.2   Blood transfusion, without reported diagnosis
V58.5   Orthodontics
V58.9   Unspecified aftercare
V72.5   Radiological examination, NEC
V72.6   Laboratory examination

19. Supplemental Classification of External Causes of Injury and Poisoning (E-codes, E800-E999)

Introduction: These guidelines are provided for those who are currently collecting E codes in order that there will be standardization in the process. If your institution plans to begin collecting E codes, these guidelines are to be applied. The use of E codes is supplemental to the application of ICD-9-CM diagnosis codes. E codes are never to be recorded as principal diagnoses (first-listed in non-inpatient setting) and are not required for reporting to CMS.

External causes of injury and poisoning codes (E codes) are intended to provide data for injury research and evaluation of injury prevention strategies. E codes capture how the injury or poisoning happened (cause), the intent (unintentional or accidental; or intentional, such as suicide or assault), and the place where the event occurred.

Some major categories of E codes include:

transport accidents

poisoning and adverse effects of drugs, medicinal substances and biologicals

accidental falls

accidents caused by fire and flames

accidents due to natural and environmental factors

late effects of accidents, assaults or self injury

assaults or purposely inflicted injury

suicide or self inflicted injury

These guidelines apply for the coding and collection of E codes from records in hospitals, outpatient clinics, emergency departments, other ambulatory care settings and provider offices, and nonacute care settings, except when other specific guidelines apply.

a. General E Code Coding Guidelines

1) Used with any code in the range of 001-V84.8

An E code may be used with any code in the range of 001-V84.8, which indicates an injury, poisoning, or adverse effect due to an external cause.

2) Assign the appropriate E code for all initial treatments

Assign the appropriate E code for the initial encounter of an injury, poisoning, or adverse effect of drugs, not for subsequent treatment.

3) Use the full range of E codes

Use the full range of E codes to completely describe the cause, the intent and the place of occurrence, if applicable, for all injuries, poisonings, and adverse effects of drugs.

4) Assign as many E codes as necessary

Assign as many E codes as necessary to fully explain each cause. If only one E code can be recorded, assign the E code most related to the principal diagnosis.

5) The selection of the appropriate E code

The selection of the appropriate E code is guided by the Index to External Causes, which is located after the alphabetical index to diseases and by Inclusion and Exclusion notes in the Tabular List.

6) E code can never be a principal diagnosis

An E code can never be a principal (first listed) diagnosis.

7) External cause code(s) with systemic inflammatory response syndrome (SIRS)

An external cause code(s) may be used with codes 995.93, Systemic inflammatory response syndrome due to noninfectious process without organ dysfunction, and 995.94, Systemic inflammatory response syndrome due to noninfectious process with organ dysfunction, if trauma was the initiating insult that precipitated the SIRS. The external cause(s) code should correspond to the most serious injury resulting from the trauma. The external cause code(s) should only be assigned if the trauma necessitated the admission in which the patient also developed SIRS. If a patient is admitted with SIRS but the trauma has been treated previously, the external cause codes should not be used.

b. Place of Occurrence Guideline

Use an additional code from category E849 to indicate the Place of Occurrence for injuries and poisonings. The Place of Occurrence describes the place where the event occurred and not the patient's activity at the time of the event.

Do not use E849.9 if the place of occurrence is not stated.

c. Adverse Effects of Drugs, Medicinal and Biological Substances Guidelines

1) Do not code directly from the Table of Drugs

Do not code directly from the Table of Drugs and Chemicals. Always refer back to the Tabular List.

2) Use as many codes as necessary to describe

Use as many codes as necessary to describe completely all drugs, medicinal or biological substances.

3) If the same E code would describe the causative agent
If the same E code would describe the causative agent for more than one adverse reaction, assign the code only once.

4) If two or more drugs, medicinal or biological substances
If two or more drugs, medicinal or biological substances are reported, code each individually unless the combination code is listed in the Table of Drugs and Chemicals. In that case, assign the E code for the combination.

5) When a reaction results from the interaction of a drug(s)
When a reaction results from the interaction of a drug(s) and alcohol, use poisoning codes and E codes for both.

6) If the reporting format limits the number of E codes
If the reporting format limits the number of E codes that can be used in reporting clinical data, code the one most related to the principal diagnosis. Include at least one from each category (cause, intent, place) if possible.

If there are different fourth digit codes in the same three digit category, use the code for "Other specified" of that category. If there is no "Other specified" code in that category, use the appropriate "Unspecified" code in that category.

If the codes are in different three digit categories, assign the appropriate E code for other multiple drugs and medicinal substances.

7) Codes from the E930-E949 series
Codes from the E930-E949 series must be used to identify the causative substance for an adverse effect of drug, medicinal and biological substances, correctly prescribed and properly administered. The effect, such as tachycardia, delirium, gastrointestinal hemorrhaging, vomiting, hypokalemia, hepatitis, renal failure, or respiratory failure, is coded and followed by the appropriate code from the E930-E949 series.

d. Multiple Cause E Code Coding Guidelines
If two or more events cause separate injuries, an E code should be assigned for each cause. The first listed E code will be selected in the following order:

E codes for child and adult abuse take priority over all other E codes. See Section I.C.19.e., Child and Adult abuse guidelines

E codes for terrorism events take priority over all other E codes except child and adult abuse

E codes for cataclysmic events take priority over all other E codes except child and adult abuse and terrorism.

E codes for transport accidents take priority over all other E codes except cataclysmic events and child and adult abuse and terrorism.

The first-listed E code should correspond to the cause of the most serious diagnosis due to an assault, accident, or self-harm, following the order of hierarchy listed above.

e. Child and Adult Abuse Guideline
1) Intentional injury
When the cause of an injury or neglect is intentional child or adult abuse, the first listed E code should be assigned from categories E960-E968, Homicide and injury purposely inflicted by other persons, (except category E967). An E code from category E967, Child and adult battering and other maltreatment, should be added as an additional code to identify the perpetrator, if known.

2) Accidental intent
In cases of neglect when the intent is determined to be accidental E code E904.0, Abandonment or neglect of infant and helpless person, should be the first listed E code.

f. Unknown or Suspected Intent Guideline
1) If the intent (accident, self-harm, assault) of the cause of an injury or poisoning is unknown
If the intent (accident, self-harm, assault) of the cause of an injury or poisoning is unknown or unspecified, code the intent as undetermined E980-E989.

2) If the intent (accident, self-harm, assault) of the cause of an injury or poisoning is questionable
If the intent (accident, self-harm, assault) of the cause of an injury or poisoning is questionable, probable or suspected, code the intent as undetermined E980-E989.

g. Undetermined Cause
When the intent of an injury or poisoning is known, but the cause is unknown, use codes: E928.9, Unspecified accident, E958.9, Suicide and self-inflicted injury by unspecified means, and E968.9, Assault by unspecified means.

These E codes should rarely be used, as the documentation in the medical record, in both the inpatient outpatient and other settings, should normally provide sufficient detail to determine the cause of the injury.

h. Late Effects of External Cause Guidelines
   1) Late effect E codes
      Late effect E codes exist for injuries and poisonings but not for adverse effects of drugs, misadventures and surgical complications.
   2) Late effect E codes (E929, E959, E969, E977, E989, or E999.1)
      A late effect E code (E929, E959, E969, E977, E989, or E999.1) should be used with any report of a late effect or sequela resulting from a previous injury or poisoning (905-909).
   3) Late effect E code with a related current injury
      A late effect E code should never be used with a related current nature of injury code.
   4) Use of late effect E codes for subsequent visits
      Use a late effect E code for subsequent visits when a late effect of the initial injury or poisoning is being treated. There is no late effect E code for adverse effects of drugs. Do not use a late effect E code for subsequent visits for follow-up care (e.g., to assess healing, to receive rehabilitative therapy) of the injury or poisoning when no late effect of the injury has been documented.

i. Misadventures and Complications of Care Guidelines
   1) Code range E870-E876
      Assign a code in the range of E870-E876 if misadventures are stated by the provider.
   2) Code range E878-E879
      Assign a code in the range of E878-E879 if the provider attributes an abnormal reaction or later complication to a surgical or medical procedure, but does not mention misadventure at the time of the procedure as the cause of the reaction.

j. Terrorism Guidelines
   1) Cause of injury identified by the Federal Government (FBI) as terrorism
      When the cause of an injury is identified by the Federal Government (FBI) as terrorism, the first-listed E-code should be a code from category E979, Terrorism. The definition of terrorism employed by the FBI is found at the inclusion note at E979. The terrorism E-code is the only E- code that should be assigned. Additional E codes from the assault categories should not be assigned.

   2) Cause of an injury is suspected to be the result of terrorism
      When the cause of an injury is suspected to be the result of terrorism a code from category E979 should not be assigned. Assign a code in the range of E codes based circumstances on the documentation of intent and mechanism.
   3) Code E979.9, Terrorism, secondary effects
      Assign code E979.9, Terrorism, secondary effects, for conditions occurring subsequent to the terrorist event. This code should not be assigned for conditions that are due to the initial terrorist act.
   4) Statistical tabulation of terrorism codes
      For statistical purposes these codes will be tabulated within the category for assault, expanding the current category from E960-E969 to include E979 and E999.1.

SECTION II. SELECTION OF PRINCIPAL DIAGNOSIS

The circumstances of inpatient admission always govern the selection of principal diagnosis. The principal diagnosis is defined in the Uniform Hospital Discharge Data Set (UHDDS) as "that condition established after study to be chiefly responsible for occasioning the admission of the patient to the hospital for care."

The UHDDS definitions are used by hospitals to report inpatient data elements in a standardized manner. These data elements and their definitions can be found in the July 31, 1985, Federal Register (Vol. 50, No, 147), pp. 31038-40.

Since that time the application of the UHDDS definitions has been expanded to include all non-outpatient settings (acute care, short term, long term care and psychiatric hospitals; home health agencies; rehab facilities; nursing homes, etc).

In determining principal diagnosis the coding conventions in the ICD-9-CM, Volumes I and II take precedence over these official coding guidelines. (See Section I.A., Conventions for the ICD-9-CM.)

The importance of consistent, complete documentation in the medical record cannot be overemphasized. Without such documentation the application of all coding guidelines is a difficult, if not impossible, task.

A. Codes for symptoms, signs, and ill-defined conditions
   Codes for symptoms, signs, and ill-defined conditions from Chapter 16 are not to be used as principal diagnosis when a related definitive diagnosis has been established.

B. Two or more interrelated conditions, each potentially meeting the definition for principal diagnosis.
   When there are two or more interrelated conditions (such as diseases in the same ICD-9-CM chapter or

manifestations characteristically associated with a certain disease) potentially meeting the definition of principal diagnosis, either condition may be sequenced first, unless the circumstances of the admission, the therapy provided, the Tabular List, or the Alphabetic Index indicate otherwise.

C. Two or more diagnoses that equally meet the definition for principal diagnosis

In the unusual instance when two or more diagnoses equally meet the criteria for principal diagnosis as determined by the circumstances of admission, diagnostic workup and/or therapy provided, and the Alphabetic Index, Tabular List, or another coding guidelines does not provide sequencing direction, any one of the diagnoses may be sequenced first.

D. Two or more comparative or contrasting conditions.

In those rare instances when two or more contrasting or comparative diagnoses are documented as "either/or" (or similar terminology), they are coded as if the diagnoses were confirmed and the diagnoses are sequenced according to the circumstances of the admission. If no further determination can be made as to which diagnosis should be principal, either diagnosis may be sequenced first.

E. A symptom(s) followed by contrasting/comparative diagnoses

When a symptom(s) is followed by contrasting/comparative diagnoses, the symptom code is sequenced first. All the contrasting/comparative diagnoses should be coded as additional diagnoses.

F. Original treatment plan not carried out

Sequence as the principal diagnosis the condition, which after study occasioned the admission to the hospital, even though treatment may not have been carried out due to unforeseen circumstances.

G. Complications of surgery and other medical care

When the admission is for treatment of a complication resulting from surgery or other medical care, the complication code is sequenced as the principal diagnosis. If the complication is classified to the 996–999 series and the code lacks the necessary specificity in describing the complication, an additional code for the specific complication should be assigned.

H. Uncertain Diagnosis

If the diagnosis documented at the time of discharge is qualified as "probable," "suspected," "likely," "questionable," "possible," or "still to be ruled out," code the condition as if it existed or was established. The bases for these guidelines are the diagnostic workup, arrangements for further workup or observation, and initial therapeutic approach that correspond most closely with the established diagnosis.

Note: This guideline is applicable only to short-term, acute, long-term care and psychiatric hospitals.

I. Admission from Observation Unit

1. Admission Following Medical Observation

When a patient is admitted to an observation unit for a medical condition, which either worsens or does not improve, and is subsequently admitted as an inpatient of the same hospital for this same medical condition, the principal diagnosis would be the medical condition which led to the hospital admission.

2. Admission Following Post-Operative Observation

When a patient is admitted to an observation unit to monitor a condition (or complication) that develops following outpatient surgery, and then is subsequently admitted as an inpatient of the same hospital, hospitals should apply the Uniform Hospital Discharge Data Set (UHDDS) definition of principal diagnosis as "that condition established after study to be chiefly responsible for occasioning the admission of the patient to the hospital for care."

J. Admission from Outpatient Surgery

When a patient receives surgery in the hospital's outpatient surgery department and is subsequently admitted for continuing inpatient care at the same hospital, the following guidelines should be followed in selecting the principal diagnosis for the inpatient admission:

• If the reason for the inpatient admission is a complication, assign the complication as the principal diagnosis.

• If no complication, or other condition, is documented as the reason for the inpatient admission, assign the reason for the outpatient surgery as the principal diagnosis.

• If the reason for the inpatient admission is another condition unrelated to the surgery, assign the unrelated condition as the principal diagnosis.

SECTION III. REPORTING ADDITIONAL DIAGNOSES

GENERAL RULES FOR OTHER (ADDITIONAL) DIAGNOSES

For reporting purposes the definition for "other diagnoses" is interpreted as additional conditions that affect patient care in terms of requiring:
clinical evaluation; or
therapeutic treatment; or
diagnostic procedures; or
extended length of hospital stay; or
increased nursing care and/or monitoring.

The UHDDS item #11-b defines Other Diagnoses as "all conditions that coexist at the time of admission, that develop subsequently, or that affect the treatment received and/or the length of stay. Diagnoses that relate to an earlier episode which have no bearing on the current hospital stay are to be excluded." UHDDS definitions apply to inpatients in acute care, short-term, long term care and psychiatric hospital setting. The UHDDS definitions are used by acute care short-term hospitals to report inpatient data elements in a standardized manner. These data elements and their definitions can be found in the July 31, 1985, Federal Register (Vol. 50, No, 147), pp. 31038-40.

Since that time the application of the UHDDS definitions has been expanded to include all non-outpatient settings (acute care, short term, long term care and psychiatric hospitals; home health agencies; rehab facilities; nursing homes, etc).

The following guidelines are to be applied in designating "other diagnoses" when neither the Alphabetic Index nor the Tabular List in ICD-9-CM provide direction. The listing of the diagnoses in the patient record is the responsibility of the attending provider.

A. Previous conditions

If the provider has included a diagnosis in the final diagnostic statement, such as the discharge summary or the face sheet, it should ordinarily be coded. Some providers include in the diagnostic statement resolved conditions or diagnoses and status-post procedures from previous admission that have no bearing on the current stay. Such conditions are not to be reported and are coded only if required by hospital policy.

However, history codes (V10-V19) may be used as secondary codes if the historical condition or family history has an impact on current care or influences treatment.

B. Abnormal findings

Abnormal findings (laboratory, x-ray, pathologic, and other diagnostic results) are not coded and reported unless the provider indicates their clinical significance. If the findings are outside the normal range and the attending provider has ordered other tests to evaluate the condition or prescribed treatment, it is appropriate to ask the provider whether the abnormal finding should be added.

Please note. This differs from the coding practices in the outpatient setting for coding encounters for diagnostic tests that have been interpreted by a provider.

C. Uncertain Diagnosis

If the diagnosis documented at the time of discharge is qualified as "probable," "suspected," "likely," "questionable," "possible," or "still to be ruled out," code the condition as if it existed or was established. The bases for these guidelines are the diagnostic workup, arrangements for further workup or observation, and initial therapeutic approach that correspond most closely with the established diagnosis. Note: This guideline is applicable only to short-term, acute, long-term care and psychiatric hospitals.

SECTION IV. DIAGNOSTIC CODING AND REPORTING GUIDELINES FOR OUTPATIENT SERVICES

These coding guidelines for outpatient diagnoses have been approved for use by hospitals/providers in coding and reporting hospital-based outpatient services and provider-based office visits.

Information about the use of certain abbreviations, punctuation, symbols, and other conventions used in the ICD-9-CM Tabular List (code numbers and titles), can be found in Section IA of these guidelines, under "Conventions Used in the Tabular List." Information about the correct sequence to use in finding a code is also described in Section I.

The terms encounter and visit are often used interchangeably in describing outpatient service contacts and, therefore, appear together in these guidelines without distinguishing one from the other.

Though the conventions and general guidelines apply to all settings, coding guidelines for outpatient and provider reporting of diagnoses will vary in a number of instances from those for inpatient diagnoses, recognizing that:

The Uniform Hospital Discharge Data Set (UHDDS) definition of principal diagnosis applies only to inpatients in acute, short-term, long-term care and psychiatric hospitals.

Coding guidelines for inconclusive diagnoses (probable, suspected, rule out, etc.) were developed for inpatient reporting and do not apply to outpatients.

A. Selection of first-listed condition

In the outpatient setting, the term first-listed diagnosis is used in lieu of principal diagnosis.

In determining the first-listed diagnosis the coding conventions of ICD-9-CM, as well as the general and disease specific guidelines take precedence over the outpatient guidelines.

Diagnoses often are not established at the time of the initial encounter/visit. It may take two or more visits before the diagnosis is confirmed.

The most critical rule involves beginning the search for the correct code assignment through the Alphabetic Index. Never begin searching initially in the Tabular List as this will lead to coding errors.

1. Outpatient Surgery

When a patient presents for outpatient surgery, code the reason for the surgery as the first-listed diagnosis (reason for the encounter), even if the surgery is not performed due to a contraindication.

2. Observation Stay

When a patient is admitted for observation for a medical condition, assign a code for the medical condition as the first-listed diagnosis.

When a patient presents for outpatient surgery and develops complications requiring admission to observation, code the reason for the surgery as the first reported diagnosis (reason for the encounter), followed by codes for the complications as secondary diagnoses.

B. Codes from 001.0 through V84.8

The appropriate code or codes from 001.0 through V84.8 must be used to identify diagnoses, symptoms, conditions, problems, complaints, or other reason(s) for the encounter/visit.

C. Accurate reporting of ICD-9-CM diagnosis codes

For accurate reporting of ICD-9-CM diagnosis codes, the documentation should describe the patient's condition, using terminology which includes specific diagnoses as well as symptoms, problems, or reasons for the encounter. There are ICD-9-CM codes to describe all of these.

D. Selection of codes 001.0 through 999.9

The selection of codes 001.0 through 999.9 will frequently be used to describe the reason for the encounter. These codes are from the section of ICD-9-CM for the classification of diseases and injuries (e.g. infectious and parasitic diseases; neoplasms; symptoms, signs, and ill-defined conditions, etc.).

E. Codes that describe symptoms and signs

Codes that describe symptoms and signs, as opposed to diagnoses, are acceptable for reporting purposes when a diagnosis has not been established (confirmed) by the provider. Chapter 16 of ICD-9-CM, Symptoms, Signs, and Ill-defined conditions (codes 780.0–799.9) contain many, but not all codes for symptoms.

F. Encounters for circumstances other than a disease or injury

ICD-9-CM provides codes to deal with encounters for circumstances other than a disease or injury. The Supplementary Classification of factors Influencing Health Status and Contact with Health Services (V01.0-V84.8) is provided to deal with occasions when circumstances other than a disease or injury are recorded as diagnosis or problems.

G. Level of Detail in Coding

1. ICD-9-CM codes with 3, 4, or 5 digits

ICD-9-CM is composed of codes with either 3, 4, or 5 digits. Codes with three digits are included in ICD-9-CM as the heading of a category of codes that may be further subdivided by the use of fourth and/or fifth digits, which provide greater specificity.

2. Use of full number of digits required for a code

A three-digit code is to be used only if it is not further subdivided. Where fourth-digit subcategories and/or fifth-digit subclassifications are provided, they must be assigned. A code is invalid if it has not been coded to the full number of digits required for that code. See also discussion under Section I.b.3., General Coding Guidelines, Level of Detail in Coding.

H. ICD-9-CM code for the diagnosis, condition, problem, or other reason for encounter/visit

List first the ICD-9-CM code for the diagnosis, condition, problem, or other reason for encounter/visit shown in the medical record to be chiefly responsible for the services provided. List additional codes that describe any coexisting conditions. In some cases the first-listed diagnosis may be a symptom when a diagnosis has not been established (confirmed) by the physician.

I. "Probable," "suspected," "questionable," "rule out," or "working diagnosis"

Do not code diagnoses documented as "probable," "suspected," "questionable," "rule out," or "working diagnosis." Rather, code the condition(s) to the highest degree of certainty for that encounter/visit, such as symptoms, signs, abnormal test results, or other reason for the visit. Please note: This differs from the coding practices used by short-term, acute care, long-term care and psychiatric hospitals.

J. Chronic diseases

Chronic diseases treated on an ongoing basis may be coded and reported as many times as the patient receives treatment and care for the condition(s)

K. Code all documented conditions that coexist

Code all documented conditions that coexist at the time of the encounter/visit, and require or affect patient care treatment or management. Do not code conditions that were previously treated and no longer exist. However, history codes (V10-V19) may be used as secondary codes if the historical condition or family history has an impact on current care or influences treatment.

L. Patients receiving diagnostic services only

For patients receiving diagnostic services only during an encounter/visit, sequence first the diagnosis, condition, problem, or other reason for encounter/visit shown in the medical record to be chiefly responsible for the outpatient services provided during the encounter/visit. Codes for other diagnoses (e.g., chronic conditions) may be sequenced as additional diagnoses.

For outpatient encounters for diagnostic tests that have been interpreted by a physician, and the final report is available at the time of coding, code any confirmed or definitive diagnosis(es) documented in the interpretation. Do not code related signs and symptoms as additional diagnoses.

Please note: This differs from the coding practice in the hospital inpatient setting regarding abnormal findings on test results.

M. Patients receiving therapeutic services only

For patients receiving therapeutic services only during an encounter/visit, sequence first the diagnosis, condition, problem, or other reason for encounter/visit shown in the medical record to be chiefly responsible for the outpatient services provided during the encounter/visit. Codes for other diagnoses (e.g., chronic conditions) may be sequenced as additional diagnoses.

The only exception to this rule is that when the primary reason for the admission/encounter is chemotherapy, radiation therapy, or rehabilitation, the appropriate V code for the service is listed first, and the diagnosis or problem for which the service is being performed listed second.

N. Patients receiving preoperative evaluations only
For patients receiving preoperative evaluations only, sequence first a code from category V72.8, Other specified examinations, to describe the pre-op consultations. Assign a code for the condition to describe the reason for the surgery as an additional diagnosis. Code also any findings related to the pre-op evaluation.

O. Ambulatory surgery
For ambulatory surgery, code the diagnosis for which the surgery was performed. If the postoperative diag-nosis is known to be different from the preoperative diagnosis at the time the diagnosis is confirmed, select the postoperative diagnosis for coding, since it is the most definitive.

P. Routine outpatient prenatal visits
For routine outpatient prenatal visits when no com-plications are present, codes V22.0, Supervision of normal first pregnancy, or V22.1, Supervision of other normal pregnancy, should be used as the principal diagnosis. These codes should not be used in con-junction with chapter 11 codes.

GODFREY REGIONAL PRACTICE INFORMATION AND FORMS

TABLE 1-1 Godfrey Regional Health Facilities and Providers

Facility Names and Addresses

Godfrey Regional Outpatient Clinic — 3122 Shannon Avenue, Aldon, FL 77712, (407) 555-7654

Godfrey Regional Hospital — 123 Main Street, Aldon, FL 77714, (407) 555-1234

Godfrey Clinical Laboratories — 465 Dogwood Court, Aldon, FL 77712, (407) 555-9876

Godfrey Medical Associates — 1532 Third Avenue, Suite 120, Aldon, FL 77713, (407) 555-4000

Provider Names

Provider	Specialty	Location(s) of Service
Maurice Doates, MD	Internal Medicine	Godfrey Regional Hospital; Godfrey Regional Outpatient Clinic; Godfrey Medical Associates
Robert Rais, MD	Emergency Department	Godfrey Regional Hospital
Stanley Krosette, MD	Internal Medicine	Godfrey Regional Hospital; Godfrey Regional Outpatient Clinic; Godfrey Medical Associates
William Obert, MD	Family Medicine	Godfrey Regional Hospital; Godfrey Medical Associates
Felix Washington, MD	Family Medicine	Godfrey Regional Hospital; Godfrey Medical Associates
Jay Corman, MD	Internal Medicine	Godfrey Regional Hospital; Godfrey Medical Associates
Nancy Connelly, MD	Emergency Department	Godfrey Regional Hospital
Adam Westgate, MD	Surgeon/General	Godfrey Regional Hospital; Godfrey Regional Outpatient Clinic; Godfrey Medical Associates
Patrick Chung, MD	Surgeon/Orthopedics	Godfrey Regional Hospital; Godfrey Regional Outpatient Clinic; Godfrey Medical Associates
Rachel Perez, MD	Surgeon/General	Godfrey Regional Hospital; Godfrey Regional Outpatient Clinic; Godfrey Medical Associates
Lisa Valhas, MD	Radiologist	Godfrey Regional Hospital; Godfrey Regional Outpatient Clinic
John Parker, MD	Internal Medicine	Godfrey Regional Hospital; Godfrey Regional Outpatient Clinic; Godfrey Medical Associates

TABLE 1-1 Godfrey Regional Health Facilities and Providers—cont'd

Provider Names

Provider	Specialty	Location(s) of Service
Nathan Brady, MD	Internal Medicine Cardiology	Godfrey Regional Hospital Godfrey Regional Outpatient Clinic Godfrey Medical Associates
Luis Perez, MD	Anesthesiologist	Godfrey Regional Hospital Godfrey Regional Outpatient Clinic
Steven Speller, MD	Pathologist	Godfrey Clinical Laboratories
Maria Callaway, MD	Surg Pathologist	Godfrey Regional Hospital Godfrey Regional Outpatient Clinic
Patrick Adams, MD	Gastroenterologist	Godfrey Regional Hospital Godfrey Medical Associates
James Ellicott, MD	Otolaryngologist	Godfrey Regional Hospital Godfrey Regional Outpatient Clinic
Linda Patrick, MD	Ophthalmologist	Godfrey Regional Hospital Godfrey Medical Associates
Vincent DiMarco, MD	Neurologist	Godfrey Regional Outpatient Clinic Godfrey Regional Hospital

TABLE 1-2 Godfrey Regional Medical Signature Log

Provider	Signature
Maurice Doates, MD	*(signature)*
Robert Rais, MD	*(signature)*
Stanley Krosette, MD	*(signature)*
William Obert, MD	*(signature)*
Felix Washington, MD	*(signature)*
Jay Corman, MD	*(signature)*
Nancy Connelly, MD	*(signature)*
Adam Westgate, MD	*(signature)*
Patrick Chung, MD	*(signature)*
Rachel Perez, MD	*(signature)*
Lisa Valhas, MD	*(signature)*
John Parker, MD	*(signature)*
Nathan Brady, MD	*(signature)*
Luis Perez, MD	*(signature)*
Steven Speller, MD	*(signature)*
Maria Callaway, MD	*(signature)*
Patrick Adams, MD	*(signature)*
James Ellicott, MD	*(signature)*
Linda Patrick, MD	*(signature)*
Vincent DiMarco, MD	*(signature)*

DIAGNOSTIC DOCUMENTATION WORKSHEET

Chart#/Patient Name:

WHAT (Service/Procedure)	WHY (MEDICAL NECESSITY) (Diagnostic Information)
Step 1 Select all words for possible use as diagnosis/diagnostic statement from the document	
Step 2 Determine which words are appropriate for inclusion: (Carry these forward) Diagnosis vs. signs/symptoms	
Step 3 Based on each service performed, determine the appropriate order of diagnosis for each service performed	
Step 4 Look up/assign the proper dx codes	

EVALUATION AND MANAGEMENT LEVEL WORKSHEET

History	1	2	3	4	5
HPI:					
PMH:					
SH/FH:					
ROS					
Level History Assigned:					

Examination	1	2	3	4	5
Body Organ(s):					
Organ System(s):					
Level Exam Assigned:					

Medical Decision Making	1	2	3	4	5
Diagnosis/Management Options:					
Amount/Complexity Data:					
Risk/Morbidity/Mortality:					
Level Medical Decision Making Assigned:					

Other Factors Documented (Time, Counseling):

LOCATION OF SERVICE (CIRCLE ONE)

Office/Outpatient	Critical Care	Prolonged	Newborn Care
Hospital	Neonatal ICU	Services	Special E&M
Observation	Nursing Facility	Case Management	Service
Hospital Inpatient	Domiciliary, Rest	Care Plan	
Consultations	Home	Oversight	
Emergency	Home Services	Preventative	
Department		Medicine	

TYPE OF SERVICE (CIRCLE ONE)

New Patient   Established Patient

Patient Name: _____   **Level Assigned:** _____

Date: _____   **Coder:** _____

Surgery Documentation Worksheet

Patient Name: _____   **Date of Procedure:** _____

Pre-Operative Information	Documented	Not Documented	Comments
Surgeon			
Resident			
Assistant			
Date of surgery			
Pre-operative diagnosis			
Post-operative diagnosis			
Procedures			

Intra-Operative Information	Documented	Not Documented	Comments
Position			
Pre/drape			
Dissection/mode of entry			
Names of structures removed/repaired			
Materials removed/inserted			
Findings			
Bilateral structures addressed/repaired			
Sponge count			
Blood loss			
Pert path findings			
Unusual findings			
Problems/complications			

Post-Operative Information	Documented	Not Documented	Comments
Post-operative findings			
Post-operative complications			

HOSPITAL INPATIENT DRG CODING WORKSHEET

Chart#/Patient Name:

List Components Here	Assign Codes Here
Step 1 - Principal/Secondary Diagnosis 1A - List diagnosis 1B - Determine primary diagnosis "Condition established after study to be chiefly responsible for admission to hospital for care" Number diagnoses in appropriate order	
Step 2 - Significant Procedures	
Step 3 - Determine whether surgical procedure performed Yes/No	
Step 4 - Assign the MDC Based on principal diagnosis	
Step 5 - Determine whether medical or surgical partition Med/Surg	
Step 6 - Check for Contributing Factors Age Sex Discharge status Presence/absence of complications or comorbidities Birthweight for neonates	
ASSIGNMENT **DRG:** Principal Dx: Addtl Dx:	

ANSWERS

CHAPTER 1

Chapter Review Exercise (p. 53)

			Location	Type of Form(s)
2.	Patient visit	Godfrey Medical Associates	Office	Office progress note
4.	Patient visit	Emergency department/ Godfrey Regional	Hospital	Emergency department note
6.	Radiology report	Hospital/ office	Either	Radiology report
8.	Staff documentation of office visit		Office	Staff/visit note
10.	Patient problem list		Office	Problem list
12.	Operative report		Hospital	Operative report
14.	Consultation	Either	Either	Consultation

CHAPTER 2

Stop and Practice Exercises

Stop and Practice (p. 59)

		Yes	No
2.	Dysuria	X	
	Probably urinary rract infection		X
4.	Femur fracture	X	
	Closed femur fracture	X	
6.	Bronchitis	X	
	Acute bronchitis	X	
8.	Shortness of breath	X	
	Asthma	X	
	Asthma, status asthmaticus	X	
10.	Upper respiratory illness (URI)		X
	Upper respiratory infection	X	

Stop and Practice (p. 61)

2.	Nausea	SS
4.	Headache	D
6.	Abdominal pain	SS
8.	Shoulder strain	D
10.	Shortness of breath	SS
12.	Ankle contusion	D
14.	Nasal congestion	SS
16.	Sore throat	SS

18. Nausea
Vomiting
Gastroenteritis

20. Angina
Coronary artery disease
Status post (S/P) bypass graft

22. Urinary retention
Urinary frequency
Urinary tract infection

24. Abdominal pain
Appendicitis

26. Fever
Urinary tract infection

Stop and Practice (p. 65)

2. Cholecystitis
Cholecystitis with cholelithiasis

Cholecystitis with cholelithiasis encompasses cholecystitis; therefore cholecystitis is not necessary.

4. Seizures
Epilepsy ruled out

Seizures
Because epilepsy was ruled out, would not be assigned code.

6. 2-year-old child with fever, rhinorrhea
Diagnosis: acute sinusitis and acute otitis media

Diagnosis was acute sinusitis and acute otitis media
Assign codes for both

Fever and rhinorrhea are signs/symptoms of either the sinusitis or otitis media and therefore do not need assigned codes.

8. Chronic heart failure (CHF) with SOB

Chronic heart failure
Shortness of breath is sign/symptom of chronic heart failure, and therefore, should not be assigned code.

10. Abdominal mass with jaundice
Consider hepatitis

Abdominal mass
Jaundice

Consider hepatitis would not be assigned code because definitive diagnosis has not been made at the time of the encounter.

Chapter Review Exercise (p. 67)

	Diagnostic Statement(s) Selected in Appropriate Order
2. Strep throat Acute pharyngitis Sore throat	Acute pharyngitis Strep throat
4. Gastroenteritis, probably viral Nausea and vomiting	Gastroenteritis only
6. Acute sinusitis Bronchitis	Acute sinusitis Bronchitis (not acute)
8. Abdominal pain RUQ due to pancreatitis or cholecystitis	Abdominal pain only (when two contrasting dx are not confirmed, cannot code)
10. Syncope with a fever in a 6-year-old child R/O meningitis	Syncope only (R/O dx are not coded)

Practical Application (p. 68)

2. Shortness of Breath versus Angina

SERVICE PROVIDED	Office visit
Diagnostic Statement #1	Angina
SERVICE PROVIDED	ECG
Diagnostic Statement #1	Angina

"Consistent with" anterior myocardial infarction cannot be used as documented.

4. Slow Heartbeat

SERVICE PROVIDED	ED visit
Diagnostic Statement #1	Bradycardia
Diagnostic Statement #2	Exacerbation COPD
SERVICE PROVIDED	ABG
Diagnostic Statement #1	Exacerbation COPD
SERVICE PROVIDED	ECG
Diagnostic Statement #1	Bradycardia
SERVICE PROVIDED	Chest x-ray
Diagnostic Statement #1	Exacerbation COPD

6. Chest Pain in an Elderly Patient

SERVICE PROVIDED	Visit
Diagnostic Statement #1	Chest pain
Diagnostic Statement #2	Dizziness/weakness
SERVICE PROVIDED	Chest x-ray
Diagnostic Statement #1	Chest pain
Diagnostic Statement #2	Dizziness/weakness
SERVICE PROVIDED	ECG
Diagnostic Statement #1	Chest pain
Diagnostic Statement #2	Dizziness/weakness
SERVICE PROVIDED	Cardiac enzymes (labs)
Diagnostic Statement #1	Chest pain
Diagnostic Statement #2	Dizziness/weakness

8. Severe Headache

SERVICE PROVIDED	Visit
Diagnostic Statement #1	Headache
Diagnostic Statement #2	Nausea, vomiting

10. Shortness of Breath

SERVICE PROVIDED	Visit
Diagnostic Statement #1	Impending ARDS
Diagnostic Statement #2	Exacerbation, COPD
SERVICE PROVIDED	Chest x-ray
Diagnostic Statement #1	Impending ARDS
Diagnostic Statement #2	Exacerbation, COPD
SERVICE PROVIDED	ABG
Diagnostic Statement #1	Impending ARDS
Diagnostic Statement #2	Exacerbation, COPD

12. Injury Trauma

SERVICE PROVIDED	Visit
Diagnostic Statement #1	Low back pain
Diagnostic Statement #2	Loss of control, vehicle
Diagnostic Statement #3	Hematuria
SERVICE PROVIDED	Back x-rays
Diagnostic Statement #1	Low back pain
Diagnostic Statement #2	Loss of control, vehicle
SERVICE PROVIDED	Urinalysis
Diagnostic Statement #1	Hematuria

14. Admitted Patient with Chills

SERVICE PROVIDED	Hospital Visit
Diagnostic Statement #1	Fever
Diagnostic Statement #2	Dysuria
SERVICE PROVIDED	IVF (intravenous fluids)
Diagnostic Statement #1	Fever
Diagnostic Statement #2	Dysuria

"Will repeat UA for symptoms"—have not performed services, therefore, not coded until service provided

16. Episode of Dyspnea

SERVICE PROVIDED	Hospital admit
Diagnostic Statement #1	Dyspnea
Diagnostic Statement #2	LLE restless leg syndrome
Diagnostic Statement #3	S/P perforated appendix with peritonitis
SERVICE PROVIDED	Chest x-ray
Diagnostic Statement #1	Dyspnea
SERVICE PROVIDED	Doppler study
Diagnostic Statement #1	LLE restless leg syndrome

Only assign diagnostic statements that relate to the service being provided.

Possible DVT cannot be coded as probably, possible, rule out not assigned codes.

SERVICE PROVIDED	Chest x-ray
Diagnostic Statement #1	Hyperinflation lung

Cannot code "possible" COPD

18. Note

SERVICE PROVIDED	Office visit
Diagnostic Statement #1	Restless leg syndrome
Diagnostic Statement #2	Dyspnea

20. Bilateral Pedal Edema

SERVICE PROVIDED	Office visit
Diagnostic Statement #1	Congestive heart failure
Diagnostic Statement #2	Pedal edema

CHAPTER 3

Examples (p. 94)

	Diagnostic Term to Reference	ICD-9-CM Code
2. Cough	Cough	786.2
Fever	Fever	780.6
Upper respiratory infection	Infection, Respiratory, Upper	465.9

Stop and Practice Exercises

Stop and Practice (p. 93)

Diagnosis	Location (Where to Look Up)
2. Finger laceration	Wound, finger, open
4. Gastrointestinal hemorrhage	Hemorrhage, gastrointestinal
6. Fractured femur	Fracture, femur
8. Senile cataract	Cataract, senile
10. Sepsis	Sepsis

Diagnosis	Location (Where to Look Up)
12. Congestive heart failure (CHF)	Failure, heart, congestive
14. Chronic obstructive pulmonary disease (COPD), with acute bronchitis	Bronchitis, acute Disease, pulmonary, obstructive, chronic
16. Acute bronchitis with URI	Bronchitis, acute Infection, respiratory, upper
18. Cough, normal chest	Cough
20. Acute URI due to pneumococcus	Infection, respiratory, upper, acute pneumococcus

Stop and Practice (p. 93)

Diagnosis	Location (Where to Look Up)
2. Closed wrist fracture	Fracture, wrist, closed
4. Abscess of right great toe	Abscess, toe
6. Streptococcal infection	Infection, streptococcal
8. Fracture of tibia/fibula	Fracture, tibia/fibula
10. Bilateral pedal edema	Edema, pedal
12. Right upper quadrant (RUQ), left lower quadrant (LLQ) abdominal pain	Pain, abdominal, RUQ Pain, abdominal, LLQ
14. Rupture, head of biceps Chronic shoulder pain with shortness of breath (SOB)	Rupture, biceps, head
16. Abdominal pain Abdominal mass Rule out (R/O) liver metastases (mets) adenotonsillar hyperplasia	Mass, abdominal Hyperplasia, adenotonsillar
18. Acute appendicitis Appendicitis with peritonitis	Appendicitis, acute with peritonitis
20. R/O endometriosis and uterine anomaly lesions, right utero ligament	Lesion, ligament, utero (uterus)

Stop and Practice (p. 95)

	Diagnostic Term to Reference	ICD-9-CM Code
2. URI	Infection, respiratory	465.9
4. Virus, varicella	None, unless use	052.9
6. Psychogenic ulcerative colitis	Colitis, ulcerative	316/556.9
8. Benign hypertension	Hypertension, benign	401.1
10. Blood loss anemia	Anemia, blood loss	280.0
12. Streptococcal pneumonia	Pneumonia, strepto	482.30
14. Gastrointestinal bleed	Bleed, gastrointestinal	578.9

16. Hepatitis C	Hepatitis C	070.51
18. Asthmatic dyspnea	Dyspnea, asthmatic	493.90
20. Fever, cough, pneumonia	Pneumonia	486

Chapter Review Exercise (p. 99)

	Diagnosis Code(s)
2. Rheumatoid arthritis, hand	714.0
4. Pelvic mass, R/O cervical neoplasm	789.30
6. Laceration of hand	882.0
8. Pendred's syndrome	243
10. *Klebsiella* pneumonia	482.0
12. Athlete's foot	110.4
14. Low back pain	724.2
16. Bell's disease	296.00
18. Bennett's fracture	815.01
20. Birthmark	757.32
22. Fever blister	054.9
24. Bradycardia	427.89
26. Burkitt's tumor	200.20
28. Degenerative spinal cord	336.8
30. Allergic eyelid dermatitis	373.32
32. Capsulitis, hip	726.5
34. Cervicitis during pregnancy	646.60
36. Ear canal cholesteatoma	385.30
38. Charcot's cirrhosis	571.6
40. Abdominal cramps	789.00
42. Forearm contusion	923.10
44. Liver contusion	864.01
46. Muscle cramps	729.82
48. Baker's cyst	727.51
50. High-frequency hearing loss	389.8
52. Clotting deficiency	286.9
54. Difficulty breast-feeding	676.80
56. Mitral valve deficiency	424.0
58. Bouillaud's disease	391.9
60. Acute gastric dilatation	536.1
62. Osteofibrocystic disease	252.0
64. Adult polycystic kidney disease	753.13
66. Stress disorder	308.9
68. Sympathetic reflux dystrophy	337.20
70. Distal end ulnar dislocation	833.09
72. Exposure to cold	991.9
74. Abnormal heart sounds	785.3
76. Anal fissure	565.0
78. Ureterosigmoidoabdominal fistula	593.82
80. Toxic goiter	242.00
82. Traumatic liver hematoma	864.01
84. Obstructed Richter's hernia	552.9
86. Adrenal hypoplasia	759.1
88. Hormonal imbalance	259.9

90. Bartholin's gland inflammation	616.8
92. Irritable bowel	564.1
94. Postpartum breast inflammation	675.24
96. Intelligence quotient (IQ) under 20	318.2
98. Spinal cord lesion	336.9
100. Myocarditis with rheumatic fever	398.0
102. Nursemaid's elbow	832.00
104. Phase of life problem	V62.89
106. Food aspiration pneumonia	507.0
108. Premature ventricular contractions	427.69
110. Rales	786.7
112. Rasmussen's aneurysm	011.20
114. Rapid respirations	786.06
116. Granulomatous rhinitis	472.0
118. Allergic reaction	995.3
120. Seborrheic wart	702.19
122. Sleeping sickness	086.5
124. Convulsions	780.39
126. Spina bifida with hydrocephalus	741.00
128. Hemoptysis	786.3
130. Cardiac bypass graft status	V45.81
132. Thyroid storm	242.91
134. Drug-induced delusional syndrome	292.11
136. Jet lag syndrome	307.45
138. Central nervous system syphilis	094.9
140. Tay-Sachs disease	330.1
142. Grinding teeth	306.8
144. Saphenous vein thrombosis	451.0
146. Omental torsion	560.2
148. CHF with mild pedal edema	428.0
	782.3
150. Cough, normal chest	786.2

Practical Application (p. 100)

2. Postpartum with Multiple Complaints

Diagnostic Statement #1: Acute bronchitis
ICD-9-CM Code: 466.0

Diagnostic Statement #2: Diarrhea
ICD-9-CM Code: 787.91

Diagnostic Statement #3: External hemorrhoids
ICD-9-CM Code: 455.3

RATIONALE:
Acute conditions are assumed to be primary

4. Abdominal Pain

Diagnostic Statement #1: Abdominal pain
ICD-9-CM Code: 789.00

Diagnostic Statement #2: Dysuria
ICD-9-CM Code: 788.1

Diagnostic Statement #3: Incontinence
ICD-9-CM Code: 788.30

RATIONALE:
Possible conditions (possible UTI) are not coded in physician coding

6. Severe Epigastric Cramping

Diagnostic Statement #1: Epigastric cramping/pain
ICD-9-CM Code: 789.06

Diagnostic Statement #2: Anxiety
ICD-9-CM Code: 300.00

RATIONALE:
Patient complaint is abdominal pain, more specifically identified during the course of the examination as epigastric abdominal pain. It is the primary reason for the encounter, with anxiety as a secondary diagnosis.

8. Garbled Speech, Gait Instability

Diagnostic Statement #1: Speech garbled
ICD-9-CM Code: 784.5

Diagnostic Statement #2: Gait instability
ICD-9-CM Code: 781.2

Diagnostic Statement #3: Chest pain
ICD-9-CM Code: 786.50

10. Knee Arthroscopy

Diagnostic Statement #1: Torn medial meniscus
ICD-9-CM Code: 836.0

CHAPTER 4

Stop and Practice Exercises

Stop and Practice (p. 116)

	Section Where Located	V Code
2. Preoperative examination	Other specified exams	V72.84
4. Visit for tetanus immunization	Need for vaccination	V03.7
6. Personal history of malignant neoplasm	Personal history malignant liver neoplasm	V10.07
8. Visit for routine child care	Related to reproduction/development	V20.2
10. General medical examination	Persons without diagnosis	V70.9
12. Dressing changes	Encounter for aftercare	V58.3
14. Chemotherapy administration	Encounter for procedural care	V58.1
16. Single liveborn birth	Related to reproduction/development	V27.0
18. Family history of malignant neoplasm of gastrointestinal (GI) tract	Related to family history	V16.0
20. Visits to the laboratory for routine blood work	Persons without diagnosis	V70.0

Stop and Practice (p. 118)

	Section Where Located	E Code
2. Auto accident, driver	Auto accident	E819.0
4. Scuba diving accident	Water/submersion	E910.1
6. Struck by fellow soccer player	Other accidents	E917.0
8. Stabbing	Homicide/injury	E966
10. Tripped and fell on stairs	Accidental falls	E880.9
12. Cut finger with piece of glass	Other accidents	E920.8
14. Accidental drowning	Accident by submersion	E910.9
16. Struck by furniture	Other accident	E917.3
18. Fall from ladder	Falls	E881.0
20. Dog bite	Due to natural/environmental factors	E906.0

Chapter Review Exercise (p. 118)

	E Code/V Code/Other
2. History of hypertension	V12.59
4. Fracture of tibia, removal of screws and pins	V54.0
6. CABG status	V45.81
8. Well-child examination	V20.2
10. Viral illness with exposure to strep throat	079.99, V01.8
12. Exposure to sexually transmitted disease (STD)	V01.6
14. Single delivery, liveborn	V27.0
16. HIV counseling	V65.44
18. History of malaria	V12.03
20. Removal of orthopedic pin	V54.8
22. Family history of mental illness	V17.0
24. Newborn, suspicion of brain damage	V29.1
26. Infant, single liveborn	V30.00
28. Adjustment of arm prosthetic	V52.0
30. Glaucoma screening	V80.1
32. History of myocardial infarction	412
34. Sterilization	V25.2
36. S/P pacemaker	V45.01
38. S/P aortic valve replacement	V42.2
40. History of allergy to penicillin	V14.0
42. History of malignant melanoma	V10.82
44. Family history of mental retardation	V18.4
46. Renal dialysis status	V45.1
48. Screening mammogram	V76.12
50. Replacement gastrostomy tube	V55.1
52. Human immunodeficiency virus (HIV) positive status	V08
54. Bicycle accident	E826.1
56. Traffic accident	E819.0

58. Fall from ladder on boat — E833.9
60. Accidental fall — E888.9
62. Injury on football field — E849.4
64. Lead poisoning, lead-based paint at home — E866.0
66. Fall into storm drain — E833.2
68. Fall out of tree — E884.9
70. Injury from colliding with another person — E917.9
72. Adverse reaction, chlorine fumes — 987.6/E869.8
74. Injury caused by foreign body, ear — E915
76. Suicide from jumping from window of home — E957.0
78. Injury from lifting heavy objects — E927
80. Accidental overdose, acetaminophen — 965.4/E866.8
82. Family history of congenital defects — V19.5
84. Need for rabies immunization — V04.5
86. Fall from tripping — E885.9
88. Injury occurring at industrial site — E849.3
90. Adverse effects, hormones taken correctly — 962.9/E932.9
92. Intentional self-inflicted knife wound — E956
94. Injured by object dropped on patient — E916
96. School physical — V70.3
98. Car versus car highway accident — E812.9
100. S/P loss of limb, below knee — V49.75

Practical Application (p. 120)
Scenario #2
ICD-9-CM Diagnosis Code(s):
V064.   Prophylactic immunization/inoculation for MMR
V04.0   Prophylactic immunization for poliomyelitis

RATIONALE:
Patient has no signs/symptoms and is being immunized only against these diseases.

Scenario #4
ICD-9-CM Diagnosis Code(s):
845.00   Ankle sprain
V22.2   Incidental pregnancy
E888.9   Fall, other

RATIONALE:
Chief reason for encounter is the diagnosed sprained ankle. A contributing factor may be the pregnancy, and the E Code is listed last to indicate how the injury occurred.

Scenario #6
ICD-9-CM Diagnosis Code(s):
470   Deviated septum
873.21   Open wound, septum
E885.9   Tripped and fell, other

RATIONALE:
The most significant injury should be listed first. Some carriers identify only the first diagnosis and that diagnosis will help in determining the level of service. Therefore the most significant injury is listed first.

The laceration repair procedure will have the following diagnosis codes in this order:

Open wound of septum
E885.9   Tripped and fell, other

Note that the deviated septum is not listed as a diagnostic code for the laceration repair because it does not contribute to that procedure.

CHAPTER 5

Stop and Practice Exercises
Stop and Practice (p. 132)

	External Cause Category	E Code
2. Digoxin toxicity	Therapeutic	E942.1
4. Suicidal ingestion of acetaminophen	Suicide	E950.0
6. Rattlesnake bite	Poisoning/ accidental	989.5/E905.0
8. Ingestion of smelter fumes	Poisoning/ undetermined	985.9/E980.9
10. Vitamin B$_{12}$ toxicity	Therapeutic	E934.1

Stop and Practice (p. 135)

	Neoplasm Behavior/Category
2. Breast cancer	Malignant (primary), 174.9
4. Breast neoplasm	Unspecified behavior, 239.3
6. Adenocarcinoma of the thyroid	Malignant (primary), 193
8. Acute myeloid leukemia	Unspecified behavior, 205.00
10. Acute lymphatic leukemia	Unspecified behavior, 204.00

Stop and Practice (p. 137)

	ICD-9-CM Code(s)
2. Postoperative hypertension	997.91
4. Postpartum hypertension	642.94
6. Myocarditis due to hypertension	429.0/401.9
8. Hypertension due to brain tumor	401.9/191.9
10. Hypertension, possibly malignant	401.9

Chapter Review Exercise (p. 138)

	Code Assigned
2. Suicide attempt by cocaine	E950.4
4. Overdose of phenobarbital, prescribed by physician, taken as directed	967.0/E937.0

6. Attempted homicide by rat poison   E962.1
8. Secondary hypertension due to   514/405.99
   pulmonary edema
10. Asbestos poisoning   989.81
12. Pulmonary hypertension   416.8
14. Accidental overdose, doxycycline   960.4/E856
16. Benign hypertension   401.1
18. Adverse effects of bupivacaine   968.5/E938.5
    hydrochloride (Marcaine),
    administered subcutaneously
20. Suicide attempt by ingestion of gas   981/E950.9
22. Adverse effects, topical   976.0/E858.7
    neomycin sulfate (Neosporin)
24. Lithium, taken as directed   969.4/E939.4
26. Elevated blood pressure reading   796.2
28. Secondary hypertension due to   405.99
    Cushing's disease
30. Intraocular hypertension   365.04
32. Metastatic malignant melanoma   196.3/195.1
    from left lateral chest wall to
    axillary lymph node
34. Adenocarcinoma, right upper lobe,   162.3/196.1
    lung, with metastases to mediastinal
    lymph nodes

Practical Application (p. 140)

2. ICD-9-CM DIAGNOSIS CODE(S):   786.6

RATIONALE:

Malignant neoplasm has not been confirmed; "suspicious for" cannot be assumed diagnostic code. Therefore, most definitive condition, lung mass, would be assigned.

4. ICD-9-CM DIAGNOSIS CODE(S):   995.2
                                 465.9
                                 E930.0

RATIONALE:

Chief reason for encounter is rash, due to penicillin.

6. ICD-9-CM DIAGNOSIS CODE(S):   780.09
                                 967.9
                                 980.9
                                 E967.9
                                 E980.9

RATIONALE:

Chief reason for encounter is nonarousable (stupor, altered level of consciousness/780.09). This was the result of drugs and chemicals; therefore the poisoning codes for alcohol (not otherwise specified) and drugs (not otherwise specified) are assigned along with the E codes (did not say whether accidental or intentional; therefore undetermined would be appropriate).

CHAPTER 6

Stop and Practice Exercises
Stop and Practice (p. 148)

	ICD-9-CM Code(s)
2. Acute streptococcal pharyngitis	034.0
4. Gastroenteritis due to *Salmonella* infection	558.9/003.9
6. Varicella	052.9
8. Encephalitis due to malaria	084.6/323.2
10. Asymptomatic HIV infection	V08

Stop and Practice (p. 149)

	ICD-9-CM code(s)
2. Diabetes, IDDM	250.01
4. Hyperthyroidism	242.9
6. Iatrogenic hypothyroidism	244.3
8. Diabetic ophthalmic neuropathy	250.50
10. Cystic fibrosis with pulmonary exacerbation	277.00

Stop and Practice (p. 150)

	ICD-9-CM Code(s)
2. Iron deficiency anemia due to blood loss	280.0
4. Sickle cell anemia in crisis	282.62
6. Acquired aplastic anemia	284.8
8. Nutritional anemia	281.9
10. Chronic lymphadenitis	289.1

Stop and Practice (p. 152)

	ICD-9-CM Code(s)
2. Bipolar disorder, manic phase, mild	296.41
4. Psychogenic paralysis	306.0
6. Depression with anxiety, dependent personality	300.4/301.6
8. Anxiety reaction manifested by tachycardia	300.00/785.1
10. Aggressive personality, adjustment reaction	309.9/301.3

Stop and Practice (p. 153)

	ICD-9-CM Code(s)
2. Chronic suppurative otitis media	382.3
4. Cataract, NOS	366.9
6. Trigeminal neuralgia	350.1
8. Bell's palsy	351.0
10. Reflex sympathetic dystrophy	337.20

Stop and Practice (p. 154)

	ICD-9-CM Code(s)
2. Old MI	412
4. Congestive heart failure	428.0
6. CVA	436
8. Unstable angina	411.1
10. Atrioventricular block, first degree	426.11

Stop and Practice (p. 155)

	ICD-9-CM Code(s)
2. Pneumonia NOS	486
4. Chronic respiratory failure	518.83
6. ARDS	518.5
8. URI	465.9
10. Sinusitis	473.9

Stop and Practice (p. 156)

	ICD-9-CM Code(s)
2. Gastroenteritis, probably viral	558.9
4. Recurrent inguinal hernia, with strangulation	550.11
6. Acute pancreatitis	577.0
8. Hematemesis	578.0
10. Anal fistula	565.1

Stop and Practice (p. 157)

	ICD-9-CM Code(s)
2. Acute renal failure	584.9
4. Polycystic kidney disease	753.12
6. Endometriosis, ovaries	617.1
8. Acute prostatitis	601.0
10. Ureter calculus	592.1

Stop and Practice (p. 160)

	ICD-9-CM Code(s)
2. Preeclampsia, delivered	642.41
4. Fetal distress, delivered	768.4
6. Poor fetal growth	764.90
8. Premature rupture of membranes, not delivered	658.13
10. False labor, not delivered	644.13

Stop and Practice (p. 160)

	ICD-9-CM Code(s)
2. Allergic urticaria	708.0
4. Decubitus ulcer	707.0
6. Abscess of the arm	682.3
8. Pilonidal cyst	685.1
10. Keloid scar	701.4

Stop and Practice (p. 161)

	ICD-9-CM Code(s)
2. Acute osteomyelitis	730.0
4. Rheumatoid arthritis, hand	714.0
6. Pain, knee	719.46
8. History of arthritis	V13.4
10. Chondromalacia, knee	717.7

Stop and Practice (p. 162)

	ICD-9-CM Code(s)
2. Abdominal pain, NOS	789.00
4. Cough	786.2
6. Dyspnea	786.09
8. Respiratory arrest	799.1
10. Urinary incontinence	788.30

Stop and Practice (p. 164)

	ICD-9-CM Code(s)
2. Nonunion of fracture, neck of femur	733.82
4. Contusions, right cheek/right forearm/right hand	920/923.10/ 923.20
6. Fracture, left hip	820.8
8. Fracture, left pelvic	808.8
10. Stab wound of abdominal wall, infected	879.3

Stop and Practice (p. 166)

	ICD-9-CM Code(s)
2. Second-degree burns in factory fire, determined to be arson	949.2/E968.0/ E849.3
4. Severe sunburn of face, neck, shoulders	692.71
6. First-degree burn of left foot, second-degree burn of toes, bonfire	945.12/945.21/ E897
8. Allergic dermatitis, face	692.9
10. Second- and third-degree burns of lower leg, house fire	945.30/E895

Chapter Review Exercise (p. 167)

	ICD-9-CM Code(s)
2. Twin pregnancy	651.00
4. Breech presentation, delivered	763.0
6. Head injury	959.01
8. Contusions to left elbow	923.11
10. Burns to left cheek from stove	941.04
12. Obsessive-compulsive disorder	300.3
14. Hyperventilation syndrome	306.1
16. Fetal disproportion	653.50
18. Four (4) rib fractures	807.04
20. Sternoclavicular joint sprain	848.41
22. Corneal foreign body	930.0
24. Antisocial personality	301.7
26. Separation anxiety	309.21
28. Cervical cancer	180.9
30. Maternal venereal disease	647.20
32. Umbilical cord around neck with compression	663.10
34. Knee laceration	891.0
36. Chemical burns of eyelids	940.0
38. Schizophrenia	295.90
40. Multiple personality disorder	300.14
42. Insect bite, leg	916.4
44. Elbow dislocation, lateral	832.04
46. Coin in nostril	932
48. Drug addiction	304.90
50. Arthritis, ankle	716.97
52. Hyperthyroidism	242.9
54. Gestational diabetes	648.80
56. Fibroadenosis of breast	610.2
58. Simple greenstick fracture, radius	813.81

60. Compound fracture, proximal end of ulna — 813.04
62. Aortic stenosis — 424.1
64. Diverticulosis of colon — 562.10
66. Fetal distress — 656.30
68. Abrasion, finger — 915.0
70. Open C1 fracture — 805.11
72. Acid burns to cornea — 940.3
74. Developmental dyslexia — 315.02
76. Hysterical paralysis — 300.11
78. Alcohol liver cirrhosis — 571.2
80. Hypoglycemia — 251.2
82. Third-degree perineal laceration — 664.20
84. Lung contusion — 861.21
86. Aggressive personality — 301.3
88. Bacterial meningitis — 320.9
90. Placenta previa — 641.00
92. Gestational hypertension — 642.30
94. Septicemia due to streptococcus — 038.0
96. Gouty arthritis — 274.0
98. Chronic alcohol abuse — 303.90
100. Separation anxiety disorder — 309.21

Practical Application (p. 168)

2. ICD-9-CM CODE(S):   794.8
                        789.00

RATIONALE:
Signs and symptoms related to abnormal liver studies (not yet diagnosed). Abdominal pain has not been proven to be associated with abnormal lab studies; therefore it, as well as a secondary diagnosis, is coded.

4. ICD-9-CM CODE(S):   250.11

RATIONALE:
Diabetes (250.00) need not be coded as included in the code for diabetic ketoacidosis.

6. ICD-9-CM CODE(S):   789.06
                        787.01

RATIONALE:
Because no definitive diagnosis was made at the conclusion of the encounter, only signs and symptoms may be coded.

8. ICD-9-CM CODE(S):   V24.2
                        V58.3

10. ICD-9-CM CODE(S):   884.0
                         913.01
                         912.0
                         923.10
                         923.03
                         E968.9

CHAPTER 7

Chapter Review Exercise (p. 181)

2. b. False
4. Type of service provided, similar to CPT, such as:
   Laboratory
   Imaging
   Chiropractic
   Obstetric

6. More digits (need to expand system)
   Physician training of documentation needs
   Alphanumerical (information systems upgrades)
   No decimals
   More codes

CHAPTER 8

Chapter Review Exercise (p. 187)

	Services	Diagnosis
2.	CBC	Anemia
4.	Injection antibiotic	Bacterial infection
6.	Bronchospasm evaluation	COPD
8.	Wrist x-ray	Wrist sprain
10.	Cardiac catheterization	Coronary artery disease

CHAPTER 9

Stop and Practice Exercises

Stop and Practice (p. 196)

		Section Found
2.	CBC w/diff	Pathology
4.	Pulmonary function testing	Medicine
6.	Endoscopy	Surgery
8.	Cast application	Surgery
10.	Allergy immunotherapy	Medicine
12.	Immunization(s)	Medicine
14.	Vaginal delivery	Surgery
16.	MRI	Radiology
18.	Allergy testing	Medicine
20.	Nursing home visit	Evaluation/management
22.	Antibiotic injection	Medicine
24.	Chemotherapy	Medicine

Chapter Review Exercise (p. 197)

		Chapter	Subsection
2.	CT scan, brain without contrast	Radiology	Diagnostic
4.	Emergency department visit	E & M	Emergency department
6.	Repair distal radius fracture	Surgery	Musculoskeletal
8.	Office visit	E & M	Office/outpatient
10.	Electrocardiogram	Medicine	Cardiography

12. Manipulation, finger   Surgery   Musculoskeletal
    joint
14. Tracheostomy,   Surgery   Respiratory
    emergency
16. Insertion of   Surgery   Cardiovascular
    pacemaker
18. Cataract extraction   Surgery   Eye
20. Hospital visit   E & M   Hospital

CHAPTER 10

Stop and Practice Exercises

Stop and Practice (p. 238)

2. Location: E & M/outpatient
   New/estab: Established
   Range of codes: 99211-99215
   Grid selected: 30
   Level of service: 99213

4. Location: E & M/office
   New/estab: Established
   Range of codes: 99211-99215
   Grid selected: 30
   Level of service: 99213

6. Location: E & M/office
   New/estab: Established
   Range of codes: 99211-99215
   Grid selected: 30
   Level of service: 99213

8. Location: E & M/office
   New/estab: Established
   Range of codes: 99211-99215
   Grid selected: 30
   Level of service: 99212

10. Location: E & M/office
    New/estab: Established
    Range of codes: 99211-99215
    Grid selected: 30
    Level of service: 99213

Chapter Review Exercise (p. 241)

2. Visit to the outpatient clinic
   Location: Outpatient
   New/established: Established
   Range of codes: 99211-99215

4. Patient requested consult
   Location: Outpatient
   New/established: New/established
   Range of codes: 99201-99205 (new)
                      99211-99215 (established)

6. Office visit, established patient
   Problem-focused history
   Problem-focused examination

Straightforward MDM
Location: Office/outpatient
New/established: Established
Range of codes: 99211-99215
Code selected: 99212

8. Outpatient consultation, established patient
   Comprehensive history
   Comprehensive examination
   Moderate medical decision making
   Location: Outpatient/office
   New/established: Established
   Range of codes: 99241-99245
   Code selected: 99244

10. Hospital observation care
    Comprehensive history
    Detailed examination
    Moderate medical decision making
    Location: Hospital
    New/established: New
    Range of codes: 99218-99220
    Code selected: 99218

Practical Application (p. 242)

2. Location: E & M/hospital/admit
   New/estab: New
   Range of codes: 99221-99223
   Grid selected: 32
   Level of service: 99221

4. Location: E & M/office
   New/estab: New
   Range of codes: 99201-99205
   Grid selected: 29
   Level of service: 99203

CHAPTER 11

Chapter Review Exercise (p. 257)

	Anesthesia CPT Code
2. Modified radical mastectomy	00846
4. Total hip replacement	01214
6. Angioplasty	01921
8. Knee arthroscopy	01382
10. Repair of hiatal hernia	00790

Practical Application (p. 258)

12. Anesthesia procedure code: 01820
    Physical status modifier: P1
    Qualifying circumstances code(s):   None
    Anesthesia modifier(s):   None
    Calculate time units (10-minute
      increments):   3

14. Anesthesia procedure code: 00120
    Physical status modifier: P1
    Qualifying circumstances code(s):   99100
    Anesthesia modifier(s):   None

Calculate time units (10-minute
increments):   5

16. Anesthesia procedure code: 01622
Physical status modifier: P1
Qualifying circumstances code(s):   None
Anesthesia modifier(s):   None
Calculate time units (10-minute
increments):   8

18. Anesthesia procedure code: 01830/
                                               01480
Physical status modifier: P1
Qualifying circumstances code(s):   None
Anesthesia modifier(s):   None
Calculate time units (10-minute   Time
increments):   not
                                           given

20. Anesthesia procedure code: 00120
Physical status modifier: P2
Qualifying circumstances code(s):   99100
Anesthesia modifier(s):   None
Calculate time units (10-minute
increments):   9

CHAPTER 12

Stop and Practice Exercises

Stop and Practice (p. 269)

		Modifier(s)
2.	Patient presents for knee arthroscopy and shoulder arthroscopy	59
4.	Patient presents for EGD (esophagogastroduodenoscopy); the scope cannot be advanced to the duodenum	52
6.	Patient has knee arthroscopy with: Arthroscopic lateral release Medial and lateral meniscectomy	51
8.	Patient has fracture of femur with preoperative and surgical care provided by surgeon at local hospital. Returns home for postoperative care only.	55
10.	Closed reduction of a distal radius fracture with application of cast was performed in the ED. Patient now returns for additional surgical intervention. The patient is taken to the OR where an open reduction of the same fracture is performed	58

Stop and Practice (p. 272)

2. Arthroscopy, knee, diagnostic
Surgery/musculoskeletal, arthroscopy, knee

4. Repair, laceration, arm, 3.5 cm, simple
Surgery/integumentary/repair/closure

6. Excision malignant lesion, 4.0 cm, arm
Surgery/integumentary/excision lesion/malignant

8. Coronary artery bypass graft, venous, 2 grafts
Surgery/cardiovascular/coronary bypass grafts/venous

10. Tonsillectomy and adenoidectomy, age 10
Surgery/digestive system/tonsils adenoids/tonsillectomy adenoidectomy

12. Salpingectomy, unilateral
Surgery/female genital system/oviduct ovary/excision

14. Extracapsular cataract removal with lens implant
Surgery/eye/cornea/cataract

16. Prostatectomy, radical, with limited pelvic lymphadenectomy
Surgery/male genital/prostate/excision

18. Bronchoscopy with brushings
Surgery/respiratory/bronchi/endoscopy

20. Closed treatment of metacarpal fracture, with manipulation
Surgery/musculoskeletal/fingers and hand/fracture

Stop and Practice (p. 274)

2. Develop such an outline specific to a particular practice and specialty. An example of a specialty-specific guideline is shown in Table 12-1. This information will prove helpful in the coding of services.

Please refer to Tool 50 and the example provided in Table 12-1.

Stop and Practice (p. 281)

		Code(s)/Modifier(s)
2.	Excision malignant lesion, arm, 2.0 cm Excision malignant lesion, face, 2.5 cm	11643/11602
4.	Laceration repair, 2.0 cm, face	12011
6.	Destruction malignant lesion, 2.0 cm, face Excision malignant lesion, 1.5 cm, face Excision benign lesion, 2.5 cm, arm	11642 17282-51 11403-51
8.	Split thickness skin graft from thigh to cheek, 2 × 3 cm	15120
10.	Adjacent tissue transfer, arm, 20 sq cm with removal of malignant lesion, arm, 16 sq cm	14021

Stop and Practice (p. 284)

Code(s)/Modifier(s)

2. Closed repair, distal radius fracture — 25600
4. Rotator cuff repair — 23410 or 23412
6. Removal FB, musculature, thigh — 27372
8. Diagnostic right knee arthroscopy with medial/lateral meniscectomy — 29880
10. Arthroscopic TMJ repair — 29804

Stop and Practice (p. 285)

Code(s)/Modifier(s)

2. Tracheostomy — 31600/31603
4. Thoracentesis with tube placement — 32002
6. Endoscopic sphenoidotomy with tissue removal — 31288
8. Emergency endotracheal intubation — 31500
10. Bronchoscopic transbronchial lung biopsy, LLL — 31628
    Bronchoscopic transbronchial lung biopsy, RUL — 31632

Stop and Practice (p. 287)

Code(s)/Modifier(s)

2. Removal of old pacemaker pulse generator — 33233/33212
   Insertion of new pacemaker pulse generator
4. CABG, venous grafting, 3 vessels — 33512
6. Aortic peripheral atherectomy, open — 35481
8. Balloon angioplasty, percutaneous, iliac vessel — 35473
10. Venipuncture, age 7 — 36415

Stop and Practice (p. 288)

Code(s)/Modifier(s)

2. T & A, age 20 — 42821
4. Esophagoscopy with FB removal — 43215
6. Initial inguinal hernia repair, age 3 — 49505
8. EGD with dilation of esophagus — 43235/43450 if not dilated through scope 43248 if thru scope
10. Diagnostic anoscopy — 46600

Stop and Practice (p. 289)

Code(s)/Modifier(s)

2. Open drainage of renal abscess — 50020
4. Needle aspiration of bladder — 51000

6. Cysto with placement of ureteral stent — 52332
8. Dilation of urethral stricture with dilator, male — 52281
10. Partial laparoscopic nephrectomy — 50549 or 50545-52

Stop and Practice (p. 291)

Code(s)/Modifier(s)

2. Cesarean delivery, antepartum, delivery, and postpartum — 59510
4. Amniocentesis — 59000
6. Simple vulvectomy — 56620
8. Vasectomy — 55250
10. Laparoscopic tubal ligation by fulguration — 58670

Stop and Practice (p. 292)

Code(s)/Modifier(s)

2. Strabismus surgery, 2 horizontal muscles, rt eye — 67312-RT
4. Elevation of simple skull fracture — 62000
6. Implantation of neurostimulator electrodes percutaneous — 64553-64565
8. Repair of carpal tunnel nerve — 64721
10. Removal of cerumen — 69210

Chapter Review Exercise (p. 293)

2. Cholecystectomy
   CPT-4 procedure code(s) — 47563
   ICD-9-CM code(s) — 574.10

4. Cataract, right eye
   CPT-4 procedure code(s) — 66984-RT
   ICD-9-CM code(s) — 366.9

Practical Application (p. 294)

2. ICD-9: — 610.3
   CPT-4: — 19125-RT/19290-RT

4. ICD-9: — 211.3/455.3/562.10/V12.72
   CPT-4: — 45385/45384-51/45380-51

CHAPTER 13

Chapter Review Exercise (p. 307)

2. CPT-4 CODE: 73090-LT   ICD-9-CM CODE: 813.21
4. CPT-4 CODE: 73600-RT, 73000   ICD-9-CM CODE: 719.47, 719.48
6. CPT-4 CODE: 76519   ICD-9-CM CODE: 366.9
8. CPT-4 CODE: 77432   ICD-9-CM CODE: V58.0
10. CPT-4 CODE: 76942   ICD-9-CM CODE: 611.72
12. CPT-4 CODE: 78300   ICD-9-CM CODE: 730.2
14. CPT-4 CODE: 76775   ICD-9-CM CODE: 593.9
16. CPT-4 CODE: 73100-50   ICD-9-CM CODE: 716.93
18. CPT-4 CODE: 71010   ICD-9-CM CODE: 491.21
20. CPT-4 CODE: 76815   ICD-9-CM CODE: V28.4

Practical Application (p. 308)

2. ICD-9-CM CODE: 789.1
   CPT-4 CODE: 74170

4. ICD-9-CM CODE: 786.2
   CPT-4 CODE: 71020

CHAPTER 14

Chapter Review Exercise (p. 320)

2. Automated hemogram and platelet count with complete white blood cell count
   CPT-4 CODE(S):   85027
4. ABO and RH blood typing
   CPT-4 CODE(S):   86900, 86901
6. Thyroid disease panel
   CPT-4 CODE(S):   none/not enough information
8. Metabolic panel
   CPT-4 CODE(S):   80048
10. Bacterial culture, urine
    CPT-4 CODE(S):   (need site/method)
12. Therapeutic assay, digoxin
    CPT-4 CODE(S):   80162
14. Potassium level
    CPT-4 CODE(S):   84132
16. Bilirubin, total
    CPT-4 CODE(S):   82247
18. Surgical pathology, oophorectomy
    CPT-4 CODE(S):   88305
20. Hemoglobin
    CPT-4 CODE(S):   85018

CHAPTER 15

Chapter Review Exercise (p. 334)

2. ECG, interpretation and report only
   CPT-4 CODE(S):   93010
4. Mumps, measles, rubella vaccine
   CPT-4 CODE(S):   90707, 90471
6. Dermatological ultraviolet light treatment
   CPT-4 CODE(S):   96900
8. Prescription and fitting of contact lenses
   CPT-4 CODE(S):   92310
10. Cardiopulmonary resuscitation
    CPT-4 CODE(S):   92950
12. Spirometry
    CPT-4 CODE(S):   94010
14. Intraoperative neurophysiology testing, 1 hour
    CPT-4 CODE(S):   95920
16. Doppler study of intracranial arteries, limited, transcranial
    CPT-4 CODE(S):   93888
18. Cardiovascular stress test, complete
    CPT-4 CODE(S):   93015

20. Comprehensive ophthalmological examination, new patient
    CPT-4 CODE(S):   92004

Practical Application (p. 335)

2.
   93510 (access was artery)
   93541/93545/93544/93543/93542 (injection codes)
   93555/93556 (imaging codes, no duplicates)

4.
   93510 (access femoral artery)
   93545/93543/93544 (injection codes)
   93555/93556 (imaging codes/no duplications)

6.
   4 motor nerves (3 F waves/1 non-F wave) 95900 X 3
                                                       95903 X 1
   4 sensory nerves   95904 X 4

8.
   Spirometry with and without bronchodilator
   ABG (arterial blood gas)
   Code: 94060
   36600 (if ABG puncture performed in office/sent to laboratory for processing)

10.
   EKG interpretation and report only
   93010 (first EKG interpretation)
   93010-76 (second EKG interpretation)

CHAPTER 16

Chapter Review Exercises (p. 357)

	Modifier Code (Examples Will Vary)
2. Services less than usually performed	52
4. Office visit **with** laceration repair, 2.5 cm, eyebrow	25
6. Office visit for postoperative complication	24
8. Repeat ECG, same day, different physician	77
10. Consult during which decision for surgery is made	57
12. Multiple procedures performed same time, same operative site	51
14. Two surgeons performing same procedures	62

16. A patient with a 1.2-cm laceration repair performed 3 days before presents for a "recheck" of suture repair.
    Service(s):   Evaluation and management
    CPT section: 99024
    Modifier?   Y (N)

Modifier code:
99024 if postoperative for global procedure

18. A laboratory service is not performed by the physician's office; however, the laboratory bills the physician's office and the physician's office bills the third-party carrier.
    Service(s): Pathology section
    CPT section: Code from pathology section 80000-89999
    Modifier? Ⓨ N   Modifier code: 90

20. Two surgical procedures are performed during the same surgical session: repair of inguinal hernia and repair of metacarpal fracture.
    Service(s): Surgery
    CPT section: 49495 (if less than 6 months); 49500 (6 months to 5 years); 49505 (more than 5 years)
    Modifier? Ⓨ N   Modifier code: 59

22. A colonoscopy scheduled to be performed is cancelled at the patient's request.
    Service(s): Surgery
    CPT section: 45378
    Modifier? Y Ⓝ   Modifier code: Procedure not started cannot be billed except for outpatient hospital/outpatient facility with use of modifier 73/74

CHAPTER 17

Chapter Review Exercise (p. 361)

		HCPCS Code
2.	Cervical or vaginal cancer screening	G0101
4.	Hospital bed, semielectric, without mattress	E0261
6.	Injection, ceftazidime, 750 mg	J0713 X 2
8.	Replacement batteries for medically necessary TENS unit	A4630
10.	Breast prosthesis, mastectomy sleeve	L8010
12.	Injection, methotrexate, 100 mg	J9260 X 2
14.	Prednisone, oral, 10 mg	J7506 X 2
16.	Repair of durable medical equipment, 30 minutes	E1340
18.	Intraoral x-rays, complete	D0210
20.	Injection, unlisted substance, 50 mg IM	J3490

Practical Application (p. 361)

2.

CODE ASSIGNMENT:

L4350	845.00
	E885.9
99213	845.00
	E885.9

4.

CODE ASSIGNMENT:

99214	276.8/414.00
93000	414.00
J3480X5	276.8
90765	276.8

CHAPTER 18

Stop and Practice Exercises

Stop and Practice (p. 383)

		ICD-9-CM Code(s)
2.	Cough Fever Probable <u>pneumonia</u>	486
4.	<u>Angina</u>, most likely <u>unstable</u>	411.1
6.	Elevated blood pressure, probably not hypertension	796.2
8.	<u>Ankle pain</u>, ankle fracture ruled out	719.47
10.	Confusional state	298.9
	Nausea and vomiting	787.01
	Dehydration	276.51
	Alzheimer's dementia	331.0, 294.1

12. 574.10 only (other diagnoses are signs/symptoms that do not need code assignment)

14. Influenza (possible diagnoses are coded for inpatient hospital as long as they have not been ruled out and are the chief reason for the admission)

Chapter Review Exercises (p. 390)

		Volume 3- ICD-9-CM Code
2.	Repair of fractured clavicle	79.00
4.	Cholecystectomy	51.22
6.	Tonsillectomy with adenoidectomy	28.3
8.	Knee arthroscopy	80.26
10.	Colonoscopy with biopsy	45.25
12.	Flexible sigmoidoscopy	45.24
14.	Cardiac catheterization	37.21
16.	Esophageal speech training	93.73
18.	Clavicular osteotomy	77.31
20.	Amputation, below the knee	84.15
22.	CPAP ventilation	93.90
24.	Vaginal delivery with episiotomy	72.1

		ICD-9-CM Code	(I), (P), (IP)
26.	Rule out pneumonia	486	I
28.	Myocardial infarction	410.90	IP
30.	Acute respiratory failure COPD	518.81	IP

		Physician	Inpatient
32.	Abdominal pain Rule out appendicitis	Abdominal pain	Appendicitis
34.	Anemia, possibly from chronic blood loss anemia	Anemia	Blood loss

CHAPTER 19

Chapter Review Exercise (p. 404)

2.

ICD-9-CM diagnostic code(s): pyelonephritis 590.80 (use 590.80 followed by 646.63 for pregnancy complication)

Dehydration:	276.5
ICD-9-CM procedure code(s):	None
MDC assignment:	11
DRG assignment:	320

2.

ICD-9-CM diagnostic code(s):	599.0
ICD-9-CM procedure code(s):	None
CPT-4 code(s):	None
APC(s) assignments:	None

Observation care is NOT reimbursable except for three conditions, one of which is not urinary tract infection. Keep in mind this service would be reimbursable on the physician side, however.

CHAPTER 20

Chapter Review Exercise (p. 413)

PHYSICIAN

	Services	Diagnoses
2.	Repair of fractured femur	Fractured femur
	Repair of fractured metacarpal	Fractured metacarpal
	Laceration repair, face, simple	Open wound, face

INPATIENT

	Services	Diagnoses
4.	Admission	Pneumonia
		Umbilical hernia
	Hernia repair	Umbilical hernia
	Arterial blood gas	Pneumonia
	Chest x-ray	Pneumonia
6.	Outpatient surgery for umbilical hernia	Umbilical hernia
	Inpatient admission for cardiac arrest during outpatient procedure	Cardiac arrest / Hypertension / CAD

Practical Application (p. 414)

2.

99213 (Limited by history of present illness <4 elements)

4.

ICD-9:   959.3 Elbow injury
          E881.0 Fall from ladder

CPT: 99213 (Expanded problem exam/history)
        A4565 Sling

6.
ICD-9:   493.10
CPT: 99212 (Visit focused only on asthma/respiratory system)

8.
ICD-9:   564.1
CPT: 99213 (Problem focused on abdominal pain; however, related systems evaluated; therefore expanded problem focused)

10.
ICD-9:   493.10
CPT: 99212 (No exam, problem focused on one system/respiratory)

12.
ICD-9:   474.02
CPT: 42820 <12 years; 42821 >12 years

14.
ICD-9:   466.0
          493.90
CPT: 99221 (Limited by review of systems)

CHAPTER 21

Chapter Review Exercise (p. 445)

(Answers to these exercises will vary considerably.)

CHAPTER 22

Chapter Review Exercise (p. 465)

2. **Give examples of abuse.**
   Overuse of medical or health services
   Billing excessive charges
   Filing claims for services not medically necessary
   Breaching assignment agreements
   Exceeding the limiting charge
   Ordering procedures more frequently than medically necessary

4. **Identify and explain what elements should be identified in a chart audit process.**
   Undercodes/overcodes
   Missing documentation/signatures
   Level of service distribution
   Ancillary service documentation/signature
   Compliance with practice/facility chart protocol

CHAPTER 23

Medical Terminology
Practice Examination 1 (p. 471)

2. tumor
4. epidermis

6. crypto
8. a and c
10. cut, section
12. through
14. atrium
16. ear
18. C1
20. spinal cord
22. speech
24. polio

Medical Terminology
Practice Examination 2 (p. 473)

2. inferior
4. gland
6. centesis
8. orrhaphy
10. surgical fixation of a testicle
12. before
14. excision of stones from gallbladder

16. protrusion of the rectum
18. cold
20. metatarsals
22. costo
24. subdural hematoma

Coding Practice Examination (p. 475)

2. 079.99, V02.52
4. 796.2
6. 784.3
8. 535.50, 995.2, E930.3
10. 99310
12. 99218, 99217
14. Patient in otherwise good health
16. 73565
18. 23410, 29826-51
20. 45385, 45380-51
22. 26608 X2
24. 69436-50

INDEX

A

Abbreviations
  ICD-9-CM, 91
  standard, 5-6
Abdominal pain, 74, 104, 107, 123
  coding exercise for, 169
Abuse, definitions of, 451-452
Accidental overdose, 130, 145
Accidents, 130
  coding exercise for, 176
  motor vehicle, 72
Acellular dermal replacement grafts, 280
Acronyms, standard, 5-6
Actinotherapy, 332
Acute renal failure, 140
Adenoidectomy, 288
Admissions
  documentation of, 15, 22f
  history and physical in, 369-370
Affective disorders, 151
Age, DRG codes for, 394
Alcohol abuse, 151
Alcohol dependence, 151
Allergies, 143
Allergy/clinical immunology, 330-331
Allogenic skin substitute, tissue-
  cultured, 280
Alzheimer's disease, 150
Ambulatory Payment Classification system.
  See APC system.
Ambulatory Payment Groups/Ambulatory
  Payment Classification, 183
American Academy of Professional Coders,
  certification examinations of, 467, 468t
American Health Information Management
  System, certification examinations of,
  467, 468t
American Medical Association, coding
  methodology of, 189
Amnesia, transient global, 150
Analgesia, types of, 254
Anatomical modifiers, 284
Ancillary records, 369
Ancillary services
  APCs for, 385, 400
  documentation of, 23, 31
  request form for, 437, 438f
Anemias, 150
Anesthesia Assistant, 253

Anesthesia services, 248-259
  calculating time units for, 256-257
  coding guidelines, 254-257
  coding steps, 249, 253
  documentation and coding guidelines,
    249, 250f, 251f-252f, 253
  global components of, 254
  modifier codes, 255-256
  monitored, 253
  practical application, 258-259
  preanesthesia evaluation for, 249, 250f
  providers of, 253
  record of, 249, 251f-252f
  types of, 253-254
Anesthesiologist, 253
Anesthesiology, CPT-4 coding for, 190-191
Angina, 69
Anxiety, 144
APC system
  ancillary services in, 385, 400
  assignment process in, 402-403, 402t
  general guidelines for, 386, 402
  hospital outpatient services and, 411
  medical visits in, 385-386, 400, 402
  payment status indicators in, 402
  significant procedures in, 385, 400
  surgical services in, 385, 400
Appendectomy, 288
  with other intraabdominal
    procedures, 290
Appendicitis, 156
Arterial grafts, 286
Arterial-venous grafts, 286
Arthritis, 161
Arthrocentesis, 282
Arthrodesis, defined, 291
Arthroscopic procedures, 283-284
  knee, 110
Assault, 130, 131
Asthma, 155
  coding exercise for, 168
Audit, chart. See Chart audit.
Auditory system, 292
  key medical terms, 292

B

Bacterial infection, leg, 103
Benefits, fraudulent receipt of, 450
Billing services. See also Hospital/facility
  billing process.
  CPT-4 and, 187
  improper practices in, 451-452
Biofeedback, 329

Bipolar disorder, 80
Birth weight, 395
Blood disorders, 149-150
Blood vessel injuries, 163
Body systems, 212
  CPT, components of, 271
  in CPT-4 physical examination
    requirements, 206
  review of, 186t
Bone grafts, 282
Brachytherapy, clinical, 306
Breast cancer, 125, 133
Breast disorders, 158
Breast mass, review exercise for, 293, 294
Breast procedures, 280
Bronchitis, 154-155
Bronchoscopy, 285
Bullet, coding significance of, 195
Bundled services, 274-277
  reimbursement for, 440
Burns, 164-165

C

Candidiasis, 148
Carcinoma in situ, 134
Cardiac catheterization, 331f
Cardiac defects, 161
Cardiac dysrhythmias, 154
Cardiovascular medicine, 330
Cardiovascular system, 286-287
Care plan oversight services, 236-237
Case management services, 236
Cast applications, 283
Cataract operation, 292
  review exercise, 294
Cataracts, diabetic (snowflake), 149
Catheterization, cardiac, 331f
Centers for Medicare and Medicaid Services
  medical reviews of, 4
  regulatory/enforcement functions of, 449
Central nervous system, assessment of,
  331-332
Cerebrovascular disease, 154
Certification examination
  practice versions, 471-476
  preparing for, 467-470
  study schedule for, 469f
Certification process, 466-476
  certifying organizations in, 467, 468t
Certification review, coding concepts in, 52
Certified Registered Nurse Anesthetist, 253
Cesarean birth, coding exercise for, 175
Charge ticket/document, 435, 436f

Page numbers followed by f indicate figures;
t, tables; b, boxes.

Chart audit, 455, 457-463
  ancillary service documentation/signature
      requirements for, 460
  compiling data from, 461
  components of, 459
  deficiency documentation and calculation
      in, 461
  events triggering, 464
  levels of service distribution in, 460
  missing documentation/signatures
      and, 460
  preparing for, 460
  protocol compliance in, 460-461
  report for, 461-463
  specific focus of, 460
  summary of findings, 463
  tools for, 460
  undercodes/overcodes in, 460
Chemicals
  documentation requirements for, 130
  ICD-9-CM coding for, 129-132, 129f
Chemistry, 318-319
Chemotherapy, 133, 332
Chest discomfort, 78
Chest pain, 70, 101
  in elderly patient, 73
Chest x-ray in physician diagnosis, 65
Childbirth, 158-160
  complaints following, 102
  V codes for, 115
Children, 223, 225. See also entries under
      Pediatric critical care services,
      inpatient.
Chills, 81
  coding exercise for, 169, 172
Chiropractic manipulative treatment,
      332-333
Cholecystectomy, review exercise, 293
Cholecystitis, 156
Cholelithiasis, 156
Chronic obstructive pulmonary disease, 155
Chronic renal failure, 157
Circulatory system disorders, 153-154
Circumcision, 289
Claims
  clean, 117
  electronic, 455
  fraudulent, 450-451
  processing of, 435
  review process for, 455
  of third-party carriers, 433
Cleft lip/palate, 162
Clinical Laboratory Improvements
      Amendments, 317
CMS. See Centers for Medicare and
      Medicaid Services.
Code 99288, 223
Code books, student notes in, 467-470
Code modifiers. See Modifier codes.
Codeable services
  concept of, 185
  documentation guidelines, 185
  matching with diagnostic codes, 185
Coders, certified, 467
Coding. See also Current Procedural
      Terminology, fourth edition; Diagnosis-
      Related Groups system; ICD-9-CM
      diagnostic codes.

Coding (Continued)
  education about, 437-438
  ethics of, 453-454
  exercise in, 99-100
  hints for, 96
  from ICD-9-CM book, 95
  monitoring and compliance in. See
      Monitoring and compliance process.
  practice examination for, 475-476
  reimbursement perspective on. See
      Reimbursement, coding and.
  review process for, 455, 457-458
  software for, 439-440
  of special complexities. See Medical
      complexities.
  steps in, 185-187
  worksheet for, 97
Coding nomenclature, computer setup
      of, 435
Coding process
  introduction to, 1
  physician documentation in, 1-53. See
      also Physician documentation.
  reference tools for, 2
Coding systems. See also Current
      Procedural Terminology, fourth
      edition; Diagnosis-Related Groups
      system; ICD-9-CM diagnostic coding.
  combining, 409-429
    example of, 412
    hospital services, 411-412
    and order of services listed, 411
    overview of, 411
    physician coding, 411
    practical applications, 414-429
    review exercise, 413-414
    steps in, 413
Colonoscopy
  defined, 287
  practical coding application, 273
Communicable disease
  childhood, 148
  health hazards related to, V codes
      for, 113
Comorbidities, 394-395
Complete blood cell count in physician
      diagnosis, 65
Compliance programs, 463-465
  advantages of, 464-465
  determining practice need for, 464
  elements triggering investigation/audit
      in, 464
  federal guidelines for, 464b
  HIPAA requirements for, 463
  JCAHO requirements for, 463-464
Complications, coding for, 394-395
Computer system
  erroneous entries in, 435
  programming of, 437
Congenital anomalies, 161-162
Consultations, 217, 222-226
  assigning diagnostic code for, 109
  in clinical pathology, 318
  crosswalk codes for, 223, 225
  documentation of, 23, 26f
  follow-up inpatient, 223
  initial inpatient, 223-224
  office/outpatient, 217, 219, 222

Contracts
  carrier coding nomenclature in, 439
  third-party
    definitions in, 433
    developing worksheets for, 441-442,
        443f, 444
    guidelines for, 433-434
Contrasts, 305
Contusions, 163
Coronary artery bypass, 286
Coronary artery disease, 153
Corpectomy, defined, 291
Counseling intervention, 237
CPT-4. See Current Procedural Terminology,
      fourth edition.
Cramping, epigastric, 106
Critical care services, 225, 228
  inpatient pediatric, 228-229
  pediatric, 223, 225
Crush injuries, 163
Current Procedural Terminology, fourth
      edition
  AMA edition of, 467
  billing services/procedures and, 187
  body systems table for, 185, 186t
  code modifiers in, 440. See also Modifier
      codes.
  code specifications of, 4
  coding book format, 195-196
  coding book layout, 189-195
  coding steps for, 185-187
  combining with other systems, 410-429.
      See also Coding systems, combining.
  definitions/concepts in, 194-195
  documentation and, 183, 189-195
  evaluation and management codes
      in, 189-190
  format of, 195-196
  future of, 196, 196b
  global procedures "package concept"
      in, 194
  guidelines for, 192, 196b
  hospital coding with, 90-91
  versus ICD-9-CM, 183
  and matching of services with diagnostic
      codes, 185
  medicine codes in, 192
  modifier codes in, 192-194
    for additional services, 193
    for bilateral services, 193
    multiple physicians/locations, 193
    professional versus technical, 193
    for repeated services, 193
    for service level, 193
    of third-party significance, 194
    for unusual circumstances/
        exceptions, 194
  pathology codes in, 191-192
  for physician services coding, 183
  preventive visits in, 440
  for procedural services, 411
  radiology codes in, 191
  reimbursement and, 439-440
  for reporting WHAT services, 411
  reviewing codes on claims, 455
  separate procedures in, 195
  services omitted from, 386
  starred procedures in, 194

Current Procedural Terminology, fourth
    edition *(Continued)*
  steps in, 190t
  surgery codes in, 191
  symbols in, 196
  terms used in, 5
  unlisted procedures and, 194-195
  using, 188-197
  WHAT and WHY elements in, 183
  WHAT services in, 185
Current Procedural Terminology, fifth
    edition, 196
  future of, 196b
Custodial services, 229, 232-233
Cystoscopy, 288
Cystourethroscopy, 288

D

Data, quantity and complexity of, 206
Data entry, monitoring of, 454
Decision making, medical, 206,
    209-210, 212
Defibrillator, 286
Depression, 152
Dermal replacement grafts, acellular, 280
Dermatological services, 332
Diabetes mellitus, 148-149
  coding exercise for, 171
  with foot ulcers, 149
  with ketoacidosis, 149
  with ophthalmic manifestations, 149
  pregnancy and, 149
  with renal manifestations, 149
Diagnoses
  with CPT-4, ICD-9-CM, and DRG
      combined, 411
  do's and don'ts for, 382
  in DRG assignment process, 399
  elements/words for possible use as, 380
  locating, in ICD-9-CM, 94
  number of, 206
  patients without, V codes for, 115
  physician. *See* Physician diagnosis.
  principal, 383-384
    in DRG system, 394
    in hospital inpatient coding, 411
  secondary, in DRG system, 394
  symptoms used in lieu of, 383
  when original treatment plans not
      completed, 384
Diagnosis-Related Groups system, 393-394
  assignment process, 399-400
    contributing factors in, 400
    medical versus surgical partition
        in, 400
  coding with, 183
    guidelines for, 395
    inpatient worksheet for, 401f
    process for, 395-396, 397b
  combining with other systems, 410-429.
      See also Coding systems, combining.
  components of, 394-395
  for reporting WHAT services, 411
  theory of, 90
Diagnostic codes. *See also* Current
    Procedural Terminology, fourth
    edition; Diagnosis-Related Groups
    system; ICD-9-CM diagnostic coding.

Diagnostic codes *(Continued)*
  for ICD-9-CM diagnoses, 380
  proper order of, 380, 382
Diagnostic infusions, 327
Diagnostic injections, 328
Diagnostic services, radiological,
    interpretation of, 305
Diagnostic statements for proper coding
    purposes, 380-382
Diagnostic studies, noninvasive
    vascular, 330
Diagnostic tests, unnecessary, 452
Dialysis, 329
Diaphragm, 287
Digestive system disorders, 155-156,
    287-288
  key medical terms, 287
  practical applications, 288
Discharge notes, 378
Discharge status, DRG codes for, 394
Discharge summary, 23, 25f, 379
Discharge summary/record, 369, 380
Diskectomy, defined, 291
Dislocations, 164, 282-283
Documentation. *See also* Physician
    documentation.
  of ancillary test findings, 23, 31
  changing role of, 4
  CPT-4 and, 183
  developing tools for, 31
  do's and don'ts list for, 49, 50
  forms and formats for, 49
  fraud and, 3
  good words/bad words list for, 49
  by health care staff, 23
  miscellaneous, 31
  monitoring procedure for, 49
  for new patients, 42f
  payment collection and, 3
  role of, 1
  signature requirements for, 49
  specialty-specific, 43f-46f
  terminology for, 31
  types of, 1
Domiciliary services, 229, 232-233
Downcoding services, 439-440
DRGs. *See* Diagnosis-Related Groups
    system.
Drug assays, therapeutic, 318
Drug overdose, 130
  flowchart for, 130-132
Drugs
  allergies to, 143
  documentation requirements for,
      130
  ICD-9-CM coding for, 129-132, 129f
  ICD-9-CM table for, 129-132, 129f
    appropriate usage of, 129-130
    documentation of, 130
    flowchart for, 130-132
Dyspnea, 83
Dysrhythmias, 154

E

E codes, 116-118
  scenarios for, 121-127
Ear, nose, and throat services. *See*
    Otorhinolaryngological services.

Edema, bilateral pedal, diagnostic coding
    for, 87
Electrocardiogram, 19f, 326f
Electromyography report, 21f, 325f
Electronic signatures, 3
Emergency department visits, 223, 227
  documentation requirements for, 36-37
Encephalopathy, metabolic, 150
Endocrine disorders, 148-149, 291
Epidural analgesia, 254
Epigastric cramping, assigning diagnostic
    code for, 106
Epigastric pain, coding exercise for, 173
Error percentage, 3
Ethics, coding, 453-454
Evaluation and Management CPT-4. *See*
    Current Procedural Terminology,
    fourth edition.
Evaluation and management services,
    198-247
  categories of
    care plan oversight services, 236-237
    case management services, 236
    consultations, 217, 222-226
    counseling/risk factor intervention, 237
    critical care services, 225, 228
    domiciliary, rest home, custodial
        services, 229, 232-233
    emergency department visits, 223, 227
    home services, 229, 234-235
    hospital inpatient services, 217,
        220, 221
    hospital observation services, 214, 217
    hospital outpatient visits, 214-216
    inpatient pediatric critical care/
        neonatal intensive care, 228-229
    newborn care, 238
    nursing facility services, 229-231
    other, 238
    pediatric critical care transport,
        223, 225
    physician standby services, 236
    preventive medicine services, 237
    prolonged services, 229, 236
    special services, 238
  coding errors, 240
  coding guidelines, 201, 204f-205f,
      205-206
  coding modifiers, 201-203, 201t
  coding problems, 241
  coding review, 240
  coding steps in, 199, 201, 212-213
  coding for third-party reimbursement,
      439-440
  component levels in, 212
  CPT-4 coding for, 189-190
  for decision for surgery, 202-203
  determination guidelines, 203, 204f-205f,
      205-206
  distinct and separate, 202
  documentation guidelines, 199-201
  history in, 206
  key terms, 199
  level of, 203, 204f-205f, 205-206
  mandated, 202
  medical decision making in, 206, 209-
      210, 212
  other, 239

Evaluation and management services
   (Continued)
   physical examination in, 206, 208
   practical applications, 238-239, 242-247
   prolonged, 201
   reduced, 202
   unrelated to global/postoperative period,
      201-202
   worksheet tables for, 211f
Evocative/suppression testing, 318
Examinations
   practice versions, 471-476
   preparing for, 467-470
Explanation of Benefits, review of,
   437-438
External causes codes. *See* E codes.
External fixation, 283
Eye/ocular adnexa, 291-292
   key medical terms, 291-292

F

Family history, health hazards related to, V
   codes for, 114
Fetal disorders, 158
Fever
   coding exercises for, 169, 172
   of unknown origin, 86
Fixation, external, 283
Foreign body removal, practical coding
   application, 272
Fracture reductions, 283
Fractures, 163, 282-283
Fraud, definitions of, 3, 450-451
Fraud and abuse
   considerations regarding, 452-453
   investigations of, events triggering, 464
   legislation on, 449-450
   reporting, 453-454
Full thickness graft, 280

G

Gait, unstable, 108
Gallbladder excision, 288
Gastroenteritis, 147, 156
Gastroenterology, 329
Gastrointestinal ulcers, 155-156
Genital system
   female, 289-290
      practical applications, 291
   male, 289
      practical applications, 291
Genitourinary system disorders, 156-157
Godfrey Regional Hospital, providers and
   facilities of, 49, 51t
Godfrey Regional Practice Information and
   Forms, 513-518
Grafts, 279-280
   arterial, 286
   arterial-venous, 286
   bone, 282
Graves' disease, 149
Gynecological disorders, 158
Gynecological procedures, common
   global, 278t

H

HCPCS. *See* Healthcare Common Procedure
   Coding System.

Headache, 75
   coding exercise for, 170
Health care costs, containment of, 5
Health care services, codeable, 184-187. *See
   also* Codeable services.
Health hazards, V codes for, 113-114
Health Insurance Portability and
   Accountability Act
   coding provisions of, 189
   monitoring compliance with, 463
Health services
   overuse of, 451
   specific procedures/aftercare in, V codes
      for, 115
Health status, conditions affecting, V codes
   for, 115
Healthcare Common Procedure Coding
   System, 189, 358-366
   format for, 359
   index for, 359-360
   Level II
      modifiers for, 354t-356t
      rules for selecting, 360
   new technology and pass through
      payments in, 402
   practical applications, 361-366
   review exercise, 361
   for services not assigned CPT-4
      codes, 386
Hearing evaluations, 292
Heart beat, slow, diagnosis coding for, 71
Heart disease
   hypertension in, 136-137
   ischemic, 153-154
Hematology, 319
Hemic system, 287
Hepatitis, viral, 148
Hernia, hiatal, review exercise, 294
Hernia repair, 288
Herpes simplex infection, 148
Herpes zoster infection, 148
Hiatal hernia, review exercise, 294
History and physical, 369-370
HIV infection, 147
Home services, 229, 234-235, 333
Hospital charge ticket/document,
   435, 436f
Hospital coding, 368-391
   definitions and inpatient guidelines,
      383-384
   documentation/coding guidelines,
      369, 380
   outpatient, 385
   versus physician coding, 90-91
   practical applications, 383
   query process in, 384-385
   steps in, 385-390
      inpatient, 380-383
   Volume 3—Procedure Index in,
      384, 384b
Hospital records, 15, 23
Hospital services
   coding for, 183
   inpatient, 217, 220, 221
   inpatient coding of, for principal
      diagnosis, 411
   observation, 214, 217
   order listed in, 411-412

Hospital services *(Continued)*
   outpatient, 214-216
      CPT-4 codes for, 411-412
Hospital/facility billing process, 392-408
   APC assignment process in, 402-
      404, 402t
   documentation/coding guidelines, 393
   inpatient billing/reimbursement methods,
      393-394
      DRG coding, 394-400
   outpatient billing/reimbursement
      methods, 400-402
   review exercises for, 404-408
Hypercholesterolemia, 68
Hyperemesis, coding exercise for, 174
Hypertension, 153, 172
   chronic, 137
   with chronic renal failure, 137
   coding for, 140
   complications of, 137
   controlled/uncontrolled, 135-136
   documentation issues, 154
   essential, 135
   with heart disease, 136-137
   ICD-9-CM table for, 135-137, 136f
   possible, assigning diagnostic code
      for, 105
   in pregnancy, 136
   transient, 136
Hyperthyroidism, 149
Hypothyroidism, 149
Hysteroscopy, 289

I

ICD. *See* International Classification of
   Diseases, versions of.
ICD-9-CM Code Book, 88-111
   abbreviations in, 91
   charts for, 101-145
   coding hints for, 96
   and differences in hospital and physician
      coding, 90-91
   documentation worksheet for, 97f
   format of, 91
   guidelines for, 93-96
   instructional notations in, 92
   medical necessity and, 90
   numerical and alphabetical index in,
      92-93
   punctuation in, 91-92
   symbols in, 92
   tabular list for, 98
   terms used in, 91
   typefaces in, 92
   uses of, 89-90
ICD-9-CM diagnostic coding, 55-181
   assigning codes from, 67
   combining with other systems, 410-429.
      See also Coding systems, combining.
   versus Current Procedural Terminology,
      fourth edition, 183
   and determining physician diagnosis, 56-
      87. *See also* Physician diagnosis.
   diagnostic statements in, 59, 61-62, 64
   versus ICD-10-CM, 180t, 181
   key elements/words in, 57, 59
   Official Guidelines for Coding and
      Reporting, 477-512

ICD-9-CM diagnostic coding (Continued)
 real case scenarios for, 89-90
 reimbursement and, 439-440
 reviewing codes on claims, 455
 standards of care and, 89
 step 1 of, 57, 59, 60f
 step 2 of, 59, 61-62, 63f, 64
 step 3 of, 64-65, 66f, 67
 steps in, 55, 57-64
 tables for, 128-145
  drugs and chemicals, 129-132, 129f
  hypertension, 135-137, 136f
  neoplasms, 132-135, 134f
  practical applications of, 140-145
 Volume 3—Procedure Index, 384, 384b
 WHAT elements in, 63f, 64, 66f,
  67, 183
 WHY elements in, 63f, 64, 66f, 67, 183
ICD-10-CM, 178-181
 code families in, 180
 expected update of, 179
 versus ICD-9-CM, 180t, 181
 implementation planning for, 181
 layout/conventions of, 179-180
 new features of, 180
 service categories in, 179
ICD-10-CM Code Book, 89
Immune globulins, 327
Immunizations, 122
Immunization/vaccination administration, 327
Immunology, 319
 allergy/clinical, 330-331
Infants, liveborn, V codes for, 115
Infectious diseases, 147-148
Infusions, therapeutic/diagnostic, 327
Injections, 282
 therapeutic/diagnostic, 327
Injuries, 79, 126, 127, 163-166
 coding exercise for, 177
 documentation of, 38f
 in ICD-10-CM, 180
Inpatient services, 217, 220
Insurance payments. See also Third-party
  carriers.
 CPT-4 codes for, 194
 documentation and, real case scenario
  of, 3-4
Integumentary system
 key medical terms, 278
 practical applications, 281
Intensive care
 versus critical care, 228
 neonatal, 228-229
International Classification of Diseases,
  versions of, 89. See also ICD-9-CM
  diagnostic coding; ICD-10-CM.
Intersex surgery, 289
Intracranial injuries, 163
Ischemic heart disease, 153-154
Isolation, V codes for, 113-114

J

Joint Commission on Accreditation of
  Healthcare Organizations
 compliance with guidelines of, 463-464
 medical record guidelines of, 15
Joint disorders, 161

K

Ketoacidosis, diabetes and, 149
Knee arthroscopy, 110

L

Laboratories
 CLIA requirements for, 317
 reference (outside), 319-320
Laboratory, CPT-4 coding for, 191-192
Laboratory report, form for, 17f
Lacerations, 279
 finger, 76
Laminectomy, defined, 291
Laminotomy, defined, 291
Laparoscopy, 289
Laryngoscopy procedures, 285
Legislation, fraud and abuse, 449-450
Lesions, 279
Lymphatic system, 287

M

Macro codes
 for dictation, 31
 for multiple services, 454
Major Diagnostic Categories, 393
 in DRG diagnosis process, 399
 listing of, 396, 397b
Malignancies, coding for, 133-134, 134f
Malpractice. See Medical malpractice.
Mammography, 305
Mastectomy, 280
Maternity care/delivery, 290-291
 key medical terms, 290
 practical applications, 291
Mediastinum, 287
Medical complexities, 146-177
 of blood and blood-forming organs,
  149-150
 of burns, 164-165
 of circulatory system, 153-154
 congenital anomalies, 161-162
 diabetes, 149
 of digestive system, 155-156
 documentation guidelines for, 147
 endocrine disorders, 148-149
 of genitourinary system, 156-157
 immunity disorders, 148-149
 infectious and parasitic diseases,
  147-148
 with injuries, poisonings, adverse effects,
  163-165
 mental disorders, 150-152
 metabolic disorders, 148-149
 of musculoskeletal system, 160-161
 of nervous system and sense organs,
  152-153
 nutritional disorders, 148-149
 in perinatal period, 161-162
 of pregnancy, birth, and puerperium,
  158-160
 of respiratory system, 154-155
 of skin/subcutaneous tissue, 160
Medical decision making, 206, 209-
  210, 212
Medical malpractice
 documentation and, 4
 medical record as defense against, 4
 real case scenario of, 4

Medical necessity
 documentation of, 3-5
 false claims involving, 451
 ICD-9-CM and, 90
 of radiological services, 303
Medical records
 ancillary, 15, 16f-21f
 components of, 5-6, 49, 52
 as defense against malpractice, 4
 formats for, 6-52
 medication record in, 9, 11f
 patient history in, 6, 7f
 problem list in, 9, 10f
 progress note/visit note in, 6, 8f
 signatures list for, 6
 SOAP format for, 9
Medical services, overuse of, 451
Medical terminology
 practice examinations for, 471-474
 variations in, 5
Medical visits, APCs for, 385-386, 400, 402
Medicare
 and evaluation and management services
  guidelines, 205
 legal rights of, 452-453
 medical necessity provision and, 4
Medicare/Medicaid Anti-Fraud and Abuse
  amendments, 449
Medicare/Medicaid False Claims Act,
  449-450
Medicare/Medicaid Patient and Program
  Protection Act of 1987, 449-450
Medication records, 9, 11f, 369
Medications, HCPCS codes for, 359
Medicine, CPT-4 coding for, 192
Medicine services, 322-345
 categories of, 323
 code modifiers for, 327
 coding guidelines for, 323, 324f, 325f,
  326f, 327
 for active wound care, 332
 for allergy/clinical immunology,
  330-331
 for biofeedback, 329
 for cardiovascular medicine, 330, 331f
 for central nervous system
  assessments, 331-332
 for chemotherapy administration, 332
 for chiropractic manipulative
  treatment, 332-333
 for conscious sedation, 333
 for dialysis, 329
 for gastroenterology, 329
 for home health services, 333
 for immune globulins, 327
 for immunization/vaccination
  administration, 327
 for neurology/neuromuscular
  procedures, 331
 for noninvasive vascular diagnostic
  studies, 330
 for ophthalmology, 329
 for osteopathic manipulative
  treatment, 332
 for other services, 333
 for physical medicine and
  rehabilitation, 332
 practical applications, 335-345

Medicine services *(Continued)*
   for psychiatry, 328
   for pulmonary medicine, 330
   review exercise, 334-335
   for special dermatological services, 332
   for special otorhinolaryngological
      services, 329
   for special supplies and services, 333
   for therapeutic/diagnostic infu-
      sions, 327
   for therapeutic/diagnostic injec-
      tions, 328
   for vaccines/toxoids, 327
  coding steps, 327
Meningitis, 147
Mental disorders, 150-152
  documentation issues in, 151-152
  in ICD-10-CM, 180
Metabolic encephalopathy, 150
Metastasis, coding of, 132
Microbiology, 319
Modifier codes, 346-357
  anatomical, 348
  for anesthesia services, 255-256
  computer entry of, errors involving,
      455-456
  in CPT-4, 192-194, 440
  description and use, for physician
      procedure coding, 350t-353t
    for E & M services, 201t
  documentation guidelines, 347
  educating about, 437
  for evaluation and management services,
      201-203, 201t
  function of, 202
  HCPCS, 348
    Level II, 354t-356t. *See also* Healthcare
      Common Procedure Coding
      System.
  for hospital coding, 386
  for indicating WHAT services were
      performed, 411
  listing of, 348
  for medicine services, 327
  for nonphysician services, 439
  for pathology services, 319-320
  for radiology services, 304
  reference tool for, 349
  review exercise, 357
  right/left, 348
  rules for, 347b
  specific issues, 348
  for surgery services, 264-269
    anesthesia by surgeon, 265
    for assistant surgeon, 268
    bilateral procedures, 265
    for decision for surgery, 266
    for discontinued procedure, 266
    for distinct procedural service, 267
    mandated services, 265
    for minimum assistant surgeon, 268
    multiple, 265-266, 268-269
    for postoperative management
      only, 266
    for preoperative management only, 266
    professional component, 265
    for reduced services, 266
    for reference, 268

Modifier codes *(Continued)*
    for repeat procedure, 267
    for return to operating room, 267
    for staged/related procedure, 266-267
    for surgical care only, 266
    for surgical team, 267
    for two surgeons, 267
    for unrelated procedure/service,
      267-268
    unusual procedures, 265
  types of, 347-348
  WHY and WHEN to use, 347b
Monitored anesthesia care, 253
Monitoring and compliance process,
    448-465
  compliance programs in, 463-465. *See
      also* Compliance programs.
  fraud/abuse legislation and, 449-454. *See
      also* Fraud and abuse.
  monitoring processes in, 454-463
    claims review, 455, 457
    coding/chart review, 455, 457-463
    data entry/techniques, 454-456
Morbidity, risks of, 206, 209
Mortality, risks of, 206, 209
Motor vehicle accidents, 72
Musculoskeletal deformities, acquired, 161
Musculoskeletal disorders, 160-161, 281-284
  key medical terms, 281
  practical applications, 284
Myocardial infarction, 153
  documentation issues, 154
Myringotomy, 292

N

NEC (not elsewhere classified), 91
Negative findings, documentation of, 9
Neonatal care, 238
Neonatal critical care services, 229
Neonatal intensive care, 228-229
Neonate
  birth weight coding for, 395
  critical care services for, 229
Neoplasms, 132-135, 135t
  table of, 134f
Nerve blocks, 254
Nerve injuries, 163
Nervous system, 291
  DRG listings for, 397b
  key medical terms, 291
  practical opportunities, 292
Nervous system disorders, 152
  documentation issues, 152
Neurology procedures, 331
Neuromuscular procedures, 331
Newborn. *See under* Neonatal entries.
NOS (not otherwise specified), 91
Nuclear medicine, 304, 306
Numerical and alphabetical index, 92-93
Nursing facility services, 229-231
  assessments and discharge, 232
Nursing notes, 23, 369, 377-378

O

Obstetrical procedures, common
    global, 278t
Office coding, education about, coder's
    role in, 437-438

Office of the Inspector General, regulatory/
    enforcement functions of, 449
Office visits, 214-216
  diagnostic statements for, 64-65
Operative reports, 262, 262f, 369
  practical applications, 294-299
Ophthalmological examinations/
    refractions, 292
Ophthalmology, 329
Organ systems, 212
  in CPT-4 physical examination
    requirements, 206
Organic brain syndrome, 150
Osteopathic manipulative treatment, 332
Otorhinolaryngological services, 329
Outpatient visits, 214-216
  billing/reimbursement methods for,
    400, 402
  codes for, 184, 214
  documentation for, 9, 12f, 13f, 14f, 15
  levels of service documentation for, 215

P

Pacemaker, 286
Pain
  abdominal, 104, 107, 123
    coding exercise for, 169
  epigastric, coding exercise for, 173
Pain management, spinal catheters in, 291
Parasitic diseases, 147-148
Pathology services, 314-321
  anatomical pathology, 319
  automated versus manual versus
    dipstick, 317
  chemistry, 318-319
  coding steps, 317, 318
  consultation, 318
  CPT-4 coding for, 191-192
  documentation/coding guidelines, 315,
    315f, 316f
  drug testing, 318
  evocative/suppression testing, 318
  general coding/billing guidelines, 317
  hematology, 319
  immunology, 319
  microbiology, 319
  modifier codes for, 319-320
  organ- or disease-oriented panels, 318
  review exercise, 320-321
  surgical pathology, 319
  therapeutic drug assays, 318
  transfusion medicine, 319
  types of, 317
  urinalysis, 318
Patient controlled analgesia, 254
Patient history, 6, 7f, 206, 207
  check-off guide for, 34-35
  levels of, 212
Payment collection, documentation and, 3
Pedal edema, bilateral, 87
Pediatric critical care services, inpatient,
    228-229
Pelvic inflammatory disorders, 158
Perinatal morbidity/mortality, maternal
    causes of, 162
Pertinent negatives, 9
Phlebitis, 154
Photochemotherapy, 332

Physical examination, 206, 208
  documentation of, 39f, 40f
  levels of, 212
Physical medicine and rehabilitation, 332
Physician assistant/extenders, coding
  for, 439
Physician coding. *See also* Physician
  diagnosis; Physician procedure coding.
  with CPT-4, ICD-9-CM, and DRG
    combined, 411
  diagnosis do's and don'ts for, 62
  versus hospital coding, 90-91
  rules for, 57
  signs and symptoms rules in, 61
  specificity level in, 62
  wording of, 67
Physician diagnosis, 56-87. *See also*
  Physician coding.
  chest x-ray in, 65
  code order rules in, 64
  complete blood cell count in, 65
  complexity of, 65
  versus signs and symptoms, 61
  specificity of, 67
  urinalysis in, 65
  WHAT elements in, 57, 59
  WHY elements in, 57, 59, 60f, 61-62
  worksheet for, 63f
Physician documentation, 2-53. *See also*
  Medical records.
  check-off format, 5
  dictated, 5
    form for, 47-48
    macros for, 31
    standardized guides for, 31-33
  in Emergency Department, 36-37
  formats for, 6-52
  handwritten, 5
  importance of, 3-4
  medical malpractice and, 4
  medical necessity and, 4-5
  for outpatient encounters, 9, 12f, 13f,
    14f, 15
  pertinent negatives in, 9
  real case scenario of, 3-4
  reimbursement and, 5
  signing of, 3
Physician procedure coding, 183-187. *See*
  also Current Procedural Terminology,
  fourth edition.
Physician standby services, 236
Physicians, malpractice suits against. *See*
  Medical malpractice
Pinch skin graft, 279
Pneumonia, 155
Poisoning, 130, 131
  flowchart for, 130-132
  in ICD-10-CM, 180
Postpartum disorders, 159-160
Pregnancy, 123, 124
  diabetes and, 149
  high-risk, 290
  hypertension in, 136
  V codes for, 114-115
Pregnancy disorders, 158-160
Preventive medicine services, 237
  reimbursement for, 440
Problem lists, 9, 10f

Procedural services, order listed in, 411
Procedures. *See also* Physician procedure
  coding.
  DRG codes for, 394, 399
  global "package concept," 194, 195f
  multiple
    macro codes for, 454
    reimbursement for, 441
  order of listing, 411
  repeated, 193
  separate, 195
  significant, APCs for, 385, 400, 402
  starred, 194
  unlisted, 194-195
Proctosigmoidoscopy, defined, 287
Progress notes, 6, 12f, 13f, 14f, 58f, 369,
  371-372, 375-376
  diagnostic coding in, 85
  hospital, 15, 23, 24f
  standardized forms for, 31
Prolonged services, 232
Prophylactic measures, V codes for, 113-114
Prospective Payment System, 393-394
Prostate procedures, 289
Prostatic hyperplasia, 158
Psychiatry, 328
Psychophysiological disorders, 151
Psychosis, substance-related, 151
Puerperium disorders, 158
Pulmonary medicine, 330
Pulmonary report, 324f

Q

Qui tam action, 4-5

R

Radiation oncology, 304, 306
Radiation physics, 306
Radiation treatment management, 306
Radiology
  CPT-4 coding for, 191
  diagnostic, 303-304, 305
Radiology report, 373-374
  diagnostic coding for, 84
  form for, 16f
Radiology services, 300-313
  categories of, 303-304
  coding guidelines, 304-305
    for contrasts, 305
    for diagnostic services, 305
    for radiopharmaceuticals, 305
    for supervision/interpretation, 304
  coding modifiers, 304
  coding steps, 301, 303, 305
  diagnostic, 305
  diagnostic ultrasound, 305-306
  documentation/coding guidelines,
    300-303
  mammography, 305
  medical necessity of, 303
  nuclear medicine, 306
  practical application, 307-313
  radiation oncology, 306
  report for, 302
  review exercise, 306-307
  technical versus professional components
    of, 304
Radiology simulation, therapeutic, 306

Radiopharmaceuticals, 305
Rash, 143
Real-time scans, 305-306
Records, ancillary, 369
Rehabilitation, 332
Reimbursement
  for anesthesia services, 253
  for bundled services, 440
  coding and, 432-445
    general third-party, 438-439
    methods of, 434-435
    overview of, 433
    practice mechanisms for, 435, 436f,
      437-438
    review exercise for, 445
    specific third-party, 439-441
    third-party contract worksheets and,
      441-445
    for third-party contracts, 433-434
  for cosurgeon/two surgeons, 440
  documentation and, 5
  E codes and, 116
  education about, coder's role in, 437-438
  fee for service, 393
  hospital billing process and, 393
  legal regulations for, 117
  methods of, 90
  for outpatient visits, 400, 402
  per diem, 393
  for preventive medicine visits, 440
  with Prospective Payment System,
    393-394
  RBRVS method for, 434-435
  UCR method for, 434
Renal disease, hypertension in, 137
Renal failure, chronic, 157
Reports, 369
Reproductive issues, V codes for, 114-115
Resistance, V codes for, 114
Resource-Based Relative Value Study,
  434-435
Respiratory system disorders, 154-155,
  284-285
  DRG listings for, 397b
  key medical terms, 284
  practical applications, 285
Respiratory testing report, 20f
Rest home services, 229, 232-233
Rheumatic fever, 153
Risk, table of, 209
Risk factor intervention, 237

S

Schizophrenic disorders, 150-151
Screening examinations, V codes for, 116
Sedation, conscious, 333
Sense organ disorders, 153
  practical applications, 292
Septicemia, 147
Services
  additional, 193
  bilateral, 193
  codeable. *See* Codeable services.
  at different than usual level, 193
  partial, 193
  repeated, 193
Sex, DRG codes for, 394
Sexually transmitted diseases, 148

Shingles, 148
Shortness of breath, 69, 77
    coding for, 141, 142
Sigmoidoscopy, defined, 287
Signatures
    electronic, 3
    reviewing requirements for, 49
    sample log, 52t
Signatures list, 6
Signs and symptoms
    coding based on, 162
    versus physician diagnosis, 61
    rules for inpatient hospital coding, 381
Sinus procedures, accessory, 285
Skin, tissue-cultured, 280
Skin disorders, 160
Skin replacement, 280
Skin replacement surgery, 279-280
Skin substitute, 280
SOAP format, 9
Social Security Act of 1966, Title XVIII
    of, 4
Sore throat, streptococcal, 147
Specimen collection, 317
Specimen drawing fees, 317
Specimen handling, 333
Speech, garbled, 108
Spina bifida, 161
Spinal catheters, 291
Spine coding, 282
Splint applications, 283
Split thickness graft, 279
Sprains/strains, 164
Staff notes, 23
Standards of care, 89
Standby services, physician, 236
Starke Anti-Kickback and Self Referral Acts
    of 1995, 1998, and 2002, 450
Strabismus operations, 292
Streptococcal sore throat, 147
Stress reactions, 151
Substance abuse disorders, 151
Substance-related psychosis, 151
Suicide attempt, 131
    coding for, 130
Supervision and interpretation codes for
    radiology services, 304
Supplies
    HCPCS codes for, 359
    for medicine services, 333
Surgeons
    assistant, reimbursement for, 440-441
    multiple, reimbursement for, 440
Surgery services, 260-299, 277-292
    APCs for, 385, 400
    coding guidelines, 263-269
        for basic layout, 263-264

Surgery services (Continued)
    for global services, 263
        modifiers in, 264-269
        for starred procedures, 263
    coding steps, 261-262, 263, 264, 269-270
    CPT-4 coding for, 191
    documentation/coding guidelines,
        261-263
    integumentary system, 278-281
    multiple, macro codes for, 454
Surgical pathology, 319
Surgical pathology report, form for, 18f
Surgical procedures
    add-on, 274
    bundled, 274-277
    common global, 278t
    documentation of, 23, 27f
    each, each additional, per, 274
    incidental, 274
    practical applications, 274
    separate, 274
Surgical tray, listing for, 276
Symbols
    CPT-4, 195
    ICD-9-CM, 92
Symptoms, used in lieu of unestablished
    diagnoses, 383
Systemic lupus erythematosus, 161

T
Team conferences, 236
Telephone calls, 236
Therapeutic drug assays, 318
Therapeutic infusions, 327
Therapeutic injections, 328
Therapeutic radiation simulation, 306
Therapeutic use, coding for, 130
Third-party carriers
    appeals process of, 433
    coding requirements for, 433
    contracts with, 433-434
        worksheets for, 441-442, 443f, 444
    CPT-4 codes for, 194
    documentation and, 4-5
    E codes and, 116
    general coding and reimbursement
        guidelines, 438-439
    ICD-9-CM and, 89
    legal rights of, 452-453
    notifying, about fraud and abuse, 453
    preventive medicine visits and, 440
    real case scenarios for, 89-90
    specific coding and reimbursement
        guidelines, 439
    time limits of, 439
Thoracentesis, 285
Thoracostomy, 285

Thrombophlebitis, 154
Tissue disorders, 160
Tissue transfers, 279
Tissue-cultured allogenic skin
    substitute, 280
Tissue-cultured skin, 280
Tonsillectomy, 288
Toxoids, 327
Transfusion medicine, 319
Transient global amnesia, 150
Trauma, 79, 164-166. See also Accidents;
    Injuries.
Triangle, coding significance of, 195
Trigger point injections, 282
Tubal ligation, 290
Tuberculosis, 147

U
Ulcers
    foot, diabetes and, 149
    gastrointestinal, 155-156
Ultrasound, diagnostic, 304, 305-306
Upper respiratory infection, diagnosis
    of, 62
Urethroscopy, 288
Urinalysis, 318
    in physician diagnosis, 65
Urinary tract disorders, 157-158, 288-289
Usual, customary, and reasonable
    method, 434

V
V codes, 112-116
Vaccines, 327
Vascular diagnostic studies,
    noninvasive, 330
Vasectomy, 289
Venous access devices, 286
Venous Doppler ultrasound, 84
Viral hepatitis, 148
Visit notes, 6, 8f

W
Whistleblower program, 453
World Health Organization, ICD of, 89. See
    also ICD-9-CM Code Book; ICD-9-CM
    diagnostic coding.
Wound care, active, 332
Wound covering, temporary, 280
Wounds, 279
    open, 163

X
X-rays, chest, in physician diagnosis, 65